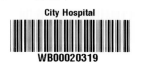

Medical Disorders in Pregnancy

Ed Howarth 1962–2010

We have dedicated this edition of the book to one of our authors who died in 2010 from complications following bone marrow transplantation for lymphoma.

Edmund Steven Howarth ('Ed' to all who knew him) qualified in Dundee in 1986 and after training in Obstetrics and Gynaecology was one of the inaugural sub-speciality trainees in Maternal and Fetal Medicine in Leicester where he was subsequently appointed as a consultant. Ed worked tirelessly to establish the Maternal Medicine Services in Leicester as well as establishing strong links with the Perinatal Epidemiology Unit at Leicester University.

Ed was a passionate teacher and always strove to raise the profile of specialist midwifery within maternal medicine services. He was an obvious choice as an author for this book and his ongoing contributions will be greatly missed. Ed will always be remembered for his enthusiasm, thoroughness and his 'matter of fact' approach to his clinical practice.

A great personality with a dry sense of humour, Ed had an excellent rapport with pregnant women and midwives. He will be remembered as a mothers' champion and a midwives' friend. Ed leaves a wife, two daughters and two granddaughters and will be sorely missed by all who knew him.

Medical Disorders in Pregnancy:
A Manual for Midwives
Second Edition

Edited by

S. Elizabeth Robson
MSc RGN RM ADM Cert(A)Ed MTD FHEA
Principal Lecturer in Midwifery
De Montfort University
Leicester

and

Jason Waugh
BSc(Hons) MB BS DA MRCOG
Consultant in Obstetrics and Maternal Medicine
Royal Victoria Infirmary
Newcastle upon Tyne

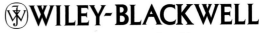
WILEY-BLACKWELL
A John Wiley & Sons, Ltd., Publication

Library of Congress Cataloging-in-Publication Data

Medical disorders in pregnancy : a manual for midwives / edited by S. Elizabeth Robson and Jason Waugh. – 2nd ed.
        p. ; cm.
    Includes bibliographical references and index.
    ISBN 978-1-4443-3748-8 (pbk. : alk. paper)
    I. Robson, S. Elizabeth.   II. Waugh, Jason.
    [DNLM: 1. Pregnancy Complications–Handbooks.   2. Midwifery–Handbooks.   3. Prenatal Care–methods–Handbooks.   WQ 39]
    618.2–dc23

                                                    2012013830

A catalogue record for this book is available from the British Library.

Wiley also publishes its books in a variety of electronic formats. Some content that appears in print may not be available in electronic books.

Cover image courtesy of S. Elizabeth Robson
Cover design by Garth Stewart

Set in 9 on 11 pt Palatino by Toppan Best-set Premedia Limited
Printed in Singapore by C.O.S. Printers Pte Ltd

3   2014

Contents

Contributors

EDITORS

S. Elizabeth Robson RGN RM ADM Cert(A)Ed MTD MSc FHEA.
Principal Lecturer in Midwifery; N&M Recruitment and Public Engagement Lead at De Montfort University

Jason Waugh MB BS BSc(Hons) MRCOG DA
Consultant in Obstetrics and Maternal Medicine at the Royal Victoria Infirmary, Newcastle upon Tyne

MIDWIFERY AND NURSING AUTHORS

Abena Addo MA , PDGE, BSc, RGN, RM
Senior Lecturer in Midwifery at De Montfort University

Eleanor Burns-Kent RM BSc(Hons)
Midwife at the University Hospitals of Leicester NHS Trust

Rhoda Cowell BSc(Hons) RGN, DipEd
Community Dermatology Specialist Nurse and Non-Medical Prescriber at County Durham and Darlington Foundation Trust

Claire Dodd RGN BA(Hons), RM BSc(Hons)
Specialist Midwife in Hypertension at the University Hospitals of Leicester NHS Trust

Rowena Doughty MSc PGDE BA(Hons) RGN RM ADM FHEA.
Senior Lecturer in Midwifery, Supervisor of Midwives and Deputy Lead Midwife for Education at De Montfort University

Daksha Elliott RGN RSCN
Lead Nurse/ Manager, Leicestershire Sickle Cell & Thalassaemia Service at the University Hospitals of Leicester NHS Trust

Caroline Farrar RGN RM BSc(Hons) PGDipEd MSC
Senior Lecturer in Midwifery at De Montfort University

Madeleine Findlay RGN RM BSc(Hons) PG Cert Education and Training
Currently Parent Education Co-ordinator Royal Victoria Infirmary, Newcastle upon Tyne

Deborah Frost RGN RM BSc(Hons) AHEA
Academic Co-ordinator, University of Leicester

Michelle Goldie
Formerly Specialist Midwife at the University Hospitals of Leicester NHS Trust

Andrea Goodlife RM Dip.Renal nursing
Specialist midwife in hypertension and renal disease at the University Hospitals of Leicester NHS Trust

Kathryn Gutteridge
RGN, RM, SoM, MSc & PG.Dip Counselling & Psychotherapy
Consultant Midwife Sandwell and West Birmingham Hospitals NHS Trust

Juliet Houghton MSc Dip RGN RSCN ENB:934
Recently the Child and Family HIV/Hepatitis Specialist Nurse at the University Hospitals of Leicester NHS Trust, and now
Programme Director of CHIVA/South Africa Support and Mentoring Initiative based in Durban, South Africa

Veronica Johnson-Roffey BA(Hons) RGN RM RHV FETC Dip.Infection control
Recently Infection Control Lead Nurse at Northamptonshire Healthcare NHS Trust. Now Infection Control Nurse at Three Shires Hospital, Northampton

Rosemary Lydall RGN RM BA(Hons)
Infant Feeding Coordinator and Supervisor of Midwives at the University Hospitals of Leicester NHS Trust

Moira McLean RGN RM ENB:402 ADM PGCEA MTD PGDip SoM
Senior Lecturer in Midwifery at De Montfort University

Jane Scullion BA(Hons) RGN MSc
Respiratory Nurse Consultant at University Hospitals of Leicester NHS Trust; Honorary Senior Lecturer at De Montfort University; Clinical Research Fellow at Aberdeen University

Diane Todd BSc(Hons) DipHE RM RGN
Specialist Midwife – Diabetes at the University Hospitals of Leicester NHS Trust

MEDICAL AUTHORS

Fionnuala McAuliffe MD, FRCOG, FRCPI, DCH
Associate Professor in Obstetrics and Gynaecology, University College Dublin, Ireland and Consultant Obstetrician and Gynaecologist and Maternal and Fetal Medicine Specialist, National Maternity Hospital, Dublin, Ireland

Christopher Brightling BSc(Hons) MBBS MRCP PhD FCCP
MRC Clinician Scientist and Honorary Consultant Respiratory Physician at the University Hospitals of Leicester NHS Trust

Nigel J. Brunskill MB ChB, PhD, FRCP
Nephrologist at the University Hospitals of Leicester NHS Trust and Professor of Renal Medicine at the University of Leicester

Frances A. Bu'Lock MD FRCP
Consultant Paediatric Cardiologist at Glenfield Hospital, Leicester

Contributors

Francis J.E. Gardner BSc MB ChB MRCOG DFFP BSCCP accredited
Consultant in Gynaecology and Gynaecological Oncology and Clinical Director for Gynaecology at the Queen Alexandra Hospital, Portsmouth Hospitals NHS Trust

Catherine Gittins BM MRCGP DCH DRCOG DFFP DPD
GP partner in Whitley Bay and Dermatology Specialty Doctor at Royal Victoria Infirmary, Newcastle upon Tyne

Julie Goddard MBBS DFFP MRCOG
Consultant Obstetrician at Calderdale Royal Hospital, Halifax

Robert Gregory BA MB BS DM FRCP
Consultant Physician and Head of Service Metabolic Medicine at the University Hospitals of Leicester NHS Trust

The late **Edmund S. Howarth** MB ChB, MRCOG
Formerly Consultant in Maternal and Fetal Medicine at the University Hospitals of Leicester NHS Trust

The late **Javed Iqbal** BSc MSc(Hons) FRCPath FRCP
Formerly Consultant in Biochemical Medicine at the University Hospitals of Leicester NHS Trust

Manjiri Khare MRCOG, MD, FCPS, DNB, Diploma in Obstetric Ultrasound
Consultant in Maternal-Fetal medicine at the University Hospitals of Leicester NHS Trust

Renuka Lazarus MBBS, MD, MRCPsych
Consultant Liaison Psychiatrist and Clinical Lead for Perinatal Psychiatry at the Leicestershire Partnership Trust

Christina Oppenheimer MA MB BS, FRCS, FRCOG
Consultant in Obstetrics and Gynaecology, Head of Service for Obstetrics at University Hospitals of Leicester NHS Trust and Honorary Senior Lecturer in Medical Education

Sue Pavord MB ChB, FRCP, FRCPath
Consultant Haematologist and Honorary Senior Lecturer in Medical Education at the University Hospitals of Leicester NHS Trust

Paul Moran BM BS BMedSci MRCOG MD
Consultant in Obstetrics and Fetal Medicine at the Royal Victoria Infirmary, Newcastle upon Tyne

Marie C. Smith MBBS MRCOG MD
Consultant Obstetrician at the Royal Victoria Infirmary in Newcastle upon Tyne and Senior Lecturer, Newcastle University

Karen Watkins MB ChB(Hons) MRCOG
Lead Obstetrician for Intrapartum Care and Maternal Medicine at The Royal Cornwall Hospital, Truro

Sophia Webster BMedSci (hons) BMBS DFFP MRCOG
Obstetric Registrar at the Royal Victoria Infirmary in Newcastle upon Tyne

Acknowledgements

In addition to the sterling work of the contributors above, we have received assistance and guidance from the practitioners below who have been generous with their time and advice in relation to specialist subjects. We are truly indebted to:

Malcolm McGregor, for work on the cardiac illustrations

Jo Matharu, Midwife at the University Hospitals of Leicester NHS Trust

Jean Johnson, Service Lead for Women's Health Physiotherapy at the University Hospitals of Leicester NHS Trust

Marie Halliday, Specialist Midwife in Diabetes at St Georges Hospital, London

Marian Parrish, Midwife at University Hospitals of Leicester NHS Trust

Trudy Boyce, recently retired Specialist Midwife in Hypertension

David Ireland, Consultant Gynaecologist at Leicester General Hospital

We would like to extend our gratitude to the many colleagues at the University Hospitals of Leicester, De Montfort University and Newcastle Royal Victoria Infirmary who have answered queries and given advice and moral support.

Furthermore, we would like to thank the associations and institutions addressed in the appendices and some of the figures for giving their assistance, and in many cases have waived a copyright fee for reproducing their material enabling the book to be kept at an affordable price for the readership.

Editing of the book had considerable impact upon domestic life, and completion would not have been possible without significant spousal support. We are truly appreciative of Kate Waugh for all her continued forbearance and support. Then to Matthew Broughton for his endless patience, culinary skills and application of his draughtsman talents when he drew figures 10.1.1 and 10.6.1 specifically for this book.

Acronyms, Abbreviations and Cardiac Terms

Abbreviations in the main narrative, or in daily use

ABO	A, B and O blood groups
AbV	Alcohol by Volume
ABU	Asymptomatic Bacteruria
ACTH	Adrenocorticotrophic Hormone
aCL	Anticardiolipin Antibodies
ADHD	Attention Deficiency Hyperactive Disorder
AFE	Amniotic Fluid Embolism
AFI	Amniotic Fluid Index
AFLP	Acute Fatty Liver of Pregnancy
AFP	Alpha Feto-protein
Ag	Antigen
AIDS	Acquired Immune Deficiency Syndrome
ALS	Advanced Life Support
ALT	Alanine Transaminase (a liver enzyme)
AN	Anorexia Nervosa
ANA	Antinuclear Antibody
ANC	Antenatal (prenatal) Clinic or Care
Anti-Ro/La	Lupus antibodies Ro and La
APA	Antiphospholipid Antibodies
APAH	Associated Pulmonary Arterial Hypertension
APD	Automated Peritoneal Dialysis
APH	Antepartum Haemorrhage
APS	Antiphospholipid (Hughes) Syndrome
AR	Aortic Regurgitation
ARDS	Acute Respiratory Distress Syndrome
ARM	Artificial Rupture of Membranes
ARVC	Arrhythmogenic Right Ventricular Cardiomyopathy
ART	Anti-Retroviral Therapy
AS	Aortic Stenosis
ASD	Atrial Septal Defect
AST	Aspartate Transaminase (a liver enzyme)
AVNRT	Atrioventricular Nodal Re-entrant Tachycardia
AVPU	Alert, Verbal, Painful, Unresponsive
βhCG	Beta Human Chorionic Gonadotrophin
BMD	Bone Mineral (measurement) Density
BMI	Body Mass Index (formally Quetelet Scale)
BN	Bulimia Nervosa
BP	Blood Pressure
BSL	British Sign Language
C1,2,etc.	Cervical vertebrae number one, two, etc.
C1,2,etc.	Complement one, two, etc. levels
CAM	Complementary and Alternative Medicine
CAPP	Continuous Ambulatory Peritoneal Dialysis
CAPS	Catastrophic Antiphospholipid Syndrome
CAT/CT	Computerised Axial Tomography (scan)
CBT	Cognitive Behaviour Therapy
CCU	Critical Care Unit
CD	Crohn's Disease
CF	Cystic Fibrosis
CFTR	Cystic Fibrosis Transmembrane Conductance Regulator
CHB	Congenital Heart Block
CHD	Coronary Heart Disease
CHF/CCF	Congestive Heart Failure (Cardiac)
CHT	Chronic Hypertension

CIN	Cervical Intraepithelial Neoplasia
CJD	Creutzfeldt–Jakob Disease
CKD	Chronic Kidney Disease
CMV	Cytomegalovirus
CNS	Central Nervous System
CO	Cardiac Output
CPR	Cardiopulmonary Resuscitation
CREST	Calcinosis, Raynaud's, Oesophageal dysmotility, Sclerodactyly & Telangiectasia
CRP	C-Reactive Protein
CS	Caesarean Section
CSF	Cerebrospinal fluid
CTG	Cardiotocograph
CTPA	Computed Tomographic Pulmonary Angiography
CTS	Carpal Tunnel Syndrome
CVA	Cerebrovascular Accident
CVP	Central Venous Pressure
CVT	Cerebral Vein Thrombosis
DCM	Dilated Cardiomyopathy
DIC	Disseminated Intravascular Coagulation
DLE	Discoid Lupus Erythematosus
DM	Diabetes Mellitus
DNA	Deoxyribonucleic Acid
DOE	Dyspnoea On Exertion
DSP	Diastasis of the Symphysis Pubis
DVT	Deep Vein Thrombosis
ECG	Electrocardiograph
ED	Eating Disorder
EDD	Expected Date of Delivery/confinement
EDTA	Ethylene-diamine-tetraacetic-acid
EEG	Electroencephalogram
EF	Ejection Fraction (heart)
EFM	Electronic Fetal Monitoring (of fetal heart)
EPDS	Edinburgh Postnatal Depression Scale
ERCP	Endoscopic Retrograde Cholangiopancreatography
ERPoC	Evacuate Retained Products of Conception
ESR	Erythrocyte Sedimentation Rate
EMDR	Eye Movement Desensitisation & Reprocessing Therapy
EWS	Early Warning Scoring
FAE	Fetal Alcohol Effects
FAS	Fetal Alcohol Syndrome
FBC	Full Blood Count
FFP	Fresh Frozen Plasma
FH	Fetal Heart
FHR	Fetal Heart Rate
FMAIT	Feto-Maternal Alloimmune Thrombocytopenia
FPAH	Familial Pulmonary Arterial Hypertension
FSE	Fetal Scalp Electrode
fT3	Free Tri-iodothyronine (a thyroid hormone)
fT4	Free Throxine (a thyroid hormone)
FVL	Factor V Leiden (a clotting factor)
FVS	Fetal Varicella Syndrome
GAS	Group A Streptococcus pyogenes
GBS	Group B Streptococcus agalactiae

GCS	Graduated Compression Stockings		MALT	Mucosa-associated lymphoid tissue
GGT	Gamma-GT (monitors alcohol)		MCH	Mean Corpuscular Haemoglobin
GD	Graves' Disease		MCM	Major Congenital Malformations
GDM	Gestational Diabetes Mellitus		MCV	Mean Cell Volume
GFD	Gluten Free Diet		MEOWS	Modified Early Obstetric Warning System
GFR	Glomerular Filtration Rate		MG	Myasthenia Gravis
GH	Genital Herpes (infection)		MI	Myocardial Infarction
GH	Gestational Hypertension		MRI	Magnetic Resonance Image (scan)
GnRH	Gonadotropin-Releasing Hormone		MS	Multiple Sclerosis
GO	Graves' Ophthalmopathy		MS	Mitral Stenosis
GORD	Gastro-oesophageal Reflux Disease		MSU	or MSSU – Midstream Specimen of Urine
GTD	Gestational Trophoblastic Disease		MVA	Mitral Valve Area
GTN	Gestational Trophoblastic Neoplasia		MVP	Mitral Valve Prolapse
GTT	Glucose Tolerance Test		NAS	Neonatal Abstinence Syndrome
GVH	Graft Versus Host (disease)		NEFA	Non Esterified Fatty Acid
HAV, HBV	Hepatitis Virus type A, type B, etc.		NHL	Non Hodgkin's Lymphoma
HAPO	Hyperglycaemic and Adverse Pregnancy Outcome Study		NICU	Neonatal Intensive Care Unit
			NNU	Neonatal Unit
Hb	Haemoglobin		NRT	Nicotine Replacement Therapy
HbA1c	Haemoglobin A1c (monitor blood glucose)		NTD	Neural Tube Defect
HBeAg	Hepatitis B e-antigen		NVP	Nausea and Vomiting in pregnancy
HBIG	Hepatitis B Immune Globulin		OASI	Obstetric Anal Sphincter Injury
HCG	Human Chorionic Gonadotrophin		OC	Obstetric Cholestasis
HCM	Hypertrophic Cardiomyopathy		OGTT	Oral Glucose Tolerance Test
HCT	Haematocrit		PAH	Pulmonary Arterial Hypertension
HD	Haemodialysis		PAPS	Primary Antiphospholipid Syndrome
HDU	High Dependency Unit		PCOS	Polycystic Ovarian Syndrome
HELLP	Haemolysis, Elevated Liver enzymes Low Platelets		PCR	Protein:Creatinine Ratio
			PET	Pre-eclampsia (formally toxaemia)
HER2	Human Epidermal Growth Factor Receptor		PD	Peritoneal Dialysis
HF	Heart Failure		PDA	Patent Ductus Arteriosus (heart)
HG	Hyperemesis Gravidarum		PE	Pulmonary Embolism
HIT	Heparin-induced Thrombocytopenia		PEA	Pulseless Electrical Activity (heart)
HIV	Human Immunodeficiency Virus		PET	Pre-eclamptic Toxaemia
HL	Hodgkin's Lymphoma		pH	Potential Hydrogen (measure acid/alkaline)
HPV	Human Papillomavirus		PH	Pulmonary Hypertension
HRT	Hormone Replacement Therapy		PIH	Pregnancy Induced Hypertension
HSV	Herpes Simplex Virus		PKU	Phenylketonuria
IBD	Inflammatory Bowel Disease		PM	Pacemaker
IBS	Irritable Bowel Syndrome		PND	Paroxysmal Nocturnal Dyspnoea
ICD	Intracardiac Device		PPCM	Peripartum Cardiomyopathy
ICP	Intrahepatic Cholestasis of Pregnancy		PPH	Postpartum Haemorrhage
Ig	Immunoglobulin (types A, E, D, G and M)		PRL	Prolactin
INR	International Normalised Ratio		PRP/SRP	Primary/Secondary Raynaud's Phenomenon
IPAH	Idiopathic Pulmonary Arterial Hypertension		PRPRG	Pregnancy related pelvis girdle pain
IQ	Intelligence Quotient		PROM	Premature Rupture of membranes
ITP	Immune Thrombocytopenic Purpura		PPROM	Pre-term Premature Rupture of the Membranes
ITU	Intensive Treatment Unit			
IUCD	Intrauterine Contraceptive Device		PS	Pulmonary Stenosis
IUFD	Intrauterine Fetal Death		PTH	Parathyroid Hormone
IUGR	Intrauterine Growth Restriction/retardation		PTSD	Post-traumatic stress disorder
IUS	Intrauterine System (contraception)		PUVA	Psoralen with Ultraviolet A light
IVF	In Vitro Fertilisation		PVD	Pulmonary Vascular Disease
IVIG	Intravenous Immunoglobulins		RA	Rheumatoid Arthritis
JIA	Juvenile Idiopathic Arthritis		RBC	Red Blood Cell (erythrocyte)
JRH	Juvenile Rheumatoid Arthritis		RCM	Restrictive Cardiomyopathy
LDH	Lactate Dehydrogenase		RCT	Randomised Control Trial
LBC	Liquid Based Cytology		RDS	Respiratory Distress Syndrome
L1,2, etc.	Lumber vertebrae one, two, etc.		Rh	Rhesus Factor (positive or negative)
LA	Lupus Anticoagulants		SAH	Sub-arachnoid Haemorrhage
LFT	Liver Function Test		SAPS	Secondary Antiphospholipid Syndrome
LHRH	Luteinising Hormone Releasing Hormone		SB	Serum Bilirubin
LMWH	Low Molecular Weight Heparin		SCBU	Special Care Baby Unit
LSCS	Lower Section Caesarean Section		SCD	Sickle Cell Disease
LV	Left Ventricle		SFH	Symphysis-fundal height
LVF	Left Ventricular Failure		SIDS	Sudden Infant Death Syndrome

SIRS	Systemic Inflammatory Response Syndrome
SLE	Systemic Lupus Erythematosus
SPD	Symphysis pubis dysfunction
SRM	Spontaneous Rupture of Membranes
STD	Sexually Transmitted Disease
STI	Sexually Transmitted Infection
SUDEP	Sudden Unexpected Death in Epilepsy
SV	Stroke Volume (heart)
SVT	Supraventricular Tachycardia
T1DM	Type 1 Diabetes Mellitus
T2DM	Type 2 Diabetes Mellitus
T3	Tri-iodothyronine (a thyroid hormone)
T4	Throxine (a thyroid hormone)
TA	Truncus Arteriosus
TB	Tuberculosis
TED	Thromboembolic Disease
TEDS	Thromboembolic Disease Stockings
TENS	Transcutaneous Electrical Nerve Stimulation
TGA	Transposition of the Great Arteries
TIA	Transient Ischaemic Attack
ToF	Tetralogy of Fallot
ToP	Termination of Pregnancy
TPR	Temperature, Pulse, Respiration
TPO	Thyroid Peroxidase
TRALI	Transfusion Related Acute Lung Injury
TSH	Thyroid Stimulating Hormone
TSHR	Thyroid Stimulating Hormone Receptor
TSIg	Thyroid Stimulating Immunoglobulin
UC	Ulcerative Colitis
UFH	Unfractionated Heparin
U&E	Urea and Electrolyte (analysis)
USS	Ultrasound Scan
UTI	Urinary Tract Infection
UVA,B,C	Ultraviolet A or B or C waves
VDRL	Venereal Disease Research Laboratory
VIN	Varicella Infection of the Newborn
VF	Ventricular Fibrillation
VQ	Ventilation Perfusion
VSD	Ventricular Septal Defect (of heart)
VTE	Venous Thrombo-embolism
VWD	Von Willebrand's Disease
WBC	White Blood Cell (leucocyte)
WPW	Wolff-Parkinson-White Syndrome
Xa	Clotting Factor Ten, sub-set A

Abbreviations of Practitioners and Institutions

BHS	British Hypertension Society
BTS	British Thoracic Society
CEMACH	Confidential Enquiry Maternal Child Health
CMACE	Centre for Maternal and Child Enquiries
COMA	Committee on Medical Aspects of Food and Nutritional Policy
DoH	Department of Health (UK)
FIGO	International Federation of Gynaecology & Obstetrics
FSA	Food Standards Agency (UK)
FSID	Foundation for the Study of Infant Deaths
GMC	General Medical Council (UK)
GP	General Practitioner
HV	Health Visitor/Public Health Nurse
IADPSG	International Association of Diabetes and Pregnancy Study Groups
ITU	Intensive Therapy Unit
MDT	Multi-disciplinary Team
NHS	National Health Service (UK)
NICE	National Institute for Clinical Excellence (UK)

NMC	Nursing and Midwifery Council (UK)
NNU	Neonatal Unit
NTPR	National Transplantation Pregnancy Registry
NTIS	National Teratology Information System (UK)
NYHA	New York Heart Association (USA)
RCM	Royal College of Midwives
RCOG	Royal College of Obstetricians & Gynaecologists
SHOT	Serious Hazards of Transfusion
SIGN	Scottish Intercollegiate Guidelines Network
WHO	World Health Organisation

Drug Administration Abbreviations (Latin in *italics*)

bd	Twice a day	(*Bis die*)
tds	Three times a day	(*Ter die sumendus*)
qds	Four times a day	(*Quatre die sumendus*)
prn	As necessary	(*Pro re nata*)
po	By mouth	(*Per orum*)
pr	Rectally	(*Per rectum*)
pv	Vaginally	(*Per vaginum*)
im	Intramuscular	
iv	Intravenous	
IVI	Intravenous infusion	
nocte	At night	
sc	Subcutaneous	
stat	At once	

Measurement Abbreviations

FL	Fluid
fl	Femtolitre
g/dl	Grams per decilitre
IU	International Units
IU/l	International Units per litre
kg	Kilogram
mg	Milligrams
mg/l	Milligrams per litre
ml	Millilitre
mmHg	Millimetres of Mercury
mmol/l	Millimoles per litre
ng/ml	Nanograms per millilitre
nM/l	Nanograms per litre

Drug and Immunisation Abbreviations

6MP	Six-Mercaptopurine
ACEI	Angiotensin Converting Enzyme Inhibitors
AED	Antiepileptic Drug
ARB	Angiotensin Receptor Blockers
ARV	Anti-Retroviral drug
AZT	Azidothymidine
BCG	Immunisation to prevent tuberculosis
CBZ	Carbimazole
CD	Controlled Drug
COCP	Combined Oral Contraceptive Pill
CSII	Continuous Subcutaneous Insulin Infusion
DMARD	Disease Modifying Anti-Rheumatic Drug
GTN	Glyceryl Trinitrate
H_2RA	Histamine$_2$-Receptor Antagonist
HBIG	Hepatitis B Immune Globulin
IVIG	Intravenous Immunoglobulin
LMWH	Low Molecular Weight Heparin
MAOI	Monoamine Oxidase Inhibitor
NSAID	Non-steroidal Anti-inflammatory Drug
OAC	Oral anticoagulant
OTC	Over-the-Counter (drug)
POM	Prescription Only Medicine
POCP	Progesterone Only Contraceptive Pill

PPI	Proton-Pump Inhibitor
PTU	Propylthiouracil
SSRI	Selective Serotonin Reuptake Inhibitor
TNF	Tumour Necrosis Factor (inhibitor)
VZIg	Varicella zoster Immunoglobulin

CARDIAC TERMS

Afterload: amount of resistance to ejection of blood from a ventricle.

Anuria: urine output of less than 50 ml per 24 hours.

Atrial fibrillation: the normal regular rhythm of the heartbeat is lost and replaced by an irregular rhythm which may be episodic (paroxysmal atrial fibrillation) or persistent. The loss of normal atrial contraction produces a risk of clot formation in the atria. Anticoagulation and drugs to slow the heart rate are required.

Cardiac failure: heart failure; cardiac output insufficient to meet the demands of the body resulting in shortness of breath, pulmonary oedema, peripheral oedema and tiredness.

Cardiac output (CO): the amount of blood pumped out of the heart in one minute.

Cardioversion: the procedure of applying electrical shock to the chest to change an abnormal heartbeat into a normal one.

Compliance: the elasticity or amount of 'give' when blood enters the ventricle.

Congestive heart failure (CHF): a fluid overload condition (congestion) that may or may not be caused by HF; often an acute presentation of HF with increased amount of fluid in the blood vessels.

Contractility: the force of ventricular contraction; related to the number and state of myocardial cells.

Diastolic heart failure: the inability of the heart to pump sufficiently because of an alteration in the ability of the heart to fill; current term used to describe a type of HF.

Dyspnoea on exertion (DOE): shortness of breath that occurs with exertion.

Ejection fraction (EF): percent of blood volume in the ventricles at the end of diastole that is ejected during systole; a measurement of contractility.

Electrical cardioversion: used to shock the heart back into normal rhythm. If this procedure is necessary, it is carried out under general anaesthesia.

Heart failure (HF): the inability of the heart to pump sufficient blood to meet the needs of the tissues for oxygen and nutrients; signs and symptoms of pulmonary and sys temic congestion may or may not be present.

Ischaemia: inability to supply adequate oxygen leading to tissue damage or death.

Left-sided heart failure (left ventricular failure): inability of the left ventricle to fill or pump (empty) sufficient blood to meet the needs of the tissues for oxygen and nutrients; traditional term used to describe patient's HF symptoms.

Oliguria: diminished urine output; less than 400 ml per 24 hours.

Orthopnoea: shortness of breath when lying flat.

Paroxysmal nocturnal dyspnoea (PND): shortness of breath that occurs suddenly during sleep.

Pericardiocentesis: procedure that involves surgically entering the pericardial sac, usually with a needle.

Pericardiotomy: surgically-created opening of the pericardium.

Pre-load: the amount of myocardial stretch just before systole caused by the pressure created by volume of blood within a ventricle.

Pulmonary hypertension: elevated blood pressure in the pulmonary arteries from constriction; causes problems with the blood flow in the lungs, and makes the heart work harder. If left untreated, this can lead to heart failure.

Pulmonary oedema: abnormal accumulation of fluid occurring in the interstitial spaces or in the alveoli of the lungs.

Pulseless electrical activity (PEA): condition in which electrical activity is present but there is not an adequate pulse or blood pressure due to ineffective cardiac contraction or circulating blood volume.

Pulsus paradoxus: systolic blood pressure that is more than 10 mmHg higher during exhalation than during inspiration; difference is normally less than 10 mmHg.

Right-sided heart failure (right ventricular failure): inability of the right ventricle to fill or pump (empty) sufficient blood to the pulmonary circulation.

Stroke volume (SV): amount of blood pumped out of the ventricle with each contraction.

Systolic heart failure: inability of the heart to pump sufficiently because of an alteration in the ability of the heart to contract; current term used to describe a type of heart failure (HF).

Thermo-dilution: method of determining cardiac output that involves injecting fluid into the pulmonary artery catheter. A thermistor measures the difference between the temperature of the fluid and the temperature of the blood ejected from the ventricle. Cardiac output is calculated from the change in temperature.

Thrombolytic therapy: Treatment to break up blood clots in the circulatory system.

Ventricular ejection fraction: (see ejection fraction).

Foreword

At a time when in the UK and around the world midwives strive to deliver high quality cost-effective care in differing but always challenging circumstances, this is a very important text.

High quality care is synonymous with safe care. Safe care has to be, at its most fundamental, about ensuring that women do not die or experience major physical disability as a result of childbirth. If care is to meet this standard of safety then midwives must have an excellent knowledge of medical disorders in pregnancy to ensure early and relevant referral and appropriate advice for women. Happily most women in the UK have a positive experience of childbirth and are fit and healthy as they start on the path of motherhood. However, despite the fact that maternal mortality rates are low in the UK, we cannot be complacent. The last Confidential Enquiry into Maternal Deaths Report for 2005–2008 demonstrated that women are still dying unnecessarily as a consequence of medical disorders in pregnancy. With more women having their babies at an older age and with women increasingly surviving to childbearing age with chronic medical disorders these tragedies risk becoming more not less common.

Worldwide the picture is very different, with a shockingly high number of women dying during pregnancy and childbirth or in the early postnatal period. In much of the world there is a pressing need to ensure healthcare workers have access to knowledge that we know can make a vast difference to their practice and to women's chances of survival.

Fortunately, safe care today is about more than just the prevention of mortality or major morbidity. It is also about reducing unnecessary medical or surgical interventions.

Assessing risk is important not just to ensure women receive the care they require but also to ensure that throughout pregnancy, labour and the postnatal period actions are taken to ensure that care keeps women as normal as is possible. The midwife who has a sound understanding of medical disorders, their physiology and their impact on pregnancy is in an ideal position to help the woman stay as 'well' as is possible and to minimise the need for intervention.

Equally, safe care is about emotional safety. Women throughout childbearing need to feel supported and respected, and to trust their caregiver. For a midwife to achieve this situation she must have a sound knowledge base from which to work. Her communication with women can only be enhanced when this is the case.

This easy to follow, well presented and highly informative text is not about turning midwives into doctors. It is about ensuring that midwives have a sound knowledge base from which they can fulfil their role. It is noteworthy that at a time when multiprofessional working has been acknowledged as one of the cornerstones of high quality care the text is authored jointly by a midwife and an obstetrician.

Cathy Warwick

Professor Cathy Warwick, CBE
Chief Executive
Royal College of Midwives

Foreword to the First Edition

Despite the considerable advances in maternity care, and world-class maternity services provided by highly trained and motivated health care professionals, good maternal health is not a given or a universal right even in countries with high quality functioning maternity services with their attendant very low maternal mortality and morbidity rates. And whilst we would all hope that pregnancy, birth and the early weeks of parenthood would be enjoyable and relatively comfortable experiences for new mothers, babies and families we know, sadly, that this is not always the case.

Not all mothers start pregnancy in the best of health, and others develop problems as they go along. The latest Confidential Enquiry into Maternal Deaths Report for 2003–2005, Saving Mothers' Lives, shows that more of our mothers died from pre-existing, or new, medical conditions aggravated by pregnancy than from the big obstetric killers of the past such as haemorrhage, sepsis and pre-eclampsia. These so-called 'indirect' maternal deaths have outnumbered those from causes directly related to pregnancy for more than 10 years. And each death is just the tip of the iceberg of severe morbidity and complications. In the last Saving Mothers' Lives report more women died from cardiac disease than from any other cause, including the leading 'directly' associated cause thrombo-embolism, and deaths from acquired heart disease brought on by unhealthy lifestyles and obesity are increasing at an alarming rate. These findings show that whilst the lessons for the management of common obstetric conditions have clearly had an impact in the past, maternity professionals need to be more aware of the impact of, and identification and management of medical conditions affecting pregnancy before conception and during and after pregnancy. This is what this book aims to achieve.

A number of factors have led to the increase in the proportion of pregnant women or new mothers who have more medically complex pregnancies. They include rising numbers of older or obese mothers, women whose lifestyles put them at risk of poorer health and a growing proportion of women with serious underlying medical conditions who would not have chosen, or have been able to become pregnant in the past. The rising numbers of births to women born outside the UK also affects the underlying general level of maternal health as these mothers often have more complicated pregnancies, more serious underlying medical conditions or may be in poorer general health.

This publication is therefore extremely timely. Its authors are to be congratulated for developing a highly readable, informative and practical book each chapter of which, in the best traditions of maternity care, has been written jointly by a midwife and obstetrician. Such partnership working is emphasised throughout the book, with a clear focus on each other's respective roles and responsibilities within the clinical team. The need for pre-pregnancy counselling and preparation for women living with conditions that are adversely affected by pregnancy, or which ideally require a change in treatment or medication prior to conception is also rightly highlighted as an important, but often overlooked aspect of obstetric medicine. Midwives, obstetricians and all other maternity team members together with those with a general interest in pregnancy and birth should find this book informative and easy to read. Acting on the important messages continued within each chapter should help lead to wider improvements in the understanding and management of mothers who need extra care to ensure they have as healthy and happy pregnancies, birth and babies as possible.

Gwyneth Lewis MBBS, MSc, MRCGP, FFPHM, FRCOG
National Director for Maternal Health, England
Director of the United Kingdom Confidential Enquiries into
Maternal Deaths

Preface

Midwives are practising in a rapidly changing world with advances in technology, increasing expectations of mothers and pressure to provide a cost-effective service in state-funded health sectors. Innovative schemes of care have been developed, such as case-holding midwifery, concentrating on normal childbearing that foster autonomy in the midwife's practice.

The nature of the child-bearing woman is also changing, with women delaying pregnancy until their thirties and forties and sometimes beyond. Whilst fertility and obstetrical aspects of such a delay are well documented, the association with medical disorders warrants attention. Advancing maternal age increases risk of chronic medical conditions. A medical disorder can subsequently complicate pregnancy, or it can present for the first time in pregnancy.

Knowledge of medical conditions is therefore necessary, first to avoid mothers being booked inappropriately for low-risk midwifery care schemes, and second for midwives to recognise the signs of deterioration in order to take principled action. The 2004 *Why Mothers Die* report found 'some midwives and junior obstetricians failed to pick up and act upon warning signs of common medical conditions unrelated to pregnancy'.

Ironically, a midwife is increasingly likely to encounter women with a medical disorder at a time when the pool of dual-qualified nurse-midwives is diminishing in the UK. This should place emphasis on inclusion of medical disorders within midwifery direct entry education programmes, although curriculum guidelines place emphasis on normality.

Until 2008, no textbook on pre-existing medical disorders written specifically for midwives existed. Our experience found student midwives unenthusiastic about standard medical textbooks, due to the lack of midwifery emphasis, and they resorted to home internet use with inherent risk of simplistic understanding. This led to the decision to create the first edition aimed specifically for midwives and student midwives, using local and national expertise from midwives, obstetricians and physicians.

This second edition of *Medical Disorders of Pregnancy: A Manual for Midwives* was created in response to the reviews from the first edition. Whilst overwhelmingly positive, this feedback indicated that extra subjects needed coverage and illustrations or algorithms were appreciated, in particular student midwives wanted more physiology. To this end, some chapters have illustrations to explain the physiology, and others have a table of physiological facts. In other chapters management-based algorithms are more appropriate and therefore included. References are now situated at the end of each chapter. Some chapters are larger than before, in particular Chapter 18 on Neoplasia which has doubled in size to recognise the increasing occurrence of cancer in child-bearing women. Topics such as cardiac transplant have been added to reflect the changing approach to conditions that were seen previously as 'no go' areas for pregnancy.

With the midwifery emphasis, there are some differences from traditional medical textbooks. In particular, differential diagnosis has not been addressed as this is very much the art of medicine. We have taken the stance that most women will already have had their medical disorder diagnosed when she meets the midwife at the booking appointment, with notable exceptions such as pre-eclampsia.

The book is divided into chapters, then into sections using a template for each medical condition. The first page of each is predominately non-pregnancy, giving an explanation of the condition (which might include investigations), complications and non-pregnancy treatment, and then pre-conception care is addressed. The second page identifies key issues pertinent to the ante-, intra- and postpartum periods in the left-hand column. Then in the right-hand column the management and care by both midwife and doctor is outlined. This allows the reader to go quickly to the access point, for all the conditions, which often suits pressurised practice circumstances. Algorithms or illustrations are inserted between or within the templates. The accompanying website allows these figures to be downloaded and used for educational purposes on an individual basis. See **www.wiley.com/go/robson**

Risk scoring is complicated but the terms low- and high-risk are used daily. Some midwives seem polarised in their view of high or low risk, perhaps branding themselves a low-risk midwife or vice versa. As the book is read it becomes apparent that many mothers have medium or variable risk, and with optimum care can still have labour managed normally by the midwife. Hence, each section identifies risk as low, variable, high or life-threatening. This allows a midwife to recognise the potential severity of a condition immediately, which will influence decisions at the booking interview.

The multi-professional authorship suits the current ethos for educating for professional pluralism. Necessity for an inter-professional culture has already been established with a need to improve teamwork in the maternity services. It is the aim of this book to contribute towards this.

Such a book may invite scrutiny, as midwives are identified as being practitioners of normality. Midwives interested in complicated pregnancy might find themselves dubbed 'medwife' rather than midwife! However, several NMC guidelines over the years indicate that midwifery responsibilities include maximising normality for women in high dependency care, recognising deviations from normal, making appropriate referral and working as equal partners in a multidisciplinary team.

The book is intended for midwives practising on British and European Union influenced models, where the midwife is part of a multidisciplinary team referring mothers with problems to a doctor and assisting the latter where appropriate. Therefore, midwives in the EU, UK, USA and throughout the British Commonwealth should find the book beneficial, with appropriate allowances for national differences.

We are proud that the first edition has been translated into Indonesian by 'EGC Medical Publisher, INDONESIA' hoping that this will contribute to the sharing of good midwifery practice to improve maternal wellbeing on an international basis.

The excitement of writing the second edition was tempered with sadness as two medical authors died suddenly and unexpectedly during the development of their respective chapters. Our sympathies go to the families of Javed Iqbal and Ed Howarth.

MIDWIFERY CARE AND MEDICAL DISORDERS

S. Elizabeth Robson

De Montfort University, Leicester, UK

Pre-conception Care
Antenatal Care
Intrapartum Care
Postnatal Care
General Considerations
Emergency Management
Preventing Maternal Mortality
Back to Basics Campaign

Medical Disorders in Pregnancy: A Manual for Midwives, Second Edition. Edited by S. Elizabeth Robson and Jason Waugh.
© 2013 John Wiley & Sons, Ltd. Published 2013 by John Wiley & Sons, Ltd.

1 Midwifery Care and Medical Disorders

INTRODUCTION

This chapter will give an overview of pre-conception, ante-natal, intrapartum and postnatal care that would be given to a woman with a medical condition that either pre-exists or presents in pregnancy. The information here will not be repeated in each subject section, which will focus on the aspects specific to that particular medical disorder.

PRE-CONCEPTION CARE

In an ideal world all women would receive state-funded pre-conception care. However, about 50% of pregnancies are unplanned[1], and most women seek medical or midwifery attention once pregnant. For certain groups such as recent immigrants this first contact may happen late in the pregnancy[2].

For a woman with an existing medical disorder, obesity or mental health problem the need for pre-conception care is more pronounced, and early booking once pregnant is of paramount importance, as the disorder can affect the pregnancy and conversely the pregnancy can affect the disorder[3]. A woman with a previously well-controlled condition can become unstable with a domino effect on the pregnancy. Hence, such women should be advised to seek pre-conception advice from 'mainstream' medical or midwifery care prior to ceasing use of contraception.

In British practice a woman contemplating pregnancy may consult her general practitioner, practice nurse or midwife. Adequate time is needed for the consultation and follow-up[4]. Practice policies vary considerably[5], but can be summarised as follows:

(1) *Nurse/midwife taking a history to ascertain:*

- Medical, surgical, psychological or infectious conditions that could complicate a future pregnancy, including any current medications or treatment
- Family history of disease and handicap, including genetic history
- Vaccination status
- Substance use, e.g. alcohol, cigarettes and street drugs
- Past obstetric and gynaecological history
- Present employment – to identify occupational hazards
- Current diet and nutritional history
- Lifestyle, including diet and exercise

(2) *Nurse/midwife observations and medical examination for:*

- Weight and height measurement for calculation of the body mass index (BMI) (see Appendix 13.1.1)
- Baseline pulse, blood pressure, urinalysis measurement
- Pelvic examination to include a cervical smear and screening for infection such as *Chlamydia*
- Respiratory and cardiac function
- Other function screening – if history indicates
- Karyotyping – if indicated by family history
- Blood samples for full blood count (FBC), Venereal Disease Research Laboratory (VDRL) and rubella
- If indicated, additional screening for TB, hepatitis B, HIV, chickenpox, cytomegalovirus and toxoplasma

- Haemoglobinopathy screening for women originating from: Africa, West Indies, Indian subcontinent, Asia, Eastern Mediterranean countries and the Middle East. If affected, partner screening should be offered with genetic counselling[6]

(3) *Interventions that are advocated:*

- Folic acid: advise 0.4 mg daily[1]
- Vaccination, such as rubella or BCG for TB, dependent upon aforementioned antibody titres. Pregnancy should be avoided for 3 months after vaccination, and this applies to 'holiday vaccinations' such as cholera, typhoid and Japanese encephalitis.
- Contraceptive cover while investigations, vaccinations and treatment are initiated

(4) *In relation to medical disorders, the doctor will usually:*

- Act upon any anomalies detected in the baseline observations and order additional tests such as a glucose tolerance test (GTT) and initiate treatment
- Refer the woman back to any specialist clinic and physician who has previously treated her; immigrant women may need referral for the first time
- Review current drug therapy to identify those on drugs associated with teratogenic effects or contraindicated in pregnancy, and initiate change
- Increase the folic acid dosage for a history of neural tube defects, haemoglobinopathies, rheumatoid arthritis, coeliac disease, diabetes or epilepsy
- Prescribe suitable contraceptive cover whilst the above is addressed
- Initiate counselling regarding prognosis for both mother and prospective child

(5) *Specific advice, from a nurse/midwife, in relation to:*

- Keeping a menstrual diary
- Pregnancy testing and need for early booking
- Perinatal diagnosis – practical aspects
- Smoking and alcohol cessation
- Street drug avoidance and cessation
- Over-the-counter medicines and therapies
- Domestic violence
- Stress avoidance
- Sport, exercise and general fitness
- Occupational hazards
- Animal contact and infection risk
- Food hygiene and hand washing
- Weight adjustment
- Health education initiatives and leaflets
- Patient organisations, e.g. *Foresight*, with additional options such as hair analysis for mineral deficiencies[7]

ANTENATAL CARE

Antenatal care on the British model has followed the same basis for much of the twentieth century[8]. A woman reports a positive pregnancy test to her general practitioner (GP) then has a 'booking history' conducted by a midwife. Options for place of care and delivery are discussed and the mother should be offered a choice of birth at a consultant unit, low-risk birth centre or at home. Risk for childbearing will be taken into consideration to avoid inappropriate bookings which are associated with maternal death (see Appendix 1.1). The mother is referred to an obstetrician and may have one appointment at a consultant clinic. Responsibility for care is shared between GP and obstetrician, hence the term *shared care*. Most appointments occur in the community at the GP premises with the midwife actually conducting the majority of the antenatal care, referring to either GP or obstetrician if problems are identified. Specialist investigations, such as ultrasonography and amniocentesis are conducted at a consultant unit, often in conjunction with an antenatal or specialist clinic.

Variations in care exist, with Domino, case-holding midwifery, and team-midwifery schemes aiming for women-centred care with continuity of carer and a focus on normality. Women on such schemes should have normal, uncomplicated pregnancies hence a significant medical condition precludes inclusion on such a low-risk scheme.

With few exceptions a mother with a medical condition will require pregnancy management and care with involvement of hospital consultants. Some mothers may need to have some of their antenatal appointments at a specialist antenatal clinic, or at other clinics that combine obstetric care with involvement from a physician. Examples of *combined clinics* are for diabetes and renal problems.

Such mothers tend to fit into a risk category of variable or high risk. Here an assumption might be made, wrongly, that no midwifery involvement is necessary, and in recent times the numbers of midwives and student midwives at high-risk clinics appears to have reduced. Whilst it might seem cost effective to have an auxiliary nurse chaperoning at a clinic and performing manual tasks, the knowledge and skills of a midwife should not be denied to a mother because she has a medical disorder and has a stereotypical label of risk.

The mother requires midwifery care and should be given the opportunity to build a rapport with a midwife and to get continuity of care as she would on a midwife-led scheme. The care that the midwife gives should be complementary to that of the obstetricians and physicians, with the mother and fetus being the cherished focus of attention.

Booking

The booking visit should be completed by 12 weeks. If on referral they are later than 12 weeks, they should be seen within a 2-week period. Migrant women will also need a full clinical examination by a doctor, to include cardio-respiratory examination.

The midwife must take and document a detailed, accurate booking history[9] which should encompass:

- Personal details – including name, address, date of birth, occupation, marital status, religion, GP, and official numbers such as National Insurance. Race is ascertained for screening of racially-specific conditions.
- Social factors – late booking, asylum seeker, drug misuse, domestic violence, known to social services, and other risk factors of consequence.
- Histories – family, medical, surgical, psychological, gynaecological and obstetric histories; cross-reference with GP case notes or hospital records if access is possible. Medical records from other geographical areas may have to be obtained.

- Identification of risk factors for mother and fetus, which should encompass biophysical factors, especially pre-existing medical disorders and current medication.
- Ascertain any hospital clinics previously attended in relation to a medical disorder or surgical operation. Determine if the mother is still attending, and discuss with the GP if the mother needs to be re-referred.
- Ascertain any pre-conception advice and care given.
- Calculate the expected date of delivery (EDD) from the menstrual history.

A mother may want certain details omitted from her hand-held records if her domestic situation entails that her records would be viewed by family members – necessitating full details in the hospital records as a 'duplicate'. Be aware that a mother might not be fully forthcoming about an existing medical condition, or prognosis, if the booking history takes place with her husband/partner or in-laws in attendance. Any language translation should be conducted by a trained interpreter rather than a friend or relative, including those who may need a British Sign Language or lip reader or documents presented in alternative formats such as Braille or DVDs with subtitles[10]

A physical examination will identify baseline observations:

- General appearance and wellbeing
- Pulse and blood pressure
- MSU and urinalysis
- Weight
- Abdominal examination – to determine if the uterus is palpable and equates to dates

The doctor may additionally examine to determine:

- Cardiac function
- Lung function

NB: Pelvic examinations are no longer performed unless there is a specific indication to do so[8].

The following serum investigations[6] will be offered to the mother after explanation and informed consent:

- Identification of blood group and Rhesus factor
- FBC
- Antibodies for rubella, hepatitis B, syphilis and HIV
- Haemoglobinopathy screening for at-risk ethnic groups

Additional screening may be discussed and offered for:

- Down's syndrome risk
- Ultrasound for gestational age assessment
- Ultrasound for fetal structural anomalies after 16 weeks

Careful consideration is given as to where the mother is booked for antenatal care and for delivery. Mothers with a medical condition may be referred for antenatal care wholly or partly at a specialist antenatal or combined clinic (Table 1.1). The midwife should share ideas with the mother on a specific model of care, and discuss and agree a realistic birth plan.

Issues specific to antenatal screening are discussed. Then further advice is given in relation to:

- Occupation hazards
- Animal contact and infection risk
- Healthy diet with vitamins (Appendix 1.2) and safe eating
- Handwashing and food hygiene
- Domestic violence
- Smoking, alcohol and street drug cessation
- Sport, exercise and stress avoidance

Table 1.1 Referral Guide for Specialist Clinics*

Maternal Medicine Clinic
Neurological disorders, especially:
Epilepsy
Multiple sclerosis
Myasthenia gravis
Myotonic dystrophy
Cardiac disease, especially:
Cardiomyopathy
Congenital heart disease
Marfan's syndrome
Rheumatic heart disease
Prosthetic valves
Gastrointestinal disease, especially:
Coeliac disease
Ulcerative colitis
Crohn's disease
Rheumatological/auto-immune disease, especially:
Rheumatoid arthritis
Systemic lupus erythematosus
Severe back problem – including kyphoscoliosis
Liver and pancreatic disease – especially
cholestasis
Malignancy (current or previous)
Substance misuse

Specialist Obstetric Clinic (Fetal Growth)
Previous small baby <2.5 kg at term
Maternal weight <45 kg
>2 first trimester miscarriages
Previous unexplained stillbirth

Diabetes and Endocrine Clinic
Diabetes mellitus
Diabetes insipidus
Thyroid disorders
Pituitary disorders
Adrenal disorders

Haematology Clinic
Immune thrombocytopenic purpura (ITP)
Von Willebrand's disease
Carriers of haemophilia
Antiphospholipid (Hughes) syndrome
Hereditary thrombophilia
Family history of thrombosis
Acute thrombosis in pregnancy
Refractory anaemia
Sickle cell disease
Thalassaemia
Low platelet count (<100 × 10^9/l) or rapidly
falling platelet count

Anaesthetic Clinic
Previous adverse drug reaction
Previous regional or general anaesthetic problems
Secondary referral from other clinic

Fetal Assessment Unit
Previous fetal abnormality (live birth or termination of
pregnancy – ToP)
Family history of genetic conditions
Monochorionic twins
Positive rhesus antibodies
Homeless women and travellers (with no GP)

General Obstetric Clinic
Grand multiparity of >5
Previous stillbirth
Previous abruption
Previous precipitate labour
Previous shoulder dystocia
Previous rotational forceps
Previous 3rd or 4th degree tear or other perineal morbidity
Previous retained placenta
Previous primary postpartum haemorrhage (PPH)
Previous difficult labour/vaginal delivery
Previous gynaecological surgery, other than fertility treatment
Previous caesarean sections

Specialist Obstetric Clinic (Prematurity Prevention)
Last pregnancy a pre-term birth (≤34 weeks)
Last pregnancy a mid-trimester miscarriage
Known uterine malformation
First pregnancy after a cone biopsy

Specialist Gynaecology/Obstetrics Clinic
Multiple pregnancy
Tubal surgery
In vitro fertilisation pregnancies
Previous myomectomy

Hypertension Clinic
Booking BP >138/85
Primigravidae with a mother or sister who had pre-eclampsia
Primigravidae with hypertension outside of pregnancy
Past obstetric history of raised blood pressure requiring
treatment

Renal Clinic
Any pre-existing renal disease
Renal transplantation or dialysis patients
History of reflux nephropathy
Recurrent urinary tract infection
Persistent first trimester proteinuria

Specialist/Consultant Midwife Referral
Age ≤16 years
Age 17–19 years with housing or social issues, or any
concerns to specialist or consultant midwife for teenage
pregnancy
Substance misuse – to drug liaison midwife
Hypertension – hypertension specialist midwife
Diabetes – to diabetic specialist midwife

*Referral guide used for University Hospitals of Leicester, adapted and used with permission

- Maternity benefits
- Attending antenatal education parentcraft classes
- Important telephone and contact details

Subsequent Antenatal Appointments

The frequency of routine antenatal visits has come under recent scrutiny, emphasising that schemes of care should be based on evidence rather than ritual[11]. However, recent research finds women actually wanting more frequent antenatal appointments, ultrasonic scans and support from their midwives[12].

Current UK recommendations[13] for routine antenatal care advocate visits at the following weeks of gestation. The regimen will vary between areas, but approximates to:

Week 8–12

- Initial booking with confirmation of pregnancy, identification of risk factors, and investigations as per previous page

Week 16

- BP and urinalysis
- AFP/serum screening for Down's risk
- Possibly ultrasound scan for fetal anomalies
- Discuss results from the booking blood tests

Week 18–20

- Discuss results from AFP or Down's risk
- Ultrasound scans for fetal anomalies, if not already done

Week 24–25

- Full antenatal examination to ascertain maternal wellbeing and to include BP, urinalysis, oedema, abdominal examination with symphysis pubis height measurement, fetal movements asked about and the fetal heart auscultated

Week 28

- Full antenatal examination as above
- FBC and antibody screen
- First dose of anti-D for rhesus negative women

Week 31–32

- Full antenatal examination as above

Week 34

- Full antenatal examination as above
- FBC and antibody screen
- Second dose of anti-D for rhesus negative women

Week 36

- Full antenatal examination as above, with emphasis on fetal position and presentation
- FBC

Week 38 (repeat at 40 weeks for nulliparae)

- Full antenatal examination as above

Week 41

- Full antenatal examination as above
- Assessment for induction of labour or increased fetal surveillance

A mother with a medical condition will require the same obstetric and midwifery care as a mother with a low-risk pregnancy on the above schedule, but with *additional* management and care from the specialists and the multidisciplinary team. Therefore midwives should consider:

- Arranging clinic appointments for both specialist clinics and antenatal clinics so that there is even spacing between them. These appointments should be made at a frequency suitable for the complexity of the medical condition and any additional fetal screening required
- If handheld notes are used the mother should be advised to keep these with her at all times
- Ensure the woman understands her condition, and the additional impact that pregnancy can have on the condition and vice versa. Further education may be necessary on a one-to-one basis
- Provide written information or leaflets to reinforce the advice given, seeking leaflets translated into other languages where necessary
- Ensure the woman understands signs and symptoms that may indicate the condition worsening, and give information on whom to contact, and what to do
- Accept that many women are fully informed about their medical condition and will be the first person to recognise an alteration in the condition
- Take the concerns of the woman and her husband/partner seriously
- Advise relatives, with the mother's consent, of acute situations that may arise, such as thrombo-embolism or an epileptic seizure, in which the mother may need emergency assistance, and give directions on first aid and whom to contact
- Be aware of, and report, any signs, symptoms and complications of a medical condition
- Carry out any treatment prescribed by the doctor, reinforcing any medical advice given. Be aware that many medical conditions have periods of remission and some mothers might be tempted to cease taking prescribed treatment if they feel their condition is stable or 'cured'. Always seek medical advice before acquiescing with any maternal decisions in relation to altering prescribed treatment
- Effective inter-disciplinary teamwork is of paramount importance for maximum feto-maternal benefit, so effective care pathways need to be established
- Normality is still possible for many aspects of the antenatal periods and labour and it is the midwife's duty to determine how best to empower the mother to achieve maximum fulfilment from her pregnancy and to make the process as natural as possible under the circumstances

INTRAPARTUM CARE

The medical condition may necessitate an elective caesarean section for many mothers. Some mothers may require induction of labour at, or before, term, dependent upon the condition and feto-maternal wellbeing during the antenatal period. Others may be able to labour normally. In these cases intrapartum care for labouring women with any other than a low-risk categorisation of a medical disorder should encompass:

- Delivery to be planned for a consultant unit with emergency facilities for both mother and baby

- The mother should have one-to-one care from a midwife, with adequate relief for breaks
- Care should be competent, compassionate and caring, with astute observation and vigilance in determining any deviations from anticipated progress
- Accurate history taking on admission to delivery suite to determine the onset and nature of the labour as well as feto-maternal wellbeing
- Baseline observations on admission of maternal temperature, pulse, blood pressure, urinalysis, oedema, and general wellbeing
- Full antenatal examination to include abdominal palpation and auscultation of the fetal heart
- Review of maternal case notes to ascertain the birth plan and care pathways for the medical and midwifery management of the medical condition in labour
- The mother would be seen by a member of the obstetric team as a matter of course, but also ascertain if a physician, paediatrician, anaesthetist or the neonatal unit needs to be informed that this mother is in labour
- Any specified treatment regimen should be implemented with full knowledge of the obstetric team on duty
- Seek medical advice before empowering the mother to eat during labour, as many such women have a high chance of operative delivery; often the mother may be on water *only* by mouth regimen
- Keep the mother well hydrated with water orally, or an iv infusion in line with medical guidance
- Prophylactic treatment to reduce acid content of the stomach, e.g. ranitidine 150 mg orally qds
- Assessment of first stage progress by abdominal palpation to assess descent, and vaginal examination at least four hourly, with results plotted on a partogram
- Abnormal progress of any of the three stages of labour must be reported to the obstetric team
- Suitable pain relief that is compatible with the planned treatment regimen
- Apt mobilisation of the mother whenever possible, or passive leg exercises if the mother has an epidural *in situ*, or is otherwise immobile
- Position should be changed regularly, and wedges placed under the mattress to prevent the mother lying *flat on her back* resulting in pressure on the inferior vena cava leading to reduced uterine blood flow
- Some mothers may require TED stockings, especially if she is obese or has a history of thrombo-embolism
- Assistance to walk to the toilet, or bedpans, should be offered every 2 hours, with the urine measured and tested on every occasion
- Regular (hourly) observations of pulse and blood pressure, with temperature recorded at least four hourly
- Additional observations may be required in relation to the specific medical condition
- Monitoring of fetal wellbeing will, in most cases, necessitate continuous fetal heart monitoring throughout the first stage of labour
- Basic hygiene and comfort should be attended to regularly; if the mother is not mobile enough to use the shower, then a bowl and towel should be brought and the mother assisted to wash
- Water immersion in labour is discouraged because the mother does not meet the low-risk criteria[14]
- A normal vertex delivery can be managed by the midwife unless additional complications result
- The cord is usually clamped twice and cut, the baby dried and given to parents for a 'cuddle', if the condition permits
- The baby should have Apgar scores calculated at one and five minutes of life, and a low score should necessitate resuscitative measures and a paediatrician being called urgently
- The baby should be weighed and examined by a midwife to determine if there are any apparent abnormalities, and if the baby is making adequate adaptation to extra-uterine life
- Identification bracelets should be applied, having first been checked with the parents
- Third stage of labour often entails *active management* as this is not a low-risk labour and the midwife should check that the drugs used are compatible with the condition, e.g. Syntometrine is contraindicated with a number of conditions because of vaso-spasm[15], and Syntocinon may be prescribed instead
- The placenta and membranes should be examined for completeness and for signs of abnormality[15]; if there is any doubt the placenta should be retained for examination by a member of the obstetric team
- Be aware that after delivery specific blood samples might be required from the placenta, and advice should be sought if in doubt
- Post-delivery umbilical cord blood pH is usually measured in high-risk pregnancy and emergencies
- Occasionally the placenta may be sent to the laboratory for histological investigation
- Ascertain if any specific care is needed for the baby at, or shortly after, delivery
- Vitamin K is given to the baby, with maternal consent, to prevent haemorrhagic disease[16]
- Perineal trauma is assessed and sutured promptly
- The midwife must report any deviations from the anticipated progress of either the labour, or the medical condition, to the obstetric team
- Measures must be taken to prevent cross-infection in the delivery suite, with especial emphasis on hand washing and meticulous aseptic techniques
- All procedures should be performed with full explanation to the mother, and with informed consent
- There must be accurate and contemporaneous record keeping throughout labour[17]
- Whilst acknowledging the necessary medical management, the midwife should still be able to give woman centred midwifery care, and many such women should still be able to have a normal vaginal birth under midwifery practice

POSTNATAL CARE

Postnatal care commences shortly after the birth and usually commences in hospital[18]. Within 6 hours of delivery the blood pressure should be recorded and the first urine void obtained and documented[19]. Gentle mobilisation is encouraged and opportunity given to talk about the birth. The midwife should be alert to life-threatening conditions in this period[19].

British midwives conduct home visits once the mother has been discharged home. These visits occur on a selective basis until the 10th postnatal day; however, the midwife can extend these visits up to or beyond the 28th day[20]. After this, care is transferred to a specialist public health nurse (health visitor), who continues child health surveillance until the child is 5 years of age, when the child commences school[18].

A physical examination of the mother is conducted by the midwife to ascertain if her body is returning to the pre-pregnant state. The examination is repeated at home, and on a selective basis, and should:

- Detemine general wellbeing of mother and child
- Determine mother's emotional state
- Include observations of pulse and blood pressure
- Determine presence of signs of infection
- Record temperature[19]
- Include breast examination to ascertain initiation of lactation and sore/cracked nipples in breast-feeding mothers, as well as other problems such as breast engorgement
- Determine uterine involution
- Determine type of lochia, and if there are any anomalies such as heavy bleeding or passing of blood clots, or offensive odour which could indicate infection
- Examine the perineum, with especial attention to wound healing, bruising and swelling
- Include other wound inspection, especially if the mother delivered by caesarean section; a dry dressing may be re-applied to protect the wound from friction
- Examine legs to see if both calves are of equal size and temperature and if there is any pain (an abnormality of which could indicate a DVT)
- Examine fingers, pre-tibial area and ankles to ascertain if oedema exists, and if excessive
- Address specific educational needs on a one-to-one basis, such as making up infant feeds

The findings of the above examination should be recorded, and preferably plotted, to determine if there is a graphic pattern of the body returning towards the pre-pregnant state.

A postnatal visit often coincides with the newborn screening (Guthrie) test at 5–7 days of milk feeding.

The following additional considerations should be given to the mother with a medical condition:

- Some mothers need to remain in hospital for a longer period postpartum
- Follow-up appointments for mother and baby may need to be made before the mother is discharged home
- Physical observations may need to be conducted more frequently than customary home 'selective visiting'
- Drug treatment may need prompt alteration
- Some conditions can destabilise rapidly postpartum

GENERAL CONSIDERATIONS

Local Protocols

Management of routine midwifery care can alter and medical management of medical conditions may need to be changed promptly, especially in light of adverse event reporting. A midwife is obliged to follow local policies and protocols[21], as this is usually part of the employment contract. It is therefore important that midwives, doctors and other health care professionals regularly review:

- **Local guidelines**, which many health authorities now put on their own intranet
- **Unit protocols** – these may be in paper or intranet form and are usually specific to a specific area or ward
- **National guidelines** – in the UK the organisations of especial relevance are the National Institute for Clinical Excellence (NICE), the Royal College of Obstetricians and Gynaecologists (RCOG), the Royal College of Midwives (RCM) and the Nursing and Midwifery Council (NMC)

Complementary Therapies

By the nature of a chronic disease many women may already have tried complementary and alternative medications (CAM), perhaps feeling that conventional medicine has failed them. A woman may be self-administering CAM when she first consults the midwife, in the mistaken belief that because they are natural they are safe[22]. Whilst some interventions have some effectiveness, others require research before they can be recommended[23].

In a tactful way the midwife needs to explain that many complementary, homeopathic and herbal medicines have not been subject to research with adequate scientific rigour to ascertain if they are safe to use in pregnancy and therefore their continued use cannot be recommended[19,24]. If the mother is firmly adherent to her beliefs in a product, then the midwife should seek additional advice from a pharmacist or doctor.

Over-the-Counter Medication

Many medicines can be purchased over the counter (OTC) at a pharmacy or shop. The midwife may be the first health professional a pregnant woman sees to seek advice about these drugs for minor ailments[25] or to alleviate symptoms of their medical condition. There is a theoretical risk of a mother choosing OTC drugs in preference to those prescribed by a doctor, as she might mistakenly believe them to be 'safer'. Therefore the midwife should advise:

- To continue taking prescribed drugs until she has sought advice from her GP or specialist clinic
- To consider OTC drugs only if absolutely necessary
- Always to ask the advice of the pharmacist before making a purchase, making it clear that she is pregnant

Some drugs can be advised by the midwife, and common examples are bowel care medications, nutritional supplements and anti-fungal preparations[25]. However, the midwife should develop adequate knowledge about the products before advising about their use within the scope of midwifery practice[24,25].

Prescribed Medication

With many medical conditions the woman is likely to be receiving prescribed drugs, some of which might be contraindicated in pregnancy as their effect upon the fetus is unknown[26]. Some drugs are known to be teratogenic in animal studies, and therefore contraindicated for use in human pregnancy[26]. A few are already known to have caused human congenital anomalies and their use is strongly contraindicated unless in emergency situations[26]. Hence, the woman should have a review of her medication conducted by a doctor experienced in pregnancy prescribing, and safer alternative drugs selected.

A mother may panic about potential effects upon the fetus and cease taking her prescribed medication. In some cases sudden withdrawal of drugs can precipitate a medical crisis, such as an epileptic fit or lupus flare, with a catastrophic effect on the pregnancy and fetal loss. For this reason a midwife should advise a woman to continue with her treatment until a medical practitioner with expertise in pregnancy prescribing has been consulted. The midwife may need to arrange an emergency appointment for the mother.

The NMC states[24] '*A practising midwife shall only supply and administer those medicines in respect of which she has received the appropriate training as to use, dosage and methods of administration.*' Therefore, a midwife may have to seek instruction or guidance in specific drugs to be able to meet the needs of certain mothers with medical conditions. She can seek recent information from reputable websites, in particular the British National Formulary or texts that specialise in prescribing in pregnancy (see Essential Reading).

Nicotine, Alcohol and Illegal Drugs

Cigarette smoking, alcohol consumption and use of illegal drugs are of concern in pregnancy or puerperium. Smoking cessation should always be promoted by the midwife. Drinking should be discouraged, or, failing this, measures taken to reduce it to a minimum. Illegal drugs are strongly contraindicated. Alcohol and illegal drugs are addressed more fully in Chapter 16.

Termination of Pregnancy

Some medical conditions can exacerbate and tragically necessitate a mother facing the emotional dilemma of having to have a termination of a wanted pregnancy. This might be for congenital anomalies or to save the mother's own life. The gynaecological terminology is 'therapeutic abortion' but when speaking to the parents 'termination' should be used in preference to 'abortion'. The Centre for Maternal and Child Enquiries (CMACE) recommendations are for *termination of pregnancy services to be readily available for women with medical conditions precluding safe pregnancy*, and *an appointment should take no longer than 3 weeks*[27].

In the UK a midwife can be a conscientious objector to termination of pregnancy. However, she cannot refuse to care for a mother if the termination is to save the life of the mother[28]. Confidentiality is also of paramount importance. The ethical, legal and emotional dilemmas cannot be addressed here, and it is strongly recommended that midwives read the RCM Position Statement No. 17 (see Essential Reading, this chapter).

Pre-term Birth

A maternal medical condition may result in pre-term induction of labour, caesarean section or a spontaneous pre-term delivery. If the presentation is cephalic the latter might be conducted by the midwife. The nature of the condition might also have caused growth restriction, and the baby may have a double set of problems. If time, surfactant prophylaxis is usually given to the mother (e.g. 12 mg betamethasone, two doses 24 h apart) to assist maturation of the fetal lungs.

The midwife should prepare for a pre-term delivery by: notifying the neonatal unit and calling an experienced paediatrician to be present at delivery[29], then:

- Preparing neonatal resuscitation equipment in advance
- Avoiding use of narcotics which suppress infant breathing[29]
- Having a warm delivery room, and calm environment
- Have bonnet and plastic bag to prevent neonatal heat loss
- Preparing detailed records; duplicates may be needed to accompany the baby to the neonatal unit (NNU)
- Preparing identity bracelets in advance, and checking these with the parents
- Giving support and clear explanations to the parents

At delivery the midwife should:

- Leave adequate length of umbilical cord below the cord clamp to allow for catheter insertion on the NNU
- Quickly dry the baby[29] and hand to the paediatrician
- Ask an assistant to apply the identity bracelets and, if the paediatrician permits, weigh the baby and pass to mother for a quick cuddle before the baby is taken to the NNU

- Neonatal vitamin K (Konakion) should be given in the delivery room or on the neonatal unit

Care of the Mother of a Baby on the Neonatal Unit

If the baby has been admitted to a specialist unit for intensive care, the mother can feel bereft on the postnatal ward[29] or at home, and will benefit from psychological support and encouragement from the midwife. Postnatal care may have to be adapted if the mother is spending a lot of time in a paediatric hospital environment. In some cases the baby may be 'out of area' and arrangements must be made for a midwife to care for the mother in a different location. Accurate communication is needed, especially in relation to specific requirements of the medical condition.

Mother–infant attachment should be fostered by allowing a 'cuddle' with the baby whenever possible[29]. A photograph of the baby should be taken and given to the mother, and arrangements for visits made. The whole family are encouraged to visit the baby with due liaison with the neonatal unit. The staff there should give the parents regular explanations as to the progress and prognosis of the baby[29]. The midwife may need to reinforce some of the explanation as tired, anxious parents might find it difficult to assimilate information of this nature.

Mothers experience tiredness with frequent visits to a neonatal unit, and might be called throughout the night. A quiet, calm environment on the ward might assist relaxation and sleeping. As there is a chance of meals and drug rounds being missed, alternative arrangements should be made. Assistance should be given with breast pump use, and arrangements made for the storage of expressed milk.

Breast-feeding

In most cases, the midwife should promote and support breast-feeding even if concern may arise over drugs passing to the baby in breast milk. Here the midwife should confer with the physician, paediatrician and pharmacist as to the best course of action. In some cases the mother may need to express and dispose of breast milk until certain drugs have 'cleared' and she is able to breast-feed as normal. Alternatively she may have to continue with her 'pregnancy drugs' and delay a return to the former treatment regimen until breast-feeding has ceased.

The midwife should address practical aspects, such as equipment for expressing breast milk, cleaning and sterilisation of that equipment and storage of the milk, which will require refrigeration and labelling to comply with food handling requirements of the individual institution. Arrangements should be made to take the milk over to the NNU if the mother is unable to go in person. Personal issues must not be forgotten, such as privacy when expressing breast milk, positive encouragement and relief of discomfort when expressing milk or breast-feeding the baby in either the postnatal ward or NNU.

Some infectious conditions, of which HIV is the most notable, could be passed on to the baby through breast-feeding, and this is expanded upon in Chapter 12.2. In these cases the midwife may have to educate the mother about formula feeding methods and sterilisation of feeding utensils. Non-pharmacological measures to suppress lactation should be taken.

Women Who Decline Blood Products or Blood Transfusion

Some mothers may decline the use of blood products or blood transfusion in pregnancy, or at any time. This may be for fear of infection, lack of understanding, religious conviction, or other reasons.

The religious group most usually associated with declining the use of blood products is the Jehovah's Witnesses. Followers accept most medical treatments, surgical and anaesthetic procedures, devices and techniques, as well as haemostatic and therapeutic agents that do not contain blood. They accept non-blood volume expanders and drugs to control haemorrhage and stimulate the production of red blood cells. However, they will *not* accept transfusions of whole blood, packed red cells, white cells, plasma and platelets. Neither are they likely to accept pre-operative autologous blood collection for later re-infusion. However, they *might* accept, on a basis of personal choice, cell salvage, haemodialysis, coagulation factors and immunoglobulins[30].

Closed loop intra-operative cell salvage may also be acceptable. Other women may consider cell salvage and autologous transfusion but need an individual care plan to be negotiated and documented.

It is important that two aspects of planning are addressed. First, as well as documenting refusal of blood products, there also must be a plan for minimisation of blood loss and for resuscitation as required. Second, women with additional risk factors for bleeding, e.g. multiple pregnancy, immune thrombocytopenic purpura (ITP) and those on anticoagulation therapy, must be delivered in a unit with experience of dealing with patients who decline blood products and expertise in alternative methods of treatment and resuscitation.

Declining blood products can pose certain challenges when caring for pregnant women with pre-existing medical conditions, because some conditions would normally require treatment with blood products. Furthermore, some conditions may predispose a mother to haemorrhagic situations, when blood products might be required in labour or emergencies. A Jehovah's Witness, is likely to produce a printed care plan at an antenatal visit and also when admitted to the delivery suite, and will ask for a copy to be kept in the obstetric notes. This care plan *must* be discussed with the most senior clinician on duty.

Whatever the mother's religion or reason for declining blood products, the midwife should establish effective two-way communication and ensure that a supportive and non-judgemental attitude is displayed throughout. It is important that the midwife *listens* to the mother and understands the rationale underpinning any stated intention to decline blood products. Informed choice is an important issue here. The midwife may have to use her educational skills to explain why some products are advisable so that the mother fully understands the choices open to her. In some cases, a clearly put explanation may result in some mothers deciding to accept the treatment. In other cases the mother and her next of kin may have thought through the issues well in advance and be aware of the potential problems, including death, and be able to make a fully informed decision. The ethical and legal dilemmas that arise cannot be addressed within the scope of this book. If a mother continues to state she wishes to decline blood products the midwife should ensure that the mother is seen by a senior doctor with due experience in haematology or obstetrics, so that the issues can be discussed to a greater extent and appropriate plans made for care. Accurate records should be kept, especially of advice given and of decisions made.

It is important that all members of the multi-disciplinary team refer to their own institution's policies and guidelines for direction. Not only will the clinical aspects need to be addressed, but there are legal aspects of considerable importance requiring the mother and next of kin to sign a declaration with appropriate witnesses.

Conflict of Interest

Some women with a medical or addictive disorder may be high risk but are insistent upon a midwifery-led scheme of care. This places the midwife in a difficult position. The midwife has a role as the mother's advocate, but the level of risk creates a conflict of interest, especially when the fetus is taken into account.

A midwife cannot refuse to care for a mother, and should work in partnership with the woman and her family[21]. Negotiating skills should be used to coax the mother to attend an appropriate specialist clinic (Table 1.1). If the mother is adamant about rejecting high-risk care the midwife should consult her named supervisor of midwives in order that a plan of action is developed to support the midwife and colleagues, to care for the mother and fetus more effectively[27].

EMERGENCY MANAGEMENT

Midwives should have the skills to identify a deviation from normality, refer[31] and initiate emergency measures in the doctor's absence, then assist the latter where appropriate[32]. Regular training is advocated on the signs and symptoms of critical illness including basic life support, with 'skills drills' for maternal resuscitation[27].

The midwife may be the first health professional to note a serious deterioration in a pregnant woman's condition and have to initiate emergency measures having called for medical aid. Midwifery management of sudden maternal collapse is outlined in Figure 1.1.

Pregnancy poses challenges for resuscitation of mothers, and there are some differences compared with standard adult resuscitation. Figure 1.2 outlines considerations that should be taken into account when resuscitating a pregnant woman.

It is not within the scope of this book to address advanced life support, and other texts give this important subject detailed attention.

PREVENTING MATERNAL MORTALITY

The seventh CMACE report, *Saving Mothers' Lives*[38] stressed individual responsibility and states that if a midwife is unhappy with a medical opinion then s/he should consult a more senior doctor and seek support from a supervisor of midwives. The eighth CMACE report[39] identified poor midwifery care with:

- Poor communication
- Inadequate documentation
- Failure to perform observations
- Failure to act when a woman reported feeling unwell
- Failure to visit or revisit during the postnatal period

The leading causes of direct and indirect maternal death have significant implications for this book, as Table 1.2 demonstrates that the four leading causes to be related to medical or psychiatric disorders. Further detail is found in Appendix 1.1.

The concept of 'low risk' needs consideration; both midwives and doctors need to be mindful that a woman who was originally deemed suitable for a low risk scheme of care

Prevention is paramount:
   (1) Recognise signs of maternal circulatory compromise using an early warning scoring (EWS) system, e.g. increasing rapid, *thready* pulse; increasing respiratory rate (early signs); falling BP (late sign); pale sweaty skin; altering consciousness.
   (2) Seek help immediately and treat any cause, e.g. haemorrhage, replace fluids, give oxygen, monitor condition[38]

Assess maternal condition:
D (danger to self and woman)
R (response – level of consciousness – AVPU scale)
A (airway – is it open?)
B (breathing – check for 10 seconds - *is it normal?*)
C (circulation – check the carotid pulse and other signs of life - *is the heart beating*?)

Shout, call or go for help:

UK hospitals – dial 2222; UK community or at home – dial 999

If conscious:
Reassure, if pregnant tilt to left side, give oxygen via non-rebreathing mask and monitor SpO$_2$ levels, observe closely, monitor vital signs, site venflon and take appropriate bloods, seek obstetric referral, involve multi-disciplinary team and treat cause[33]

If unconscious, but breathing norma lly with adequate circulation:
Tilt to left side, give oxygen via non-rebreathing mask and monitor SpO$_2$ levels, observe closely, monitor vital signs, monitor AVPU, site venflon and take appropriate bloods, seek obstetric referral, involve multidisciplinary team and treat cause[33]

If breathing is absent or abnormal* and carotid pulse is absent[34]:
- Ensure help is on its way (see above) and ask for/collect equipment/resuscitation trolley
- In hospital, while waiting for equipment, commence continuous chest compressions – these are only effective for around 5 minutes, so if in the community and if skilled help is delayed commence CPR 30:2 immediately[34].
- Treat where found, unless in immediate danger
- If pregnant, or recently given birth, tilt to left side to reduce aortal–caval compression
- Once equipment is available, commence CPR - 30 chest compressions to a depth of 5–6 cms at a rate of 100–120 per minute[34]
- Open airway using head tilt/chin lift manoeuvres and using a pocket mask or bag-valve-mask system give two breaths, each lasting 1 second[34]
- Give oxygen, when available, at 15 l/min with the pocket mask (60% O$_2$ concentration) or via a reservoir bag on the bag-valve-mask system (100% O$_2$ concentration)
- If available, consider use of oropharyngeal/nasopharyngeal airways and suction to maintain airway until intubation is achieved
- Continue at a rate of 30:2 until advanced skilled help arrives, the woman starts to breathe spontaneously or shows signs of regaining consciousness[35]
    *less than 10 times a minute/gasping/agonal breathing - if breathing is absent/abnormal, but circulation is intact this is a re spiratory arrest and management consists of respiratory ventilatory support - 1 breath every 6 seconds, reassessing after every minute

Once help arrives:
Hand over to the medical team or paramedic, depending on environment, including recent and relevant medical/obstetric history.

Support the medical team or paramedic with advance life support (ALS) algorithms, i.e.:
- Gaining iv access and administration of drugs, i.e. *adrenaline and amiodarone*
- Early assistance to achieve a secure airway – intubation is the preferred method in pregnancy
- Assist with capnography – if available
- Attaching ECG leads, analysing the cardiac rhythm and using the defibrillator, if the rhythm dictates
- Consider obstetric causes, e.g. eclampsia and amniotic fluid embolism (AFE) and manage any reversible causes – those particularly relevant to childbirth may include hypovolaemia, metabolic disorders, toxins and thrombosis[35]
- If in the community, travel with the woman to a consultant-led unit with NNU facilities

If still pregnant, the woman's condition will usually be stabilised before considering operative delivery. However, perimortem lower section caesarean section (LSCS) may improve maternal survival by increasing maternal cardiac output and venous return, especially if the woman is >20 weeks gestation and there is no response to management after 5 minutes.

After the event:
- Provide support to relatives
- Liaise with other departments and professionals, e.g. ICU, as appropriate,
- Ensure records are comprehensive and complete; complete critical incident and risk management reports.
- Midwives should seek personal support post-event from a Supervisor of Midwives

Figure 1.1 Midwife management of sudden collapse in pregnancy. This figure is downloadable from the book companion website at www.wiley.com/go/robson

may develop complications. Table 1.3 shows maternal death by type of antenatal care.

From both reports 'back to basics' recommendations arise:

Improve basic medical and midwifery practice
Skills need to be developed with:

- history taking
  - basic observations
  - understanding normality

Signs and symptoms
A red flag scheme is advocated for midwives and doctors to attribute signs and symptoms to an emerging serious illness, in order to make speedy referrals and take appropriate action. This is outlined in Box 1.1.

Improved communication and referral
This is outlined in Table 1.1.

Similar as for non-pregnant individuals, but important additions are:

Left lateral position
Use a wedge/pillow to avoid vena caval compression, and improve cardiac output and venous return. Ensure the direction of compressions remains perpendicular when a tilt is used

↓

Oxygen
Due to increased risk of hypoxia during pregnancy high flow oxygen (100%) is required whenever ventilation is assisted

↓

Stabilising airway
Take care as the risk of aspiration during resuscitation is more likely due to increased gastric emptying/decreased motility and relaxation of the cardiac sphincter

↓

Drugs
Consider increased drug dosages during resuscitation if the standard dosages do not have desired effects due to the increased maternal fluid volume[36]

↓

Blood volume
Restore circulating blood volume
Blood products
These may improve oxygen delivery to vital organs[36]

↓

Surgery
If >20 weeks gestation and resuscitation is not successful within 5 minutes a *perimortem caesarean section* is advocated to assist with resuscitation of the mother[37]

Figure 1.2 Basic and advanced life support in pregnancy. This figure is downloadable from the book companion website at www.wiley.com/go/robson

Table 1.2 Leading Causes of UK Maternal Death 2006–2008[39]

Rank	Direct	Indirect
1st	Sepsis	Cardiac disorders
2nd	Pre-eclampsia and eclampsia	Neurological disorders
3rd	Thrombosis and thrombo-embolism	Psychiatric disorders
4th	Amniotic fluid embolism	Indirect malignancies

Table 1.3 Maternal Death by Type of Antenatal Care, United Kingdom 2006–2008[39]

Type of Antenatal Care	Classification of Death					
	Direct (*n*)	Indirect (*n*)	Direct and Indirect (*n* ~ %)	Coincidental (*n*)	Late (*n*)	Total (*n* ~ %)
Team-based or 'shared' care	42	68	110 ~ 42%	16	1	127 ~ 40%
Midwife only	27	25	52 ~ 20%	12	2	66 ~ 21%
Consultant-led unit only	11	32	43 ~ 17%	7	3	53 ~ 17%
Midwife and GP	6	4	10 ~ 4%	2	1	13 ~ 4%
Other	2	1	3 ~ 1%	1	0	4 ~1%
Private	0	1	1 ~ 0%	0	0	1 ~ 0%
No antenatal care (death before booking; ToP; miscarriage; concealed pregnancy; not known)	18	23	41 ~ 16%	12	2	55 ~ 17%
Total	107	154	261 ~ 100%	50	9	320 ~ 100%

Box 1.1 Back to Basics Campaign

Communication
- Midwives should notify a GP that a woman is pregnant
- Midwives should seek additional information from the GP if risk factors are identified
- GPs should inform midwives of prior mental/medical problems

Signs and symptoms 'Red Flags' – for prompt identification of a potentially life threatening condition

Blood Pressure
▶ Systolic blood pressure of over 160 mmHg
▶ Systolic blood pressure of *under* 90 mmHg
▶ Diastolic blood pressure of over 80 mmHg

Sepsis
▶ Sore throat (take a throat swab)
▶ Pyrexia >38 °C
▶ Sustained tachycardia >100 bpm
▶ Breathlessness (RR >20)
▶ Abdominal or chest pain
▶ Diarrhoea and/or vomiting
▶ Reduced or absent fetal movements
▶ Reduced or absent fetal heart
▶ Spontaneous rupture of membranes (SOM) or significant vaginal discharge
▶ Uterine or renal angle pain and tenderness
▶ Generally unwell, unduly anxious or panicking

Breathlessness
▶ Breathlessness of sudden onset
▶ Breathlessness associated with chest pain
▶ Orthopnoea (severe difficulty in breathing)
▶ Paroxysmal nocturnal dyspnoea (wake suddenly with breathing difficulties)

Headache
▶ Headache of sudden onset
▶ Headache with neck stiffness
▶ Headache described 'the worse she has ever had'
▶ Headache with any abnormal signs on neurological examination

Mental Health
▶ Ideas of suicide
▶ Marked change from normal functioning
▶ Mental health deterioration
▶ Persistent symptoms in late pregnancy or 6 weeks postpartum
▶ Association with panic attacks and/or obtrusive, obsessional thoughts
▶ Morbid fears that are difficult to reassure
▶ Profound low mood or ideas of guilt and worthlessness, insomnia and weight loss
▶ Personal or family history of serious affective disorder

Referrals
- Explain the importance of keeping the appointment
- Check that the appointment has been made and the woman seen
- If urgent, phone a senior clinician
- Reinforce the referral with a written letter (copy to midwife/GP) including details of:
  ○ current problem and reason for referral
  ○ details of past medical and mental history
  ○ past and present medications
  ○ investigations so far
- Remember that referral is not treatment

Box 1.1 may be copied and placed in clinical areas (Robson S.E. and Waugh J. 2012 Medical Disorders in Pregnancy: A Manual for Midwives, 2nd Edn, © 2013 by John Wiley & Sons, Ltd.)

1 Midwifery Care and Medical Disorders

PATIENT ORGANISATIONS

Association for the Promotion of Preconceptual Care – Foresight.
178 Hawthorn Road
West Bognor
West Sussex PO21 2UY
www.foresight-preconception.org.uk

Association for Improvements in the Maternity Services (AIMS)
5 Ann's Court
Grove Road
Surbiton
Surrey KT6 4BE
www.aims.org.uk

Antenatal Results and Choices (ARC)
73–75 Charlotte Street
London W1T 4PN
www.arc-uk.org

Centre for Pregnancy Nutrition
University of Sheffield
Jessop Wing
Hallamshire Hospital
Tree Root Walk
Sheffield S10 2SF
www.shef.ac.uk/pregnancy_nutrition

La Leche League
PO Box 29
West Bridgford
Nottingham NG2 7NP
www.laleche.org.uk

Maternity Alliance
3rd Floor West
2–6 Northburgh Street
London EC1V 0AY
www.maternityalliance.org.uk

National Childbirth Trust (NCT)
Alexandra House
Oldham Terrace
London W3 6NH
www.nct.org.uk

Tommy's – The Baby Charity
Nicholas House
3 Laurence Pountney Hill
London EC4R 0BB
www.tommys.org

ESSENTIAL READING

Billington M and Stevenson M 2006 **Critical Care in Childbearing for Midwives**. Oxford; Blackwell Publishing Ltd.

BMJ books – Wiley-Blackwell/Blackwell Publishing Ltd. *ABC series:* **ABC of Antenatal Care, ABC of Labour Care, ABC of Alcohol, ABC of Hypertension, ABC of Smoking Cessation, ABC of Sexual Health, ABC of Nutrition**

Briggs GG, Freeman RK and Yaffe SJ 2011 **Drugs in Pregnancy and Lactation**, 9th Edn. USA; Lippincott.

British National Formulary www.bnf.org

Chan KL and Kean LH 2004 Routine antenatal management in later pregnancy. **Current Obstetrics and Gynaecology**, 14:86–91

Glenville M 2007 **Health Professional's Guide to Pre-Conception Care** (booklet) www.foresight-preconception.org.uk/booklet_healthproguide.htm

James D. (Ed.) 2011 **High Risk Pregnancy: Management Options**, 4th Edn. London; Elsevier

Fraser D and Cooper M 2009 (Eds) **Myles Textbook for Midwives**, 15th Edn. London; Elsevier

Lewis G. (Ed.) 2011 **Saving Mothers' Lives: Reviewing Maternal Deaths to Make Motherhood Safer**. 2006–2008. 8th CEMACH Report. London; BJOG

NICE http://www.nice.org.uk/guidance/CG/guidelines.asp *Clinical guidelines:* **CG46 Antenatal Care, CG45 Antenatal and Postnatal Mental Health, CG13 Caesarean Section, CG37 Routine Postnatal Care of Women and Babies**. London; National Institute for Health and Clinical Excellence. www.nice.org.uk

Redshaw M 2006 **Recorded Delivery: Women's Perception of Maternity Care from a National Survey**. National Perinatal Epidemiology Unit www.npeu.ox.ac.uk/maternitysurveys/maternitysurveys_downloads/maternity_survey_report.pdf

RCM 1997 **Position Paper No.17 Conscientious Objection**. London; Royal College of Midwives http://www.rcm.org.uk

Royal College of Obstetricians and Gynaecologists (RCOG) http://www.rcog.org.uk *Green Top Clinical Guidelines:* 40 listed

References

1. Schrander-Stumpel C 1999 Pre-conception care: challenge of the new millennium? **American Journal of Medical Genetics**, 89:58–61

2. Treacy A, Byrne P, Collins C and Geary M 2006 Pregnancy outcome in immigrant women. **Irish Medical Journal**, 99:22–23

3. Nelson-Piercy C 2002 **Handbook of Obstetric Medicine**. London; Martin Dunitz

4. Barrowclough D 2009 Chapt 13 *Preparing for pregnancy* in Fraser D and Cooper M **Myles Textbook for Midwives**. 15th Edn. London; Elsevier 173–188

5. Heyes T, Long S and Mathers N 2002 Preconception care – practice and beliefs of primary care workers. **Family Practice**, 21: 22–27

6. Chan KL and Kean LH 2004 Routine antenatal management at the booking clinic. **Current Obstetrics and Gynaecology**, 14: 79–85

7. Glenville M 2007 **Health Professional's Guide To Pre-Conception Care** (booklet) Bognor; Foresight www.foresight–preconception.org.uk/booklet_healthproguide.htm

8. Enkin M, Keirse MJNC, Neilson J, Crowther C, Duley L, Hodnett E and Hofmeyr J 2000 **A Guide to Effective care in Pregnancy and Childbirth**. Oxford; Oxford University Press Chapters 3 and 18

9. NMC 2005 **Guidelines for Records and Record Keeping**. London; Nursing and Midwifery Council

10. Gregory B 2011 Deaf parents: breaking through the barriers. **Midwives**, 3; 30–32

11. Chan KL and Kean LH 2004 Routine antenatal management in later pregnancy. **Current Obstetrics and Gynaecology**, 14:86–91

12. Janssen B and Wiegers T 2006 Strengths and weaknesses of midwifery care from the perspective of women. **Evidence Based Midwifery**, 4:53–59

13. NICE 2008 **Clinical Guideline: Antenatal care**. London; National Institute for Clinical Excellence http://www.nice.org.uk/ nicemedia/live/11947/40115/40115.pdf

14. Alfirevic Z 2006 **RCOG/RCM Joint Statement No.1: Immersion in Water during Labour and Birth**. London; Royal College of Obstetricians and Gynaecologists and Royal College of Midwives www.rcm.org.uk/info/docs/RCOG_RCM_Birth_in_ Water_FINAL_COPY_1.pdf

15. Harris T 2011 Chapt.39 *Care in the third stage of labour* in Mcdonald S and Magill-Cuerden J (Eds) **Mayes' Midwifery: A Textbook for Midwives**, 14th Edn. London; Elsevier 535–550

16. Speidel B, Fleming P, Henderson J, Leaf A, Marlow N, Russell G and Dunn P 1998 Chapt.4 *Routine care of the newborn infant* in **A Neonatal Vade-mecum**, 3rd Edn. London; Arnold 47–53

17. NMC 2010 **Midwives Rules and Standards** *Rule 9: Records*. London; Nursing and Midwifery Council http://www.nmc-uk.org/ Documents/Standards/nmcMidwivesRulesandStandards.pdf

18. MacArthur C 1999 What does postnatal care do for women's health? **Lancet**, 353(9150):343–344

19. NICE 2006 **Clinical Guideline No. 37: Routine postnatal care of women and their babies**. London; National Institute for Clinical Excellence http://www.nice.org.uk/CG037

20. NMC 2010 **Midwives Rules and Standards** *Rule 2: Interpretation*. London; Nursing and Midwifery Council

21. NMC 2010 **Midwives Rules and Standards** *Rule 6: Responsibility and sphere of practice*. London; Nursing and Midwifery Council

22. Tiran D 2006 Complementary therapies in pregnancy: midwives' and obstetricians' appreciation of risk. **Complementary Therapies in Clinical Practice**, 12:126–131

23. Anderson F and Johnson C 2005 Complementary and alternative medicine in obstetrics. **International Journal of Gynaecology and Obstetrics**, 91:116–124

24. NMC 2010 **Midwives Rules and Standards** *Rule 7: Administration of Medicines*. London; Nursing and Midwifery Council

25. Young F 2001 Using over the counter medication in pregnancy. **British Journal of Midwifery**, 9:613–616

26. Briggs GG, Freeman RK and Yaffe SJ 2011 **Drugs in Pregnancy and Lactation**, 9th Ed. Philadelphia, USA; Lippincott

27. Lewis G and Drife J 2004 **Why Mothers Die 2000–2002 6th Report. Confidential Enquiries into Maternal and Child Health**. London; RCOG Press

28. RCM 1997 **Position Paper 17 Conscientious Objection**. London; Royal College of Midwives

29. Simpson C 2004 Chapt.34 *The pre-term baby and the small baby* in Henderson C and Mcdonald S (Eds) **Mayes' Midwifery: A Textbook for Midwives**, 13th Edn. London; Baillière Tindall 637

30. Hospital Liaison Committee Network for Jehovah's Witnesses Leaflet – An information and Referral Service, London; HIS www.his@wtbs.org.uk

31. RCM 2006 **Position Paper 26 Refocusing the Role of the Midwife**. London; Royal College of Midwives

32. NMC 2010 **Midwives Rules and Standards** *EU Activities of a Midwife*. London; Nursing and Midwifery Council 36

33. Boyle M (Ed) 2002 **Emergencies Around Childbirth: A Handbook For Midwives**. UK; Radcliffe Medical Press

34. Resuscitation Council (UK) 2010 **Adult Basic Life Support**. www.resus.org

35. RCOG (2011) **Maternal Collapse in Pregnancy and the Puerperium**. Green Top Guideline No. 56.

36. Whitty JE 2002 Maternal cardiac arrest in pregnancy. **Clinical Obstetrics and Gynaecology**, 45:377–392

37. De Sweit M 2002 **Medical Disorders in Obstetric Practice**. Oxford; Blackwell Publishing Ltd. 135

38. Edwards G 2007 Chapt.16 *Midwifery* in Lewis G (Ed.) **Saving Mothers' Lives: Reviewing Maternal Deaths to Make Motherhood Safer. 7th Report of the Confidential Enquiries into Maternal and Child Health**. London; CMACE 199–212

39. Lewis G (Ed.) 2011 **Saving Mothers' Lives: Reviewing Maternal Deaths to Make Motherhood Safer. 8th Report of the Confidential Enquiries into Maternal and Child Health**. London; CMACE

Appendices References

Appendix 1.1 UK Maternal Deaths: Causes and Risk Factors

1. Lewis G (Ed.) 2011 **Saving Mothers' Lives: Reviewing Maternal Deaths to Make Motherhood Safer. 8th Report of the Confidential Enquiries into Maternal and Child Health**. London; CMACE

Appendix 1.2 Daily Vitamin and Mineral Dietary Intake for Pregnancy and Lactation

1. Food Standards Agency (UK) Website www.eatwell.gov.uk/ healthydiet/nutritionessentials/vitaminsandminerals/folicacid/ [Accessed 1–06–2012]

2. Rutherford D 2007 **Vitamins and Minerals – What Do They Do?** www.netdoctor.co.uk/health_advice/facts/vitamins_which.htm [Accessed 1–6–2012]

3. Briggs GG, Freeman RK and Yaffe SJ 2005 **Drugs in Pregnancy and Lactation**, 7th Ed. Philadelphia; Lippincott

4. National Academy of Sciences (USA) 2012 **Dietary Reference Intakes** http://fnic.nal.usda.gov/dietary-guidance/dietary-reference-intakes/dri-tables [Accessed 1–6-2012]

5. Nowson CA and Margerison C 2002 Vitamin D intake and vitamin D status of Australians. **Medical Journal of Australia**, 177:149–152

Appendix 1.1 UK Maternal Deaths – Causes and Risk Factors

Number of Deaths from Consecutive UK Confidential Enquiries into Maternal Mortality[1]

Type of Cause of Death	Triennial Report				
	1994–1996	1997–1999	2000–2002	2003–2005	2006–2008
Direct Causes					
Sepsis	16	18	13	18	26
Pre-eclampsia and eclampsia	20	16	14	18	19
Thrombosis and thrombo-embolism	48	35	30	41	18
Amniotic fluid embolism	17	8	5	17	13
Early pregnancy deaths:	15	17	15	14	11
Ectopic pregnancy	12	13	11	10	6
Spontaneous miscarriage	2	2	1	1	5
Legal termination of pregnancy	1	2	3	2	0
Other early pregnancy deaths	0	0	0	1	0
Haemorrhage	12	7	17	14	9
Anaesthesia	1	3	6	6	7
Other direct causes:	7	7	8	4	4
Genital tract trauma	5	2	1	3	0
Fatty liver	2	4	3	1	3
Other causes	0	1	4	0	1
Total number of direct deaths	**134**	**106**	**106**	**132**	**107**
Indirect Causes					
Cardiac	39	35	44	48	53
Indirect neurological conditions	47	34	40	37	36
Psychiatric	9	15	16	18	13
Indirect malignancies	N/A	11	5	10	3
Other indirect causes	39	41	50	50	49
Total number of indirect deaths	**134**	**136**	**155**	**163**	**154**
Coincidental Deaths	36	29	36	55	50
Late Deaths (42–365 days postpartum)					
Direct causes	4	7	4	11	9
Indirect causes	32	39	45	71	24
Total number of late deaths	**72**	**107**	**94**	**82**	**33**
Total of all deaths	**376**	**378**	**391**	**432**	**344**

Appendix 1.2 Daily Vitamin and Mineral Dietary Intake for Pregnancy and Lactation

Vitamin[1,2]	RDA (Recommended Daily Dietary Amount/ Allowance)*	Sources[1,2]	Overdose[2]	Notes
A Retinol	Pregnancy 2700– 8000 IU[3] Lactation 3–4000 IU[3,4]	Liver, fish liver oil, green leafy vegetables, carrots, yellow fruits, egg yolks, enriched margarine, milk products	A fat soluble vitamin which accumulates in the body[2]. Overdose in pregnancy can be dangerous[3]. 8000 IU is the maximum dose. High doses may be teratogenic[3]	Pregnant women should not take supplements, and should avoid eating liver[3]
B$_1$ Thiamine	Pregnancy 1.5 mg[3] Lactation 1.6 mg[3]	Yeast products, liver, rice, wholemeal products, peanuts, pork, milk	A water-soluble vitamin that is excreted in urine, so overdose unlikely[2]	Destroyed by alcohol[2]
B$_2$ Riboflavin	Pregnancy 1.6 mg[3] Lactation 1.8 mg[3]	Yeast products, milk, liver, fish, cheese, green leafy vegetables	A water-soluble vitamin that is excreted in urine, so no danger of overdose	Destroyed by alcohol[2]
B$_6$ Pyridoxine	Pregnancy 2.2 mg[3] Lactation 2.1 mg[3]	Fish, bananas, chicken, pork, wholegrains, dried beans	May cause nerve problems in large doses. Conflicting evidence about maximum safe dose	Destroyed by alcohol and the contraceptive pill[2]
B$_{12}$ Cobalamin	Pregnancy 2.2 µg[3] Lactation 2.6 µg[3]	Fish, liver, beef, pork, milk and cheese	A water-soluble vitamin that is excreted in urine, so no danger of overdose.	
C Ascorbic Acid	Pregnancy 70 mg[3] Lactation 95 mg[3]	Citrus fruits, berries, tomatoes, cauliflower, green leafy vegetables, peppers	Large doses can cause diarrhoea. Excessive doses, ≥1000 mg, *might* damage DNA	
D	Pregnancy 400 IU[3] Lactation 400 IU[3]	80% from sunlight 20% from cod liver oil, sardines, herrings, salmon, tuna, and milk products	A fat-soluble vitamin which accumulates in the body[2]. High doses are teratogenic in animals[3]	Australia advocates daily sunlight exposure 15 min to prevent deficiency[5]; no data for the UK
E Tocopherol	Pregnancy 10 mg[3] Lactation 12 mg[3]	Eggs, nuts, soya, wholemeal products, beans, vegetable oil, broccoli, sprouts, spinach	A fat-soluble vitamin with a slight risk of overdose	
Folic Acid	Pre-conception 0.4 mg[3] Pregnancy 0.4 mg[3] Lactation 0.28 mg[3] NB: Higher doses are given for folate deficiency[3]	Liver, yeast products, egg yolk, carrots, melon, apricots, avocado, beans, whole wheat, green leafy vegetables	A water-soluble vitamin that is excreted in urine, so no danger of overdose	Essential for production of erythrocytes and other body cells. Use in periconception period reduces risk of neural tube defects
Mineral	RDA	Sources[1,2]	Overdose[2]	Notes
Calcium	Pregnancy 1000 mg[4] Lactation 1000 mg[4]	Dairy products and green leafy vegetables	High doses lead to hypertension, headaches, renal or gall bladder stones[2]	
Iron	Pregnancy 27 mg[†] Lactation 9 mg[4]	Red meat, oily fish, egg yolk, green leafy vegetables, dried apricots, nuts, wholegrain foods	Iron accumulates in the body. High doses lead to nausea and constipation and can be fatal	Deficiency leads to anaemia. Best taken with folic acid to aid absorption
Magnesium	Pregnancy 350 mg[4] Lactation 310 mg[4]	Green leafy vegetables, wholegrain foods, nuts	High dose causes diarrhoea	
Zinc	Pregnancy 11 mg[4] Lactation 12 mg[4]	Meat, shellfish, milk, brown rice and wholegrain foods	High dose results in nausea and vomiting	

*RDA figures are based on the USA National Academy of Sciences Recommendations[3,4]
†This figure is lower in the UK, and the exact dosage is debated in the midwifery press

SKIN DISORDERS

Catherine Gittins[1] and Rhoda Cowell[2]

[1]Royal Victoria Infirmary, Newcastle upon Tyne, UK
[2]County Durham and Darlington Foundation Trust, UK

2.1 Physiological Skin Changes in Pregnancy
2.2 Dermatoses Specific to Pregnancy
2.3 Eczema
2.4 Psoriasis

Medical Disorders in Pregnancy: A Manual for Midwives, Second Edition. Edited by S. Elizabeth Robson and Jason Waugh.
© 2013 John Wiley & Sons, Ltd. Published 2013 by John Wiley & Sons, Ltd.

2.1 Physiological Skin Changes in Pregnancy

Skin changes occur during pregnancy under hormonal influence. Usually reassurance by the midwife or GP is all that is required, but further investigation and referral may be indicated in some cases.

Hyperpigmentation

The areola, nipples, genital skin, axillae, linea alba (becomes the linea nigra) and inner thighs can darken. Sometimes moles, freckles and scars also become darker. Hyperpigmentation usually fades postpartum[1].

Melasma (chloasma)

Melasma (mask of pregnancy) is very common, affecting 75% pregnant women[1], and consists of symmetrical increased pigmentation over the cheeks, jaw line, brow or upper lip. Melasma is worsened by sunlight so sun protection should be advised. It usually fades postpartum (see Figure 2.1.1)

Hair

It is common to have some degree of hirsutism during pregnancy. This resolves 6 months after delivery. Postpartum there is often an increased loss of hair (telogen effluvium) which lasts for up to 15 months. (It may be worth checking for other causes of generalised hair loss, e.g. ferritin levels and thyroid function tests.)

Striae Gravidarum

These appear in the sixth and seventh month on the abdomen, breasts, thighs or inguinal areas, they gradually fade postpartum but do not resolve (see Figure 2.1.2).

Skin Tags

May occur after the first trimester in the flexures, on the face chest and neck. They may regress postpartum.

Vascular Changes

Spider naevi (Figure 2.1.3), facial flushing, varicose veins, red swollen gums and palmar erythema can all occur and resolve postpartum.

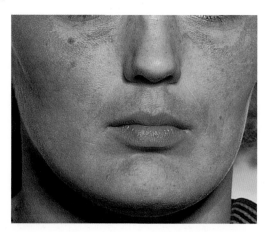

Figure 2.1.1 Melasma (Burns 2010). This figure is downloadable from the book companion website at www.wiley.com/go/robson

Pruritus

Itching without a rash can occur in up to 20% of pregnant women; it resolves spontaneously. Moisturisers and 1% menthol in aqueous cream may help.

Moles (naevi)

Significant changes to moles during pregnancy need referral to dermatology/GP for further evaluation. Women who develop malignant melanoma during pregnancy do not have a worsened prognosis (see Chapter 18.8).

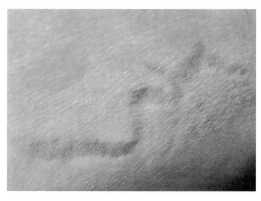

Figure 2.1.2 Striae gravidarum (Buxton 2009). This figure is downloadable from the book companion website at www.wiley.com/go/robson

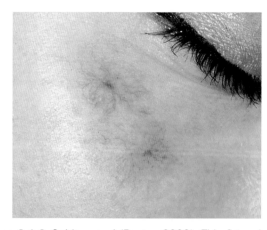

Figure 2.1.3 Spider naevi (Buxton 2009). This figure is downloadable from the book companion website at www.wiley.com/go/robson

2.2 Dermatoses Specific to Pregnancy

Atopic Eruption of Pregnancy (AEP)

This is the commonest pregnancy related rash; 20% have eczema and there is often a family history of atopy. It occurs on the face, neck, chest and flexures, as red scaly itchy patches, with some papules and nodules from scratching, in the second and third trimesters. Treat as eczema. UVB can be helpful. Rarely oral steroids are needed (Figure 2.2.1). There is no adverse effect for the mother or baby.

Pruritic Urticarial Papules and Plaques of Pregnancy (PUPP)

This occurs in 1 in 160 pregnancies and predominantly affects primiparous women in the third trimester. The rash usually starts in the abdominal striae and spares the umbilicus (Figure 2.2.2). It consists of urticarial papules and plaques but also vesicular, eczematous, annular and target lesions. The rash is usually itchy and disappears 10 days after delivery. There is no risk to mother and baby. Recurrence in subsequent pregnancies is unusual. Treatment is with topical steroids, moisturisers, 1% menthol in aqueous cream and if severe oral steroids. Appendix 2.2.1 outlines the use of emollients and steroid creams.

Pemphigoid Gestationis (PG)

This is a rare autoimmune blistering disease occurring in 1 in 40 000 pregnancies. It starts in the second and third trimesters (occasionally postpartum), with an itch, followed by urticarial lesions, then large blisters (bullae) develop often around the umbilicus, which spread and can involve hands, soles and face. It will often quieten in late pregnancy but can flare badly postpartum. Referral to dermatology is necessary for a skin biopsy and further management with moisturisers, topical steroids, antihistamines, and oral steroids. Risk of premature delivery, low birth weight and small for gestational age is increased. Occasionally there are transient bullous lesions in the baby (10% of babies)[1]. It frequently recurs in future pregnancies (Figure 2.2.3).

Pustular Psoriasis of Pregnancy

This is rare; most patients do not have a history of psoriasis. It can occur during any trimester, presents as itchy plaques surrounded by rings of sterile pustules, often starts in flexures and may spread all over. The patient feels unwell with diarrhoea, vomiting, fever and malaise. There is an increased risk of miscarriage, still birth and low birth weight. The rash resolves quickly postpartum (occasional flare). Recurrences can occur in future pregnancies. Urgent referral to dermatology is indicated. Treatment is with high dose steroids and an early delivery.

Intrahepatic Cholestasis of Pregnancy (ICP)

See Chapter 10.8.

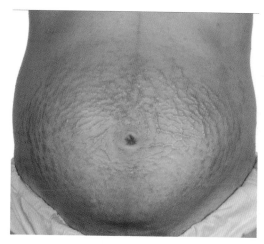

Figure 2.2.2 Pruritic urticarial papules and plaques of pregnancy (PUPP) (Buxton 2009). This figure is downloadable from the book companion website at www.wiley.com/go/robson

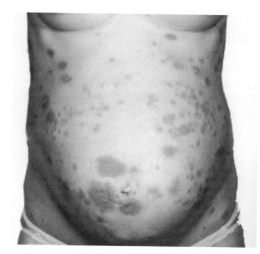

Figure 2.2.3 Pemphigoid gestationis (PG) (Buxton 2009). This figure is downloadable from the book companion website at www.wiley.com/go/robson

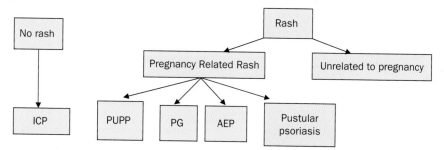

Figure 2.2.1 Dermatoses specific to pregnancy. Any blistering rash in pregnancy requires urgent referral for a dermatology opinion (Buxton 2009). AEP, Atopic eruption of pregnancy. PUPP, Pruritic urticarial papules and plaques of pregnancy. PG, pemphigoid gestationis. ICP, Intrahepatic cholestasis of pregnancy. This figure is downloadable from the book companion website at www.wiley.com/go/robson

2.3 Eczema

Incidence	Risk for Childbearing
Atopic eczema affects 18–20 % of school children and 2–10% of adults[1]. The incidence increases with affected parents.	None

EXPLANATION OF CONDITION

Eczema is an itchy, dry, erythematous, skin condition. It can develop anywhere on the body but typically is found in the flexures (Figure 2.3.1).

Acute eczema usually displays all the clinical signs of infection, heat, pain, and redness, with scaling and excoriations. If infected it is accompanied by a clear discharge which dries to form a crust (Figure 2.3.2).

Chronic eczema is due to constant scratching; the skin becomes thick and leathery (lichenification), with scaling, fissuring and redness.

Dermatitis – the terms dermatitis and eczema are now used interchangeably by most dermatologists.

COMPLICATIONS

- Bacterial infections: These are common, are caused by reduced waterproofing of the skin and *Staphylococcus* and/or *Streptococcus*. The eczema is usually weepy, crusted and yellow. Only swab if resistance is suspected or if you suspect a micro-organism other than *Staphylococcus*.
- Viral infections: The presence of the herpes virus (cold sore) in patients with eczema can lead to widespread skin infection with the virus (eczema herpeticum). This needs immediate referral to the dermatology team.

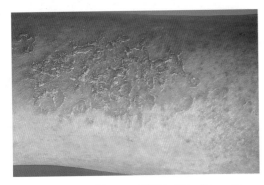

Figure 2.3.1 Eczema (Buxton 2009). This figure is downloadable from the book companion website at www.wiley.com/go/robson

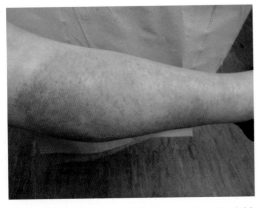

Figure 2.3.2 Infected eczema. This figure is downloadable from the book companion website at www.wiley.com/go/robson

NON-PREGNANCY TREATMENT AND CARE

All skin conditions have the potential to lower an individual's quality of daily life and the psychosocial impact of this condition must always be considered when treatment is discussed.

General advice

- Education plays an important role in the management of eczema. Advice about allergens, explanation about eczema and its management should be given[2].

Topical treatment (1st line therapy)

- Daily lukewarm baths with a bath oil help to relieve symptoms, e.g. Oilatum bath or Dermol 600.
- Shower gels or soap should not be used. Suitable soap substitutes include, e.g. Hydromol bath/shower emollient or Hydromol ointment.
- Topical emollients should be applied after bathing when skin is still moist. Emollients can be applied as frequently as required during the day.
- Topical steroids: The correct potency for the severity of the eczema should be prescribed (a mild steroid, e.g. 1% hydrocortisone for mild eczema , a moderate steroid, e.g. Eumovate for moderate eczema and a potent steroid, e.g. Betnovate for severe eczema). Steroids can be stepped up and down according to severity[3]. Only hydrocortisone 1% should be used on the face.
- Antihistamines: May not help itching but may aid sleep if a sedating antihistamine is taken at night.
- Generalised secondary bacterial infection is treated with systemic antibiotics, e.g. flucloxacillin or erythromycin.
- Localised bacterial infections can be treated with topical creams, e.g. Trimovate or Betnovate C.

2nd line therapy

- Topical calcineurin inhibitors: Tacrolimus or pimecrolimus are only used for difficult to treat eczema where there is no infection.
- Oral prednisolone, methotrexate, azathioprine, ciclosporin, UVB or PUVA (psoralen with long-wave UVA) light treatment can be used to treat severe cases of eczema.

PRE-CONCEPTION ISSUES AND CARE

Atopic eczema generally worsens in pregnancy. However, improvement has been reported in up to 24% of cases[2].

Emollients, topical steroids and antihistamines are all safe to use.

Topical tacrolimus/pimecrolimus are not to be used in pregnancy.

Azathioprine is not proven to be teratogenic, however there have been reports of low birth weight babies, spontaneous abortion and premature labour/birth. Ciclosporin is not considered to be any more harmful than azathioprine[4]. It would be advisable for any woman on these medications to seek preconception advice (see Appendix 11.1.1). Methotrexate should be stopped at least 3 months prior to conception.

Pregnancy Issues

- Of all the skin conditions during pregnancy, eczema is the most prevalent (36% of total cases)
- As pregnancy progresses women may have difficulty applying topical treatments to some areas
- No reports have been found to prove any adverse fetal affects due to eczema
- Of babies born to mothers with eczema, 19% may develop the condition.

Medical Management and Care

- All soap substitutes, bath oils and emollients are suitable and safe to use in pregnancy
- Difficult to reach areas, e.g. back, sides, back of legs can be reached using a new long-handled radiator paint roller covered in emollient. (for more information about application of emollients see: eczpert.co.uk-eTutorials)
- The lowest potency of topical steroid should be used when required for any inflamed eczema
- For severe generalised eczema a short course of oral steroid can be used[4]
- For bacterial infections, flucloxacillin or erythromycin can be used or localised infections can be treated with topical creams
- UVB treatment is safe and is occasionally used for eczema in pregnancy

Midwifery Management and Care

- Women not taking immune-modulating drugs can be booked for low risk care
- Emollients and other first line treatments should be encouraged. If the condition deteriorates the woman should be advised to see her GP or specialist dermatology nurse/doctor
- Normal general advice should be given, especially the use of cotton clothes to keep the skin as cool as possible

Labour Issues

- Eczema is not a contraindication to siting an epidural unless infection is present

Medical Management and Care

- Topical treatments should be continued, as above

Midwifery Management and Care

- Keeping the environment cool and wearing cotton clothing may help keep eczema more comfortable during labour. Emollients which are kept cool (refrigerated) can be applied at any time[6]
- Low risk guidelines and protocols can be followed during labour[6]

Postpartum Issues

- There is inconclusive evidence that breast-feeding may prevent atopic eczema. The overall evidence does suggest that babies exclusively breast fed for at least 4 months may have some protection against atopic eczema[5]
- Postpartum hand dermatitis and nipple eczema may occur

Medical Management and Care

- Breast-feeding should be supported and encouraged
- Hand dermatitis and nipple eczema can be treated with emollients, steroid creams, and avoidance of irritants (see Non-pregnancy treatment and care)
- Secondary infection with *Staphylococcus* is often a problem with nipple eczema and should be treated with flucloxacillin or erythromycin.
- Tacrolimus, pimecrolimus, azathioprine, methotrexate and ciclosporin should be avoided when breast-feeding[4] (see Appendix 11.1.1)

Midwifery Management and Care

- Support, information and reassurance as above[6]

2.4 Psoriasis

Incidence	Risk for Childbearing
2–3% of the UK population[1]	Low Risk
No gender differentiation	
Usual onset is in early adulthood but can occur at any age[2]	

INTRODUCTION

Psoriasis is a common skin disease presenting with well demarcated red plaques with silvery scales which bleed easily. Psoriasis appears symmetrically, often involving the scalp, elbows, knees, sacral area, umbilicus and lower legs. Any part of the body can be affected including the flexures, hands, feet and nails (Figure 2.4.1).

There is a genetic susceptibility to psoriasis. It can be triggered by infection (streptococcal sore throat), hormonal changes, trauma and stress.

More recent research suggests that psoriasis is an autoimmune disease.

COMPLICATIONS

Of people with psoriasis, 5–10% suffer from psoriatic arthropathy. This resembles rheumatoid arthritis.

If a severe flare of psoriasis involves over more than 90% of the body surface (erythroderma), then immediate admission to hospital is required for treatment and observation.

Rarely generalised pustular psoriasis can occur. This condition is often precipitated by oral or potent topical steroids and also requires emergency admission.

NON-PREGNANCY TREATMENT AND CARE

General Advice

- Daily bathing/showering with soap substitutes
- Stop smoking and reduce/stop alcohol intake

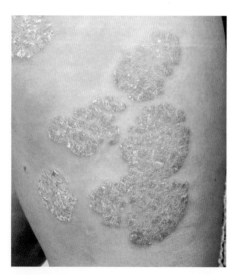

Figure 2.4.1 Psoriasis (Buxton 2009). This figure is downloadable from the book companion website at www.wiley.com/go/robson

Topical Treatments

First-line Therapy

- Emollients: at least twice a day
- Vitamin D analogues: Dovobet[3]
- Tar preparations: Alphosyl HC or Exorex
- Topical steroids: for face, flexures, scalp, hands and feet

Less Frequently Used

- Dithranol cream
- Vitamin A derivative: Zorac
- Diprosalic ointment for thick scale
- Calcineurin inhibitors (pimecrolimus and tacrolimus) for facial psoriasis.

Second-line Therapy

- UVB light treatment
- PUVA (photosensitising medication topically or orally with long-wave ultraviolet light treatment)
- Oral methotrexate, acitretin, ciclosporin and azathioprine

Third-line Therapy
Biologic Agents: These agents interfere with specific components of the autoimmune response and are licensed for severe plaque psoriasis unresponsive to second line treatments[4].

PRE-CONCEPTION ISSUES AND CARE

The familial tendency for psorasis is variable, but there is approximately a 10% chance of a child developing psoriasis if one parent is affected[5].

In the pre-conception period vitamin D analogues (Dovobet), retinoid creams and PUVA should be avoided. Acitretin should be discontinued 2 years before conception and all other systemic treatments should be stopped at least 3 months before conception (see Section 2.3 Eczema)

Partners being treated with methotrexate should stop 3 months before conception[6].

Pregnancy Issues
- As pregnancy progresses women may have difficulty applying topical treatments to some areas
- Excessive weight gain can cause the plaques to crack and bleed

Medical Management and Care
- The condition and effectiveness of treatments requires regular reviews throughout the pregnancy
- First line treatments, e.g. emollients, tar preparations, topical steroids, dithranol and UVB light therapy are all safe to use during pregnancy[8]

Midwifery Management and Care[9]
- Good skin care routines established pre-conception should be promoted, to maintain the skin in a soft and flexible condition
- Reassurance should be given that vulval psoriasis does not exclude vaginal delivery
- The midwife should be able to demonstrate sensitivity to the needs of the woman with psoriasis. She should palpate the abdomen in the normal way and be aware of the need of privacy during examination if affected areas are to be exposed

Labour Issues
- A warm, dry environment can irritate dry, scaly skin
- The belts to secure transducers for fetal monitoring may rub causing aggravation to the skin
- Psoriatic plaques do not exclude the use of epidural analgesia

Medical Management and Care
- Continue all topical treatment as above

Midwifery Management and Care[9]
- Humidification of a warm dry environment (a small bowl of water on a radiator will suffice) may help to minimise environmental effects
- If monitoring is required, gauze swabs under the belt may help to protect tender skin
- Help to apply emollients frequently (as often as wanted)
- Cool, loose cotton clothing should be encouraged

Postpartum Issues
- In more than 50% of women, psoriasis will deteriorate within 4 months postpartum[7]

Medical Management and Care
- Treatment may need to be reviewed if there is any change in condition
- If breast-feeding, retinoids, PUVA, ciclosporin, methotrexate and acitretin should all be avoided.
- Emollients, vitamin D analogues, tar preparations, topical steroids, dithranol and UVB light therapy are all safe to use whilst breast-feeding[6]

Midwifery Management and Care[9]
- Reassure and explain that psoriasis may deteriorate postpartum
- Support the woman to establish successful breast-feeding
- Encourage the use of emollients on and around any plaques on the breast and nipples to prevent the skin cracking

2 Skin Disorders

PATIENT ORGANISATIONS

National Eczema Society
Hill House
Highgate Hill
London N19 5NA
Tel: 0870 2413604 (Helpline)
Tel: 0207 2813553
Fax: 0207 816395
www.eczema.org

The Psoriasis Association
Milton House
7 Milton Street
Northampton NN2 7JG
Tel: 0845 6760076
www.psoriasis-association.org.uk

Psoriatic Arthropathy Alliance
PO Box 111
St Albans
Hertfordshire AL2 3JQ
Tel: 0870 703212
www.paalliance.org

British Association of Dermatologists
BAD House
19 Fitzroy Square
London W1P 5HQ
Tel: 0171 383 0266
www.bad.org.uk

The Skin Care Campaign
www.skincarecampaign.org

British Dermatology Nurses Group
4 Fitzroy Square
London W1T 5HQ
www.bdng.org.uk

Changing Faces
The Squire Centre
33–37 University Street
London WC1E 6JN
www.changingfaces.org.uk

ESSENTIAL READING

Ashton R and Leppard B 2005 **Differential Diagnosis in Dermatology** 3rd Edn. Oxford; Radcliffe Publishing Ltd

Berth-Jones J, Tan E and Mailbach H 2004 **Fast Facts: Eczema and Contact Dermatitis**. Oxford; Health Press Ltd

Best Practice in Emollient Therapy A Statement for Healthcare Professionals 2007 International Skin Care Nursing Group and the British Dermatological Nursing Group

eczpert.co.uk-eTutorials (for advice on applying emollients)

Mitchell T and Kennedy C 2006 **Your Questions Answered: Common Skin Disorders**. London; Elsevier

Smith C, Barker S and Munter A 2004 **Fast Facts: Psoriasis**. Oxford; Health Press Ltd

The NHS Skin Disorders library on http://www.library.nhs.uk/skin/Default.aspx?pagename=HOME

References

2.1 Physiological Skin Changes in Pregnancy
1. Geraghty LN and Pomeranz MK 2011 Physiological changes and dermatoses of pregnancy. **International Journal of Dermatology**, 50:771–782

2.2 Dermatoses Specific to Pregnancy
1. Geraghty LN and Pomeranz MK 2011 Physiological changes and dermatoses of pregnancy. **International Journal of Dermatology**, 50:771–782

2.3 Eczema
1. Diepgen TL 2000 *Is the prevalence of atopic dermatitis increasing?* in Williams HC (Ed.) **Atopic Dermatitis**. Cambridge; Cambridge University Press
2. Kroumpouzos G and Cohen LM 2001 Dermatoses of pregnancy. **Journal of the American Academy of Dermatology**, 45:1–19
3. NICE Clinical Guideline 57: Atopic eczema in children. Developed by the National Collaborating Centre for Women's and Children's Health December 2007. London; National Institute for Health and Clinical Excellence. www.nice.org.uk
4. Reed BR 1997 Dermatological drug use during pregnancy and lactation. **Dermatologic Clinics**, 15:197–206
5. Snijders BE, Thijs C, Kummeling I, Penders J and van den Brandt PA 2007 Breastfeeding and infant eczema in the first year of life in the KOALA birth cohort study: a risk period-specific analysis. **Pediatrics**, 119:e137–141
6. Gittins C and Parrish M 2008 Chapt. 2 in Robson S. E. and Waugh J **Medical Disorders of Pregnancy: A Manual for Midwives**. Oxford; Blackwell Publishing Ltd.

2.4 Psoriasis
1. Krueger GG, Bergstresser PR, Lowe NJ, *et al.* 1984 Psoriasis. **Journal of the American Academy of Dermatology**, 11:937–974
2. Rees JL and Farr PM 1997 Psoriasis. **Journal of the Royal College of Physicians of London**, 31:238–240
3. Diagnosis and management of psoriasis and psoriatic arthritis in adults. *A National Clinical Guideline*: SIGN Guideline No 121 ISBN 978 1 905813 67 4, October 2010
4. NICE technology appraisal TA 199: Etanercept, infliximab and adalimumab for the treatment of psoriatic arthritis. August 2010
5. Murase J, Chan K, Garite T, Cooper D and Weinstein G 2005 Hormonal effect on psoriasis in pregnancy and post partum. **Archives of Dermatology**, 141:601–606
6. BNF 2010 **British National Formulary No: 60**. London; BMA and RPSGB
7. McHugh NJ and Laurent MR 1989 The effect of pregnancy on the onset of psoriatic arthritis. **British Journal of Rheumatology**, 28:50–52
8. Tauscher AE, Fleischer AB Jr, Phelps KC and Feldman SR 2002 Psoriasis and pregnancy. **Journal of Cutaneous Medicine and Surgery**, 6:561–570
9. Gittins C and Parrish M 2008 Chapt. 2 in Robson SE and Waugh J **Medical Disorders of Pregnancy: A Manual for Midwives**. Oxford; Blackwell Publishing Ltd.

Figure References
Burns T, Breathnach S, Cox N and Griffiths C 2010 **Rook's Textbook of Dermatology**, 8th Edn. Oxford; Wiley-Blackwell
Buxton PK and Morris-Jones R 2009 **ABC of Dermatology** 5th Edn. Oxford; BMJ Books/Wiley-Blackwell

Appendix 2.2.1 Emollients and Steroid Creams

Emollients (moisturisers)

- Emollients come as lotions, creams and ointments
- Lotions are water based, and not suitable for dry skin as they need to be applied frequently
- Creams are thicker but are still easy to apply, are cosmetically acceptable and should be applied at least twice a day
- Ointments are thick and greasy, are used to treat very dry skin and can be used as soap substitutes
- Most patients use too little
- When reviewing, check compliance and frequency of application. If no improvement try a different preparation

Steroid Creams/Ointments

- Steroids are used to take the inflammation (redness and itching) out of the skin
- They are applied daily
- They are stopped when the skin is clear of inflammation
- Steroid strength is dependent on the site used and the severity of the condition
- 1% hydrocortisone is mild, is used for mild conditions anywhere on the skin and is the only steroid suitable for the face
- Eumovate/betnovate rd are moderate topical steroids used for moderate skin conditions and suitable for flexures
- Betnovate is potent and used for more severe skin inflammation
- Dermovate is very potent, used for very severe skin inflammation and for short periods only unless under dermatology supervision
- Topical steroids can be stepped up and down according to the severity of the condition

Advice For Patients

Emollients

- Apply creams as often as possible. Emollients cannot be over-used
- Always treat the whole skin surface. Not just the affected area
- Use bath emollients when bathing, air or pat dry the skin (do not rub with a towel) and then apply emollients
- Always use emollients, even when the skin improves
- Always have emollients in stock (ensure the patient is prescribed sufficient quantities of 250–500 g per week)
- Emollients can be cooled or warmed to make them more acceptable
- Always apply in the direction of the hair growth, never rub into the skin
- Ointments can be mixed with water to make them easier to apply
- After skin infection discard all old creams and prescribe new

How Much Steroid to Use: the Finger Tip Unit

One fingertip unit (FTU) is the amount of topical steroid that is squeezed out from a standard tube, from the very end of an adult finger to the first crease in the finger. See Figure 2.2.1.1. One FTU is enough to treat an area of skin twice the size of the flat of an adult's hand with the fingers together.

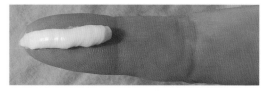

Figure 2.2.1.1 Finger tip unit of topical steroid. This figure is downloadable from the book companion website at www.wiley.com/go/robson

Finger Tip Unit (FTU) Dosage

Area of Skin to be Treated (adults)	Rough Size	FTU each Dose (adults)
1 hand and fingers (front and back)	2 adult hands	1 FTU
Front of chest and abdomen	14 adult hands	7 FTUs
Back and buttocks	14 adult hands	7 FTUs
Face and neck	5 adult hands	2.5 FTUs
1 entire arm and hand	8 adult hands	4 FTUs
1 entire leg and foot	16 adult hands	8 FTUs

NB, For more information about application of emollients see: eczpert.co.uk-eTutorials

HYPERTENSIVE DISORDERS

Sophia Webster[1], Claire Dodd[2] and Jason Waugh[1]

[1]Royal Victoria Infirmary, Newcastle upon Tyne, UK
[2]University Hospitals of Leicester NHS Trust, UK

3.1 Chronic Hypertension
3.2 Pre-eclampsia
3.3 Severe Pre-eclampsia and Eclampsia
3.4 HELLP Syndrome

Medical Disorders in Pregnancy: A Manual for Midwives, Second Edition. Edited by S. Elizabeth Robson and Jason Waugh.
© 2013 John Wiley & Sons, Ltd. Published 2013 by John Wiley & Sons, Ltd.

3.1 Chronic Hypertension

Incidence	Risk for Childbearing
2% of pregnancies	High Risk

INTRODUCTION

Hypertension in pregnancy is defined as a systolic blood pressure of ≥140 mmHg and/or a diastolic blood pressure of ≥90 mmHg[1] (Box 3.1.1). The significance of any blood pressure measurement is related to gestation and, in general terms, the earlier in pregnancy that hypertension is found the more likely it is to be pre-existing, chronic hypertension.

Chronic hypertension (CHT) describes all hypertension that exists before pregnancy. Most women in this group have *essential hypertension* and have no apparent underlying cause. Many go undiagnosed until booking due to infrequent medical encounters. The development of CHT is poorly understood, but risk factors are clearly described and include advanced age, a strong family history, black ethnicity, obesity, low rates of exercise and high cholesterol.

Renal hypertension can complicate kidney disease of any kind and the reason for its development depends on the type of renal disease and its duration as a problem. Sodium retention by the kidney leading to water retention and an increased blood volume is usually a factor. Early delivery may become necessary to prevent long-term kidney damage.

Other rarer but important causes of hypertension in pregnancy are:

- **Phaeochromocytoma,** an adrenal gland tumour secreting the 'fight or flight' hormones dopamine, adrenaline and/or noradrenaline
- **Coarctation of the aorta,** a narrowing of the aorta more common in patients with congenital heart disease
- **Cushing's syndrome,** an excess of glucocorticoid hormones
- **Conn's syndrome,** and excess of aldosterone hormone causing sodium retention and associated hypokalaemia

Chronic Hypertension *versus* Pregnancy Induced Hypertension (PIH)

In the first trimester of pregnancy, marked vasodilatation causes a drop in systemic vascular resistance which sees blood pressure fall in both normotensive and hypertensive women, with an exaggerated effect in those with CHT[2]. Knowing this, it should be remembered that a patient with CHT may not actually be hypertensive until late in the second trimester and therefore CHT cannot be diagnosed with certainty unless non-pregnant blood pressure (BP) readings are available for reference. In the absence of such readings, diagnoses of CHT and PIH are difficult to differentiate and postnatal follow-up should involve medical review of BP at 6 weeks to determine this. Clinical management of a newly discovered hypertensive patient in the latter stages of pregnancy who in fact has either CHT or PIH is identical, in the absence of proteinuria, and so pregnancy care is unaffected by the potential inaccuracy in diagnosis.

COMPLICATIONS

Most women can expect a relatively uncomplicated pregnancy with a good outcome; however, the following potential complications should be kept in mind.

Fetal Growth Restriction

Poor placentation can lead to fetal growth restriction in women with CHT. NICE advocates ultrasound scans (USS) at 28–30 weeks and 32–34 weeks to identify and monitor small for gestational age fetuses[3] and clinical assessment of symphysis–fundal height (SFH) should be continued at every visit up until delivery.

Placental Abruption

Placental abruption affects only 1% of pregnancies complicated by CHT[4] but carries significant risk to mother and fetus. Smoking adds significantly to this risk and smoking cessation support (see Chapter 16.3) should be offered to those with the habit.

Severe Hypertension

Episodes of acute severe hypertension (≥160/110 mmHg) can occur. Some women may stop their antihypertensive medication when they conceive despite medical advice for fear of harming the pregnancy. For some their hypertensive disease may progress, with a requirement for additional medication. Such patients in the community should be referred urgently for hospital assessment. Acute pharmacological management may be with oral or intravenous (iv) labetalol, iv hydralazine or oral nifedipine and after stabilisation longer term antihypertensive medications can be altered to maintain BP <150/100 mmHg (<140/90 mmHg in diabetic patients)[3].

Superimposed Pre-Eclampsia

These women are at high risk of developing superimposed pre-eclampsia[5]. Symptoms and signs are the same as may be seen for all patients with pre-eclampsia (Section 3.3) but the BP profile may be more difficult to interpret due to higher baseline BPs and medication effects. Development of significant proteinuria (urinary protein:creatinine ratio >30 mg/mmol or 24 hour urine collection >300 mg protein) is suggestive of pre-eclampsia[3] and is often associated with fetal growth restriction. Urate (uric acid) will often be raised at diagnosis even if the rest of the blood picture is normal.

NON-PREGNANCY TREATMENT AND CARE

Extensive guidelines by the British Hypertension Society outline the management of hypertension in all patient groups[6]. The majority of women of child-bearing age with proven essential hypertension will be on one or more antihypertensive drugs, most commonly an ACE inhibitor (e.g.

enalapril or lisinopril) or an angiotensin receptor blocker (e.g. losartan or irbesartan) and/or a beta-blocker (e.g. atenolol). In addition, there may be other medications such as statins (e.g. atorvastatin or simvastatin) to lower cholesterol levels. Women with diabetes have lower target BPs than women with essential hypertension alone as their risk of cardiovascular disease is greater.

Lifestyle factors to address includes weight reduction, smoking cessation and dietary advice (see Pre-conception care).

Low-dose aspirin (75 mg once daily) and statins may feature in the care of some women thought to be at significant risk of cardiovascular disease (age over 50 years +/− ≥10 year history of type 2 diabetes +/− cholesterol >3.5 mmol/l)[6] all of which, although rare, in the obstetric population are more frequently encountered.

PRE-CONCEPTION ISSUES AND CARE

Ideally patients with medicated CHT together with significant co-morbidities, e.g. diabetes or renal disease, should be referred to a consultant Obstetrician for pre-pregnancy counselling prior to discontinuing contraception so that pregnancy risks can be discussed and antihypertensive medication changed to, most commonly, labetalol or nifedipine. Co-morbid factors would also be addressed and statins stopped as these are contraindicated in pregnancy.

Women should be advised on lifestyle factors and their importance in minimising pregnancy risk. Such factors include the encouragement of weight reduction to BMI <30, smoking cessation and the lowering of dietary sodium intake or use of a sodium substitute[3]. A BMI calculation chart is found in Appendix 13.1.1.

Box 3.1.1 Physiology of Blood Pressure

Blood pressure is an important concept worth understanding at a physiological level. Put simply, blood pressure is the pressure exerted by blood volume on the blood vessel walls.

As the heart pumps blood, it causes a change in its speed of flow, and this blood exerts a pushing force when it encounters blood vessel walls, creating a pressure. The following variable factors determine the degree of this pressure:

- The volume of blood in the vessel, which is influenced by the body's total blood volume and the volume pumped by the heart (cardiac output)
- The strength of heart contractions and how often the heart beats, which influence cardiac output
- The degree of stretch of the vessel wall
- The resistance to blood flow downstream from the vessel in question, which depends on the size of the downstream blood vessels, their length, the blood viscosity ('stickiness') and vessel wall contour ('smoothness')

Blood flows from an area of higher pressure to an area of lower pressure and pressure is always higher in the first part of a vessel than the end.

The cardiovascular system contains several different types of blood vessels. Venules and small and large veins make up the venous system and all serve to carry blood back to the heart only, whereas the arterial system, made up of arteries, arterioles and capillaries, not only serves to carry blood from the heart to the tissues but exhibits other functions in addition (see table below).

Vessel type	Size	Number	Vessel Wall Features	Function
Arteries	Large	Few	Thick and elastic ('balloon-like')	· Rapid transfer of blood from heart to organs and tissues · Creation of forward pressure during heart relaxation to maintain blood flow
Arterioles	Small	Many	Muscular with many nerve connections	· Main determinant of resistance to blood flow which affects blood distribution to individual organs and regulates overall blood pressure
Capillaries	Very small	Very many	Thin	· Exchange of materials between blood and tissues

'Blood pressure' generally refers to arterial pressure – the pressure within the systemic arteries. Its value varies throughout each contraction–relaxation cycle of the heart:

- During systole (contraction) more blood enters the arteries from the ventricle than leaves them through the arterioles (highest pressure)
- During diastole (relaxation) no new blood enters the arteries from the ventricle but blood leaves under pressure (much like air escapes from a balloon if the seal is broken) from elastic force in the wall of the arteries (lowest pressure)

Blood pressure is never 0 (except in the event of cardiac arrest) as there is always forward blood flow within the arteries caused by ongoing heart contractions continuing to fill the arteries before they have fully emptied.

S.

30

Pr
•
•
•
•
•

See
alg
hyp
in p

Medical Management and Care

All women with CHT should be referred for specialist input in the first trimester.

This will include risk assessment and treatment review[7].

Blood pressure – BP medication is commonly reduced or stopped in the first 20 weeks of pregnancy and may then become required, often in increasing doses, towards term. The following oral preparations are used:

• **Labetalol** is a combined alpha- and beta-blocker and the current first line antihypertensive medication in pregnancy[3]. It should be avoided in asthmatic patients as it can precipitate bronchospasm. It is used in iv form for the acute treatment of severe hypertension.

• **Nifedipine** is a calcium-channel blocker and is available in short (e.g. adalat) and long-acting (e.g. adalat retard and coracten XL) formulations. It can also be used as a tocolytic agent.

• **Methyldopa** is a centrally active antihypertensive which was previously used extensively in pregnancy due to its long established safety record. It has fallen out of favour but may still be used for selected patients.

• **Diuretics** such as bendroflumethiazide are used with combination therapy for patients with complex disorders such as concurrent heart or renal disease

Midwifery Management and Care

Nulliparae schedule of antenatal care with visits at 16, 25, 28, 31, 34, 36, 38 and 40 weeks[8] (see Chapter 1). At every visit perform:
• SFH measurement
• BP
• Urine dipstick for proteinuria
• Ask about symptoms of pre-eclampsia

Labour Issues
• Induction of labour from 37 weeks
• Earlier delivery in event of severe uncontrolled BP or other significant antenatal complications
• Usual antihypertensive medications during labour
• Caesarean section for usual obstetric indications only
• Avoidance of syntometrine or ergometrine for third stage

Medical Management and Care
• NICE and the RCOG recommend continuous fetal monitoring in labour[9,10]
• Consider epidural to aid BP control

Midwifery Management and Care
• Hourly BP in labour
• Do not routinely limit length of second stage unless severe hypertension when operative birth may become necessary
• Oxytocin for active management of the third stage

Postpartum Issues[8]
• Continue antenatal antihypertensives
• Stop methyldopa if used and change to pre-pregnancy regime
• Ensure appropriate midwifery and medical follow-up

Medical Management and Care
• There are no known adverse effects on breast-fed babies of mothers taking labetalol, nifedipine, enalapril, captopril, atenolol and metoprolol
• There is insufficient evidence regarding safety with breast-feeding with amlodipine and losartan, which should therefore be avoided
• Methyldopa should be changed to an alternative antihypertensive
• Ongoing antihypertensive treatment should be reviewed at 2 weeks by the GP who will also follow-up long term as required
• Offer obstetric review at 6–8 weeks

Midwifery Management and Care
• Target BP <140/90 mmHg
• Daily BP check days 1 and 2 postnatal
• BP check once days 3–5 or more often if otherwise indicated/requested
• Encourage compliance with antihypertensive medication
• Contraceptive advice (consider referral to family planning or GP)
• Remind the mother of lifestyle factors

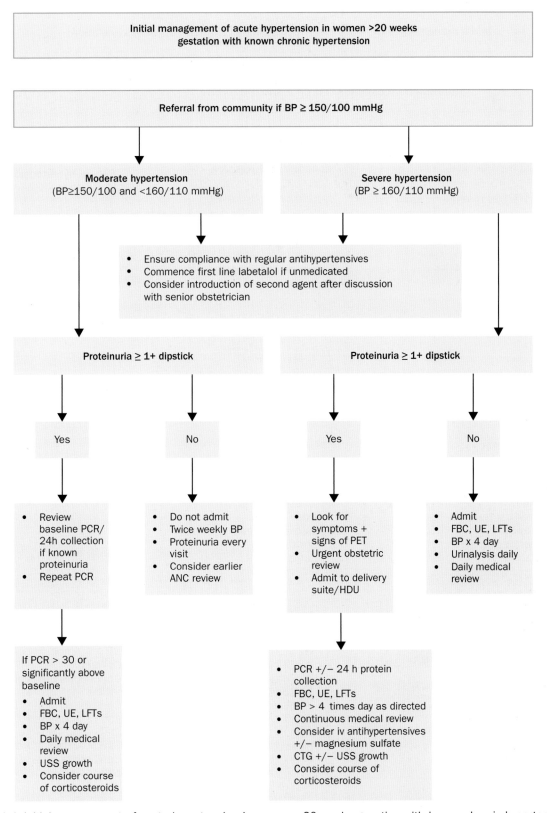

Figure 3.1.1 Initial management of acute hypertension in women >20 weeks gesation with known chronic hypertension. PCR, Protein: creatinine ratio. ANC, Antenatal clinic. PET, Pre-eclamptic toxaemia. HDU, High dependency unit. FBC, Full blood count. U&E, Urea and electrolytes. LFTs, liver function tests. USS, Ultrasound scan. CTG, Cardiotocograph. Data from NICE: Hypertension in Pregnancy CG107. This figure is downloadable from the book companion website at www.wiley.com/go/robson

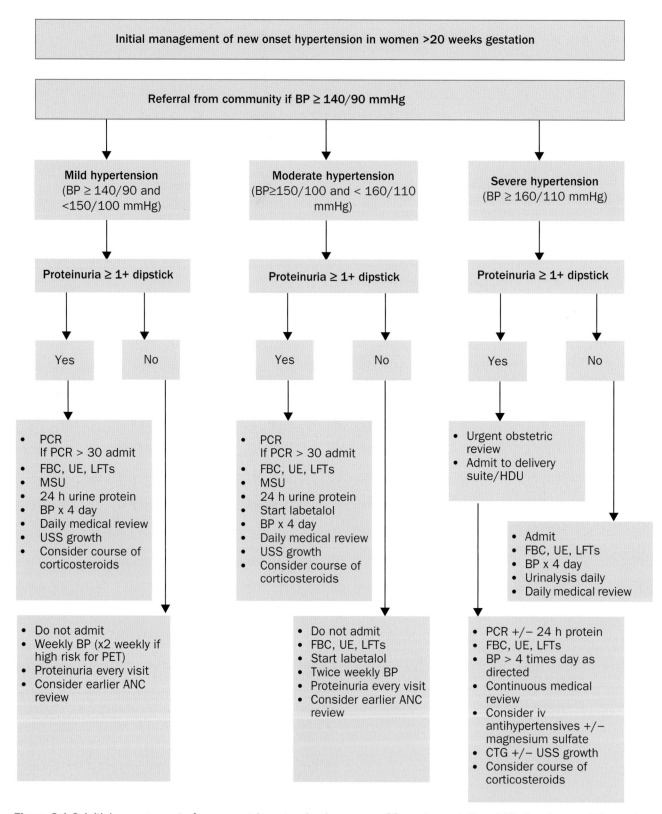

Figure 3.1.2 Initial management of new onset hypertension in women >20 weeks gestation. PCR, Protein: creatinine ratio. PET, Pre-eclamptic toxaemia. FBC, Full blood count. U&E, Urea and electrolytes. LFTs, liver function tests. USS, Ultrasound scan. CTG, Cardiotocograph. MSU, Midstream urine specimen. Data from NICE: Hypertension in Pregnancy CG107. This figure is downloadable from the book companion website at www.wiley.com/go/robson

Box 3.1.2 British Hypertension Society's Blood Pressure Measurement Recommendations

With Mercury Blood Pressure Monitors[11]
* The patient should be seated for at least 5 minutes, relaxed and not moving or speaking
* The arm must be supported at the level of the heart
* Ensure no tight clothing constricts the arm
* Place the cuff on neatly, with the centre of the bladder over the brachial artery
* The bladder should encircle at least 80% of the arm (but not more than 100%)
* The column of mercury must be vertical, and at observer's eye level
* Estimate the systolic pressure beforehand:
    * palpate the brachial artery
    * inflate cuff until pulsation disappears
    * deflate cuff
    * estimate systolic pressure
* Then inflate to 30 mmHg above the estimated systolic level needed to occlude the pulse
* Place the stethoscope diaphragm over the brachial artery and deflate at a rate of 2–3 mm/s until you hear regular tapping sounds
* Measure systolic (first sound) and diastolic (disappearance) to the nearest 2 mmHg

Cuff Sizes	Width (cm)	Length (cm)	Bladder width and length (cm)	Arm circumference (cm)
Small adult/child	10–12	18–24	12 × 18	<23
Standard adult	12–13	23–35	12 × 26	<33
Large adult	12–16	35–40	12 × 40	<50
Adult thigh cuff	20	42		<53

Points to Note
* The date of next servicing should be clearly marked on the sphygmomanometer (6 monthly)
* All maintenance necessitating handling of mercury should be conducted by the manufacturer or specialised service units
* Aneroid manometers tend to deteriorate and need regular checking
* In many instances aneroid monitors cannot be corrected accurately, therefore they should not be used as a substitute for mercury sphygmomanometers

With Electronic Blood Pressure Monitors[12]
* The patient should be seated for at least 5 minutes, relaxed and not moving or speaking
* The arm must be supported at the level of the heart
* Ensure no tight clothing constricts the arm
* Place the cuff on neatly, with the centre of the bladder over the brachial artery
* The bladder should encircle at least 80% of the arm (but not more than 100%)
* Most monitors allow manual blood pressure setting selection where you chose the appropriate setting; other monitors will automatically inflate and re-inflate to the next setting if required
* Repeat three times and record measurement as displayed
* Initially test blood pressure in both arms, and use arm with highest reading for subsequent measurement

Cuff Sizes	Width (cm)	Length (cm)	Bladder width and length (cm)	Arm circumference (cm)
Small adult/child	10–12	18–24	12 × 18	<23
Standard adult	12–13	23–35	12 × 26	<33
Large adult	12–16	35–40	12 × 40	<50
Adult thigh cuff	20	42		<53

Points to Note
* If checking against a mercury sphygmomanometer the blood pressure may differ slightly between devices
* It is good practice to occasionally check the monitor against a mercury sphygmomanometer or another validated device
* It is important to have a monitor calibrated according to the manufacturer's instructions

NB: A4-size colour posters of both of these columns can be downloaded from the BHS website as
www.bhsoc/bp_monitors/BLOOD_PRESSURE_1784a.pdf
www.bhsoc/bp_monitors/BLOOD_PRESSURE_1784b.pdf

Reproduced with kind permission of the British Hypertension Society.

Please check the BHS website www.bhsoc.org for updates on these guidelines.

3.2 Pre-eclampsia

Incidence	Risk for Childbearing
2–7% of all pregnancies[1]	High Risk

EXPLANATION OF CONDITION

Pre-eclampsia, or pre-eclamptic toxaemia (PET), is a major cause of maternal and fetal mortality and morbidity. It is a pregnancy-specific syndrome characterised by variable degrees of placental dysfunction and a maternal response featuring systemic inflammation[1] and by the development of new hypertension and significant proteinuria in the second half of pregnancy. It always resolves postnatally[2].

Pregnancy induced hypertension (PIH) or **gestational hypertension** (GH) are terms used to describe new hypertension occurring in the second half of pregnancy in the absence of significant proteinuria, and which resolves postnatally. Risk to the mother and fetus is less than with pre-eclampsia. Approximately 10% of all women will have hypertension during their pregnancy. Within this group 3–4% will have pre-eclampsia, 5% PIH and 1–2% chronic hypertension.

The exact aetiology of the condition remains unclear. There are placentation problems including inappropriate activation of endothelial cells in the walls of placental blood vessels which leads to various biochemical substances being released into the systemic circulation. This can manifest clinically as a primarily maternal problem (hypertension + proteinuria +/− systemic involvement) or a primarily fetal problem (growth restriction and hypoxia).

Pre-eclampsia once established will always progress as long as the pregnancy continues. Disease progression can be gradual (1–2 weeks) or fulminant (24 hours). Delivery is the only cure and cannot usually be delayed for more than 2 weeks. Pre-eclampsia can first manifest during the antenatal, intrapartum or postnatal periods.

Risk factors for pre-eclampsia include[3]:

- Extremes of maternal age
- Primiparity
- Chronic hypertension
- Family history
- Previous pre-eclampsia

COMPLICATIONS

It is imperative to diagnose and closely monitor pre-eclampsia because of the associated maternal and fetal risks. Pre-eclampsia can progress to severe pre-eclampsia and eclampsia (see Section 3.3). Complications include, for the fetus, growth restriction, prematurity, placental abruption and intrauterine death, and, for the mother, renal and liver failure, intracerebral bleeds, eclampsia, HELLP syndrome (**H**aemolysis, **E**levated **L**iver enzymes, **L**ow **P**latelets) (see Section 3.4), disseminated intravascular coagulation (DIC), liver rupture and even death.

NON-PREGNANCY TREATMENT AND CARE

Pre-eclampsia is a disease unique to human pregnancy. Important issues for women who have had pre-eclampsia are:

- Has the condition completely resolved postnatally, or is there an element of chronic hypertension or renal disease on which the pre-eclampsia was superimposed which needs to be further investigated and treated?
- Will it recur in subsequent pregnancies? Recurrence risk is about 16% (25% if severe pre-eclampsia, HELLP or eclampsia with birth <34 weeks)[4].
- Does a history of pre-eclampsia provide insight into potential cardiovascular disease in later life, for example heart disease and stroke? This is currently the subject of considerable research[5].
- Women should be advised regarding other factors contributing to cardiovascular risk:
  - maintaining BMI 18–25
  - smoking cessation
  - regular exercise

PRE-CONCEPTION ISSUES AND CARE

Many risk factors that predispose to pre-eclampsia have been recently clearly defined in the NICE guideline 'Hypertension in Pregnancy'.[4] These risk factors can usually be found by taking a thorough history.

The interaction of risk factors is not fully understood but it seems logical that an increasing number of risk factors in any individual woman increases her risk of developing pre-eclampsia and at an earlier gestation.

Aspirin (75 mg once daily) has been found to make a small impact in lowering the risk of developing pre-eclampsia in women with risk factors and it is safe[6]. It is now advised from 12 weeks until delivery for women with two moderate or one high risk factor[4].

No other pharmaceutical or dietary treatment is currently recommended.

Pregnancy Issues
- Surveillance is a major component of ante-/intrapartum care to ensure early diagnosis with appropriate intervention, and the reader is directed to more detailed accounts (see Essential Reading)
- Risk factor assessment +/− aspirin at booking
- Follow NICE routine antenatal care guidelines in the absence of risk factors[7]
- Follow nulliparae schedule of care (see Chapter 1)
- Individualised plan if risk factors present
- Refer to obstetric day unit according to local guidelines, usually if BP ≥140/90 mmHg with any degree of proteinuria (see algorithm)
- Detailed fetal assessment should be made at time of diagnosis of pre-eclampsia and blood tests taken

Medical Management and Care
- Women identified as at increased risk of developing pre-eclampsia should be referred for specialist input. This may involve investigation of underlying medical problems. They will normally be started on aspirin from 12 weeks until delivery

If Pre-eclampsia Develops[4]
- Inpatient care is the norm
- BP should be treated with first-line oral labetalol if ≥150/100 mmHg (see Section 3.1 for details of other antihypertensive medications)
- FBC, U&E, LFTs should be measured 2–3 times per week
- USS should be performed for growth, amniotic fluid index and umbilical artery Doppler
- Corticosteroids should be given if gestation <34 weeks at diagnosis
- Consider thromboprophylaxis with thromboembolic deterrent (TED) stockings and low molecular weight heparin
- An individualised care plan should be made including thresholds for delivery

Midwifery Management and Care
- If low risk for pre-eclampsia, BP and proteinuria assessments should be made at 16, 28, 34, 36, 38 and 41 weeks in parous women, with additional visits at 25 and 31 weeks for nulliparous women[7]
- Measurement of BP: see Box 3.1.2 for technique. When measuring BP in pregnancy it is essential to use Korotkof sound 1 – sound appears (for systolic BP) and 5 – sound disappears (for diastolic BP). Accurate blood pressure measurement is essential for correct diagnosis. Many automated devices are not accurate in pregnancy
- Measurement of proteinuria: urine dipsticks remain the preferred method of choice for the assessment of proteinuria. These are prone to observer error and the use of automated dipstick readers has been shown to improve accuracy[8]. With proteinuria ≥1+ a urinary protein : creatinine ratio (PCR) or 24 hour urine protein collection should be performed to quantify proteinuria
- If symptoms or signs of pre-eclampsia develop the midwife MUST refer the mother to an obstetrician promptly, and support any medical treatment
- Psychological support and advice regarding the condition should be given and any reassurance should be realistic

Labour Issues[9,10]
- Corticosteroids for fetal lung maturity will be given if delivery planned <34 weeks and often between 34 and 36 + 6 weeks if LSCS is expected
- Blood tests depending on previous results and clinical picture
- Severe pre-eclampsia may prompt delivery or develop intrapartum and all obstetric units should all have specific guidelines
- Avoid syntometrine/ergometrine for third stage, as these increase blood pressure acutely
- Caesarean section may be performed if delivery is very urgent or pre-term
- BP should be closely observed postnatally
- Some women will require intensive HDU monitoring for 24–48 hours

Medical Management and Care[4] (see also Section 3.3 Eclampsia)
- Timing and mode of delivery determined by consultant Obstetrician (individualised plan)
- Continuous fetal monitoring in labour[10,11]
- Consider epidural to aid BP control (recent platelet count mandatory)
- FBC, U&E, LFTs if not performed in last 2–3 days, or if severe pre-eclampsia develops
- Continue antihypertensive medications started antenatally

Midwifery Management and Care
- Hourly BP in labour
- Do not limit length of second stage unless severe hypertension develops
- Observe for signs and symptoms of severe pre-eclampsia (see Section 3.3) and call for urgent medical review if concerned
- Oxytocin for active management of the third stage
- Midwife may have to prepare for a pre-term delivery (see Chapter 1)

Postpartum Issues
- Close observation of BP until antihypertensive medication is stopped, therefore midwives may need to extend the period of postnatal visiting ≥10 days
- Obstetric review should be offered at 6–8 weeks (see Section 3.1 regarding antihypertensives and breastfeeding)

Medical Management and Care[4]
- Continue antihypertensive medication if started antenatally with reduction once BP <130/80 mmHg
- If still required, methyldopa should be changed to an alternative
- Start antihypertensive medication if never medicated and if BP rises to ≥150/100 mmHg
- Repeat bloods at 48–72 hours and after that only as clinically indicated
- Ongoing antihypertensive treatment should be reviewed at 2 weeks by the GP who will also follow-up long term as required
- Offer obstetric review at 6–8 weeks

Midwifery Care
- BP check four times daily whilst an inpatient
- BP at least once days 3–5 postnatal
- Refer for medical care if BP ≥150/100 mmHg
- Ensure 6–8 week medical review

3.3 Severe Pre-eclampsia and Eclampsia

Incidence	Risk for Childbearing
Severe pre-eclampsia 0.5% of all pregnancies	High Risk
Eclampsia 0.05% of all pregnancies[1]	

INTRODUCTION

Severe pre-eclampsia (aka severe PET) is generally defined by systolic blood pressure ≥160 mmHg or diastolic blood pressure ≥110 mmHg on two occasions, together with significant proteinuria and the possible presence of other defined clinical features (see below)[1]. Women who have more moderate hypertension and who exhibit two or more of these features may also be described as having severe pre-eclampsia:

- Severe headache
- Visual disturbances (blurring or flashing)
- Epigastric pain +/− vomiting
- Liver tenderness
- Clonus
- Papilloedema
- Platelet count <100 × 10⁶/l
- Abnormal liver function (ALT or AST >70 IU/l)
- HELLP syndrome (Haemolysis, Elevated Liver enzymes, Low Platelets, see Section 3.4)

Severe pre-eclampsia can lead to **eclampsia,** which is the occurrence of one or more generalised convulsions on the background of pre-eclampsia. A case fatality rate of 1.8% has been reported and up to 35% of women suffer a major complication[2].

Whilst severe pre-eclampsia and eclampsia can occur at any time after 20 weeks gestation including up to 6 weeks postpartum, it should be remembered that up to 44% of cases of eclampsia occur postnatally, especially at term[2].

Strategy

- Local and/or regional guidelines should usually be in place for the management of severe pre-eclampsia and eclampsia and closely adhered to
- During diagnosis, there should be careful assessment of BP and proteinuria with consideration of potential organ involvement (including the feto-placental unit)
- Following the diagnosis of severe pre-eclampsia, intensive monitoring of BP and fluid balance is required, as well as regular FBC, U&E and LFTs to monitor for changes in renal function and HELLP syndrome
- Delivery is dependent upon the woman being stable
- Eclamptic convulsions are an obstetric emergency and require senior obstetric involvement, but do not necessitate immediate delivery
- Attempts should be made to manage severe early onset pre-eclampsia conservatively to prolong pregnancy for fetal maturation. This requires inpatient care in a unit with adequate neonatal facilities for pre-term infants. On average, 7–15 days of additional gestation can be obtained

COMPLICATIONS

As for pre-eclampsia (see Section 3.2).

NON-PREGNANCY TREATMENT AND CARE

As for pre-eclampsia (see Section 3.2).

PRE-CONCEPTION ISSUES AND CARE

Pre-conception counselling and care are as for pre-eclampsia (see section 3.2).

Obstetric follow-up of women who suffered severe pre-eclampsia is important so that delivery debriefing can occur, any underlying renal pathology can be excluded and plans for subsequent pregnancies can be made.

Pregnancy and Labour Issues

(1) Blood pressure control

As for pre-eclampsia (Section 3.2)

There should be urgent review by the obstetric team if severe pre-eclampsia suspected by midwifery staff

(2) Fluid management

(3) Prevention of seizures

(4) Control of seizures

Medical Management and Care[1]
- As for pre-eclampsia (Section 3.2)
- Blood pressures of >160/110 mmHg require urgent intervention
- At presentation, it may be possible to manage severe hypertension with oral agents (labetalol or nifedipine)
- Intravenous (iv) administration of labetalol or hydralazine often becomes necessary and use should follow local guidelines. In general, labetalol is first line except in asthmatics. Both are given initially in bolus doses to lower blood pressure and then as infusions for BP maintenance.
- Fluid restriction is advised to reduce the risk of fluid overload (leading to pulmonary and cerebral oedema)
- Usual regimes are 1 ml/kg/h or 80–85 ml/h
- Restriction is usually maintained until there is evidence of a postpartum diuresis
- If haemorrhage or other fluid loss occurs, more iv fluid may be required and this is sometimes guided by invasive central venous pressure monitoring and anaesthetic advice
- Intravenous magnesium sulfate should be given to all women with severe preeclampsia, as it halves the risk of an eclampsia and has a proven safety record[3]
- Consider giving magnesium sulfate 24 h prior to delivery to allow a course of corticosteriods for fetal lung maturity
- Give 4 g by slow iv infusion for 5 min followed by infusion of 1 g/h for 24 h
- Magnesium sulfate should be continued for either 24 h post-delivery or 24 h after the last eclamptic seizure
- For recurrent seizures, either give a further bolus of 2–4 g or increase the infusion rate to 1.5–2 g/h
- Signs of magnesium toxicity are reduced urine output (<20 ml/h), the loss of deep tendon reflexes and decreased respiratory rate, and if any of these are apparent the magnesium sulfate infusion should normally be stopped. Calcium gluconate 1 g (10 ml) over 10 minutes can be given to reverse the effects if respiratory depression is significant
- If seizures persist, other agents such as diazepam and thiopentone can be used but this is rare and would be in the ITU setting with the woman ventilated

Team Approach

Good teamwork is essential, and this can be rehearsed in skills-drills

Remember the basic principal of ABC (Airway, Breathing, Circulation)

Midwifery Management and Care
- One-on-one care with HDU/ITU monitoring and documentation, including hourly urine output, reflex assessment and respiratory rate and continual BP checks
- Target BP <150/80–100 mmHg
- Careful and well-documented fluid balance
- Management of iv infusions
- Six 12-hourly blood tests
- Close liaison with medical team

Labour Issues
- It is imperative to remember that standard midwifery care and support for a woman in labour are essential in addition to the special measures described
- Avoidance of syntometrine or ergometrine for the third stage

Medical Management and Care
- Mode of delivery individualised in view of clinical picture and woman's preferences
- Continuous fetal monitoring in labour
- Consider epidural to aid BP control (recent platelet count mandatory)

Midwifery Management and Care
- Continue with above high dependency care in labour
- Prepare for a potentially pre-term birth
- Length of second stage may be shortened depending on level of hypertension
- Oxytocin for active management of the third stage
- Prepare for a potentially pre-term birth

Postpartum Issues
- Remember the possibility of postpartum pre-eclampsia
- Close observation of BP until antihypertensive medication stopped

Medical Management and Care

As for pre-eclampsia (see Section 3.2)
- The woman may require continued HDU care for 24–48 h postnatally, and should not be transferred to the postnatal ward in this time
- Magnesium sulfate will usually be stopped 24 h after birth or the last seizure
- Intrapartum events should be debriefed with the patient and midwifery staff

Midwifery Management and Care
- As for pre-eclampsia (Section 3.2)
- Women will remain in-patients for approximately 4 days, and the baby may be on the special care baby unit, with women requiring additional psychological support
- Breast-feeding should be encouraged

S. E. Robson and J. Waugh

3.4 HELLP Syndrome

Incidence	Risk for Childbearing
0.6% of all pregnancies	High Risk

INTRODUCTION

HELLP syndrome was first described in 1982[1] and probably represents a severe form of pre-eclampsia (PET). The exact relationship between the two remains uncertain and it can develop in women showing no signs or symptoms of pre-eclampsia. Proteinuric hypertension is evident in up to 85% of cases[2]. Maternal complications can be serious and perinatal infant mortality high[3]. The diagnosis is suspected when the following are present on blood testing:

- *Haemolysis* (red blood cell rupture demonstrated on blood film and leading to a drop in haemoglobin level)
- *Elevated Liver Enzymes* (raised alanine transaminase (ALT) or aspartate transaminase (AST) indicating liver damage)
- *Low Platelets* (cell fragments involved in the clotting process)

HELLP is a multi-system disorder characterised by activation of the coagulation system leading to increased deposition of the protein fibrin throughout the body. In the blood system, deposited fibrin causes damage to red blood cell membranes leading to fragmentation of cells. In the liver, fibrin deposited within the organ's blood vessels decreases the vessel diameter and therefore lowers the blood volume reaching liver cells and increases the pressure of blood flow, leading to injury and death of liver cells. Fibrin deposits on the walls of any blood vessel damage the vessel lining (endothelium), leading to activation and clumping together of platelets which forms blood clots and lowers the platelet count.

Women will often present in the second or third trimester of pregnancy with signs and symptoms of severe pre-eclampsia, and in particular they may have abdominal pain (usually right upper quadrant or epigastric), liver tenderness and/or nausea and vomiting. HELLP can also occur postnatally. Ten to twenty percent of those women with severe pre-eclampsia or eclampsia will develop HELLP and risk factors include older childbearing women, multiparity and Caucasian origin[2].

Important differential diagnoses to consider are:

- **Acute fatty liver of pregnancy**, where the predominant symptom is nausea and vomiting and where there is fatty liver change leading to acute liver failure with severe blood clotting problems (see Chapter 13.4)
- **Haemolytic uraemic syndrome-thrombotic thrombocytopenic pupura**, which is a complex disorder involving multiple organ systems, characterized by haemolytic anaemia, low platelets, renal failure and/or severe headache for which there is no other explanation and which requires treatment with plasma exchange (see Chapter 14.5 for thrombocytopenic purpura)
- Exacerbation of **systemic lupus erythematosus** (SLE), a chronic inflammatory disease affecting multiple organs including the kidneys, lungs and neurological system and which can be exacerbated by pregnancy (see Chapter 11.3).

HELLP-related epigastric pain can be confused with the common problem of heart burn in pregnancy (see Chapter 10.1). However, the pain associated with HELLP syndrome is not relieved by antacid preparations and does not radiate upwards towards the throat as with heartburn.

The diagnosis of HELLP is an obstetric and medical emergency that requires prompt and appropriate care in an obstetric-led unit with access to intensive care facilities and liver, renal and haematological specialists. Delivery is the only cure and should be conducted promptly with senior staff on hand.

COMPLICATIONS

The most important complications which may be apparent at, or shortly after, presentation, are:

- Disseminated intravascular coagulation (DIC) (abnormal clotting – see Chapter 14.3)
- Placental abruption
- Acute renal failure
- Pulmonary oedema
- Liver haematoma and rupture

NON-PREGNANCY TREATMENT AND CARE

HELLP syndrome is unique to human pregnancy. Given its association with pre-eclampsia, non-pregnancy care is as for pre-eclampsia (Section 3.3). Biochemical abnormalities usually normalize within 2 weeks of delivery.

PRE-CONCEPTION ISSUES AND CARE

Women who have suffered with severe pre-eclampsia, HELLP or eclampsia in a previous pregnancy are at an increased risk of the condition re-occurring in subsequent pregnancies. The reoccurrence risk of pre-eclampsia is 25% if birth was <34 weeks and 55% if birth was <28 weeks[4].

This highlights the need for early specialist referral and increased surveillance in the next and subsequent pregnancies. A plan may well have been made at the postnatal follow-up of the previous pregnancy.

Pregnancy Issues
- As for pre-eclampsia (Sections 3.2 and 3.3)
- There should be urgent review by the obstetric team if there are abnormalities on FBC, U&E or LFTs in a patient with or without hypertension

Medical Management and Care
- As for pre-eclampsia (Sections 3.2 and 3.3)
- Stabilise[6]
- Perform an USS for fetal growth, and CTG to assess fetal wellbeing[6]
- Involve senior obstetricians; make a delivery plan including timing

Midwifery Management and Care
- As for pre-eclampsia (Sections 3.2 and 3.3)
- Liaise closely with medical staff

Labour Issues
As for severe pre-eclampsia (Section 3.3)
- One-on-one care in labour with regular obstetric review and HDU monitoring
- Blood pressure control
- Fluid management
- Prevention and control of seizures
- Consider ITU based on anaesthetic and obstetric opinion

Medical Management and Care
- HELLP should be managed as for severe pre-eclampsia (Section 3.3) with good control of BP (antihypertensives not always necessary) and strict fluid balance
- Senior obstetricians should be involved from the outset
- Other specialist teams should be involved as necessary, such as anaesthetics, haematology and the renal physicians
- Magnesium sulfate should be given for seizure prophylaxis[6]
- If <34 weeks at diagnosis, corticosteroids should be given to encourage fetal lung maturity as early delivery is expected
- Mode of delivery is individualised and thresholds for delivery should be clearly documented

Midwifery Management and Care
- HDU care by experienced senior midwifery staff or junior staff under supervision (as for severe pre-eclampsia, see Section 3.3)
- Accurate fluid balance recording with hourly urine measurement
- Blood tests as clinically indicated but often 6–12 hourly
- Observe for unexpected bleeding from nose, gums and wounds
- Continuous support should be offered to the woman and her partner as this situation is often anxiety provoking

Postpartum Issues
- Be aware of the possibility of HELLP syndrome developing in the postnatal period[5]
- Close observation of BP and symptoms in patients with a history of ante/intrapartum pre-eclampsia
- Abnormal blood results need to be reviewed by obstetric staff and a monitoring plan made
- De-briefing, counselling and obstetric follow-up should be ensured

Medical Management and Care
- Regular medical reviews in the postnatal period (at least daily for the first 3 days following birth)
- The woman will usually require continued HDU care for 24–48h postnatally
- Obstetric review at 6–8 weeks

Midwifery Management and Care
- Continued HDU care until 'discharged' to the postnatal ward
- BP and symptom checks four times a day whilst an inpatient and at least once on days 3–5
- Continued BP and symptom checks until blood results normalise and until any antihypertensive medication is stopped
- Ensure breast-feeding and psychological support

3 Hypertensive Disorders

PATIENT ORGANISATIONS

British Hypertension Society
BHS Administrative Officer
Clinical Sciences Building Level 5
PO Box 65
Leicester Royal Infirmary
Leicester LE2 7LX
www.bhsoc.org

Action on Pre-eclampsia – APEC
84–88 Pinner Road
Harrow
Middlesex HA1 4HZ
www.apec.org.uk

The Pre-eclampsia Society – PETS
Rhianfa
Carmel LL54 7RL
www.pre-eclampsia-society.org.uk

Blood Pressure Association
60 Cranmer Terrace
London SW17 0QS
www.bpassoc.org.uk

Australian Action on Pre-eclampsia
P.O. Box 29 Carlton South
Vic. 3053
Australia
www.aapec.org.au

New Zealand Action on Pre-eclampsia
34 Ridge Rd
Howick
Auckland
New Zealand
info@nzapec.com

The Pre-eclampsia Foundation
5353 Wayzata Blvd.
Suite 207
Minneapolis, MN 55416
United States of America
www.preeclampsia.org

The HELLP Syndrome Society
P.O. Box 44
Bethany
West Virginia 26032
United States of America
www.hellpsyndrome.org

ESSENTIAL READING

Billington M and Stevenson M 2006 *Hypertensive disorders and the critically ill woman* in **Critical Care in Childbearing for Midwives**. Oxford; Blackwell Publishing Ltd.

Gilbert ES 2007 *Hypertensive disorders* in **Manual of High Risk Pregnancy and Delivery**, 4th Edn. St Louis, MO; Mosby/Elsevier

Johnson R and Taylor W 2006 Assessment of maternal and neonatal vital signs – blood pressure measurement. In: **Skills for Midwifery Practice**, 2nd Edn. Edinburgh; Elsevier Churchill Livingstone

Joshi D, James A, Quaglia A, *et al.* 2010. Liver disease in pregnancy. **Lancet**, 375:594–605

Lip G, Beevers YH, O'Brien G, Beevers E and Gareth D 2007 **ABC of Hypertension**, 5th Edn. Oxford; BMJ books/Blackwell Publishing Ltd.

Macdonald S and Magill-Cuerden J 2011 *Hypertensive disorders of pregnancy* in **Mayes Midwifery: A Textbook for Midwives**, 14th Edn. Baillière Tindall

NICE 2008: Antenatal Care: routine care for the healthy pregnant woman CG62. On line as: http://www.nice.org.uk/CG62

NICE 2010. Hypertension in Pregnancy CG107. On line as: http://www.nice.org.uk/cg107

RCOG 2006 **Clinical Guideline No. 10a: The management of severe pre-eclampsia/eclampsia**. London; Royal College of Obstetricians and Gynaecologists. On line as: www.rcog.org.uk/resources/Public/pdf/management_pre_eclampsia_mar06.pdf

Sibai B, Dekker G and Kupferminc M 2005 Pre-eclampsia. **Lancet**, 365(9461):785–799

References

3.1 Chronic Hypertension

1. Nelson TR 1995. A clinical study of pre-eclampsia (parts 1 & 2). **Journal of Obstetrics and Gynaecology of the British Empire**, 62:48–62
2. Chesley LC 1978 **Hypertensive Disorders in Pregnancy**. New York; Appleton-Century-Crofts 478
3. NICE 2010 **Hypertension in Pregnancy** CG107. London; National Institute for Health and Clinical Excellence. www.nice.org.uk
4. Williams MA, Lieberman E, Mittendirf R, Monson RR and Schoenbaum SC 1991 Risk factors for abruptio placentae. **American Journal of Epidemiology**, 134:965–972
5. Sibai BM 2002 Chronic Hypertension in Pregnancy. **Obstetrics and Gynecology**, 100:369–377
6. Williams B, Poulter NR, Brown MJ, et al. 2004 British Hypertension Society guidelines for hypertension management (BHS–IV) summary. **British Medical Journal**, 328:634–640
7. Milne F, Redman C, Walker J, et al. 2005 The pre-eclampsia community guideline. PRECOG: how to screen for and detect onset of pre-eclampsia in the community. **British Medical Journal**, 330:576–580
8. NICE 2008 **Antenatal Care: Routine Care for the Healthy Pregnant woman** CG62. London; National Institute for Health and Clinical Excellence. www.nice.org.uk
9. NICE 2008 **Intrapartum Care** CG55. London; National Institute for Health and Clinical Excellence. www.nice.org.uk
10. RCOG 2001 Evidence Based Clinical Guideline No 8. **The Use of Electronic Fetal Monitoring**. London; RCOG Press.
11. British Hypertension Society 2007 Factsheet: **Blood Pressure Measurement with Mercury Blood Pressure Monitors** www.bhsoc/bp_monitors/BLOOD_PRESSURE_1784a.pdf [accessed 08-06-2007]
12. British Hypertension Society 2007 Factsheet: **Blood Pressure Measurement with Electronic Blood Pressure Monitors** www.bhsoc/bp_monitors/BLOOD_PRESSURE_1784b.pdf [accessed 08-06-2007]

3.2 Pre-Eclampsia

1. James, Steer et al. 2011. **High Risk Pregnancy: Management Options**. 35: 600. Saunders, Elsevier Inc
2. Shennan AH and Waugh JJS 2003 **Pre-eclampsia**. London; RCOG Press
3. Joshi D, James A, Quaglia A et al. 2010 Liver disease in pregnancy. **Lancet**, 375:594–605
4. NICE 2010 **Hypertension in Pregnancy** CG107. London; National Institute for Health and Clinical Excellence. www.nice.org.uk
5. Clifton VL, Stark MJ, Osei-Kumah A, et al. 2012 Review: the feto-placental unit, pregnancy pathology and impact on long term maternal health. **Placenta**, 33:S37–S41
6. Askie LM, Duley L, Henderson-Smart DJ and Stewart LA 2007 PARIS Collaborative Group: Antiplatelet agents for the prevention of preeclampsia: a meta-analysis of individual patient data. **Lancet**, 369:1791–1798
7. NICE 2008 **Antenatal Care: Routine Care for the Healthy Pregnant Woman** CG62. London; National Institute for Health and Clinical Excellence. www.nice.org.uk
8. Waugh JJS, Bell SC, Kilby MD, et al. 2005 Optimal bedside urinalysis for the detection of proteinuria in hypertensive pregnancy: a study of diagnostic accuracy. **British Journal of Obstetrics and Gynaecology**, 112:412–417
9. Tuffnell DJ, Shennan AH, Waugh JJS and Walker JJ 2006 **RCOG Guideline No. 10(A):The Management of Severe preeclampsia/eclampsia**. London; Royal College of Obstetricians and Gynaecologists
10. NICE 2008 **Intrapartum care** CG55. London; National Institute for Health and Clinical Excellence. www.nice.org.uk
11. RCOG 2001 Evidence Based Clinical Guideline No 8. **The Use of Electronic Fetal Monitoring**. London; RCOG Press

3.3 Severe Pre-eclampsia/Eclampsia

1. Tuffnell DJ, Shennan AH, Waugh JJS, Walker JJ 2006 **RCOG Guideline 10(A) The Management of Severe preeclampsia/eclampsia**. London; Royal College of Obstetricians and Gynaecologists
2. Douglas KA, Redman CW 1994 Eclampsia in the United Kingdom. **BMJ**, 309:1395–400
3. Altman D, Carroli G, Duley L, Farrell B, Moodley J et al. 2002 Do women with pre-eclampsia, and their babies, benefit from magnesium sulphate? The Magpie Trial: a randomised placebo-controlled trial. **Lancet**, 359(9321): 1877–1890

3.4 HELLP

1. Weinstein L 1982 Syndrome of hemolysis, elevated liver enzymes, and low platelet count: a severe consequence of hypertension in pregnancy. **American Journal of Obstetrics and Gynecology**, 142:159–67
2. Joshi D, James A, Quaglia A, et al. 2010 Liver Disease in Pregnancy. **Lancet**, 375:594–605
3. Mihu D, Costin N, Mihu CM et al. 2007 HELLP syndrome – a multisystemic disorder. **Journal of Gastrointestinal and Liver Diseases**, 16:419–424
4. NICE 2010 **Hypertension in Pregnancy** CG107. London; National Institute for Health and Clinical Excellence. www.nice.org.uk
5. Egerman RS, Sibai BM 1999 HELLP syndrome. **Clinical and Obstetric Gynecology**, 42:381–89
6. RCOG 2010 Guideline No. 10a **The Management of Severe Pre-eclampsia/eclampsia** 2006. Reviewed 2010 London; RCOG http://www.rcog.org.uk/files/rcog-corp/GTG10a230611.pdf

HEART DISEASE

Moira McLean[1], Frances A. Bu'Lock[2]
and S. Elizabeth Robson[1]

[1]De Montfort University, Leicester, UK
[2]Glenfield Hospital, Leicester, UK

4.1 Mild Structural Heart Disease
4.2 Moderate Structural Heart Disease
4.3 Severe Structural Heart Disease
4.4 Rheumatic and Valvular Heart Disease
4.5 Marfan's Syndrome
4.6 Functional Heart Disease: Cardiomyopathy
4.7 Functional Heart Disease: Arrhythmias
4.8 Ischaemic Heart Disease: Angina and
Myocardial Infarction
4.9 Pulmonary Hypertension and
Eisenmenger's Syndrome
4.10 Heart Transplant

Medical Disorders in Pregnancy: A Manual for Midwives, Second Edition. Edited by S. Elizabeth Robson and Jason Waugh.
© 2013 John Wiley & Sons, Ltd. Published 2013 by John Wiley & Sons, Ltd.

4.1 Mild Structural Heart Disease

Incidence	Risk for Childbearing
Affects 1% of live births[1]	Variable Risk (dependent upon repair and condition)
2500 adults present with congenital heart disease a year[2]	
0.8% pregnant women have congenital heart disease[3]	

EXPLANATION OF CONDITIONS

Of children born with congenital heart disease, 85% now survive to adulthood[1,3–5]. There are a wide range of lesions. Isolated valve lesions are dealt with separately. Other cardiac abnormalities are associated with shunts, missing chambers +/− abnormal connections. Mild conditions are outlined below, moderate and complex conditions in the next sections. Some conditions, especially atrial septal defect, may present or be detected for the first time in pregnancy. Most have previously been repaired but all require consideration and some require further management. Recurrence risks must also be addressed. Congenital heart disease is the most frequent cardiovascular disease presenting in pregnancy with shunt lesions predominating[6,7]. Figure 4.1.1 shows a normal heart, against which the structural defects can be compared.

Shunts

A shunt is passage of blood through a channel that is not its normal one. Severity is determined not only by the size of the shunt but also the complexity and repairability of associated lesions.

Atrial Septal Defect (ASD)

This is an incomplete closure of the wall between the upper chambers of the heart (left and right atria). It is commoner in women and may be associated with valve problems (see Figure 4.1.2). It is generally repaired in childhood; transcatheter umbrella closure is now common.

Ventricular Septal Defect (VSD)

Ventricular septal defect is one or more openings in the wall separating the right and left ventricles (see Figure 4.1.2).

It is one of the most common congenital heart defects. About 60% of these close spontaneously or are too small to need surgery; the remaining 40% require open heart surgery, usually in infancy.

Patent Ductus Arteriosus (PDA)

This is the persistence of a normal fetal structure between the left pulmonary artery and the descending aorta. Persistence of this fetal structure beyond 10 days of life is considered abnormal. It is commoner in pre-term infants and is generally closed either surgically or with a transcatheter umbrella-type device (see Figure 4.1.2).

Tetralogy of Fallot

Tetralogy of Fallot has four components:

1. Ventricular septal defect (VSD)
2. Aorta dextroposition, which overrides a VSD
3. Right ventricular outflow tract obstruction
4. Right ventricular hypertrophy

Tetralogy of Fallot is the most common cyanotic heart defect, representing 5–7% of congenital heart defects. It can be associated with chromosome 22 deletion[8], and is generally repaired in infancy or early childhood (see Figure 4.1.3).

COMPLICATIONS

Atrial Septal Defect

- Atrial fibrillation
- Heart failure
- Stroke

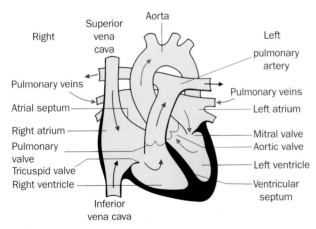

Figure 4.1.1 Normal heart (adapted from Meeks 2010). This figure is downloadable from the book companion website at www.wiley.com/go/robson

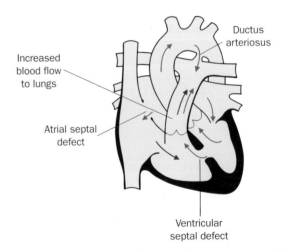

Figure 4.1.2 Atrial septal defect, ventricular septal defect and patent ductus arteriosus (adapted from Meeks 2010). This figure is downloadable from the book companion website at www.wiley.com/go/robson

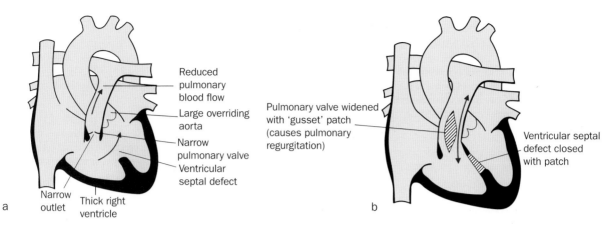

Figure 4.1.3 (a) Tetralogy of Fallot (adapted from Meeks 2010). (b) Tetralogy of Fallot post trans-annular patch (adapted from Meeks 2010). This figure is downloadable from the book companion website at www.wiley.com/go/robson

Ventricular Septal Defect

- Congestive heart failure and failure to thrive in infancy and early childhood
- Damage to the heart's electrical conduction system during surgery (requiring pacemaker or causing late arrhythmias)
- Infective endocarditis
- Aortic insufficiency (leaking of the valve that separates the left ventricle from the aorta)
- Pulmonary hypertension (high blood pressure in the lungs) leading to failure of the right side of the heart[9,10] (see Section 4.9 Pulmonary Hypertension)

Patent Ductus Arteriosus

Closure is usually completely successful, but there is an increased recurrence risk for the fetus.

Tetralogy of Fallot

- Post-repair, residual lesions are frequent
- Pulmonary regurgitation is common +/− stenosis, and the valve may need replacement
- Regular cardiological follow-up is essential
- Late arrhythmias also occur
- 22q deletion may not have been recognised previously and has 50% recurrence risk[11]

NON-PREGNANCY TREATMENT AND CARE

See above

PRE-CONCEPTION ISSUES AND CARE

- Seek expert congenital heart disease specialist advice as to whether further assessment required, e.g. PDA/ASD device closure relatively new
- Assess the requirement for endocarditis prophylaxis (only fully-closed defects are low risk)
- Consideration of pre-pregnancy interventions to optimise maternal and fetal wellbeing in pregnancy for ongoing/residual haemodynamic problems

- Clinical genetics referral for recurrence risk and need for fetal surveillance
- PDA and secundum ASD are **normal** *in utero*, hence fetal screening is not prognostic and postnatal echocardiography is recommended
- Other types of ASD (such as partial AVSD), VSD and Tetralogy of Fallot can be detected *in utero*; mild forms cannot be completely excluded

Pregnancy Issues

Low risk if closed or repaired with surgery

- Increased recurrence risk in the baby, so specialised cardiac ultrasound screening may be indicated at specialist centres, some as early as 13 weeks[12] (see pre-pregnancy counselling)
- Fetal nuchal translucency screening may also be helpful[13]

Atrial septal defect

- May be newly diagnosed in pregnancy; if repaired, problems are unlikely[14]
- Open ASD increases risks of arrhythmia, thrombo-embolic stroke and right heart failure

Ventricular septal defect

- Previously closed defects very low risk; occasional arrhythmia issues, possible increased risk of pre-eclampsia[15]
- Small defects near valves have increased endocarditis risks
- Large untreated defects are high risk (see Section 4.9 Eisenmenger's Syndrome)

Patent ductus arteriosus

- Previously closed/asymptomatic small shunts behave normally
- Large shunts' ducts can lead to pulmonary hypertension (see Section 4.9 Eisenmenger's Syndrome)
- 4% recurrence risk postnatally[16]

Tetralogy of Fallot

- If repaired, pregnancy generally tolerated well but needs cardiological supervision
- For unrepaired defects, see Section 4.3, Severe Structural Heart Disease

Medical Management and Care

- Maternal risk assessment should be carried out according to the modified World Health Organization (WHO) risk classification (see Box 4.1.1)
- Endocarditis prophylaxis no longer routinely required[19] but should be discussed on a per patient basis.

Atrial septal defect

- Routine care if previously successfully closed, otherwise consider aspirin thrombo-prophylaxis

Ventricular septal defect

- Routine care if previously successfully closed; usual pre-eclampsia screening[15]
- Small shunts treated as normal, plus endocarditis prophylaxis
- Larger shunts need cardiological supervision
- Co-existing pulmonary hypertension: counselling for ToP etc. (see Section 4.9 Eisenmenger's Syndrome)
- Arrhythmias may occur

Patent ductus arteriosus

- Closed – treat as normal
- Open or newly diagnosed –follow cardiological advice

Tetralogy of Fallot

- Assess for right outflow obstruction/pulmonary regurgitation, right ventricular function and other residual lesions
- Arrhythmia monitoring and treatment may be required
- Diuretics may be helpful but bed-rest is rarely necessary[22]
- In the absence of problems a normal vaginal birth is anticipated[17]

Midwifery Management and Care

All will require:

- Early booking with immediate referral to specialist
- Accurate and careful personal and family booking history and baseline observations including respiratory rate and pulse
- Advice on diet and iron supplements to maintain a normal Hb level
- Ascertain need for antibiotic prophylaxis for dental/surgical/obstetric procedures
- Observation for worsening tiredness and breathlessness
- If right ventricular failure develops prepare for a pre-term delivery

Labour issues

Symptomatic patients and those with open ASD have a higher risk of thrombo-embolic disease, are likely to require compression stockings[17] and anticoagulation considered if immobile[14].

Patients with active problems will require:

- Anaesthetic review prior to labour
- Plan of care drawn up, to include a strategy for oxytoxic drugs[18] – generally as normal
- Antibiotic prophylaxis for rupture of membranes or active labour no longer routinely[19] required, but should be considered on an individual basis

Medical Management and Care

- Assess individual requirements for antibiotic prophylaxis
- Consider epidural for pain relief
- Define monitoring needs, such as oximetry and ECG
- Define thromboprophylaxis needs, including TED stockings

Midwifery Management and Care

- Read and follow the care plan thoroughly
- Assist with TED stockings
- Careful monitoring of materno-fetal wellbeing including oximetry as above
- Assess progress in labour, with prompt referral if concerned
- Oxytocin is usually the drug of choice for third-stage management

Postpartum Issues

The neonate is at risk of cardiac disease and requires screening according to cardiological advice[20].

Standard contraceptive advice is appropriate unless open ASD/concerns re pulmonary hypertension (see Section 4.9 on Eisenmenger's Syndrome). Combined oral contraceptives are commonly used. Intrauterine devices may be appropriate but consider if endocarditis prophylaxis is warranted[21].

Medical Management and Care

- ASD – routine care if no complications
- VSD/corrected ToF – monitor fluid balance if potential for congestive cardiac failure (CCF)
- Discuss contraceptive options
- Consider multi-disciplinary follow-up for 6 weeks after delivery[23]

Midwifery Management and Care

- Encourage ambulation to reduce risk of thrombo-embolic disease
- Ascertain if maintenance of fluid balance is to be continued
- Reinforce contraceptive advice as above
- Be alert for signs of cardiac disease in the neonate, which might initially present as lethargy or as a feeding problem
- The neonatal examination prior to discharge home is best performed by a paediatrician, not a midwife, due to the risk of cardiac disease

Box 4.1.1 New York Heart Association and WHO Classifications of Heart Disease

In 1928 the New York Heart Association published a classification of patients with cardiac disease based on clinical severity and prognosis. This classification has been updated in subsequent editions of *Nomenclature and Criteria for Diagnosis of Diseases of the Heart and Great Vessels* (Little, Brown & Co.). The ninth edition, revised by the Criteria Committee of the American Heart Association, New York City Affiliate, was released in 1994 and is summarised below[1].

NYHA Functional Capacity Classification

Class	Description
I	Patients with cardiac disease but without resulting limitation of physical activity Ordinary physical activity does not cause undue fatigue, palpitation, dyspnoea or anginal pain
II	Patients with cardiac disease resulting in slight limitation of physical activity They are comfortable at rest Ordinary physical activity results in fatigue, palpitation, dyspnoea or anginal pain
III	Patients with cardiac disease resulting in marked limitation of physical activity They are comfortable at rest Less than ordinary activity causes fatigue, palpitation, dyspnoea or anginal pain
IV	Patients with cardiac disease resulting in inability to carry on any physical activity without discomfort Symptoms of heart failure or the anginal syndrome may be present even at rest If any physical activity is undertaken, discomfort increases

NYHA Objective Assessment

A	No objective evidence of cardiovascular disease
B	Objective evidence of minimal cardiovascular disease
C	Objective evidence of moderately severe cardiovascular disease
D	Objective evidence of severe cardiovascular disease

Reprinted with permission www.heart.org © 2012 American Heart Association, Inc

Principles of WHO classification of cardiovascular risk in pregnancy[2]

Risk class	Risk of pregnancy by medical condition
I	No detectable increased risk of maternal mortality and No, or mild, increase in morbidity
II	Small increased risk of maternal mortality or moderate increase in morbidity
III	Significantly increased risk of maternal mortality or severe morbidity. Expert counselling required. If pregnancy is decided upon, intensive specialist cardiac and obstetric monitoring needed throughout pregnancy, childbirth, and the puerperium
IV	Extremely high risk of maternal mortality or severe morbidity; pregnancy contraindicated. If pregnancy occurs termination should be discussed. If pregnancy continues, care as for class III

Application of WHO classification of cardiovascular risk in pregnancy[2]

WHO I
- Uncomplicated, small or mild
  - pulmonary stenosis
  - patent ductus arteriosus
  - mitral valve prolapse
- Successfully repaired simple lesions (atrial or ventricular septal defect, patent ductus arteriosus, anomalous pulmonary venous drainage)
- Atrial or ventricular ectopic beats, isolated

WHO II (*if otherwise well and uncomplicated*)
- Unoperated atrial or ventricular septal defect
- Repaired tetralogy of Fallot
- Most arrhythmias

WHO II–III (*depending on individual*)
- Mild left ventricular impairment
- Hypertrophic cardiomyopathy
- Native or tissue valvular heart disease not considered WHO I or IV
- Marfan syndrome without aortic dilatation
- Aorta <45 mm in aortic disease associated with bicuspid aortic valve
- Repaired coarctation

WHO III
- Mechanical valve
- Systemic right ventricle
- Fontan circulation
- Cyanotic heart disease (unrepaired)
- Other complex congenital heart disease
- Aortic dilatation 40–45 mm in Marfan syndrome
- Aortic dilatation 45–50 mm in aortic disease associated with bicuspid aortic valve

WHO IV (*pregnancy contraindicated*)
- Pulmonary arterial hypertension of any cause
- Severe systemic ventricular dysfunction (LVEF <30%, NYHA III–IV)
- Previous peripartum cardiomyopathy with any residual impairment of left ventricular function
- Severe mitral stenosis, severe symptomatic aortic stenosis
- Marfan syndrome with aorta dilated >45 mm
- Aortic dilatation >50 mm in aortic disease associated with bicuspid aortic valve
- Active severe coarctation

REFERENCES

1. American Heart Association 2007 **Classification of Functional Capacity and Objective Assessment** www.americanheart.org/presenter.jhtml?identifier=4569
2. Thorne S, MacGregor A, Nelson-Piercy C 2006 Risks of contraception and pregnancy in heart disease. **Heart**, 92:1520–1525

S. E. Robson and J. Waugh

4.2 Moderate Structural Heart Disease

Incidence	Risk for Childbearing
5–8% of congenital heart disease (CHD)1	Variable and High Risk (dependent upon repair and
Transpostion of great vessels <1% CHD	condition)

EXPLANATION OF CONDITIONS

Coarctation of the Aorta

- Congenital narrowing of the aorta, generally at the site of ductal insertion, resulting in upper body hypertension and lower body hypoperfusion (see Figure 4.2.1). Aortic wall is often more diffusely abnormal; even with complete and timely repair there is a life-long risk of aneurysm formation and aortic dissection[2]
- Up to 50% have other heart defects, e.g. VSD, aortic or mitral valve disease (including bicuspid aortic valve)
- Up to 10% of older patients may have cerebral aneurysms at presentation[2]
- Most coarctations are detected and repaired in infancy or childhood; however, diagnosis in adulthood and even during pregnancy is not uncommon

After coarctation repair many children were considered 'cured' and were discharged, but there is increasing appreciation of their premature morbidity and mortality[3,4] and the need for long-term cardiological supervision.

Transposition of the Great Vessels

Like Tetralogy of Fallot, it has been successfully treated for more than 30 years, so there are significant numbers of women with it now entering reproductive life. The right ventricle gives rise to the aorta and the left ventricle the pulmonary artery[4] (see Figure 4.2.2a). Initial long-term survivors have generally undergone *Senning* or *Mustard* repairs[5,6] in which the venous blood is rerouted within the atrial chambers (see Figure 4.2.2b). Current techniques 'switch' the great arteries, and coronary arteries to the correct chambers (see Figure 4.2.2c).

COMPLICATIONS

Coarctation of the Aorta

- Residual/re-coarctation after repair
- Associated aortic/mitral valve disease
- Hypertension
- Impaired left ventricle function and CCF[7]
- Thoracic aortic aneurysm/dissection (higher risk in pregnancy)
- Cerebral aneurysm rupture (higher risk in pregnancy)
- Reduced life expectancy[7,8]
- Infective endocarditis[6,9]

Transposition of the Great Vessels

Of patients with atrial diversion operations, 30–50% have a degree of systemic ventricular dysfunction and systemic atrio-ventricular valve regurgitation, because the morphologic right ventricle and tricuspid valve are in the systemic circulation[10]. They are prone to atrial arrhythmias; both tachycardia and sinus node disease can be life threatening and need drugs or pacemaker. *Baffle obstruction* can occur, and can exacerbate problems from arrhythmias. Following the arterial switch operation there is a potential for coronary artery ostial stenosis and early coronary artery disease. Many patients have branch pulmonary artery stenosis and some have required pulmonary or aortic valve replacement.

NON-PREGNANCY TREATMENT AND CARE

Coarctation of the Aorta

Generally, infants/children are treated surgically, with primary balloon dilatation or stenting used for older children or young adults, as is residual coarctation. Surgery in adulthood entails higher risk, often requiring conduit bypass of the narrowed segment. Hypertension requires aggressive treatment. Aneurysms are increasingly recognised, being managed with surgery or covered stents.

Transposition of the Great Vessels

Post-Mustard (Figure 4.2.2b) or Senning repair, many patients will be on ACE inhibitors +/− diuretics for ventricular dysfunction and systemic A-V valve regurgitation. Stenting for baffle obstruction, the use of atrial pacemakers and antiarrhythmic medication are common. Residual intracardiac shunts, and also pulmonary hypertension, need to be detected and managed.

PRE-CONCEPTION ISSUES AND CARE

Appropriate counselling regarding pregnancy should:

- Start in adolescence
- Give accurate, individual advice correcting misinformation about both contraception and pregnancy
- Identify potential effects of the defect on pregnancy in terms of maternal and fetal risks
- Discuss the effects of cardiac disease including risks of long-term deterioration, and even dying, and whether these will change with time or treatment

Coarctation of the Aorta

- MRI scan prior to pregnancy to exclude aneurysm[11] or significant obstruction; deal with if present
- Genetic referral for abnormalities such as 22q deletion
- Recurrence risk is around 4%, and fetal cardiac surveillance is recommended

Transposition of the Great Vessels

- MRI scan and echocardiogram to assess baffles and systemic ventricle or valve function
- Stent baffles if narrowed
- Holter monitoring for rhythm, and drugs/pacemaker initiated if required
- Cease ACE inhibitors

Pregnancy Issues

Coarctation of the Aorta

Most women reach childbearing age. Untreated coarctation carries a 3–8% increased feto-maternal risk[1]. Hypertension occurs in 30%, with additional risk of pre-eclampsia[12]. Uncorrected coarctation carries a risk of **aortic dissection** and cerebral haemorrhage in pregnancy, as well as fetal hypoperfusion. Only patients with evidence of dissection should undergo surgical repair during pregnancy[12]. However, most adult coarctation is now treated with percutaneous dilatation and stenting. This can be performed in pregnancy with a much lower risk to mother and fetus than surgery, particularly in the second trimester if there are problems with blood pressure control or concerns re fetal compromise. There is at least a 4% risk of recurrence.

Transposition of the Great Vessels

Well tolerated if good systemic ventricular function and competent valves[13]. May require diuretics, anti-arrhythmics +/− pacemaker. Pregnancy may exacerbate or unmask systemic ventricular dysfunction, baffle obstruction or arrhythmia. Recurrence risk for the fetus is probably low.

Medical Management and Care

Coarctation of the Aorta

- Control BP with beta-blockers and avoid ACE inhibitors[12]
- Consider elective caesarean section before term in case of aortic aneurysm formation or uncontrollable hypertension[14]
- Avoid balloon angioplasty in pregnancy[12], but stenting is probably safe

Transposition of the Great Vessels

- Monitor for signs of heart failure and arrhythmia[15]
- Diuretics for oedema
- Beta-blockers for tachycardias but may then need pacing
- Systemic venous baffle obstruction may need stenting

Midwifery Management and Care

- Early booking with immediate referral to a maternal medicine clinic and re-referral to the cardiologist
- Accurate booking history with baseline observations, especially pulse
- Check blood pressure is correct (usually right) arm as the left subclavian artery is often involved in coarctation repair
- Monitor blood pressure regularly for prompt identification of hypertensive disease, especially with coarctation of the aorta
- Maintain Hb levels, so give advice on diet and iron supplementation
- Advise on antibiotic treatment for any dental or other procedures
- Prepare the mother for the possibility of a pre-term delivery

Labour Issues

Labour is a risk period for acute cardiac decompensation or pulmonary oedema, and also for increased aortic wall stress. However, this may still be managed successfully in the majority of these women.

- Antibiotic prophylaxis for rupture of membranes or active labour is no longer routinely required, but should be considered on an individual basis
- Epidural analgesia may be useful as tachycardia secondary to pain increases cardiac work. Care with blood pressure and cardiac rhythm management is important
- Pushing increases vagal tone and may worsen bradycardia

Medical Management and Care

- Assessment for antibiotic prophylaxis
- Antihypertensive drugs may be needed to treat hypertension
- Prophylactic (even temporary) pacemaker may be considered for some transposition of the great arteries (TGA) patients
- If normal birth anticipated consider shortening the second stage
- If there is evidence of aneurysm formation, caesarean section is preferable for delivery[13]
- Epidural use is recommended

Midwifery Management and Care

- The midwife *might* be able to conduct a normal delivery in uncomplicated cases, with an emphasis on a short second stage, which could require an episiotomy
- Alternatively the role might be to assist with an operative delivery, which may well be pre-term
- Otherwise the care is as in Section 4.1

Postpartum Issues

- As with mild structural defects (see Section 4.1) the neonate risks heart disease and requires screening
- The mother with TGA may be at increased risk of venous thrombo-embolism, but for most the risk is normal
- The same contraceptive issues arise as in Section 4.1

Medical Management and Care

- Review medications prior to discharge: some beta-blockers are excreted less in breast milk
- Blood pressure often settles rapidly
- Systemic ventricular dysfunction may continue or worsen postpartum so careful review pre-discharge is required
- ACE inhibitors may be restarted
- Cardiac follow-up 4–6 weeks post-delivery for problematic patients

Midwifery Management and Care

- This mother is not for discharge until reviewed by the medical team
- Basic post-operative care is required if post-caesarean section
- Basic observations might need to be continued for longer than usual, with an emphasis on blood pressure and fluid balance
- Advise and support specific to the needs of a mother with a baby on a neonatal unit if the delivery was pre-term (see Chapter 1)
- The basic care is the same as in Section 4.1

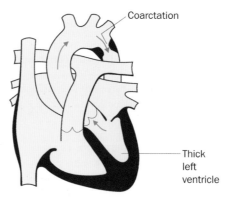

Figure 4.2.1 Coarctation of the aorta (adapted from Meeks 2010). This figure is downloadable from the book companion website at www.wiley.com/go/robson

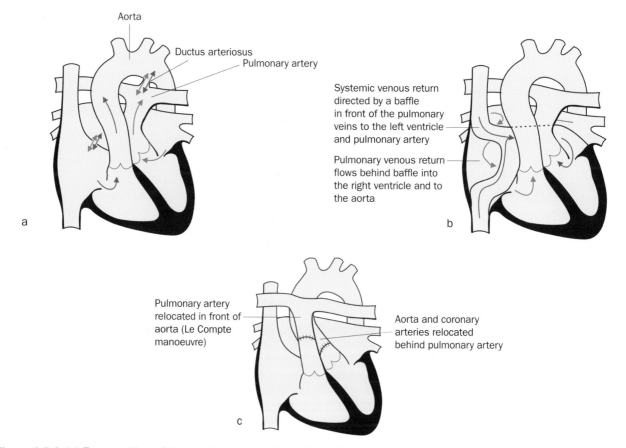

Figure 4.2.2 (a) Transposition of the great arteries (adapted from Meeks 2010). (b) Transposition of the great arteries post mustard repair (adapted from Meeks 2010). (c) Transposition post 'switch' (adapted from Meeks 2010). This figure is downloadable from the book companion website at www.wiley.com/go/robson

4.3 Severe Structural Heart Disease

Incidence	Risk for Childbearing
Varies as per individual condition	High Risk: life threatening; ≥5% maternal mortality[1]

EXPLANATION OF CONDITIONS

These are conditions in which pregnancy carries a significant risk (≥2–5%) for mother and/or fetus, i.e. pregnancy is either high/very high risk or contraindicated. Inevitably, despite counselling, some women will become/wish to remain pregnant. These women require intensive supervision, with which some will achieve an acceptable outcome. This includes women with:

- Unoperated/palliated cyanotic or complex congenital heart disease, including single ventricle conditions
- Women with poor systemic ventricular function (see Section 4.6 Cardiomyopathy)
- Women with Eisenmenger's syndrome (see Section 4.9)
- Women with Marfan's syndrome (see Section 4.5)

Unoperated Cyanotic Heart Disease

Many women will be recent immigrants. Rarely, cyanotic heart disease may not be diagnosed until adulthood, including in the UK. Some conditions are balanced and may have been managed conservatively deliberately. Lesions include uncorrected Tetralogy of Fallot, pulmonary stenosis/atresia with ventricular septal defect, functionally univentricular heart conditions such as tricuspid atresia (Figure 4.3.1a) and Ebstein's anomaly with ASD (Figure 4.3.1b).

Palliated Complex Heart Disease

Increasing numbers of children with complex cardiac abnormalities, including both single ventricle conditions and non-septatable VSD, +/– transposition, are surviving to adulthood with a Fontan circulation (see Figure 4.3.1c). This is a 'final common pathway' of surgeries for conditions in which the heart pumps blood solely around the systemic circulation, with the systemic venous return passing to the pulmonary arteries without being pumped by a ventricle. It permits separation of the arterial and venous sides of the circulation (hence most are 'pink'), and also offloads the heart, but pulmonary blood flow is dependent on the venous pump (from the calf muscles), respiratory 'suction' and

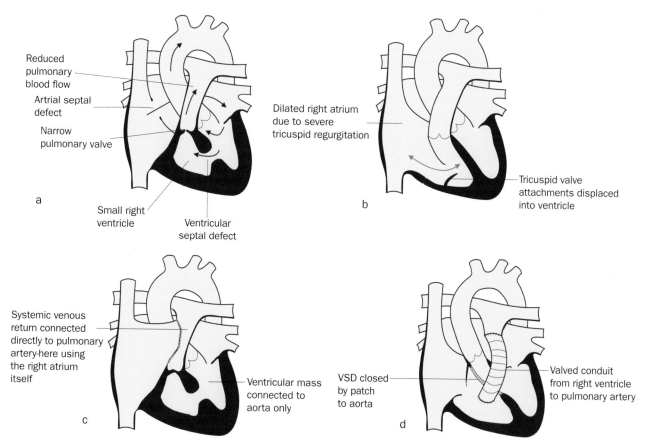

Figure 4.3.1 (a) Complex – tricuspid atresia (adapted from Meeks 2010). (b) Complex – Ebstein's anomaly (adapted from Meeks 2010). (c) Complex – tricuspid atresia post-Fontan operation (adapted from Meeks 2010). (d) Transposition, VSD post Rastelli (adapted from Meeks 2010). This figure is downloadable from the book companion website at www.wiley.com/go/robson

gravity as well as a low-resistance circuit. Many of these patients are anticoagulated to reduce the possibility of thrombosis of rather sluggish pulmonary arterial circulation and increasing numbers are taking diuretics +/− ACE inhibitors. Atrial arrhythmias are common, and some will have pacemakers +/− anti-arrhythmic drugs. Some may have had palliative shunt operations or intermediate/partial Fontan surgery, and hence remain hypoxic to some degree. Some patients will have had repairs involving conduits from the right ventricle to the pulmonary artery (e.g. Rastelli repair for transposition; Figure 4.3.1d) which may become stenosed or regurgitant and require replacement.

COMPLICATIONS

During pregnancy the fall in systemic vascular resistance and rise in cardiac output exacerbates any right-to-left shunting, worsening pre-existing cyanosis and hypoxia. The required increase in cardiac rate and output may also worsen the effects of valvular lesions and ventricular dysfunction.

Maternal complications depend mainly on functional classification of the mother (NYHA classification is in glossary). NYHA classes I–II have a maternal mortality rate of <1%, whilst NYHA classes III–IV have a maternal mortality rate of 7% or greater[2]. This is largely determined by the degree of cyanosis, ventricular dysfunction and prior cardiac events, such as pulmonary oedema, arrhythmia, stroke, etc.[3] Complications include heart failure, arrhythmia, pulmonary/paradoxical embolism and haemorrhage. The effects on the fetus are marked, with a high incidence of spontaneous abortion, a 30–50% risk of premature delivery and low birth weight. The degree of maternal hypoxaemia is the most important predictor of neonatal outcome; oxygen saturations <85% give only a 12% chance of live birth[4]. NYHA class IV mothers also have a fetal mortality rate of around 30%. Recurrence risks are generally around 4% but may be up to 50% for patients with 22q deletion, which may not have been recognised previously.

NON-PREGNANCY TREATMENT AND CARE

These women should be under regular, careful supervision of cardiologists in tertiary centres specialising in the care of adults with congenital heart disease. They are monitored:

- Clinically, including oxygen saturation, and Hb estimation
- Functionally, with cardio-pulmonary exercise testing etc.
- By echocardiograph, plus CT or MRI as required
- Regular Holter monitoring for occult arrhythmia

Many will require trans-catheter or surgical interventions and indeed may benefit from new technology as time progresses.

PRE-CONCEPTION ISSUES AND CARE

Ideally, all women should be able to make an informed choice about pregnancy based on both maternal and fetal risks, long-term prognosis and alternative options such as contraception, termination of pregnancy, adoption, surrogacy and IVF. Encourage realistic expectations, and advocate active preparation for pregnancy. This includes:

- Ensuring easy access to multidisciplinary care
- Genetic counselling
- Pre-pregnancy surgery or intervention: e.g. change of valve type; consider risk of surgery versus reduction in pregnancy risk; catheter interventions; ablation of arrhythmia; and optimisation of cardiac function
- Optimal timing of pregnancy (pregnancy at a younger age is lower risk for some complex conditions)
- Avoidance of teratogens (medication may need to be changed prior to pregnancy, e.g. anticoagulants, ACEI, anti-arrhythmics) (see Cardiac Drugs in Appendix 4.3.1)
- Prompt initiation of iron supplementation
- General measures: smoking cessation and folic acid supplementation

Pregnancy Issues

Each woman will need management according to individual anatomical and functional status. Close liaison between cardiologists and obstetricians is essential.

- Admission for bed-rest +/− oxygen therapy may be required
- Anaemia should be avoided
- Fetal echocardiography is required as well as regular fetal wellbeing and growth monitoring
- Appropriate timing for delivery is crucial to balance maternal and neonatal morbidity and mortality
- A clear plan of management for labour and delivery should be established in advance, clearly documented and widely available

Medical Management and Care

- Iron deficiency – monitor red cell indices plus Hb, because cyanotic patients can be functionally anaemic even with a 'normal' Hb
- Warfarin may not be essential especially for Fontan patients; change to aspirin, or low-molecular-weight heparin
- Stop ACE inhibitors if not done pre-conceptually
- Regular outpatient review, echocardiography +/− Holter monitoring
- Beta-blockers for arrhythmia +/− pacemaker if indicated
- Diuretics for heart failure/breathlessness[5]
- Oxygen therapy may help severely cyanosed patients, especially if they have a reduced respiratory capacity

Midwifery Management and Care

- Early booking, with thorough history taking, and immediate referral to a maternal medicine clinic, then liaison with tertiary cardiologist
- Baseline observations, including oxygen saturation
- Maintain Hb levels as above, with additional dietary advice[5]
- Advise on antibiotic treatment for any dental or other procedures
- Teach the mother to keep a fetal movement chart after 24 weeks
- Prepare parents for potential pre-term/IUGR baby or fetal loss

Labour Issues

Labour requires careful monitoring of both mother and fetus. Pre-load and blood pressure should be monitored carefully and blood loss minimised.

Antibiotic prophylaxis for rupture of membranes or active labour is no longer routinely required, but should be considered on an individual basis with a lower threshold for antibiotics for these patients

In general, vaginal delivery with low dose epidural is the mode of choice. Forceps or ventouse delivery may be used to shorten maternal expulsive effort in the second stage. Cardiac indications for caesarean section include aortic dilatation >40 mm, warfarin treatment and important systemic ventricular dysfunction.

Bolus doses of syntocinon should be avoided in the third stage, as they can cause severe hypotension. Low dose oxytocin infusions are safer. Ergometrine is best avoided in most cases as it can cause acute hypertension. Uterine compression sutures are the most effective treatment in the management of uterine atony at caesarean section. The safety of misoprostol is yet to be determined.

Medical Management and Care

- Prophylactic (even temporary) pacemaker is considered for some women as pushing is vagotonic
- If normal birth is anticipated consider shortening the second stage
- If there is evidence of aneurysm formation, or major ventricular dysfunction, caesarean section is preferable[6]
- Epidural use is recommended
- Avoid supine position, especially for Fontan patients, because caval compression restricts pulmonary blood flow
- Invasive arterial +/− venous pressure monitoring may benefit vaginal delivery
- Cyanotic patients may require intravenous hydration, especially if nauseated
- Prescribe antibiotic prophylaxis as indicated

Midwifery Management and Care

- Intensive care setting is likely[5]; experienced staff required
- Administer the antibiotics and any other prescribed drugs as above
- Keep the mother in left lateral position throughout the first stage[7]
- The midwife may well be required to conduct a normal delivery under close medical supervision, with an emphasis on a short second stage, which could require an episiotomy.
- Low dose oxytocin infusion for the third stage.
- Alternatively the role might be to assist with an instrumental/operative delivery, which may well be pre-term
- Otherwise the care is as in Section 4.1

Postpartum Issues

Following delivery, the return of the uterine blood flow into the systemic circulation results in an increase of cardiac output. Stroke volume, heart rate and cardiac output remain high for 24 hours post-delivery with rapid intravascular volume shifts in the first 2 weeks postpartum, thus the later stages of labour and early postpartum period are times of high risk for pulmonary oedema[1].

- The neonate may require intensive care in addition to heart screening
- Contraceptive issues are similar to the previous section
- Most require progesterone-only methods

Medical Management and Care

- Close medical supervision is still required after delivery with monitoring for at least 48 hours
- Review medications prior to discharge: restart ACE inhibitors and warfarin; some beta-blockers are excreted less in breast milk
- Systemic ventricular dysfunction may continue or worsen postpartum so careful review pre-discharge is required
- Cardiac follow-up 4–6 weeks post-delivery for almost all patients

Midwifery Management and Care

- This mother is not for discharge until reviewed by the medical team
- Basic post-operative care is required if post-caesarean section
- Basic observations may need continuation for longer than usual with emphasis on oxygen saturation, blood pressure and fluid balance
- Advise and support specific to the needs of a mother with a baby on a neonatal unit if delivery was pre-term (see Chapter 1)
- Bereavement care if a stillbirth occurred
- The basic care is as in Section 4.1

4.4 Rheumatic and Valvular Heart Disease

Incidence	Risk for Childbearing
5–30 million children/young adults have rheumatic heart disease 90 000 individuals die each year; mortality rate of disease is 1–10%[1]	High Risk[4]

EXPLANATION OF CONDITIONS

Rheumatic heart disease is a complication of rheumatic fever in which acute cardiac valve damage (mainly aortic or mitral) arises from immunologic injury in group A haemolytic streptococcal infection (GAS) – see Chapter 12.8. Incidence remains high in developing countries and the UK immigrant population, hence it is re-emerging as a cause of maternal death[2]. Chronic sequelae include valve stenosis/regurgitation, arrhythmias +/− ventricular dysfunction. **Stenosis** is the narrowing of a valve restricting forward flow, commonly affecting the mitral, aortic and pulmonary valves. The latter is rarely problematic. Stenosis may be congenital or acquired as with rheumatic fever or SLE[3].

Regurgitation/insufficiency/incompetence results from incomplete valve closure that allows regurgitation of blood back to the preceding chamber. It can be congenital or acquired as with rheumatic fever, Marfan's syndrome or Ehlers-Danlos syndrome.

Prosthetic heart valves are replacements for diseased heart valves. These can be *bioprostheses* (donor/animal tissue) or *mechanical*. They are mainly used on the left side and need lifelong anticoagulation; this complicates pregnancy.

COMPLICATIONS

Mitral valve disease: atrial fibrillation, heart failure, endocarditis or thrombosis may develop. Risk of stroke is increased and increased left atrial pressure may cause pulmonary oedema. Mitral regurgitation causes LV volume overload which may impair function.

Aortic valve disease: stenosis restricts the cardiac output increase required in pregnancy and may cause effort restriction, angina or syncope. Symptoms must be taken very seriously as they indicate a high risk of sudden death. Regurgitation is better tolerated but also leads to LV volume overload, myocardial failure and arrhythmia.

Pulmonary valve problems: isolated mild stenosis is common and of little consequence but more severe stenosis may be revealed during pregnancy by increased cardiac output. Pulmonary regurgitation is mainly post-intervention. Residual stenosis and regurgitation are common as part of more complex congenital heart disease.

Ebstein's anomaly: the tricuspid valve leaflets are displaced into the right ventricle (see Figure 4.3.1b). The valve is regurgitant and malformed. It is associated with other structural cardiac abnormalities. Incidence of arrhythmia is high[3].

Mixed disease is common (multiple valves +/− stenosis and regurgitation) complicating care and worsening prognosis.

Infective endocarditis during pregnancy is rare, with an estimated overall incidence of 0.006% (1 per 100 000 pregnancies) and an incidence of 0.5% in patients with known valvular or congenital heart disease. The incidence is higher in drug addicts. Patients with the highest risk for infective endocarditis are those with a prosthetic valve or prosthetic material

used for cardiac valve repair, a history of previous infective endocarditis, and some special patients with congenital heart disease. Bacterial infection, especially in pregnancy, of heart valves/structures can initiate systemic or pulmonary embolism, so antibiotic prophylaxis is given within 2–3 hours of unexpected exposure and for predictable bacteraemia.

Antibiotic prophylaxis is no longer routinely advised advisable for valvular disease unless there are other maternal or obstetric indications such as pre-term rupture of membranes or Caesarean section[5,6]. However, it is probably still advisable for patients with mechanical valves[7].

NON-PREGNANCY TREATMENT AND CARE

- **Medication** might ease symptoms
- **Balloon dilatation** of valves may be performed safely for non-calcified valves (preferably after first trimester)
- **Surgical repair**, or replacement, requires cardio pulmonary bypass and is high risk in pregnancy (especially for the fetus) but can be life-saving

Rheumatic Heart Disease

- Can deteriorate with time
- High index of suspicion with newly arrived immigrant women
- Regular cardiologist review
- Earlier surgery if pregnancy is contemplated

Metal Prosthetic Heart Valves

- Patients require long-term anticoagulation and antibiotic prophylaxis as above

PRE-CONCEPTION ISSUES AND CARE

- Expert clinical and echocardiographic assessment of:
  - functional status
  - previous cardiac events
  - ventricular and valvular function
  - pulmonary artery pressure
  - current medication[8]
- Discussion of risks associated with pregnancy[9]
- Discuss risks and benefits of anticoagulant therapy
- Pre-pregnancy interventions, with contraceptive cover, to plan and optimise wellbeing for pregnancy[10]
- Identify if pregnancy is contraindicated, with either pulmonary hypertension or >2 risk factors below:
  - reduced LV systolic function (ejection fraction <40%)
  - left heart obstruction: aortic or mitral stenosis with valve areas of <1.5 cm or <2.0 cm[2], respectively
  - past cardiovascular events (heart failure, TIA, stroke)
  - reduced functional capacity with a disease score of NYHA class II or higher[11] (Box 4.1.1) as the maternal death rate is 30–60%[1]

Pregnancy Issues

Newly arrived immigrants require a full GP examination and referral if signs of cardiovascular disease are found[1]. Consider risk of pregnancy continuation versus termination. Most valvular heart disease is manageable with expert input. Anticoagulation regimens carry increased risk of miscarriage and of haemorrhagic complications, including retroplacental bleeding leading to premature birth and fetal death[4].

Mitral stenosis may cause pulmonary oedema or atrial arrhythmias in pregnancy or soon after delivery[12]. May present for the first time in pregnancy, with poor toleration because the increased stroke volume of pregnancy cannot be supported through the narrowed valve. Left atrial pressure rises, causing pulmonary oedema[4,13,14]. Risk factors relate to severity:

- Decompensation (third trimester risk)[15]
- Death increases with left heart obstruction or NYHA class II disease[16] (Box 4.1.1). Mortality from 0 to 3%[4]
- Pre-term delivery and IUGR

Aortic stenosis becomes more significant during pregnancy if the valve area is severely compromised, as above. However, symptoms appear late due to left atrial capacitance. Pulmonary oedema, angina from reduced coronary flow and effort syncope are all ominous signs and urgent intervention is required.

Mitral and aortic regurgitation are usually well tolerated due to reduced systemic vascular resistance[17], but peripheral/pulmonary oedema benefits from diuretics.

Prosthetic heart valves are managed individually dependent on type and position of valve and cardiac function[12]. Immediate echocardiography is indicated in women with mechanical valves presenting with dyspnoea and/or an embolic event [4].

Medical Management and Care

- Regular appointments at a combined obst
- ECG, echocardiography, USS, electrolytes, ɑ indicated
- Diuretics and beta-blockers may be helpful, +/− b
- Risk of systemic emboli if atrial fibrillation, so anticoagɑ usually with low-molecular-weight heparin[4]
- Heart rate control with digoxin, beta-blocker, calcium channɛ a combination of these[19]
- Pulmonary oedema – treat with oxygen and diuretics[13], cɔ intervention.
- Balloon dilatation of mitral or aortic valve should be considered in pregnant patients with severe symptoms or systolic pulmonary artery pressure >50 mmHg despite medical therapy[4], preferably after the first trimester[13]
- If surgery is required, careful monitoring of fetal wellbeing is necessary throughout[13]; increased risk of preterm delivery +/− IUGR[13], cardiopulmonary bypass with increased flow, if needed, to respond to fetal distress
- Anaesthetic agents used in the first trimester may have teratogenic effects[11]

Metal Prosthetic Valves and Anticoagulation

- Conception to week 12: consider the use of monitored and dose adjusted heparin if on >5 mg/day of warfarin; discuss drug teratogenicity versus the risk of valve thrombosis[4,12]
- Weeks 12–36: generally warfarin therapy is used[4]
- If labour starts while on oral anticoagulants (OAC), caesarean delivery is indicated[4]
- Week 36 Hospital: discontinue warfarin; start heparin titrated to a therapeutic activated partial-thromboplastin time, or anti-factor Xa level[20] and check weekly.
- Low molecular weight heparin (LMWH) should be replaced by intravenous unfractured heparin (UFH) at least 36 hours before planned delivery. UFH should be continued until 4–6 hours before planned delivery and restarted 4–6 hours after delivery if there are no bleeding complications[4]
- Valve thrombosis: thrombolytic treatment first line as risks of embolism, bleeding or placental abruption are less than surgery risk

Midwifery Management and Care

- At/before booking, refer for combined obstetric/cardiology care
- Re-refer promptly if palpitations or breathlessness are reported, because it is difficult to differentiate cardiac decompensation from the physiological symptoms of pregnancy[1,8,21]
- Social support, and interpreters can improve outcomes[1]
- Hospital admission for bed-rest, oxygen therapy, saturation monitoring and fluid balance estimation

Labour Issues

Labour is a risk period for acute decompensation, pulmonary oedema and thromboembolism.

Epidural analgesia may be useful, because tachycardia secondary to pain increases cardiac work, predisposing to pulmonary oedema. However, excessive vasodilatation reduces coronary perfusion in aortic stenosis and must be prevented, e.g. with adrenaline/epinephrine [13].

Avoid vaginal delivery if possible due to the increased risk of fetal and maternal bleeding[4].

If anticoagulated, reverse warfarin with fresh frozen plasma/vitamin K. Protamine sulfate reverses heparin [12].

Medical Management and Care

- Vaginal delivery anticipated and clear plan of care documented including shortened second stage, caesarean section for obstetric indications[13]
- Antibiotics as indicated[12]
- Heparin is discontinued for labour and delivery
- ECG, intravenous infusion (IV) plus invasive monitoring for moderate or severe disease[13]
- Avoid fluid overload

Midwifery Management and Care

- High dependency care, with observations of fluid balance, oximetry and electronic fetal monitoring (EFM)[13]
- TED stockings and early ambulation[4]
- Avoid supine and lithotomy positions, left lateral position is recommended[13]
- Avoid active directed pushing[12] (heart rate increase might not be tolerated)
- Syntocinon NOT Syntometrine[4]; uterine massage reduces blood loss[13]

Postpartum Issues

Early puerperium is associated with increased venous return to the heart which can lead to heart failure[16], continued haemodynamic monitoring being required.

Breast-feeding is not contraindicated when using warfarin, as its high protein binding in the maternal circulation leads to very small amounts secreted into breast milk. Advise letting the baby empty the breasts when feeding because hind milk has a higher vitamin K level[18]

Medical Management and Care

- Night after delivery – resume warfarin in the absence of bleeding complications [20]
- Haemodynamic monitoring >24 h, treat any pulmonary oedema rapidly with 02 diuretic beta-blockers or diamorphine[13]
- Contraception counselling[13], with emphasis on progesterone implants

Midwifery Management and Care

- Careful fluid balance surveillance as pulmonary oedema is a serious risk
- Gentle mobilization; supportive assistance with baby care to inspire confidence
- Encourage neonatal vitamin K administration
- Liaison with the multidisciplinary team in readiness for discharge

4.5 Marfan's Syndrome

Incidence	Risk for Childbearing
Prevalence of 5 per 100 000 of population[1] 5000 UK cases per annum, 10% being severely affected[2]	High Risk

EXPLANATION OF CONDITION

Marfan's syndrome was first described in Paris by Bernard Marfan in 1896[3]. It is an autosomal dominant condition on chromosome 15[3]. It is inherited in 50–75% of cases, and also occurs as a spontaneous mutation. Fibrillin (a fine fibre found in connective tissue) production is affected[3–5]. This connective tissue disorder presents in various body systems: musculoskeletal, ocular, cardiovascular, respiratory and integumentary[6].

Typically, there is a disproportionate length of long bones and little subcutaneous fat, presenting as a tall, thin physique with long fingers and toes and hyperflexibility of joints. Further signs of the condition vary considerably between individuals, who may have one or more of:

- Narrow 'pigeon' chest[3]
- Scoliosis[3] (curvature of the spine)
- Flat feet[3]
- Myopia (short-sighted)[2] and lens problems[3]
- High arched dental palate with overcrowding of teeth

Although the condition affects men and women equally[3,7] this appearance may be more exaggerated in men, with some women being undiagnosed[8].

The valve between the left chambers of the heart is defective and may be large and floppy, resulting in an abnormal valve motion when the heart beats. In some cases, the valve may leak, creating a heart murmur. Small leaks may not cause any symptoms, but larger ones can result in shortness of breath, fatigue, and palpitations.

Due to faulty connective tissue, the wall of the aorta is weakened and stretches causing **aortic dilatation**. This increases the risk that the aorta will tear (**aortic dissection**), or rupture. The rupture causes serious complications of mitral-valve prolapse, aortic-root dilatation or sometimes sudden death[5].

COMPLICATIONS

General Complications

- Joint pain and dislocations, due to joint laxity[3,7]
- Scoliosis (curvature) of the spine and consequent back pain and mobility restrictions[2,3,7]
- Spontaneous pneumothorax in >10%[3]
- Bronchiectasis, asthma and emphysema[3]
- Hernias[3,7]
- Fatigue[3]

Cardiac Complications

- Aortic dissection – accounting for 20% of maternal cardiac fatalities[8]
- Aortic aneurysm formation
- Dilatation of the aortic root can cause the aortic valve to become stretched and leak

- Aortic or mitral valve regurgitation may worsen leading to increased breathlessness, pulmonary oedema or arrhythmias
- New heart murmurs may present
- Cardiomyopathy may develop
- Arrhythmia may occur

NON-PREGNANCY TREATMENT AND CARE

General Treatment

Early diagnosis, meticulous echocardiographic follow-up and multidisciplinary assessment are essential[9]. Restrictive lifestyle advice and drugs may be necessary, but should be counterbalanced with the need for a child to develop and mature as normally as possible[9]. Exercise and a healthy, vitamin-rich diet is encouraged, and smoking strongly discouraged as it destroys elastin[3].

Cardiac Treatment

- Beta-blockers might be used[9] to reduce aortic root dilatation[7]. If the aortic root is greater than 45 mm, root replacement may be considered, especially if pregnancy is contemplated[10]
- Following elective aortic root replacement, patients remain at risk for dissection in the residual aorta[11]
- Increasingly patients may have been on Losartan or other angiotensin receptor blockers (ARB). These are NOT currently viewed as safe in pregnancy.

PRE-CONCEPTION ISSUES AND CARE

- Start advice in adolescence, reinforced by effective contraception
- Genetic counselling as there is a 50% chance the prospective child could inherit the gene[3]
  - the implications for reproductive choices and relationships should be sensitively discussed alongside genetic counselling[12]
  - feelings of guilt about passing on the condition to children, or of being a family member who has been found not to have the condition, have been reported[12]
- There should be access to expert pre-pregnancy care and implications for pregnancy should be discussed
- Echocardiography is essential
- If aortic root <40 mm reassure about the lesser (1%) risk of dissection[13,14]
- If aortic root >40 mm advise about increased risk of adverse outcome[13,14]
- If aortic root >45 mm, suggest elective root replacement prior to pregnancy[4,13]
- If taking ARBs (e.g. Losartan) change to beta-blockers. Otherwise continue beta-blockers. Consider starting beta-blockers if not already on medication.
- Discussion of pregnancy care and possible need for hospitalisation[15]

Pregnancy Issues

Pregnancy in women with Marfan's syndrome carries a lethal risk of acute aortic dissection[16]. All Marfan's pregnancies are therefore high risk throughout and multidisciplinary team management is needed at a specialist centre caring for high cardiac risk pregnancy.

If no pre-pregnancy assessment took place, it should be undertaken at first booking. Here counselling is vital. Antenatal staff should be made aware that the pregnancy is high risk, and management guidelines and emergency contact numbers should be clearly recorded.

There is a 50% chance of the woman having an affected child[16]. Pre-natal diagnoses may be offered, in particular a detailed ultrasound at 20–24 weeks including echocardiography and careful limb measurement. Molecular diagnosis is only available if the family mutation is known.

- Premature labour and ruptured membranes are common[8,17]
- Pelvic instability and backache increase

Close monitoring for hypertension is necessary, being aware that there may be a disparity between reading in the right and left arms.

Vigilance for aortic dissection, which presents as intermittent 'tearing' chest pain radiating to back, which can mimic labour.

Emergency imaging essential even if presentation not typical[4,18]

Medical Management and Care

- Care plan devised and updated as delivery may occur at short notice[8]
- Monitor aortic root diameter with serial echocardiograms
- Consider surgical repair if dilation greatly increasing, but consider gestation and elective delivery by LSCS prior to surgery (association with fetal loss)[4,13]
- Those with an aortic root diameter of <40 mm historically tolerate pregnancy well, though no evidence for safe diameter [5,14,19,21]
- Close monitoring for hypertension which should be treated aggressively[8]
- Beta-blockers are continued throughout pregnancy, maintain heart rate <110 [4,8,21]
- Regular monitoring of fetal growth by ultrasound[14]
- A pre-delivery anaesthetic assessment is advised[8,20]
- MRI of the pelvis (to detect dural ectasia) may be useful to guide epidural catheter placement[8]
- Steroids if delivery likely <34 weeks, but this risks fluid retention and cardiac failure, hence diuretics should also be considered[22]
- Anticoagulants need reviewing
- Aortic-root dilatation may be a risk predictor, but aortic dissection may occur without a clinically significant dilatation[5]
- Surgery in pregnancy is possible if root dilatation presents[14,19]

Midwifery Management and Care

- Astute booking history, refer promptly to obstetric cardiology clinic
- Monitor pulse and respiration alongside normal antenatal observation at each antenatal appointment
- Be alert for signs of hypertension and pre-eclampsia
- Encourage iron and vitamins to reduce anaemia
- Limitation of physical activity[4] and prepare woman/family for possibility of third trimester bed-rest
- Provide pelvic support girdle and teach techniques for safe movement, because of pelvic pain and laxity (see Section 9.2)
- Prepare the mother for early labour and a small baby

Labour Issues

If there are no cardiac complications and no obstetric risk factors, vaginal delivery is possible[14,19,20], with an assisted second stage. However, most specialist units recommend caesarean section for higher-risk women. Elective caesarean section if the aortic root exceeds 40 mm.

Epidural anaesthesia is recommended; however this should only be performed after the possibilities of dural ectasia or an arachnoid cyst have been excluded, as these can result in dilution of anaesthetic.

There is a higher risk of postpartum haemorrhage and inversion of the uterus[19].

If LSCS required due to aortic root dilation consider doing in cardiac theatre with neonatal facilities available[14].

The neonate is at increased risk of mild IUGR, bradycardia and hypoglycaemia due to maternal beta-blockers[13].

Medical Management and Care

- Continue beta-blockers in labour[14]
- Prostaglandins should be used with caution
- Instrumental delivery likely[20] and active pushing avoided
- Syntocinon via slow IVI for active management of third stage[14]
- Ergometrine should be avoided if possible[22]
- Avoid carboprost and misoprostol and consider bimanual compression, uterine sutures or intrauterine balloons to reduce bleeding rather than pharmacological agents; careful risk–benefit assessment is required[22]
- Cardiac and invasive monitoring with an arterial line[8,23], but beware risks of endocarditis and emboli

Midwifery Management and Care

- Intensive care/support needed; rigorous monitoring of feto-maternal condition and fluid balance; avoid fluctuating BP which increases risk of dissection[14]
- TED stockings
- Left lateral/supported sitting position to assist placental oxygenation
- EFM as the fetus is dependent on maternal oxygenation when the mother is haemodynamically unstable; hypoxaemic reduced variability of fetal heart may be an initial sign prior to maternal signs[24]
- Effective communication and adept interpersonal skills are necessary to maintain a positive atmosphere
- Ensure paediatric presence at, or shortly after, birth

Postpartum Issues

- Maternal risk continues
- Contraception is essential, as further pregnancy poses further risk to the mother
- 7% fetal/neonatal mortality[17] hence neonatal examination/investigations to be performed by a paediatrician, for early diagnosis
- Neonate risks hyperbilirubinaemia and hypoglycaemia[13] so monitoring is required
- Breast-feeding is possible

Medical Management and Care

- Arrange cardiac assessment whilst still in hospital
- Surveillance should continue until 8 weeks postpartum
- Review suitability for contraceptive pill or intrauterine system (IUS), especially if a risk of hypertension or thrombo-embolism[20]. Sterilisation carries anaesthetic risk[25]

Midwifery Management and Care

- Continue with blood pressure monitoring until otherwise directed
- Reinforce the need for contraception
- Ensure regular paediatric review of the neonate
- Note that this mother is not for early discharge from hospital

4.6 Functional Heart Disease: Cardiomyopathy

Incidence	Risk for Childbearing
1:5000[1]	High Risk
Peripartum cardiomyopathy 1:10 000[2]; 1:3000–4000 live births[3]	

EXPLANATION OF CONDITIONS

The term 'cardiomyopathy' is derived from the Latin, meaning *disease of the heart muscle*. Characterised by ventricular dysfunction and eventual development of cardiac failure, this rare and potentially lethal condition has five manifestations.

Dilated Cardiomyopathy (DCM)

Progressive loss or damage of cardiac myocytes leads to chamber dilatation, cardiac enlargement and reduced systolic function. This leads to venous stasis in the lungs, pulmonary oedema, breathlessness, and eventually reduced cardiac output becoming **left heart failure. Right heart failure** can also follow, with fluid accumulation in the soft tissues, ankle/leg oedema, liver enlargement and ascites (abdominal fluid). The cause can be genetic in 25–30% of cases, with both autosomal dominant and recessive types. It can follow viral myocarditis, and be associated with other muscle diseases, collagen disorders, metabolic disorders, chemotherapy[4], autoimmune disease (Chapter 11), haemoglobinopathies, hypothyroidism and hyperthyroidism[2].

Hypertrophic Cardiomyopathy (HCM)

There is enlargement and abnormal fibre orientation of the cardiac myocytes. Impaired diastolic relaxation results, the heart does not fill properly and there may be left ventricular outflow obstruction. It can present in childhood but may manifest at any age. There may be no symptoms, or there may be:

- Chest pain (angina) due to increased cardiac muscle oxygen requirements and reduced coronary blood flow
- Dyspnoea (breathlessness)
- Syncope (fainting due to fall in blood pressure)
- Atrial or ventricular arrhythmias
- Heart failure[5]
- Sudden death

At least 70% of cases have a genetic basis[2]. Inheritance is generally autosomal dominant and it affects 0.2–0.5% of the population[6,7].

Restrictive Cardiomyopathy (RCM)

The ventricular walls are stiff and filling is markedly impaired. Pressure in both atria then rises, the atria dilate to compensate and fibrillation results[8]. Symptoms occur late and include: heart failure, arrhythmias, syncope and sudden death. Prognosis is very poor.

Arrhythmogenic Right Ventricular Cardiomyopathy (ARVC)

Right (and eventually left) ventricular muscle is replaced by fatty and fibrous tissue. Early symptoms are mainly palpitations/sudden death; heart failure develops late. The condition may present in pregnancy with arrhythmias, and the ECG is characteristic. Inheritance is frequently autosomal dominant.

Peripartum Cardiomyopathy (PPCM)

This refers to the onset of cardiac failure between the last month of pregnancy and 6 months postpartum[9], in the absence of a prior cause[2]. Differentiation from normal pregnancy-associated dyspnoea, ankle oedema and tiredness can be difficult initially[3]. Although rare, onset of heart failure can be rapid and is frequently fatal[10], accounting for around 25% of maternal cardiac deaths[9,11]. Of uncertain aetiology[12] it is associated with higher maternal age, parity or gestation, black race, family history, smoking, diabetes, hypertension, malnutrition, teenage pregnancy, and prolonged use of beta-agonists[13].

Presenting features include:

- Orthopnoea, dyspnoea and nocturnal cough[14]
- Chest pain and palpitations
- New regurgitant murmurs, and pulmonary crackles
- Raised jugular venous pressure
- Third trimester or postnatal, signs of heart failure[2]

Guidelines for the acute management of heart failure apply[15].

Sudden collapse may occur in fluid overload situations, e.g. multiple pregnancy, Syntocinon infusion and epidural. Chest X-ray may reveal an enlarged heart, pulmonary oedema and pleural effusion.

COMPLICATIONS

- Dilated cardiomyopathy – heart failure, sudden death[5]
- Hypertrophic cardiomyopathy – angina, sudden death
- Restrictive cardiomyopathy – arrhythmias, sudden death
- ARVC – palpitations, sudden death
- Peripartum cardiomyopathy – heart failure, sudden death[3]

NON-PREGNANCY TREATMENT AND CARE

- Drug therapy:
  - diuretics
  - ACE inhibitors
  - beta-blockers
  - anti-arrhythmics
  - warfarin and aspirin
- Cardioversion to stabilise heart rhythm
- Pacemakers/implantable defibrillators
- Heart transplant for severe cases

PRE-CONCEPTION ISSUES AND CARE

- History taking to identify a significant family history
- Genetic counselling
- Refer to cardiologist with experience of cardiomyopathy
- Echocardiogram
- Stop or change drugs, e.g. ACE inhibitors, warfarin
- Explain the physiological impact of pregnancy upon the heart with risk of sudden death
- The woman may be advised against pregnancy as it can result in cardiac failure and death
- Increased risk of recurrent PPCM in future pregnancies, for survivors of PPCM, prophalactic use of dopamine antagonist bromocriptine in being trialled[14]
- Termination of pregnancy may be advised

Pregnancy Issues

Breathlessness (see Chapter 5.1) is common in pregnancy, therefore cardiomyopathy often presents late. Risk factors include multiparity, black race, pre-eclampsia and multiple pregnancy[14].

Puerperal cardiomyopathy manifests in the third trimester, the fetus is relatively mature and can be delivered reasonably safely prior to treatment.

There is an increased thromboembolic risk.

Labour should be induced, or a caesarean section performed if left ventricle function is poor or deteriorating rapidly[16].

Medical Management and Care

- Refer/collaborate with cardiologist, obstetric, anaesthetic and paediatric teams
- Clear care pathways to be documented and agreed antenatally
- Acute care may need to be in critical care unit[14]
- Beta-blockers may prevent arrhythmias and improve long-term outcome[16]

Midwifery Management and Care

- At booking, or if it presents later, refer immediately to maternal medicine clinic
- Sensitivity – this is a major, life-threatening illness
- Supportive advice about fluid and salt intake restriction[16]
- Side effects of drugs include IUGR; regular ultrasound monitoring is required[16]
- Support with thromboprohylaxis administration

Labour Issues

As PPCM poses high risks to both mother and fetus, intense fetal and maternal monitoring is required during delivery[16]

First Stage
- Invasive monitoring, guided by individual case details, is generally recommended
- Pain relief may relieve cardiac stress

Second Stage
- Aim to minimise cardiovascular stresses whilst maintaining adequate analgesia
- Vaginal delivery safe in most women[17]; advantages of reduced blood loss, greater haemodynamic stability, avoidance of surgical stress, less chance of post-operative infection and pulmonary complications
- Short second stage by instrumental delivery can minimise cardiovascular compromise[18]

Third Stage
- Intravenous oxytocin produces a small reduction in arterial BP followed by an increase in cardiac output[10,19]
- Oxytocin is associated with decreased cardiac contractility and heart rate[20], so ergometrine should be avoided[21]
- Carboprost and misoprostol are also contraindicated; use if benefit outweighs risk
- Consider compression/intrauterine balloons for PPH rather than pharmacological solutions[20]

Medical Management and Care

- Plan the location and timing of induction of labour with extreme caution[20]
- Regional analgesia[18], with careful monitoring, unless anticoagulated
- Stabilisation of condition by multi-disciplinary team aim to improve symptoms
- Monitoring for cardiac failure, e.g. ischaemia, atrial fibrillation, infarction[14]
- Avoid fluid overload, consider diuretic use[14]
- Avoid hypotension; consider inotropes.
- Ensure adequate oxygenation, which may require ventilatory support[14]
- Consider pulmonary arterial catheterisation
- ECG monitoring for cardiac arrhythmias
- Consider elective, instrumental, vaginal delivery
- Planned caesarean section is preferred for women who are critically ill and in need of inotropic therapy or mechanical support[12]
- Consider diuretic immediately following third stage[13]
- Recommence thromboprophylaxis when risk of bleeding subsides[13]
- Vaginal birth is preferable if maternal and fetal condition are stable[18]
- Once delivered, if condition unstable, transfer to the ICU[18]

Midwifery Management and Care

- Labour may need to be induced. Oxytocin should be finely titrated, administered in low dosage to avoid hypotension, arrhythmia and tachycardia[18,20]
- Care of the IVI throughout labour and maintain a strict fluid balance[18]
- Vigilant monitoring and documentation of: BP, pulse, respiratory rate, ECG, oxygen therapy and oxygen saturation monitoring, MEOWS scoring[10]
- Continuous EFM
- Maintain adequate pain relief having conferred with anaesthetist
- Monitor progress of labour, and refer slow progress promptly
- Left lateral position for labour, or sitting up if in cardiac failure[13]
- TED stockings and passive leg exercises if immobile
- Avoid ergometrine and syntometrine in the third stage[21]
- Care of the (pre-term) baby at birth and possible transfer to NNU

Postpartum Issues

- Major changes in cardiac output and plasma volumes continue >2 weeks postpartum, so ongoing cardiological surveillance required[22]
- Maternal condition usually returns to baseline by 6 months postpartum
- Cardiac function returns to normal in 50% women with PPCM but risk reoccurrence[16,23,24]
- Increased risks of pulmonary oedema, thrombo-embolism and rhythm disturbances
- Treatment with angiotensin-converting enzyme inhibitors (ACEI), beta-blockers and full anticoagulation is appropriate[9,14]
- Prognosis for PPCM is dependent on recovery of left-sided ventricular function; if left ventricular dysfunction is on-going, mortality rates are 85% over 5 years
- If myocardial dysfunction is severe, a cardiac transplant may be required[14,22]
- Neonate may be admitted to NICU/special care baby unit (SCBU) to identify potential bradycardia, hypoglycaemia, and respiratory depression secondary to maternal medication[18]; treatment as required.

Medical Management and Care

- Multi-disciplinary care plan, prior to discharge, addressing dynamic disease change with treatment modification and recovery potential[12]
- Life-long treatment may be required if condition does not recede, so enlist the cardiologist's support and promote outpatient attendance
- Advise on need for future pre-conception care, with contraceptive cover
- Prescribe contraception, avoiding combined oral contraceptive pill (COCP). Progesterone only pill, intrauterine contraceptive device and injected/subdermal progesterone only preparations are safe[12]

Midwifery Management and Care

- Continue observation of vital signs, reporting any anomalies
- Breast-feeding not recommended with PPCM [13] due to prolactin levels
- Plan care and counsel the mother in caring for infant and own health – seeking assistance from family, and social services for household and other support
- Advice in avoiding stress and anxiety and adequate rest
- Avoidance of extreme exertion – advise the family on adjustments to the baby's room and movement of equipment, to minimise exertion
- Extensive education regarding medications and their side effects
- Advice to mother/family of heart failure signs (weight gain, dyspnoea, cough, pallor, chest pain, arrhythmias) and reporting thereof
- Promote a healthy, low sodium, iron-rich diet
- Reiterate contraception advice[16]

4.7 Functional Heart Disease: Arrhythmias

Incidence	**Risk for Childbearing**
2–4% simple arrhythmias in school girls and women >40 years[1] Incidence of each type of arrhythmia in pregnancy unknown[1]	Variable Risk

EXPLANATION OF CONDITIONS

Cardiac arrhythmia is any variation from the normal regular rhythm of the heart beat[2]. It is more common when pre-existing structural, functional or ischaemic heart disease interferes with the mechanisms controlling heart rhythm[1]. Arrhythmia can manifest as: tachycardia, palpitations (heart rate >100 beats per minute [bpm]) or bradycardia (heart rate <60 bpm).

Tachycardia

This is a commoner problem during pregnancy. Pregnancy itself causes a physiological increase in heart rate, predisposes to atrial arrhythmias and exacerbates pre-existing arrhythmic tendencies[3]. If the rate is very high or the arrhythmia is sustained then chest pain (angina), dizziness (pre-syncope) or fainting (syncope) may occur.

Supraventricular Tachycardia (SVT)

This is a rapid heart rate emanating from the atria (upper chambers) of the heart.

Atrial Ectopy

Extra beats may be perceived as missed beats/chest thumping. The condition is benign, requiring no treatment above reassurance.

Atrio-Ventricular Re-Entrant Tachycardias: Wolff-Parkinson-White Syndrome (WPW) and Atrioventricular Nodal Re-entrant Tachycardia (AVNRT)

There is a congenital deficiency in the 'electrical insulation' between the atria and ventricles which allows short-circuiting of the normal conduction pathway. Atrial ectopy can allow initiation of an atrio-ventricular electrical re-entry circuit producing a rapid heart rate. If atrial fibrillation occurs this can be life threatening. Many people have a predisposition to pre-excitation which may be unmasked during pregnancy.

Non-Pregnancy Treatment

- Vagal stimulation – induced by swallowing ice, the Valsalva manoeuvre, eyeball pressure or carotid sinus massage[4,5] may terminate tachycardia but often iv adenosine is required
- DC cardioversion is rarely needed[5]
- Catheter ablation of re-entry pathway now treatment of choice, ideally before pregnancy[6]
- Risk of heart block from AVNRT ablation may mean medical therapy is preferred
- Maintenance drugs: beta-blockers, flecainide, amiodarone[5]

Atrial Flutter

- Associated with significant heart disease
- Atrial rates 240–400 bpm
- Generally ventricular rate about half atrial rate
- Can impede cardiac output, allow atrial thrombus formation and risks systemic embolisation[7]

Non-Pregnancy Treatment

- Catheter ablation if possible

- Anticoagulation and rate control with digoxin or beta-blocker for chronic flutter
- Amiodarone for cardioversion and prevention[6,8]

Atrial Fibrillation

Rapid, chaotic depolarisation of the atria (300–500 bpm) with variable atrio-ventricular conduction.

- May be idiopathic or related to underlying cardiac disease
- Increased risk of thrombo-embolism[1]
- May be asymptomatic with low-ventricular-rate response

Treatment is as per atrial flutter.

Ventricular Tachycardia (VT)

Rapid rhythm emanating directly from the ventricles.

- More common in women with structural/ischaemic heart disease or long QT syndrome[3]
- Rarely asymptomatic
- Palpitations, dyspnoea and syncope
- Increased risk of sudden death[1]
- Long QT syndrome hereditable

Non-Pregnancy Treatment

- Treatment of underlying disease
- Catheter ablation if possible
- Anti-arrhythmic medication tailored to cause
- Implantable pacemaker or defibrillator

Treatment in pregnancy is as for pre-pregnancy, but avoid amiodarone and excessive radiation exposure if possible.

Bradycardia

- May be sinus bradycardia
- Present in otherwise normal individuals
- Common in well-trained athletes and during deep sleep[9]
- Rarely, it may be related to myocardial disease
- Can be vagally induced[5]

Non-pregnancy treatment: ignore if asymptomatic, otherwise it generally responds to atropine or adrenaline[9] and rarely needs a pacemaker[5]. Treatment in pregnancy generally consists of pacemaker insertion.

PRE-CONCEPTION ISSUES AND CARE

- Many conditions now amenable to catheter ablation which should be performed pre-pregnancy if possible[10]
- Avoid amiodarone if possible due to fetal thyroid disease and its long half-life[11,12]
- Discuss hereditable conditions, e.g. long QT syndrome
- Beta-blockers may cause slight reduction in fetal weight
- Discuss risks/benefits of warfarin individually
- Optimise treatment of underlying heart disease but avoid ACE inhibitors
- Balance between symptoms and fetal risk
- General health promotion: smoking cessation, weight loss, healthy diet, BP measurements, cholesterol level, encourage exercise and avoiding stress

Pregnancy Issues
- New onset arrhythmias are common in pregnancy[13]
- Pre-existing arrhythmias increase
- Low incidence of serious arrhythmia[14]

Supraventricular tachycardia
- Premature atrial beats are present in 50% pregnant women, being generally well tolerated[14]
- WPW, AVNRT may worsen with catheter ablation required for uncontrollable, or life-threatening, symptoms
- Digoxin, adenosine and beta-blockers are generally safe, but amiodarone best avoided due to fetal thyroid toxicity

Ventricular arrhythmia, atrial fibrillation/flutter
- Frequently indicates underlying heart disease needing to be excluded or treated, e.g. hypertrophic cardiomyopathy, ischaemic heart disease; these are high risk indicators for sudden death[15,16]
- Long QT syndrome and Brugada syndrome are also life threatening and need accurate diagnosis and treatment[3,17]

Atrial flutter/fibrillation is commoner in patients with atrial septal defects and atrial scars from surgical repair. Catheter ablation for this is possible, but complex, with prolonged X-ray exposure. Therefore, it is generally managed medically with rate control and anticoagulation during pregnancy.

Automatic implantable cardio-defibrillators:
- Limited literature but no device or therapy complications are reported
- Implantation is possible during pregnancy if indicated, such as ARVD

Bradycardia
Pathological bradycardia is rare in pregnancy. It is usually benign, but heart block may require pacemaker insertion[18].

Medical Management and Care
For new onset arrhythmias:
- ECG – note that arrhythmia might have subsided by the time an ECG is done!
- Symptom diary and 24-hour Holter monitor
- Serum investigations in order to exclude metabolic abnormalities, particularly hyperkalaemia, acidosis and hypoxaemia
- Try simple measures first, such as vagal stimulation for tachycardia[16]
- Asymptomatic arrhythmia should not be treated unless life threatening
- Recurrence of arrhythmias has adverse fetal or neonatal effects[14]
- Digoxin or beta-blockers for first line management[10,16,19]. Although beta-blockers cross the placenta and can potentially result in fetal bradycardia, hypoglycaemia, premature labour, low birth weight and metabolic abnormalities, they are usually well tolerated during pregnancy and are widely used[20]
- Adenosine is safe in second and third trimesters[21] but needs to be given by experienced practitioners in a monitored area with equipment ready for resuscitation; continual EFM to observe for fetal bradycardia[14,15]
- DC cardioversion if haemodynamically unstable (this is safe in all phases of pregnancy)[16]
- EFM throughout due to the small risk of fetal arrhythmia
- If catheter ablation required, safest period is third trimester[1]
- Exclude hyperthyroidism
- Be alert to risk of thrombo-embolism especially with atrial fibrillation or flutter[22]

Midwifery Management and Care
- Recognise signs and symptoms (breathlessness, chest pain, pre-syncope)
- Take accurate history of onset, frequency and duration to differentiate from physiological symptoms of advancing pregnancy
- Rule out pre-existing anaemia
- Give advice about avoiding stimulants such as caffeine, cigarettes and alcohol and illicit drug use
- Remember may be more symptomatic in third trimester and refer
- Women with severe arrhythmia and who are unstable should be on coronary care unit where more familiar with drugs and treatments
- Assist with vagal manoeuvres – educate woman that the Valsalva manoeuvre, or cold drink, may terminate the episode
- Assess fetal growth if woman on beta-blockers

Labour Issues
- **Tachycardia** – manage according to symptoms and haemodynamics
- **Bradycardia** – usually transient and due to vagal stimulation; atropine/adrenaline useful[16]

Medical Management and Care
- Monitor with ECG, only treat if symptomatic[13]
- Blood samples for U&E and cardiac enzymes

Midwifery Management and Care
- Avoid Valsalva manoeuvre as this can worsen bradycardia
- Care with epidural
- PO$_2$ monitoring
- Continual pulse and blood pressure monitoring
- Continual EFM for fetal bradycardia secondary to beta-blockers

Postpartum Issues
- If occurrence was for first time in pregnancy, postnatal follow-up is required

Medical Management and Care
- If condition persists, or worsens, initiate ongoing ECG monitoring
- Referral for investigation

Midwifery Management and Care
- Neonatal care – monitor carefully for metabolic abnormalities especially hypoglycaemia and thyroid function[12]

4.8 Ischaemic Heart Disease: Angina and Myocardial Infarction

Incidence	Risk for Childbearing
1:10 000–1:30 000; incidence is increasing significantly according to the 2006–2008 Saving Mothers Lives report[1-3]	High Risk – maternal mortality rate of 37% 33% maternal cardiac disease deaths are ischaemic[2,8]

EXPLANATION OF CONDITION

Ischaemic heart disease is due to inadequate myocardial blood flow related to coronary arterial narrowing. This may be temporary – **angina pectoris** (angina), or permanent – **myocardial infarction** (MI). It manifests as chest pain or discomfort, and may radiate to the left arm or jaw. It is accompanied by feelings of constriction/suffocation. Angina is generally precipitated by exertion or stress, but more severe cases may present at rest. The pain of myocardial infarction is generally more severe and may be accompanied by sweating, nausea and a feeling of impending death or collapse.

Coronary artery disease is due to gradual and incomplete occlusion of the coronary vessels by fatty deposits (atheromatous plaques) accumulating in the endothelial cells lining the arterial walls. Symptoms occur when myocardial oxygen demands exceed possible supply.

Complete occlusion of a diseased coronary artery may occur suddenly due to clot formation within the narrowing (**coronary thrombosis**). It may also arise from coronary artery spasm, or dissection of coronary arteries[2]. The supplied myocardium will infarct (die) unless the obstruction is relieved rapidly.

Risk Factors for Ischaemic Heart Disease in Women

- Age >35 years – but 10% women with MI are under 35[1]
- Cigarette smoking; cardiac effects exacerbated by pregnancy[4,5]
- Obesity, diabetes or cocaine abuse
- Family history of cardiovascular disease and dyslipidaemia[3,6]
- Hypertension
- Ethnicity – Black and Asian women have higher risk[3]
- In pregnancy, risk is increased by:
  - increased parity[3]
  - pre-eclampsia, eclampsia and phaeochromocytoma
  - sickle cell and collagen vascular disease[4,6]
  - infection and postpartum haemorrhage (PPH)[7]

Presentation in Pregnancy

- Can be confusing as chest discomfort, nausea and breathlessness are common in pregnancy and may be confused with gastro-oesophageal reflux (heartburn)
- Typical presentation – dizziness, vomiting, abdominal pain and ischaemic chest pain with an abnormal ECG and elevated cardiac enzymes (MI) (NB: ECG may be normal if not in pain)[3]
- Symptoms may be masked/unclear during labour or delivery
- ECG and cardiac enzymes can be insensitive
- Cardiac specific troponin I >0.15 ng/ml is a more specific indicator of myocardial infarction than creatinine kinase muscle–bone (CK–MB) levels, which increase during normal labour[7,8]
- Differential diagnosis of ischaemic chest pain includes haemorrhage, sickle crisis, pre-eclampsia, acute pulmonary embolism and aortic dissection – beware systolic hypertension[2]
- There may be no symptoms at all (especially in diabetics) with the presentation as for cardiomyopathy

COMPLICATIONS

Associated with exacerbation of angina in pregnancy or progression to *de novo* myocardial infarction are:

- **Arrhythmias**
  - ventricular tachycardia/fibrillation
  - heart block
- **Haemodynamic problems**
  - pericarditis
  - tamponade
  - LVF
  - cardiogenic shock
  - acute mitral regurgitation
- **Mortality** is 37–50% in pregnancy, with greatest risk if:
  - the infarct occurs late in pregnancy[3]
  - the woman is *under* 35 years of age
  - pulmonary/amniotic fluid embolism, haemorrhage, placental abruption, eclampsia, or drug toxicity arise

Sudden severe chest pain in a previously fit pregnant woman may be caused by dissection of the aorta +/− coronary arterial dissection. If suspected, withhold thrombolytics and perform immediate CT/coronary angiography.

- The indication for coronary intervention depends on the site and apparent size of the evolving infarct
- Acute aortic dissection itself requires urgent surgery

NON-PREGNANCY TREATMENT AND CARE

- Reduction of obesity, smoking cessation and statins
- Glyceryl trinitrate (GTN) spray or tablets – administered under the tongue
- Early recognition and treatment of MI by history taking, ECG results and raised cardiac enzymes
- Drug therapy includes aspirin, beta-blockers, ACEI, calcium channel blockers and statins
- Treat pain, nausea and vomiting
- Early thrombolysis/intervention improves outcome in MI
- Basic and advanced life support
- Angioplasty[2]

PRE-CONCEPTION ISSUES AND CARE

- Previous coronary bypass surgery does not of itself contraindicate pregnancy
- Impaired LVF is one of the main determinants of maternal and neonatal outcome[1]
- Seek expert cardiological input:
  - echocardiography to evaluate left ventricular ejection fraction and exclude structural anomalies
  - coronary angiography to ascertain disease severity +/− angioplasty/stenting
  - echocardiography and exercise testing 3 months prior to stopping contraception is helpful
- Optimise medication prior to cessation of contraception: aspirin[9], beta-blockers and GTN to be encouraged as directed
  - ACE inhibitors are strongly contraindicated[10]
- Promote smoking cessation
- Encourage daily exercise and weight reduction/control[11]
- Advocate diet low in fat, salt and cholesterol
- Advise on stress avoidance, including control measures, e.g. deep breathing, muscle relaxation and imagery

Pregnancy Issues

Ischaemic heart disease has a rising incidence[1-3], with midwives increasingly likely to see women with angina or myocardial infarction. Smoking, obesity, diabetes mellitus, increasing maternal age and familial lipid disorders are responsible[3].

Recent myocardial infarction:
- Low dose aspirin advised[12]
- Risk of complications high: cardiac arrhythmias (premature ventricular contraction [PVC]), ventricular tachycardia or fibrillation, bradycardia, pericarditis, tamponade, left ventricular failure (LVF), mitral regurgitation, ventricular septal defect, free wall rupture, systemic or pulmonary embolism and cardiogenic shock[13]
- Some women may develop symptoms *during pregnancy* and need investigation and treatment to maintain sufficient coronary flow reserve to survive the pregnancy; timely and expert cardiological input are crucial
- Severe chest pain requiring opiate analgesia must be investigated by CT chest/MRI/echocardiogram[2]
- Diabetic women require attention as they may have 'silent' myocardial ischaemia
- Discuss genetic consequences of having a child with a hereditary genetic predisposition to premature ischaemic heart disease

Medical Management and Care

- Close cardiological supervision is essential[10]
- Beta-blockers, aspirin/heparin, nitrates and calcium antagonists are reasonably safe[12]; statins in 2nd and 3rd trimester can be recommenced[11] (Appendix 4.3.1)
- If acute MI suspected, diagnosis based on ECG and troponin I levels (as CK–MB unreliable peripartum)
- Echocardiography helpful to assess LV function, regional wall motion and valvar abnormalities and guide management
- Coronary angiography/angioplasty/stenting may be needed[8,10]
- Thrombolytic therapy for life-threatening massive, acute MI has been used to favourable effect, but risks haemorrhagic complications[1,8,10]

Midwifery Management and Care

- Careful booking history, noting drug regime and symptoms
- Book at a consultant unit, premature birth common in antenatal MI[10]
- Refer to maternal medicine clinic, and re-refer to the cardiologist those with known disease or risk factors and ischaemic-sounding chest pain
- Advise limited physical activity +/– salt and fluid intake; self-weigh
- Monitor BP (manual[3]), pulse, oedema etc. for pre-eclampsia/CCF
- Remember angina can present for the first time in pregnancy, hence chest discomfort or abdominal pain should not be dismissed as 'heartburn'
- Counselling and support re challenges of motherhood with an underlying cardiac condition, and any potential interventions
- Effective communication with the multi-disciplinary team
- Support smoking cessation programmes
- Clinical assessment of fetal growth and wellbeing supplemented by ultrasound growth, liquor volume and Doppler to exclude IUGR linked to drug regimes[12]
- If the mother reports angina symptoms associated with driving, report to the medical team and advise the mother that she should cease driving until the cardiologist has reviewed her condition[17]

Labour Issues

- Vaginal delivery avoids surgical stress, reduces blood loss and risk of infection and permits early ambulation
- Use of instrument delivery and regional analgesia reduce the second stage and some elements of unpredictability
- Recent MI – if possible delay delivery until the infarct has time to heal, as mortality is higher within 2 weeks of event[10,13]
- Ergometrine is best avoided as it can cause coronary artery spasm[14]
- Caesarean section with an epidural may be more appropriate if the infarct is recent[15]

Medical Management and Care

- Agree care plan between mother and all team members
- Carefully document in records: delivery options, drug, fluid and monitoring regimes and methods
- Anticoagulants discontinued 12–24 hours prior to regional anaesthesia
- Plan a strategy for potential primary or secondary haemorrhage

Midwifery Management and Care

- Immediate referral for medical review
- Feto-maternal monitoring by: EFM, ECG, BP, pulse, respirations, oximetry
- Iv access, strict fluid balance recorded and MEOWS scoring recorded
- Supplementary oxygen and saturation monitoring if indicated
- Left or right lateral position advised
- Review thromboprophylaxis; use compression (TED) stockings[3]
- Monitoring of analgesia requirement and effectiveness
- Careful use of oxytoxic drugs[3], **avoid ergometrine** (coronary spasm)
- Resuscitation skills and equipment to hand
- Avoid active closed glottis 'pushing'; passive descent is beneficial[18,19]
- Anticipate and assist with operative delivery and support the mother

Postpartum Issues

- Spontaneous coronary artery dissection most common cause of MI in postnatal period[16]
- Avoid ergometrine, as it can cause coronary artery spasm[14]
- Thrombolysis is generally contraindicated with acute MI, as it increases the risk of haemorrhage
- Oestrogen-based contraception is contraindicated due to risk of venous thrombo-embolism (VTE)

Medical Management and Care

- Observe for exacerbation of the underlying condition and arrhythmia
- Consider drug regimes and breast-feeding (Appendix 4.3.1)
- Advise on future pregnancy options, and contraception choice

Midwifery Management and Care

- Continue vital signs observations every 15 minutes post-birth until stable
- Continue with fluid volume assessment and watch for bleeding
- Avoid ergometrine for PPH, unless life threatening
- TED stockings, and administer prescribed anticoagulants
- Encourage rest and avoiding exertion
- Diet – well balanced, high iron and fibre content (avoid constipation)
- Consider social support issues
- Reinforce contraceptive advice, explaining use of progestogen-only contraceptive pill or intrauterine contraceptive device
- Encourage rest and gentle mobilisation

S. E. Robson and J. Waugh

4.9 Pulmonary Hypertension and Eisenmenger's Syndrome

Incidence	**Risk for Childbearing**
1:20000 of which approximately 6% appears to be familial[1,2]	High Risk – maternal mortality 36%-56%[9]

EXPLANATION OF CONDITION

Pulmonary hypertension (PH) is progressive elevation of pulmonary artery pressure leading to right ventricular failure and death. It is due to increased pulmonary vascular resistance impeding blood flow through the lungs. It is defined as an elevated mean pulmonary artery pressure of 25 mmHg or greater at rest or 30 mmHg with exercise. This is commoner in women, aged 30–40, with a ratio of female to male of 1.7–3.5:1[3].

Classification[4]

- Pulmonary arterial hypertension (PAH)
- PH with left heart disease
- PH with lung disease and hypoxaemia
- PH due to thrombotic/embolic disease
- Miscellaneous

Pulmonary Arterial Hypertension

Pulmonary arterial hypertension is due mainly to changes in the pulmonary arterioles. It may be **idiopathic** (IPAH) or **familial** (FPAH), often with autosomal dominant inheritance, and there may be worsening of the disease in subsequent generations[5]. PAH is often **associated** (APAH) with one or more triggering factors (+/– a genetic pre-disposition), resulting in endothelial injury, vasoconstriction and vascular remodelling. The main triggers are:

- Connective tissue diseases such as scleroderma, CREST (Calcinosis, Raynaud's, Oesophageal dysmotility, Sclerodactyly, Telangiectasia), rheumatoid arthritis, and SLE
- Congenital systemic to pulmonary shunts (mainly cardiac)
- Portal hypertension[6,7]
- Viral infection – especially HIV
- Drugs and toxins, especially appetite suppressants
- Pulmonary veno-occlusive disease
- Persistent pulmonary hypertension of the newborn
- Miscellaneous triggers, e.g. autoimmune and storage diseases

Signs and Symptoms

The signs and symptoms are usually insidious, with advanced presentation, with several years elapsing prior to diagnosis.

- Dyspnoea main symptom until late in the disease
- Pre-syncope or syncope
- Chest pain and palpitations
- Cyanosis if atrial shunting present
- Raised jugular venous pressure, right-ventricular heave, loud pulmonary component of the second heart sound, tricuspid or pulmonary regurgitant murmurs and right heart failure (see above) occurs late[8]

Eisenmenger's Syndrome

Eisenmenger's syndrome is the end-stage reaction of the pulmonary vasculature to the increased pulmonary blood flow (and pressure) from systemic to pulmonary shunting in congenital heart disease. There is usually severe cyanosis and restricted effort tolerance.

COMPLICATIONS

- Mortality from PAH is high[9], with <3 year from diagnosis to death, mainly from right ventricular (RV) failure or sudden death; some treatments now available which may improve this
- Pregnancy is very poorly tolerated, irrespective of cause of PAH, with maternal mortality >36%[10] and miscarriage rate 40%[10]
- Patients with Eisenmenger's syndrome generally survive longer due to preserved RV function

NON-PREGNANCY TREATMENT AND CARE

Screening, with ECG and echocardiography, should be offered to women with a family history of PAH, as well as those with HIV, scleroderma or other known triggers.

Drug Treatment

- Pulmonary vasodilator therapy – nifedipine of benefit in a small group with reactive pulmonary vasculature; intravenous or inhaled prostanoids may also be of long-term benefit but are very expensive and have major lifestyle implications
- Anticoagulants – warfarin reduces risk of pulmonary thrombosis and may be life prolonging[11]
- Phosphodiesterase 5 inhibitors, such as sildenafil (Viagra), and endothelin receptor antagonists, such as bosentan (Tracleer), are more recent therapies (Appendix 4.3.1)
- Diuretic therapy reduces breathlessness and oedema
- Oxygen therapy may be required, often overnight

Interventions

- Atrial septostomy may be life saving when there is severe PAH: enlargement of the *foramen ovale* (between the atria) permits right-to-left shunting which augments cardiac output, albeit at the expense of cyanosis
- Heart–lung or double lung transplant, once drugs and therapy become ineffective

PRE-CONCEPTION ISSUES AND CARE

- Advise strongly **against** pregnancy[12]
- Contraception: sterilisation, partner sterilisation, progesterone only contraceptive pill, Mirena intrauterine system (progestogen eluting)
- Genetic counselling
- Management of underlying diseases

If Pregnancy Occurs

- Prompt liaison with specialist PAH unit (most patients are already under their care but denial can be a problem)
- Termination of pregnancy – rapid referral with specialist anaesthesia if instrumentation required
- Supportive treatment with nebulised iloprost, oxygen therapy, anticoagulation, etc. is possible but carries a very high risk to mother and fetus (Appendix 4.3.1)
- Bosentan is contraindicated as it is teratogenic

Pregnancy Issues

Consider termination of pregnancy:

- Risk of death, especially in the last trimester or puerperium, due to pulmonary hypertensive crises, pulmonary thrombosis, or refractory right heart failure. Can occur in patients with little disability before or during pregnancy. Risk factors for maternal death are: late hospitalization, severe pulmonary hypertension, and general anaesthetic[13]
- Ensure women have made informed choice if they plan to continue with pregnancy
- Clearly document all discussions[10]
- Prior treatment with pulmonary vascular therapy for over a year with improved right ventricular function slightly improves outcome but there is still considerable risk
- Limited experiences of newer therapies with pregnant women especially first trimester (some cases teratogenic in animal studies)[8]
- Low cardiac output state entails poor coping with physiological changes of pregnancy
- Fetal morbidity and mortality are considerable; premature delivery and restricted fetal growth occur in 50% of cases[10]
- Only 15–25% pregnancies reach term

Medical Management and Care

- Contact and refer to the national designated specialist centre
- Drug therapies: prostaglandin therapy, e.g. iv or nebulised iloprost
- Newer treatments may be teratogenic, but calcium channel blockers, e.g. nifedipine, may be helpful
- Monthly specialist appointments; as pregnancy progresses more frequent – exercise capacity, oxygen saturation, 'echo', etc.
- Multidisciplinary team approach
- Early hospital admission may be appropriate with early, elective LSCS[10]
- Fetal growth and development – clinical assessment and ultrasound and Doppler studies
- Anticoagulant therapy on individual basis[10]

Midwifery Management and Care

- **Urgent** referral to consultant unit and cardiologist team; should be referred to **specialist referral centre** or own team contacted
- Support of family and woman
- Consider legal issues, especially guardians for the baby if the parents are unmarried and there is an adverse outcome
- Support if needed for additional appointments, especially if travelling to regional centres
- Preparation for early hospital admission and prolonged stay
- Recognition of signs and symptoms of heart failure[10]
- Promote a healthy and nutritious diet, avoid anaemia[10]
- Preparation for a growth restricted and pre-term baby

Labour Issues

- **One of the times most at risk**
- **Cardiac intensive care** setting – if on delivery unit skilled professionals at hand, close team work essential
- Pulmonary artery pressure monitoring may be useful during delivery and several days afterwards
- Prepare resuscitation equipment, plus ventilation with inhaled nitric oxide
- **Dangers:**
    - post-operative or delivery fluid shifts
    - **high-risk time** for sudden death
- *Spontaneous labour is preferred,* but induction is safe using prostaglandins[14]
- Operative delivery may be indicated
- Regional analgesia is advantageous, but not spinal analgesia alone due to hypotension risk from inadequate response of right ventricle. Low-dose sequential combined spinal–epidural or incremental spinal anaesthesia is preferred[8,15]

Medical Management and Care

- Labour birth plan made early in collaboration with the combined team and woman/family, documented clearly in the case notes and *adhered to;* an ITU bed must be booked
- Pre-term birth is likely for worsening maternal condition
- Planned LSCS from 30 weeks gestation in many cases with team available[8,10]
- LSCS may be in general/cardiac theatres; closer to ITU if needed
- Invasive monitoring arterial line central venous pressure (CVP)
- Stop anticoagulants pre-delivery/regional anaesthesia

Midwifery Management and Care

- Intensive monitoring of ECG, CVP, BP, pulse, respirations and oxygen therapy with saturation monitoring and arterial blood gases
- Foley catheter hourly readings; accurate fluid balance, avoid overload and early recognition of reduced urine output
- Continual EFM, risks of IUGR and/or pre-term birth
- Vaginal birth may be possible but elective LSCS is more usual as early induction of labour is often not possible
- Lateral tilt for labour, compression stockings, passive exercises
- Second stage – avoid 'bearing down'; forceps/ventouse electively[17,18]
- Third stage – avoid or minimise oxytoxic drugs; either physiological third stage or carefully titrated oxytocin with careful monitoring[19] to minimise blood loss

Postpartum Issues

- **Mortality high in the postnatal period**[13]
- Care in intensive care for at least a week
- Risk of pulmonary oedema
- **Sudden death** risk due to right heart failure
- Follow-up with cardiology team is essential to assess heart function
- Providing information to family members frequently, concisely and honestly[16]
- Counselling re risks of another pregnancy
- Contraception – advise about sterilisation (but risks with surgery): intrauterine system or subdermal implant are as effective[12]

Medical Management and Care

- Oxygen therapy, thrombo-embolism prophylaxis, fluid balance, and observations remain vital[10]
- Inhaled nitric acid and/or iv prostacyclin is continued or initiated[8]

Midwifery Management and Care

Immediate – close monitoring continues, plus:

- Regular visits from the midwifery team while the mother is on ITU
- Advice re maternal–infant interaction, photos/video of baby (may be in SCBU or NICU dependent on gestation)
- Lactation – advice with support re breast-feeding/pumping/timing related to drug therapy

Longer term:

- Support with recovery and the practical aspects of baby care

4.10 Heart Transplant

Incidence	Risk for Childbearing
1 in 190 USA[1] and 1 in 140 French women[2] with heart, or heart/lung, transplants become pregnant	Moderate to High Risk

EXPLANATION OF CONDITION

Cardiac transplantation is the procedure by which the failing heart is replaced with another heart from a suitable donor. The procedure is generally reserved for patients who have end-stage congestive heart failure with a prognosis of less than a year to live without the transplant, who are not candidates for conventional medical therapy, or have not been helped by conventional medical therapy.

Reasons for transplant are:

- Idiopathic cardiomyopathy – 54%
- Ischemic cardiomyopathy – 45%
- Congenital heart disease and other diseases – 1% [3]

The one year survival rate after cardiac transplantation is as high as 81.8%, with a 5-year survival rate of 69.8%. A significant number of recipients survive more than 10 years after the procedure[4].

A growing number of heart, heart–lung, or lung transplant recipients are women of reproductive age[5]. Most often, fertility is restored with successful organ transplantation and good overall health[6,7]. Over an 18-year period 9831 USA women had heart, and 534 heart/lung, transplants of whom 54 became pregnant[1] who subsequently posed complex medical, psychosocial, and ethical problems[5]. In the UK 2010/11, 131 heart, 169 lung and three heart/lung transplants were performed[8]. Increasing numbers of younger patients are being transplanted for end stage congenital heart disease.

COMPLICATIONS

- Organ rejection (no more common during pregnancy[9])
- Side effects of immunosuppressive therapy are common, including systemic hypertension and hyperlipidemia[10]
- Infection (may be less obvious with immunosuppressant therapy and must not be overlooked)
- Premature coronary artery disease is common in the transplanted heart and may be asymptomatic. Most transplant recipients undergo regular intravascular ultrasound assessments as well as coronary angiography and are receiving statins.
- Malignancies are common after heart and heart lung transplantation with 6% affected by one year rising to 14% by ten years, with lymphoma the most common[10]. One case of choriocarcinoma transferred from a pregnant donor to four recipients has also been reported[11]

NON-PREGNANCY TREATMENT AND CARE

- Lifelong treatment with immunosuppressant drugs, such as ciclosporin, to avoid tissue rejection; often multiple drug combinations are used[3]
- Regular hospital appointments to monitor progress
- Prompt identification and treatment of hypertension
- Statins to reduce risks of atheroma
- Advice on a healthy lifestyle (diet, weight, smoking cessation, regular exercise, and to seek medical treatment if feeling unwell)
- Prompt identification and treatment of infection
- Recognition of co-morbidities, such as previous congenital heart disease and recurrence risk

PRE-CONCEPTION ISSUES AND CARE

- Should be introduced at least at the pre-transplant evaluation
- Should be followed up throughout the post-transplant process
- Should be offered to both the patient and her partner

Pregnancy may be considered if:

- At least 1 year post-transplant
- No rejection in the past year[4]
- Adequate and stable graft function
- No acute infections that might impact the fetus
- Maintenance immunosuppression at stable dosing.

Special circumstances that impact on recommendations:

- Rejection within the first year
- Maternal age
- Comorbid factors that may impact pregnancy or graft function
- Established medical noncompliance.
- Genetic counselling regarding genetic factors associated with transplant, e.g. peripartum cardiomyopathy, and recurrence risk
- Management of underlying diseases
- Ideally, patients should be vaccinated pre-transplant, but if not, should be vaccinated pre-pregnancy – influenza, pneumococcus, hepatitis B, tetanus[4]
- Counselling[12], to include consequences of pre-term birth and long-term consequences of pre-term birth for both the mother and child with both prospective parents[4]

Potential Teratogenesis of Drug Therapy

To date, the outcomes of children exposed to immunosuppressant drugs *in utero* have been encouraging, as specific effects have not been identified. Continued surveillance is still paramount. Of concern are new immunosuppressives, specifically **mycophenolate mofetil**, where data reported to the National Transplantation Pregnancy Registry (NTPR) have shown an increased incidence of non-viable outcomes and increased incidence of malformation in the newborn, resulting in a pregnancy category change[13].

In children born to transplanted women taking ciclosporin, renal function developed normally despite prolonged exposure *in utero*[14] and neurocognitive and behavioral development were normal[15]. Any co-morbidity is associated with prematurity and consequently poorer neurocognitive and behavioural outcomes[13].

If Pregnancy Occurs

- Contact the patients transplant physician
- In conjunction with them, assess current risk states
- Formulate a management plan; whether ToP or to continue
- Management by high-risk obstetrician (because of IUGR and pre-eclampsia) in conjunction with transplant physician[4]
- Graft dysfunction during pregnancy warrants appropriate investigation (by biopsy if necessary)[4]
- Maintain immunosuppression in pregnancy to avoid rejection
- Balance of risks of teratogenesis and rejection; less available information on newer drugs[4,16]

Pregnancy Issues

The physiological changes occurring in pregnancy are generally well tolerated by mothers who have undergone transplant[5]. Management should be shared between transplant physicians and specialists in high-risk pregnancies because good multidisciplinary team working improves a favourable outcome[3].

Prevention of maternal and fetal complications secondary to graft rejection[6], is paramount. Benefits of immunosuppressant drugs outweigh fetal risks[17].

Whilst many successful pregnancy outcomes have been reported, there are risks of[4,5,18]:

- Hypertension and pre-eclampsia
- Infection
- Miscarriage
- Prematurity and growth restriction
- Theoretical coronary artery disease risk

Complicating factors:

- Sequelae of original disease (e.g. renal)
- Chronic allograft dysfunction
- Cardiovascular status and pulmonary status
- Diabetes mellitus (or history of DM)
- Hypertension
- Inherited diseases in mother and or father (genetic versus chromosomal)
- Infection, such as hepatits B and C (HBV, HCV) and cytomegalovirus (CMV)[16]
- Obesity
- Hyperemesis gravidarum may lead to decreased absorption or inadequate immunosuppression[1,4,18]

Medical Management and Care

- Contact and confer with the mother's designated specialist centre
- Goals are to ensure that mothers maintain graft function using appropriate immunosuppressive dosing during gestation and immediately after delivery
- Optimise maternal health including graft function
- Maintain a normal metabolic environment
- Immunosuppressant drugs should be continued in pregnancy; dosage may need increasing as maternal blood volume increases during the pregnancy[3]
- Minimise complications associated with underlying disease and ongoing treatment
- Detect and manage hypertensive complications especially pre-eclampsia
- Ensure adequate fetal growth
- Monitor closely for rejection and require regular right ventricular biopsies that may even increase in frequency during pregnancy, exposing the fetus to radiation
- Be aware of and alert for:
  - likely baseline tachycardia (vagal denervation)[17]
  - asymptomatic myocardial ischemia (sensory denervation)[17]
  - tachyarrhythmias[17]
  - signs of rejection leading to maternal death[17]
- Possible need for pre-term delivery
- Caesarean section is indicated only for obstetric reasons

Midwifery Management and Care

- **Urgent** referral to consultant unit and cardiologist team (see above)[3]
- Support of family and woman
- Be alert for early signs of hyperemesis gravidarum; refer to a doctor sooner than later
- Established baseline normal heart rate and BP for this mother + acceptable variation
- Ensure pulse and BP measured at each antenatal visit
- Monitor for gestational diabetes if taking prednisolone[4]
- Be alert to possible rejection symptoms which include fever, flu-like symptoms, malaise, chest pain, breathlessness, cough, peripheral oedema (especially early in pregnancy), cough, diarrhoea, elevated blood sugars, etc.

Labour Issues

- Labour and delivery should be planned
- Vaginal birth attempted
- Invasive monitoring only needed if mother is in heart failure
- Regional anaesthesia appears to be safe[19]
- Response to vasoactive drugs may be unpredictable due to cardiac denervation[19]
- Possible reduced cough reflex
- Intravenous fluid should be administered carefully due to risk of fluid overload and pulmonary oedema[19]

Medical Management and Care

- Labour birth plan made early in collaboration with the combined team and woman/family, documented clearly in the case notes[3]
- Consider need for peripheral/central venous access, and level of monitoring
- Pre-term birth is more common[18], so advise and prepare accordingly

Midwifery Management and Care

- Intensive monitoring of ECG, BP, pulse, respirations
- Low threshold for siting an IVI.
- Continual EFM, risks of IUGR and/or pre-term birth
- Vaginal birth should be anticipated
- Lateral tilt for labour, compression stockings, passive exercises
- Third stage – as normal
- If delivered pre-term prepare for a premature baby and alert paediatrician

Postpartum Issues

- Postnatal follow-up with specialists
- Good prognosis[18]
- Breast-feeding is possible, although some immunosuppressants are contraindicated[1]
- Immunosuppressive drugs decrease the effectiveness of intrauterine contraceptive devices; immunocompromised women using such devices have increased risk for infection
- Progesterone only pill is not associated with adverse medical consequences
- If BP well controlled the combined contraceptive pill may be safe
- Barrier methods may be necessary

Medical Management and Care

- Continue on anti-rejection drugs, monitor levels frequently for first month, especially if doses have been altered during pregnancy
- Counselling about the risks of another pregnancy
- Risk–benefit evaluation on safety of contraception; prescribe as indicated

Midwifery Management and Care

- Encourage mobility as soon as possible
- Continue with regular observations
- If breast-feeding consult pharmacist as to drug safety; support breast-feeding
- Reinforce contraceptive advice, including advice on barrier methods
- Book follow-up appointments including transplant team and any necessary surveillance for the baby
- Increased risk to mother from postpartum mood changes or depression (or just being too busy) as may forget to take their anti-rejection medication[16]

S. E. Robson and J. Waugh

4 Heart Disease

PATIENT ORGANISATIONS

Antenatal Results and Choices
73–75 Charlotte Street
London W1T 4PN
www.ARC-UK.org

Birth Defects Foundation
BDF Centre
Hemlock Way
Cannock
Staffordshire WS11 2GF
www.BDFcharity.co.uk

British Heart Foundation
14 Fitzhardinge Street
London W1H 6DH
www.bhf.org.uk/default.aspx

Children's Heart Federation
Level One
2–4 Great Eastern Street
London EC2A 3NW
www.childrens-heart-fed.org.uk/

Arrhythmia Alliance
PO Box 3697
Stratford upon Avon
Warwickshire CV37 8YL
www.arrhythmiaalliance.org.uk

Cardiomyopathy Association
40 The Metro Centre
Tolpits Lane
Watford WD18 9SB
www.cardiomyopathy.org

Echo UK
www.echocharity.org.uk

Grown Up Congenital Heart Patients Association
http://www.guch.org.uk

Marfan Association UK
Rochester House
5 Aldershot Road
Fleet
Hampshire GU51 3NG
http://marfan.org.uk

Max Appeal
Supporting families affected by DiGeorge syndrome VCFS
and 22q11.2 deletion
http://www.maxappeal.org.uk

ESSENTIAL READING

Billington M and Stevenson M (Eds) 2007 **Critical Care in Childbearing for Midwives**. Oxford; Blackwell Publishing Ltd.

Edwards G 2004 **Adverse Outcomes in Maternity Care – Implications for Practice, Applying the Recommendations of the Confidential Enquiries**. London; BFM/Elsevier

The European Society of Cardiology 2011 ESC Guidelines on the management of cardiovascular diseases during pregnancy. **European Heart Journal**; doi:10.1093/eurheartj/ehr218

Gilbert ES 2007 Cardiac disease. In: **High Risk Pregnancy and Delivery**, 4th Edn. London; Mosby/Elsevier

James D (Ed) 2011 Chapt.36 Cardiac disease in **High Risk Pregnancy Management Options** 4th Edn. London; Elsevier 627–656

Jason D, Christie M, Leah B *et al.* 2011 The Registry of the International Society for Heart and Lung Transplantation: Twenty-eighth Adult Lung and Heart-Lung Transplant Report 2011. **The Journal of Heart Lung Transplantation**, 10:1104–1122

Meeks M, Hallsworth M and Yeo H 2010 Chapt.11 *Nursing newborn babies with congenital heart disease* in Bu'Lock F, Currie A and Kairamkona (Eds) **Nursing the Neonate**, 2nd Edn. Oxford; Wiley-Blackwell 172–206

Mukherjee S 2009 **Transplantation and Pregnancy**. http://emedicine.medscape.com/article/429932-overview#showall

Nelson-Piercy C 2005 *Heart disease* in **Handbook of Obstetric Medicine**, 2nd Edn. London; Martin Dunitz

Powrie R, Greene M and Camman W (Eds) 2010 Chapt.5 *Heart disease in pregnancy* in **de Swiet's Medical Disorders in Obstetric Practice**, 5th Edn. Oxford: Wiley-Blackwell 118–152

RCOG 2002 **Maternal Morbidity and Mortality** Study Group Statement. www.rcog.org.uk/index.asp?PageID=1738

RCOG 2011 **Cardiac Disease and Pregnancy** Good Practice Guideline 13 London; Royal College of Obstetricians and Gynaecologists. www.rcog.org.uk/files/rcog-corp/GoodPractice13CardiacDiseaseandPregnancy.pdf

Steer PJ, Gatzoulis MA and Baker P (Eds) 2006 **Heart Disease and Pregnancy**. London; RCOG Press

Thorne S, Nelson-Piercy C, MacGregor A *et al.* 2006 Pregnancy and contraception in heart disease and pulmonary arterial hypertension. **Journal of Family Planning and Reproductive Health Care**, 32:75–81

References

4.1 Mild Structural Heart Disease

1. Walker F 2006 Chapt.5 *Antenatal care of women with cardiac disease: a cardiologist's perspective* in Steer PJ, Gatzoulis M and Baker P (Eds) **Heart Disease in Pregnancy**. London; RCOG Press 55–66
2. Wren C and O'Sullivan JJ 2001 Survival with congenital heart disease and need to follow-up in adult life. **Heart**, 85:438–443
3. Khairy P, Ionescu-Ittu R, Mackie AS, *et al.* 2010 Changing mortality in congenital heart disease. **J Am Coll Cardiol**, 56:1149–1157
4. Vause S, Thorne S and Clarke B 2006 Chapt.1 *Preconceptual counselling for women with cardiac disease* in Steer PJ, Gatzoulis M and Baker P (Eds) **Heart Disease in Pregnancy**. London; RCOG Press 3–8
5. Stout K 2005 Pregnancy in women with congenital heart disease: the importance of evaluation and counselling. **Heart**, 91:713–714
6. Stangl V, Schad J, Gossing G, *et al.* 2008 Maternal heart disease and pregnancy outcome: a single-centre experience. **Eur J Heart Fail**, 10:855–860.
7. Siu SC, Sermer M, Colman JM, *et al.* 2001 Prospective multicenter study of pregnancy outcomes in women with heart disease. **Circulation**, 104 515–521
8. Shinebourne EA, Babu-Narayan SV and Carvalho JS 2006 Tetralogy of Fallot: from fetus to adult. **Heart**, 92:1353–1359
9. Perloff J and Warnes C 2001 Challenges posed by adults with repaired congenital heart disease. **Circulation**, 103:2637
10. Neumayer U, Stone S and Somerville J 1998 Small ventricular septal defects in adults. **European Heart Journal**, 19:1573–1582
11. Siu SC and Colman J 2001 Heart disease in pregnancy. **Heart**, 85:710–715
12. Rasiah SV, Publicover M, Ewer AK, *et al.* 2006 J. A systematic review of the accuracy of first-trimester ultrasound examination for detecting major congenital heart disease. **Ultrasound in Obstetrics and Gynecology**,28:110–116
13. Hyett J, Perdu M, Sharland G, Snijders R and Nicolaides KH 1999 Using fetal nuchal translucency to screen for major congenital cardiac defects at 10–14 weeks of gestation: population based cohort study. **British Medical Journal**, 318:81–85
14. Zuber M, Gautschi N and Oechslin E 1999 Outcome of pregnancy with congenital shunt lesions. **Heart**, 81:271–275
15. Yap SC, Drenthen W, Pieper PG *et al.* on behalf of ZAHARA investigators 2010 Pregnancy Outcome in women with repaired versus unrepaired isolated ventricular septal defect **BJOG** DOI:10.1111/j.1471-0528.2010.02512x
16. Pitkin RM, Perloff JK, Kos BJ and Beall MH 1990 Pregnancy and congenital heart disease. **Annals of Internal Medicine**, 112:445–454
17. Thorne SA 2004 Pregnancy in heart disease. **Heart**, 90:450–456
18. Nelson-Piercy C 2011 Chapt.9 *Cardiac disease* in Lewis G (Ed) 2011 **Saving Mothers Lives: Reviewing Maternal Deaths to Make Motherhood Safer. 2006–2008 BJOG** 118(supplement 1)
19. Habib G, Hoen B, Tornos P, *et al.* 2009 Guidelines on the prevention, diagnosis, and treatment of infective endocarditis (new version 2009): the Task Force on the Prevention, Diagnosis, and Treatment of Infective Endocarditis of the European Society of Cardiology (ESC). **European Heart Journal**, 30:2369–2413
20. Tomlinson M 2006 Chapt.37 *Cardiac disease* in James DK, Steer PJ, Weiner CP and Gonik B (Eds) 2006 **High Risk Pregnancy: Management Options**, 3rd Edn. London; Elsevier 790–827
21. Thorne S 2006 Chapt.13 *Mitral and aortic stenosis* in Steer PJ, Gatzoulis M and Baker P (Eds) **Heart Disease in Pregnancy**. London; RCOG Press 183–190
22. Khairy P, Quyang DW and Fernandes S 2006 Pregnancy outcomes in women with congenital heart disease. **Circulation**, 113:1564–1571
23. Gelson E, Johnson M, Gatzoulis M and Uebing A 2007 Cardiac disease in pregnancy. Part 1: congenital heart disease. **The Obstetrician and Gynaecologist**, 9:15–20

4.2 Moderate Structural Heart Disease

1. Swan L 2006 *Aortopathies including Marfan's syndrome and coarctation* in Steer PJ, Gatzoulis M and Baker P (Eds) **Heart Disease in Pregnancy**. London; RCOG Press
2. Warnes C 2005 The adult with congenital heart disease – born to be bad? **Journal of the American College of Cardiology**, 46:1–8
3. Cohen M, Fuster V, Steele PM, Driscoll D and McGoon DC 1989 Coarctation of the aorta. Long-term follow-up and prediction of outcome after surgical correction. **Circulation**, 80:840–845
4. Raja SG and Basu D 2005 Pulmonary hypertension in congenital heart disease. **Nursing Standard**, 19(50):41–49
5. Presbitero P, Somerville J, Rabajoli F, *et al.* 1995 Corrected transposition of the great arteries without associated defects in adult patients: clinical profile and follow-up. **British Heart Journal**, 74:57–59
6. Serfontein SJ and Kron IL 2002 Complications of coarctation repair. **Seminars in Thoracic and Cardiovascular Surgery: Pediatric Cardiac Surgery Annual**, 5:206–211
7. Shah S and Calderon D 2005 **Aortic Coarctation**. www.emedicine.com/med/topic154.htm [Accessed 30-08-2007]
8. Celermajer D and Greaves K 2002 Survivors of coarctation repair: fixed but not cured. **Heart**, 88:113–114
9. Gatzoulis MA, Balaji S, Webber SA, *et al.* 2000 Risk factors for arrhythmia and sudden cardiac death late after repair of tetralogy of Fallot: a multicentre study. **Lancet**, 356:975–981
10. Connolly HM, Grogan M and Warnes CA 1999 Pregnancy among women with congenitally corrected transposition of great arteries. **Journal of the American College of Cardiology**, 33:1692–1695
11. Adamson D, Dhanjal C, Nelson-Piercy C and Collis R 2007 *Cardiac disease in pregnancy* in Geer I, Nelson-Piercy C and Walters B (Eds) **Maternal Medicine – Medical Problems in Pregnancy**. Edinburgh; Churchill/Elsevier
12. Nelson-Piercy C 2007 Chapt.9 *Cardiac Disease* in Lewis G (Ed) 2007 **Saving Mothers' Lives: Reviewing Maternal Deaths to Make Motherhood Safer. 7th Report of the Confidential Enquiries into Maternal and Child Health**. London; CEMACH 117–130
13. Thorne SA 2004 Pregnancy in heart disease. **Heart**, 90:450–456
14. Siu SC, Sermer M, Colman JM, *et al.* 2001 Prospective multicentre study of pregnancy outcomes in women with heart disease. **Circulation**, 104:515–521
15. Guedes A, Mercier L, Leduc L, Berube L and Marcotte F 2004 Impact of pregnancy on the systemic right ventricle after a Mustard operation for transposition of the great arteries. **American College of Cardiology**, 21:44:433–437

4.3 Severe Structural Heart Disease

1. Abbas AE, Lester SJ and Connolly H 2005 Pregnancy and the cardiovascular system. **International Journal of Cardiology**, 98:179–189
2. Gatzoulis MA, Webb GD and Daubeny PEF (Eds) 2003 **Diagnosis and Management of Adult Congenital Heart Disease**. London; Churchill Livingstone/Elsevier 136
3. Siu SC, Sermer M, Colman JM, *et al.* 2001 Prospective multicentre study of pregnancy outcomes in women with heart disease. **Circulation**, 104:515–521
4. Presbitero P, Somerville J, Sone S, *et al.* 1994 Pregnancy in cyanotic congenital heart disease – outcome of mother and fetus. **Circulation**, 89:2673–2676

5. Tomlinson M 2006 Chapt.37 *Cardiac disease* in James DK, Steer PJ, Weiner CP and Gonik B (Eds) 2006 **High Risk Pregnancy: Management Options**, 3rd Edn. London; Elsevier 790–827
6. Thorne SA 2004 Pregnancy in heart disease. **Heart**, 90:450–456
7. Gilbert ES 2007 Chapt.11 *Cardiac disease* in **High Risk Pregnancy and Delivery**, 4th Edn. London; Mosby/Elsevier 270–285

4.4 Rheumatic and Valvular Heart Disease

1. Nelson-Piercy C 2011 Chapt.9 *Cardiac disease* in Lewis G (Ed) 2011 **Saving Mothers Lives: Reviewing Maternal Deaths to Make Motherhood Safer. 2006–2008 BJOG** 118 (supplement 1)
2. Tomlinson M 2006 Chapt.37 *Cardiac disease* in James DK, Steer PJ, Weiner CP and Gonik B (Eds) 2006 **High Risk Pregnancy**, 3rd Edn. London; Elsevier 790–827
3. Braunwald E 2001 *Valvular heart disease* in Braunwald E and Zipes DP (Eds) **Heart Disease: A Textbook of Cardiovascular Medicine**, 6th Edn. London; Saunders/Elsevier
4. Regitz-Zagrosek V, Blomstrom Lundqvist C, Borghi C, *et al.* ESC Guidelines on the management of cardiovascular diseases during Pregnancy; The Task Force on the Management of Cardiovascular Diseases during Pregnancy of the European Society of Cardiology (ESC) **European Heart Journal** doi:10.1093/eurheartj/ehr218www.escardio.org/guidelines-surveys/esc-guidelines/Pages/cardiovascular-diseases-during-pregnancy.aspx [Accessed 27-8-2011]
5. Habib G, Hoen B, Tornos P, *et al.* 2009 Guidelines on the prevention, diagnosis,and treatment of infective endocarditis (new version 2009): the Task Force on the Prevention, Diagnosis, and Treatment of Infective Endocarditis of the European Society of Cardiology (ESC). **European Heart Journal**,30:2369–2413
6. Warnes CA, Williams RG, Bashore TM, *et al.* 2008 Guidelines for the management of adults with congenital heart disease: a report of the American College of Cardiology/American Heart Association Task Force on Practice Guidelines. **Journal of the American College of Cardiology 2008**;52:e1–e121
7. Saratain J (2008) Obstetric patients with rheumatic heart disease. **O&G Magazine**, 10:18-20
8. Elkayam U 2005 Valvular heart disease and pregnancy part 11 prosthetic valves. **Journal of the American College of Cardiology**, 46:403–410
9. **WHO** Rheumatic fever and rheumatic heart disease – report of a WHO Expert ConsultationWHO technical report series 923 http://whqlibdoc.who.int/hq/2000/WHO_CVD_00.1.pdf [Accessed 31-8-11]
10. Reimold S and Rutherford J 2003 Valvular heart disease in pregnancy. **New England Journal of Medicine**, 349:52–59
11. Prasad A and Ventura H 2001 Valvular heart disease and pregnancy. **Post Graduate Medicine**, 110:69–88
12. Nelson-Piercy C 2010 **Handbook of Obstetric Medicine**, 4th Edn. Abingdon; Informa Health Care
13. Vasu S and Stergiopoulos K 2009 Valvular heart disease in pregnancy. **Hellenic Journal of Cardiology**, 50:498–510
14. Silversides CK, Coleman JM, Sermer M and Siu SC 2003 Cardiac risk in pregnant women with rheumatic mitral stenosis. **American Journal of Cardiology**, 91:182–185
15. Ray P, Murphy GJ and Shutt LE 2004 Recognition and management of maternal cardiac disease in pregnancy. **British Journal of Anaesthesia**, 93:428–439
16. Hameed A, Karaalp I, Tummala P, *et al.* 2001 The effect of valvular heart disease on maternal and fetal outcome of pregnancy. **Journal of the American College of Cardiology**, 37:893–899
17. Tucker D, Liu D and Ramoutar P 1996 Myocardial infarction at term – a case report to consider management options. **Journal of Obstetrics and Gynaecology**, 16:522–524
18. Breast-feeding Network 2007 www.breast-feedingnetwork.org.uk/supporterline/medication.php
19. Niwa K and Tateno S 2006 Chapt.18 *Maternal cardiac arrhythmias* in Steer PJ, Gatzoulis M and Baker P (Eds) **Heart Disease in Pregnancy**. London; RCOG Press 251–265
20. Chan WS, Anand S and Ginsberg JS 2000 Anticoagulation of pregnant women with mechanical heart valves a systematic review of the literature. **Archives of Internal Medicine**, 160:191–196
21. Gilbert ES 2007 Chapt.11 *Cardiac disease* in Gilbert ES **High Risk Pregnancy and Delivery**; 4th Edn. London; Mosby/Elsevier 270–285

4.5 Marfan's syndrome

1. Lalchandani S and Wingfield M 2003 Pregnancy in women with Marfan's syndrome. **European Journal of Obstetrics Gynaecology and Reproductive Biology**, 110:125–130
2. Rubenstein D, Wayne D and Bradley J 2003 **Lecture Notes on Clinical Medicine**, 6th Edn. Oxford; Blackwell Publishing Ltd. 280–281
3. Marfan's Association 2007 Factsheet online marfan.org.uk/content/view/14/31/ [Accessed 02-09-2007]
4. Maxwell C, Poppas A, Sermer M and McGrady E 2010 Heart Disease in Pregnancy in Powie R, Greene M , Camann W (Eds) **De Sweit's Medical Disorders in Obstetric Practice**, 5th Edn. Oxford: Wiley-Blackwell 118-151
5. Chen H 2006 Marfan's Syndrome. www.emedicine.com/ped/topic1372.htm [Accessed 30-06-2007]
6. Pyeritz R 2000 The Marfan's syndrome. **Annual Review of Medicine**, 51:481–510
7. Kumar P and Clarke M 2002 **Clinical Medicine**, 5th Edn. London; Saunders/Elsevier 803–804
8. Swan L 2006 *Aortopathies including Marfan's syndrome and coarctation* in Steer P, Gatzoulis M and Baker P (Eds) **Heart Disease in Pregnancy**. London; RCOG Press
9. Stuart AG and Williams A 2007 Marfan's syndrome and the heart. **Archives of Disease in Childhood**, 92:351–356
10. Nelson-Piercy C 2010 **Handbook of Obstetric Medicine**, 2nd Edn. London; Martin Dunitz 27–28
11. Pacini L, Digne F, Boumendil A *et al.* 2009 Maternal complication of pregnancy in Marfan syndrome. **International Journal of Cardiology**, 136: 156–161
12. Ryan-Krause P 2002 Identify and manage Marfan's syndrome in children. **Nurse Practitioner**, 27:26–37
13. Gorland S,Barakat M, Khatri N ,Elkayam U 2009 Pregnancy in Marfan Syndrome. **Cardiology in Review**, 17:253–261
14. Regitz-Zagrosek V, Blomstrom Lundqvist C, Borghi C *et al.* 2011 ESC Guidelines on the management of cardiovascular diseases during pregnancy The Task Force on the Management of Cardiovascular Diseases during Pregnancy of the European Society of Cardiology (ESC) **European Heart Journal** doi:10.1093/eurheartj/ehr218 http://www.escardio.org/guidelines-surveys/esc-guidelines/Pages/cardiovascular-diseases-during-pregnancy.aspx [Accessed 27-8-2011]
15. Uebing A, Steer PJ, Yentis SM and Gatzoulis MA 2006 Pregnancy and congenital heart disease. **British Medical Journal**, 332:401–406
16. Elkayam U and Googdwin TM 1995 Adenosine therapy for supraventricular tachycardia during pregnancy. **American Journal of Cardiology**, 75:521–523
17. MEIJBOOM LI, Drenthen W, Pieper PG, *et al.* 2006 Obstetric complications in Marfan's syndrome. **International Journal of Cardiology**, 110:53–59
18. Nelson-Piercy C 2011 Chapt.9 *Cardiac disease* in Lewis G (Ed) 2011 **Saving Mothers Lives: Reviewing Maternal Deaths to Make Motherhood Safer. 2006–2008 BJOG** 118(supplement 1)
19. Rahman J, Rahman FZ, Rahman W, *et al.* 2003 Obstetric and gynecologic complications in women with Marfan's syndrome. **The Journal of Reproductive Medicine**, 48:723–728
20. Thorne S, Nelson-Piercy C, MacGregor A, *et al.* 2006 Pregnancy and contraception in heart disease and pulmonary arterial hypertension. **Journal of Family Planning and Reproductive Health Care**, 32:75–81
21. Oakley C, Child A, Jung B, *et al.* 2003 The task force on the management of cardiovascular disease during pregnancy of the European Society of Cardiology. **European Heart Journal**, 24:761–781
22. Durbridge J, Dresner M, Harding K and Yentis S 2006 Chapt.20 *Pregnancy and cardiac disease – peripartum aspects* in Steer P, Gatzoulis M and Baker P (Eds) **Heart Disease in Pregnancy**. London; RCOG Press 285–298

23. Fujitani S and Baldisseri M 2005 Hemodynamic assessment in a pregnant and peripartum patient. **Critical Care Medicine**, 33(Suppl. 10):S354–361
24. Witcher P and Harvey C 2006 Modifying labor routines for the woman with cardiac disease. **Journal of Perinatal and Neonatal Nursing**, 20:303–310
25. Dhanjal MK 2006 Chapt.2 Contraception in women with heart disease in Steer P, Gatzoulis M and Baker P (Eds) **Heart Disease in Pregnancy**. London; RCOG Press 9–28

4.6 Functional Heart Disease: Cardiomyopathy

1. Maron BJ 2002 Hypertrophic cardiomyopathy: a systematic review. **Journal of the American Medical Association**, 287:1308–1320
2. Nelson-Piercy C 2006 Chapt.16 *Cardiomyopathy* in Steer P, Gatzoulis M and Baker P (Eds) **Heart Disease in Pregnancy**. London; RCOG Press 231–242
3. Tan J 2004 Cardiovascular disease in pregnancy. **Current Obstetrics and Gynaecology**, 14:155–165
4. Valeriano C, Simbre VC II, Jacob Adams M, *et al.* 2001 Current treatment options. **Cardiovascular Medicine**, 3:493–505
5. Matthews T and Dickinson JE 2005 Considerations for delivery in pregnancies complicated by maternal hypertrophic obstructive cardiomyopathy. **Australian and New Zealand Journal of Obstetrics and Gynaecology**, 45:526–528
6. Autore C, Conte MR, Piccininno M, *et al.* 2002 Risk associated with pregnancy in hypertrophic cardiomyopathy. **Journal of the American College of Cardiology**, 40:1864–1869
7. Paix B, Cyna A, Belperio P and Simmons S 1999 Epidural analgesia for labour and delivery in a parturient with congenital hypertrophic obstructive cardiomyopathy. **Anaesthesia and Intensive Care**, 27:59–62
8. Macpherson G 2004 **Black's Student Medical Dictionary**. London; A and C Black Publishers
9. Nelson-Piercy C 2011 Chapt.9 *Cardiac disease* in Lewis G (Ed.) **Saving Mothers Lives: Reviewing Maternal Deaths to Make Motherhood Safer. 2006–2008 BJOG** 118(supplement 1)
10. Yacoub A and Martel MJ 2002 Pregnancy with primary dilated cardiomyopathy. **Obstetrics and Gynaecology**, 99:928–930
11. Elkayam U 2005 Valvular heart disease and pregnancy part 11: prosthetic valves. **Journal of the American College Cardiology**, 46:403–410
12. Murali S and Baldisseri M 2005 Peripartum cardiomyopathy. **Critical Care Medicine**, 33(Suppl.):S340–S346
13. Sliwa K, Hilfiker-Kleiner D, Petrie MC, *et al.* 2010 Current state of knowledge on aetiology, diagnosis management, and therapy of peripartum cardiomyopathy: a position statement from the Heart Failure Association of the European Society of Cardiology Working Group on peripartum cardiomyopathy. **European Journal of Heart Failure**, 12:767–778
14. Calin AJ, Alfievic Z and Gyte G 2010 interventions for treating peripartum cardiomyopathy to improve outcomes for mothers and babies **Cochrane Data Base of systematic Reviews** issue 9 art no CD008589.doi: 10.1002/14651858.CD008589.pub2
15. Dickstein K, Cohen-Solal A, Filippatos G *et al.* 2008 ESC guidelines for the diagnosis and treatment of acute and chronic heart failure. European Society of Cardiology. **European Jounral of Heart Failure**, 10:933–989.
16. Pyatt J and Dubey G (2011) Peripartum cardiomyopathy: current understanding,comprehensive management review and new developments. **Postgraduate Medical Journal**, 87:34e39. doi: 10.1136/pgmj.2009.096594
17. Ray P, Murphy GJ and Shutt LE 2004 Recognition and management of maternal cardiac disease in pregnancy. **British Journal of Anaesthesia**, 93:428–439
18. Regitz-Zagrosek V, Blomstrom Lundqvist C, Borghi C *et al.* 2011 ESC Guidelines on the management of cardiovascular diseases during pregnancy The Task Force on the Management of Cardiovascular Diseases during Pregnancy of the European Society of Cardiology (ESC). **European Heart Journal** doi:10.1093/eurheartj/ehr218
19. Hendricks CH and Brenner WE 1970 Cardiovascular effects of oxytocic drugs used post partum. **American Journal of Obstetrics and Gynecology**, 108:751–760

20. Durbridge J, Dresner M, Harding K and Yentis S 2006 *Pregnancy and cardiac disease – peripartum aspects* in Steer P, Gatzoulis M and Baker P (Eds) **Heart Disease in Pregnancy**. London; RCOG Press
21. Jordan S 2010 **Pharmacology for Midwives: The Evidence Base**, 2nd edition. London; Palgrave Macmillan
22. Ramsay M 2006 *Management of the puerperium in women with heart disease* in Steer P, Gatzoulis M and Baker P (Eds) **Heart Disease in Pregnancy**. London; RCOG Press 299–312
23. Elkayam U, Tummala P and Rao K 2001 Maternal and fetal outcomes of subsequent pregnancies in women with peripartum cardiomyopathy. **New England Journal of Medicine**, 344: 1567–1571
24. Elkayam U 2003 Pregnant again after peripartum cardiomyopathy: to be or not to be. **European Heart Journal**, 23:753–756

4.7 Functional Heart Disease: Arrhythmias

1. Niwa K and Tateno S 2006 Chapt.18 *Maternal cardiac arrhythmias* in Steer P, Gatzoulis M and Baker P (Eds) **Heart Disease in Pregnancy**. London; RCOG Press 251–265
2. Macpherson G 2004 **Black's Student Medical Dictionary**. London; A and C Black Publishers
3. Brodsky M, Doria R, Allen B, *et al.* 1992 New-onset ventricular tachycardia during pregnancy. **American Heart Journal**, 123:933–941
4. Ferrero S, Colombo BM and Ragni N 2004 Maternal arrhythmias in pregnancy. **Archives of Gynecology and Obstetrics**, 269:244–253
5. Trappe H 2006 Acute therapy maternal and fetal arrhythmias during pregnancy. **Journal of Intensive Care Medicine**, 21:305–315
6. Zevitz ME 2006 Ventricular Fibrillation www.emedicine.com/med/topic2363.htm [Accessed 27-6-2007]
7. Waldo A 2000 Electrophysiology: treatment of atrial flutter. **Heart**, 84:227
8. Conway D and Yip G 2003 **Atrial Physiology in Cardiac Arrhythmias – A Clinical Approach**. London; Mosby/Elsevier
9. Cox D and Dougall H 2001 Understanding ECGs – bradycardia. **Student BMJ**, 09:443–848 www.studentbmj.com/issues01/12/education /453;php
10. Blomstrom-Lundqvist C, Scheinman MM, Aliot EM, *et al.* 2003 ACC/AHA/ESC Guidelines for the management of patients with supraventricular arrhythmias – executive summary: a report of the American College of Cardiology/American Heart Association Task Force on Practice Guidelines and the European Society of Cardiology Committee for Practice Guidelines. **Circulation**, 108:1871–1909
11. Rotmensch H, Rotmensch S and Elkayam U 1987 Management of cardiac arrhythmias during pregnancy, current concepts. **Drugs**, 33:623–633
12. Bartalena L, Bogazzi F, Braverman LE and Martino E 2001 Effects of amiodarone administration during pregnancy on neonatal thyroid function and subsequent neurodevelopment. **Journal of Endocrinological Investigation**, 1:116–130
13. Devendra K, Ching CK, Tan LK, Tan HK and Yu SL 2006 Intrapartum maternal sinus bradycardia with spontaneous resolution following delivery. **Singapore Medical Journal**, 47:971–974
14. Silversides CK, Coleman JM, Sermer M and Siu SC 2003 Cardiac risk in pregnant women with rheumatic mitral stenosis. **American Journal of Cardiology**, 91:182–185
15. Elkayam U, Googdwin TM 1995 Adenosine therapy for supraventricular tachycardia during pregnancy. **American Journal of Cardiology**, 75: 521–523
16. Regitz-Zagrosek V, Blomstrom Lundqvist C, Borghi C *et al.* 2011 ESC Guidelines on the management of cardiovascular diseases during pregnancy The Task Force on the Management of Cardiovascular Diseases during Pregnancy of the European Society of Cardiology (ESC) **European Heart Journal** doi:10.1093/eurheartj/ehr218http://www.escardio.org/guidelines-surveys/esc-guidelines/Pages/cardiovascular-diseases-during-pregnancy.aspx [Accessed 27-8-2011]
17. Mark S and Harris L 2002 *Arrhythmias in pregnancy* in Wilansky S (Ed.) **Heart Disease in Women**. Philadelphia; Churchill/Elsevier 497–514

18. Lee S, Chen SA, Wu TJ, *et al.* 1995 Effects of pregnancy on first onset and symptoms of paroxysmal supraventricular tachycardia. **American Journal of Cardiology**, 76; 675–678

19. Fuster V, Ryden LE, Asinger RW, *et al.* 2001 ACC/AHA/ESC Guidelines for the management of patients with atrial fibrillation: executive summary – a report of the American College of Cardiology/American Heart Association Task Force on Practice Guidelines. **Circulation**, 104:2118–2150

20. Tomlinson M 2006 Chapt.37 *Cardiac disease* in James D, Steer P, Weiner C and Gonik B (Eds) **High Risk Pregnancy: Management Options**, 3rd Edn. London; Elsevier 790–827

21. Wolbrette D 2005 Arrhythmias during pregnancy a therapeutic challenge – business briefing. **Women's Health Care**, 51–55

22. Lip G, Hart RG and Conway DSG 2002 ABC of antithrombotic therapy: antithrombotic therapy for atrial fibrillation. **British Medical Journal**, 325(7371):1022–1025

4.8 Ischaemic Heart Disease: Angina and Myocardial Infarction

1. Roos-Hesselink JW 2006 *Ischaemic heart disease* in Steer P, Gatzoulis M and Baker P (Eds) **Heart Disease in Pregnancy**. London; RCOG Press 243–250

2. Nelson-Piercy C 2011 Chapt.9 *Cardiac disease* in Lewis G (Ed) 2011 **Saving Mothers Lives: Reviewing Maternal Deaths to Make Motherhood Safer. 2006–2008 BJOG** 118(supplement 1)

3. RCOG 2011 **Cardiac Disease and Pregnancy Good Practice Guideline No 13** London; RCOG

4. James AH, Abel DE and Brancazio LR 2006 Anticoagulants in pregnancy. **Obstetrical and Gynecological Survey**, 61;59–69

5. Anderson C 2007 Pre-eclampsia: exposing future cardiovascular risk in mothers and their children. **Journal of Obstetric, Gynecologic and Neonatal Nursing**, 36:3–8

6. Roth A and Elkayam U 1996 Acute myocardial infarction associated with pregnancy. **Annals of Internal Medicine**, 125:751–762

7. James AH, Jamison MG, Biswas MS, Brancazio LR, Swamy JK, Myers ER 2006 Acute myocardial infarction in pregnancy – a United States population based study. **Circulation**, 133: 1564–1571

8. Maxwell C, Poppas A, Sermer M ,McGrady E. 2010 *Heart disease in pregnancy* in Powie R, Greene M, Camann W (Eds) **De Sweit's Medical Disorders in Obstetric Practice** 5th Edn. Oxford; Wiley Blackwell 118–151

9. Ray P, Murphy GJ and Shutt LE 2004 Recognition and management of maternal cardiac disease in pregnancy. **British Journal of Anaesthesia**, 93: 428–439

10. Tomlinson M 2010 Chapt.36 *Cardiac disease* in James DK, Steer PJ, Weiner CP, Gonik B, Crowther C and Robson S (Eds) **High Risk Pregnancy Management Options**, 4th Edn. London; Elsevier 790–827

11. Gelson E, Gatzoulis MA, Steer P, Johnson MR 2009 Heart disease: why is maternal mortality increasing? **BJOG**, 116:609-611

12. Neilson Piercy C, Chakravarti S 2007 Cardiac disease and pregnancy. **Anaesthesia and Intensive Care Medicine**, 8:312–316

13. Marini J and Wheeler A 2006 **Critical Care Medicine**, 3rd Edn. Philadelphia; Lippincott/Williams and Wilkins

14. Tsui BC, Stewart B, Fitzmaurice A and Williams R 2001 Cardiac arrest and myocardial infarction induced by post partum intravenous ergonovine administration. **Anaesthesiology**, 94: 363–364

15. Shieikh AU and Harper MA 1993 Myocardial infarction during pregnancy management and outcome of two pregnancies. **American Journal of Obstetrics and Gynecology**, 169:279–284

16. McKechnie RS, Patel D, Eitzman DT, Rajagopalan S and Murthy TH 2001 Spontaneous coronary artery dissection in a pregnant woman. **Obstetrics and Gynaecology**, 98:899–902

17. Rubenstein D, Wayne D and Bradley J 2003 **Lecture Notes on Clinical Medicine**, 6th Edn. Oxford; Blackwell Publishing Ltd. 264

18. Blake MJ, Martin A, Manktelow BN *et al.* 2000 Changes in baroreceptor sensitivity for heart rate during normotensive pregnancy and the puerperium. **Clin Sci (Lond)**, 98: 259–268

19. Foley M, Lockwood C, Gersh B and Bass V 2010 **Maternal cardiovascular and hemodynamic adaptation to pregnancy. Uptodate**

4.9 Pulmonary Hypertension and Eisenmenger's Syndrome

1. D'Alonzo GE, Barst RJ, Ayres SM, *et al.* 1991 Survival in patients with primary pulmonary hypertension: results from a national prospective registry. **Annals of Internal Medicine**, 115:343–349

2. Simon J and Gibbs R 2001 Recommendations on the management of pulmonary hypertension in clinical practice. **Heart**, 86(Suppl. 1):i1–i13

3. Rich S, Dantzker DR, Ayres SM, *et al.* 1987 Primary pulmonary hypertension. A national perspective study. **Annals of Internal Medicine**, 197:216–223

4. Simonneau G, Galie N, Rubin LJ, Langleben D, Seeger W, *et al.* 2004 Clinical classification of pulmonary hypertension. **Journal of the American College of Cardiology**, 43(12 supplements): 5s–12s

5. Nichols WC, Koller DL, Slovis B, *et al.* 1997 Localization of the gene for familial primary pulmonary hypertension to chromosome 2q31–32. **Nature Genetics**, 15:277–280

6. Gaille N, Ghofrani HA, Torbicki A, *et al.* 2005 Sildenafil citrate therapy for pulmonary arterial hypertension. **New England Journal of Medicine**, 353:2148–2157

7. Abenhaim L, Moride Y, Brenot F, *et al.* 1996 Appetite-suppressant drugs and the risk of primary pulmonary hypertension. International Primary Pulmonary Hypertension Study Group. **New England Journal of Medicine**, 335:609–661

8. Kiely D, Elliot C, Webster V and Stewart P 2006 *Pregnancy and pulmonary hypertension: new approaches to management* in Steer P, Gatzoulis M and Baker P (Eds) **Heart Disease in Pregnancy**. London; RCOG Press

9. Bedard E, Dimopoulos K, Gatzoulis MA 2009 Has there been any progress made on pregnancy outcomes among women with pulmonary hypertension? **European Heart Journal**, 30:256–265

10. Naguib MA, Dob DP and Gatzoulis MA 2010 A functional understanding of moderate to complex congenital heart disease and the impact of pregnancy. Part II: Tetralogy of Fallot, Eisenmenger's syndrome and the Fontan operation. **International Journal of Obstetric Anesthesia**, 19;306–312

11. **Pulmonary Hypertension Association** www.pha–uk.com/ [Accessed 17-05-2007]

12. Thorne S, Nelson-Piercy C, MacGregor A, *et al.* 2006 Pregnancy and contraception in heart disease and pulmonary arterial hypertension. **Journal of Family Planning and Reproductive Health Care**, 32:75–81

13. Bedard E, Dimopoulos K and Gatzoulis MA.2009 Has there been any progress made on pregnancy outcomes among women with pulmonary arterial hypertension? **European Heart Journal**, 30:256–265

14. Tomlinson M 2006 Chapt.37 *Cardiac disease* in James DK, Steer PJ, Weiner CP and Gonik B (Eds) **High Risk Pregnancy**, 3rd Edn. London; Elsevier 790–827

15. Parneix M, Faonou L, Morau E and Colson P 2009 Low-dose combined spinal-epidural anaesthesia for caesarean section in a patient with Eisenmenger's syndrome. **International Journal of Obstetric Anaesthesia**, 18:81–84

16. Campbell P and Rudisill P 2006 Psychological needs of the critically ill obstetric patient. **Critical Care Nursing**, 29:77–80

17. Blake MJ, Martin A, Manktelow BN *et al.* 2000 Changes in baroreceptor sensitivity for heart rate during normotensive pregnancy and the puerperium. **Clinical Science (London)**, 98:259–268

18. Foley M, Lockwood C, Gersh B and Barss V **2010 Maternal cardiovascular and hemodynamic adaptation to pregnancy. Uptodate**

19. Weiss BM, Zemp L, Seifert B and Hess OM 1998 Outcome of pulmonary vascular disease in pregnancy: a systematic overview from 1978 through to 1996. **Journal of the American College of Cardiology**, 31:1650–1657

4.10 Heart Transplant

1. Mukherjee S and Shapiro R 2009 Transplantation and Pregnancy. http://emedicine.medscape.com/article/429932-overview #aw2aab6b5 [Accessed 1-9-2011]

2. Troché V, Ville Y, Frydman R and Fernandez H 1997 Pregnancy after heart and heart-lung transplantation. A series of 10 cases

and a review of the literature. **Journal de Gynecologie Obstetrique et Biologie de la Reproduction**, 26;597–605

3. Miniero R, Tardivo I. Centofanti P *et al.* 2004 Pregnancy in heart transplant recipients. **The Journal of Heart and Lung Transplantation**, 23;898–901

4. Subramaniam P and Robson R 2008 Heart transplant and Pregnancy. **O&G Magazine** 10:832–34

5. Wu DW, Wilt J and Restaino S 2007 Pregnancy after thoracic organ transplantation. **Seminars in Perinatology**, 31;354–362

6. Alston PK, Kuller JA and McMahon MJ 2001 Pregnancy in transplant recipients. **Obstetrical and Gynecological Survey**, 56:289–295

7. Douglas NC, Shah M and Sauer MV 2007 Fertility and reproductive disorders in female solid organ transplant recipients. **Seminars in Perinatology**, 31;332–338

8. UK transplant organization [Accessed 7-12-2011] http://www.uktransplant.org.uk/ukt/statistics/transplant_activity_report/current_activity_reports/ukt/cardiothoracic_activity.pdf

9. Sibanda N, Briggs JD, Davison JM *et al.* 2007 Pregnancy after organ transplantation: a report from the UK. Transplant Pregnancy Registry. **Transplantation**, 83:1301–1307

10. Jason D, Christie LB *et al.* 2011 The Registry of the International Society for Heart and Lung Transplantation: Twenty-eighth Adult Lung and Heart-Lung Transplant Report; **The Journal of Heart and Lung Transplantation**, 30:1104–1122

11. Braun-Parvez L, Charlin E, Caillard S *et al.* 2010 Gestational choriocarcinoma transmission following multiorgan donation. **American Journal of Transplantation**, 10:2541–2546

12. Estensen M, Gude E, Ekmehag B *et al.* 2011 Pregnancy in heart- and heart/lung recipients can be problematic. **Scandinavian Cardiovascular Journal**, 45;349–353

13. Armenti VT, Constantinescu S, Moritz MJ and Davison JM 2008 Pregnancy after transplantation. **Transplant Review**, 22:223–240

14. Lo Giudice P, Dubourg L, Hadj-Aïssa A, Saïd *et al.* 2000 Renal function of children exposed to cyclosporin in utero. **Nephrology Dialysis Transplantation**, 150:1575–1579

15. Nulman I, Sgro M, Barrera M *et al.* 2010 Long-term neurodevelopment of children exposed in utero to ciclosporin after maternal renal transplant. **Pediatric Drugs**, 12:113–122

16. Armenti V, Moritz M and Davison J 2011 Chapt. 53 Pregnancy after transplantation in James D (Ed.) **High Risk Pregnancy Management Options** 4th Edn. London; Elsevier 961–972

17. Dashe JS, Ramin KD and Ramin SM 1998 Pregnancy following cardiac transplantation. **Primary Care Update for Ob/Gyns**, 5:257–262

18. Maxwell C, Poppas A, Sermer M, McGrady E 2010 Heart disease in pregnancy in Powie R, Greene M and Camann W (Eds) **De Sweit's Medical Disorders in Obstetric Practice** 5th Edn. Oxford: Wiley-Blackwell 118–151

19. Rigg CD, Bythell VE, Bryson MR and Davidson JM (2000) Caesarean section in patients with heart-lung transplants: a report of three cases and review. **International Journal of Obstetric Anesthesia**, 9:125–132

Figure Reference

All figures in this chapter were adapted, with permission from Wiley-Blackwell, from Meeks M, Hallsworth M and Yeo H 2010 **Nursing the Neonate,** 2nd Edn.

Appendix References

Appendix 4.3.1 Drugs for Cardiac Disease – an Overview for Midwives

1. Briggs GG, Freeman RK and Yaffe SJ 2008 **Drugs in Pregnancy and Lactation**, 8th Edn. USA; Lippincott

2. Ostensen M, Khamashta M, Lockshin M, *et al.* 2006 Anti-inflammatory and immunosuppressive drugs and reproduction. **Arthritis Research and Therapy**, 8:209–228 http://arthritis-research.com/content/8/3/209

3. MIMS 2011 **Monthly Index of Medical Specialities**, March.. London; Haymarket Medical Publications

4. Steer PJ, Gatzoulis MA and Barker P (Eds) 2006 **Heart Disease and Pregnancy**. London; RCOG Press

5. **British National Formulary** 2011 online www.bnf.org

Appendix 4.3.1 Drugs for Cardiac Disease – An Overview for Midwives

This table is to give the midwife an **overview** of cardiac drug use and the implications for pregnancy. These drugs are prescribed, by a doctor, if the expected benefit to the mother outweighs any effect upon the fetus (see legend).

Type of Drug	Name	Risk		Notes
		Pregnancy[1]	Breast-feeding	
Diuretics to reduce fluid retention	Amiloride	B	Probably compatible[1]	
	Bumetanide	C	Probably compatible[1]	Used for prompt diuresis[3]
	Chlorothiazide	C	Compatible[1]	
	Furosemide/frusemide	C	Probably compatible[1]	
	Spironolactone	C	Probably compatible[1]	
ACE inhibitors to lower BP and treat heart failure	Captopril	C	Compatible[1]	Teratogenic risk in first trimester (animal studies) and fetal renal toxicity in second and third trimesters (human data)[1,3,5]. Most cardiologists stop ACE inhibitors promptly pre-conception and restart them post delivery
	Enalapril	C	Probably compatible[1]	
	Lisinopril	C	Probably compatible[1]	
	Losartan	C	Probably compatible[1]	
	Ramipril	C	Probably compatible[1]	
	Valsartan	C	Probably compatible[1]	
Beta-blockers to reduce frequency/force of the heartbeat, treat heart failure, lower BP	Atenolol	D	Potential toxicity[1]	All may cause minor growth restriction[1,3,5] in second and third trimesters, but this is rarely of clinical significance. Some are excreted to a lesser extent than others in breast milk, hence a prescriber should seek individual drug details
	Carvedilol	C	Potential toxicity[1]	
	Metoprolol	C	Potential toxicity[1]	
	Nadolol	C	Potential toxicity[1]	
	Propranolol	C	Potential toxicity[1]	
	Sotalol	B	Potential toxicity[1]	
Nitrates to dilate coronary arteries	Glyceryl trinitrate/nitroglycerin	B	Probably compatible[1]	
	Isosorbide mono-/dinitrate	C	Probably compatible[1]	
Anti-arrhythmics to steady an irregular heartbeat	Adenosine	C	Probably compatible[1]	Maternal benefit >> fetal risk[1]
	Amiodarone	**D**	**Contraindicated**[1]	Pregnancy risk
	Bretylium	C	Hold breast-feeding[1]	No pregnancy data[1]
	Digoxin/digitalis	C	Compatible[1]	
	Disopyramide	C	Probably compatible[1]	Risk in 3rd trimester[1]
	Flecainide	C	Probably compatible[1]	Moderate risk[1]
	Verapamil	C	Probably compatible[1]	
Anticoagulants	Aspirin – low dose	Safe[2]	Safe[2]	See NSAIDs in Appendix 11.1.1
	Aspirin – standard	C	Use with caution[1]	
	Heparin	C	Compatible[1]	Does not pass to placenta or breast[1]
	Dalteparin	B	Compatible[1]	Low molecular weight heparins
	Enoxaparin	B		
	Warfarin	**D** or **X**	Compatible[1]	One manufacturer rates X[1] Contraindicated in first trimester[1]
Antihypertensives to lower blood pressure	Doxazocin	C	Potential toxicity[1]	
	Methyldopa	B	Probably compatible[1]	
	Nifedipine	C	Probably compatible[1]	See vasodilators in Appendix 11.1.1
	Nicardipine	C	Probably compatible[1]	
Others to treat pulmonary hypertension	Prostacycline/epoprostenol	B	Probably compatible[1]	
	Sildenafil (Viagra; Revatio)	No data	No data	
	Bosentan	X	**Contraindicated**[5]	Contraindicated pregnancy/lactation[3,5]

Key: Pregnancy risk factors[1]: **A** = Little or no risk (human studies)[1]; **B** = Little risk (animal studies)[1]; **C** = Some adverse effects (animal studies); used if benefit outweighs risk[1]; **D** = Positive evidence of risk (human studies); used with serious conditions[1]; **X** = Risk outweighs possible benefits, contraindicated in pregnancy[1]

Midwives: Mothers should be advised to continue with existing medication until a doctor with experience of prescribing such medications in pregnancy has been consulted, because sudden cessation of any medication without careful thought for substitution can be associated with adverse feto-maternal outcome.

Doctors: This simple table cannot address factors for prescribing, and a more authoritative source **must** be used, e.g.

- **British National Formulary**, latest issue from the BMA, or on-line www.bnf.org.
- Briggs GG, Freeman RK and Yaffe SJ (2008) **Drugs in Pregnancy and Lactation**, 8th Edn. USA; Lippincott.

RESPIRATORY DISORDERS

Jane Scullion[1], Christopher Brightling[2] and Michelle Goldie

[1,2]University Hospitals of Leicester NHS Trust, Leicester, UK

5.1 The Breathless Pregnant Woman

5.2 Asthma

5.3 Pneumonia and Chest Infections

5.4 Tuberculosis

5.5 Cystic Fibrosis

5.6 Sarcoidosis

Medical Disorders in Pregnancy: A Manual for Midwives, Second Edition. Edited by S. Elizabeth Robson and Jason Waugh.
© 2013 John Wiley & Sons, Ltd. Published 2013 by John Wiley & Sons, Ltd.

5.1 The Breathless Pregnant Woman

Incidence/prevalence	Risk for Childbearing
60–70% pregnant women, either as a normal physiological response or due to underlying pathology	Low Risk – physiological causes Variable Risk – pathological causes

EXPLANATION OF CONDITION

Breathlessness is the sensation of feeling *out-of-breath* or unable to *catch your breath*. The normal respiratory rate is 12–20 breaths/minute at rest. A persistent respiratory rate at rest >24 breaths/minute is abnormal[1].

Breathlessness in pregnancy is extremely common and may reflect the normal anatomical and physiological changes that occur in pregnancy or may be a consequence of an underlying pathology.

The normal changes of pregnancy that may influence the respiratory rate, perception of breathlessness and decreased exercise capacity comprise:

- Increase in weight
- Elevation of the diaphragm by up to 4 cm, although its excursion is not impaired
- Capillary enlargement throughout the respiratory tract with increased mucosal oedema and hyperaemia
- Increased transverse and antero-posterior diameter leading to an increase in the sub-costal angle and up to 7 cm increase in chest circumference
- 20% increase in oxygen consumption
- 15% increase in maternal metabolic rate
- Increased tidal volume but normal respiratory rate
- Increased progesterone leading to hyperventilation
- Increased free cortisol

Pathological Causes of Breathlessness

- Respiratory disease:
  - asthma
  - chest infection and/or pneumonia
  - thrombo-embolic disease
  - interstitial lung disease, e.g. sarcoid or secondary to a connective tissue disorder
  - pneumothorax
  - amniotic fluid embolism
- Cardiac disease:
  - arrhythmias
  - ischaemic heart disease
  - cardiomyopathy
- Endocrine disease:
  - diabetes mellitus leading to hyperventilation in the setting of acute ketoacidosis
  - acute thyrotoxicosis
- Haematological:
  - chronic anaemia
  - acute haemorrhage
- Renal disease:
  - hyperventilation to compensate for metabolic acidosis secondary to acute renal failure

This list is not exhaustive and further details on all of these conditions are outlined in the relevant chapters.

COMPLICATIONS

Breathlessness is experienced by 60–70% of women during pregnancy, especially in the second and third trimesters. Physiological breathlessness does not cause complications.

Breathlessness due to a pathological cause can result in complications and these are detailed in the chapters relating to specific conditions.

NON-PREGNANCY TREATMENT AND CARE

Breathlessness is a normal physiological response to exercise. However, breathlessness at rest and breathlessness in response to minimal exercise out of proportion to an individual's normal level of fitness needs to be investigated. When a pathological cause of breathlessness is suspected, a detailed history and examination need to be taken.

First line investigations should include:

- Full blood count
- Renal function
- Glucose
- Simple lung function tests
- Urine dipstick
- Chest radiograph

Additional tests may include:

- D-dimers
- ECG
- Full lung function tests
- Thyroid function tests
- Computed tomography of the chest, with or without pulmonary angiography
- Echocardiogram
- Detailed cardiopulmonary exercise testing

Treatment should be directed at the specific cause. In the setting of hyperventilation, physiotherapy to instruct patients in breathing control techniques may be of benefit.

PRE-CONCEPTION ISSUES AND CARE

Whether the cause of breathlessness has pre-conception implications is dependent upon the cause of the breathlessness, and the reader needs to refer to the individual chapters on the management of specific conditions that can cause breathlessness.

Strongly encourage smoking cessation.

Pregnancy Issues

In most cases breathlessness in pregnancy is due to a normal physiological response[2]. Pathological causes need to be considered when there is a clinical suspicion.

The risk–benefit ratio of investigations for breathlessness needs to be evaluated. Most radiological investigations expose the woman and baby to radiation, which needs to be minimised, but chest radiography is generally regarded as safe.

In extreme circumstances, in the setting of respiratory failure, whether the woman and baby are sufficiently oxygenated needs to be considered.

Medical Management and Care

- If a pathological cause is suspected the woman needs to be investigated[2] and, in particular, conditions that are more common in pregnancy, e.g. pulmonary emboli, need to be considered
- Treatment needs to be specific for the cause of breathlessness but the potential risks of treatment need to be considered, e.g. antibiotic choice for pneumonia
- Details of the management of specific conditions are outlined in the other relevant chapters

Midwifery Management and Care

- The midwifery care needs to be tailored to the woman's needs[3]. This should be focused on education through antenatal care and support for physiological breathlessness. With pathological breathlessness this will involve referral to a consultant obstetrician to assess the woman's case and need for further investigations
- Regular antenatal appointments with the community midwife to ensure that the baby is not compromised and to ensure the woman's health does not deteriorate
- At all stages of pregnancy, whether at the booking visit or mid-trimester the midwife must recognise any complications and give full explanations of these and potential consequences to the mother. This is important in order for her to make informed decisions about where she may want to give birth. If she had intended to give birth at home or in a midwifery-led unit this may not be the most appropriate place

Labour Issues

Breathlessness is very common in labour, but breathlessness in early labour that is not associated with contractions is unusual. This, together with other symptoms or abnormal vital signs should alert the carer to potential pathological causes of breathlessness.

Early referral to a doctor is indicated in the setting of pathological breathlessness because delivery options need review.

Medical Management and Care

- In the setting of pathological breathlessness, augmented labour or early caesarean section may need to be considered

Midwifery Management and Care

- On admission to delivery suite the midwife needs to make an initial assessment of her immediate condition and needs
- This should involve basic observations – recording of maternal pulse, blood pressure, temperature and respiratory rate
- Take a detailed history taking into account any investigations which may recently have been carried out
- Carry out abdominal palpation and auscultation of the fetal heart. If maternal or fetal observations are outside of normal parameters then the midwife should refer to a doctor for further advice. This is also true if the woman has been admitted to a midwifery-led unit or is labouring at home
- If pathological breathlessness is suspected then the baby needs to be continuously monitored with maternal vital signs recorded at more frequent intervals

Postpartum Issues

Breathlessness in the postpartum period is unusual and is likely to reflect a pathological cause such as pulmonary emboli or haemorrhage.

Breathlessness in combination with changes in vital signs is suggestive of a serious complication. The move towards early discharge after delivery places even more importance on the postnatal examination by the midwife in the community.

Medical Management and Care

- Postpartum breathlessness should be taken seriously
- It is important to be mindful of the potential pathological causes of postpartum breathlessness, e.g. pulmonary emboli or anaemia
- A low threshold for seeking further medical advice is required

Midwifery Management and Care

- The midwife needs to be mindful of the potential seriousness of a woman with postpartum breathlessness
- A mother with signs of breathlessness should not be discharged from hospital without having first had a medical review
- Once home, thorough postnatal examinations with astute observation of the physical condition should be conducted. Where necessary instigate appropriate investigations and refer to the primary care physician, or as an emergency to hospital, as warranted

5.2 Asthma

Incidence	Risk for Childbearing
10–15% of UK children and 5–10% of UK adults[1] 3–12% of pregnant women[2]	Variable Risk

EXPLANATION OF CONDITION

Asthma is a common condition in western societies, affecting 5–15% of the population and its prevalence and incidence are increasing.

Asthma is a chronic inflammatory disease of the airways, which is characterised by intermittent episodes of wheeze, shortness of breath, chest tightness and cough. It is a variable disease in which, in response to certain stimuli, or triggers, inflammation and structural changes occur in the lungs. This causes airway hyper-responsiveness and variable airflow obstruction leading to the symptoms described. Symptoms of asthma tend to be variable, intermittent and worse at night.

Patients suffer from *flare-ups* or exacerbations of their disease either in response to an acute infection, which is usually viral in origin, or due to poor control of their airway inflammation.

Triggers for Asthma

- Smoking
- Allergens, e.g. house dust mite, pollen, etc.
- Exercise
- Occupational exposure
- Pollution
- Drugs, e.g. aspirin, beta-blockers, including eye drops and as part of an anaphylactic response to other drugs
- Food and drinks such as dairy produce, alcohol, peanuts and orange juice
- Additives such as monosodium glutamate and tartrazine
- Medical conditions, e.g. rhinitis and gastric reflux
- Hormonal, e.g. pre-menstrual conditions and pregnancy

There is a strong link between asthma and atopy (the tendency to become sensitised to allergens and to develop allergic disease).

COMPLICATIONS

Asthma is a major burden not only on the patient, but also for health care provision and on society, causing time off work.

There are currently around 1500 asthma deaths per year. Many factors are believed to be responsible for these, including:

- A long history of asthma
- Marked peak flow variability
- Non-adherence to medication, especially inhaled corticosteroids
- Psychosocial problems
- Previous admissions with asthma, particularly if ventilated or if life-threatening features were present

The majority of asthma deaths occur in patients who present late for treatment, often despite having symptoms. Poor patient education, an underestimation of the severity of the asthma by both the patient and the health care professional, and inappropriate treatments have also been implicated in asthma deaths. On occasion, fatal attacks occur rapidly with little time for intervention, but this is uncommon[3].

NON-PREGNANCY TREATMENT AND CARE

British Thoracic Society (BTS) guidelines for the management of asthma have been in existence since the 1990s. These are now living guidelines and can be accessed through the BTS website (www.brit-thoracic.org.uk).

Aims of Asthma Management

- Control of symptoms
- Prevention of exacerbation
- Achievement of the best pulmonary function for the patient with minimal side effects

Good Asthma Care[4]

- Correct diagnosis: a history consistent with a diagnosis of asthma, supported by objective tests and after consideration of possible differential diagnoses
- Control of symptoms
- Pharmacological management – in a stepwise manner
- Non-pharmacological management: avoidance of triggers[3,5]
- Smoking cessation advice: to avoid fixed airway obstruction in later life[6]
- Self-management: essential for any chronic disease[5]

In a third of patients symptoms will get better, in a third symptoms will worsen and in a third they will stay the same.

PRE-CONCEPTION ISSUES AND CARE

It is important that women with asthma are optimally managed in the pre-conception period. The treatment may require review, and the woman might need to be re-referred to a specialist clinic. The Royal College of Physicians suggests three questions[3], which can be incorporated as part of the woman's assessment:

- Have you had difficulty sleeping because of your asthma symptoms, including a cough?
- Have you had your usual asthma symptoms during the day, such as a cough, wheeze, chest tightness or breathlessness?
- Has your asthma interfered with your usual activities, e.g. housework, work, school, etc.?

Pregnancy Issues
- Poorly-controlled asthma confers an increased risk to the mother and fetus[2,6]
- Asthmatic women are more at risk of low birth weight neonates, pre-term delivery and complications such as pre-eclampsia, especially in the absence of actively managed asthma treated with inhaled corticosteroids[2]
- There is no contraindication to most first-line treatments for asthma when used in pregnancy
- Smoking cessation is an important part of general obstetric advice, but is important in asthma to reduce symptoms and the efficacy of inhaled corticosteroids is reduced in asthmatics who smoke
- Carrying a female fetus has been associated with worse maternal asthma. (Kwon HL, Belanger K, Holford TR et al. in BTS Sign)
- Studies reported in the BTS guidance suggest 11–18% of pregnant women with asthma will have at least one emergency department visit for acute asthma and of these 62% will require admission

Medical Management and Care
Details about the management of asthma are available in the BTS/SIGN guidelines (see Essential Reading this chapter).
- It is important to optimise the control of the woman's asthma, as this will reduce the potential of asthma-related morbidity during pregnancy. This includes addressing issues related to trigger factors and adherence to medication
- Inhaled corticosteroids alone or in combination with long-acting bronchodilators are safe in pregnancy
- Leukotriene antagonists are relatively contraindicated in pregnancy due to the lack of information about possible teratogenic effects. These medications are rarely a critical part of asthma care and therefore should not be initiated in pregnancy. Alternative therapy should be considered
- Oral corticosteroids should be used for acute severe exacerbations
- Maintenance systemic corticosteroids should be reserved for women with severe refractory asthma and need to be reviewed by respiratory and obstetric specialists

Midwifery Management and Care
- Pregnancy does not appear to have a consistent effect on asthma control, which can either worsen or improve. Hence, it should be stressed to the woman that well-controlled asthma is *better for baby* and pregnancy outcomes
- Explain that asthma medication is generally safe in pregnancy
- Education about good control and adherence to medication is an essential part of early antenatal care[8]
- In unstable asthma, shared care with obstetrician, midwife and GP is advisable
- Advise women who smoke about the dangers and give appropriate advice about smoking cessation
- Encourage attendance at parent-craft and relaxation classes
- Reinforce health education advice with appropriate leaflets (see Appendix 5.2.1 for an example)

Labour Issues
- Acute, severe or life-threatening exacerbations of asthma during labour are extremely rare
- Women who have been on regular oral steroids may require hydrocortisone during labour
- Ergometrine[6], Syntometrine and prostaglandin may cause bronchoconstriction and should be used with caution

Medical Management and care
- In the absence of acute asthma, caesarean section should only be carried out when indicated
- If anaesthesia is required then an epidural is preferential to a general anaesthetic[6]

Midwifery Management and Care
- Advise women that acute asthma is rare in labour
- Women should continue their usual asthma medications in labour
- A mother who has well-controlled asthma should be able to have low risk care, with labour managed normally by the midwife
- Normal pain relief can be given and Entonox is considered safe[6]
- Syntocinon is the preferable drug for active third stage management

Postpartum Issues
Primary care physicians (GPs) can manage most women with asthma, but women with severe disease, particularly if systemic corticosteroids are considered, need to be managed by respiratory physicians.

WHO recommends women should exclusively breast-feed for at least 6 months[7]. Whether breast-fed children have a reduced risk of developing allergic disease including asthma is contentious, but this does not detract from the overwhelming benefit of breast-feeding.

Medical Management and Care
- Women need to continue on their regular medication
- It is unusual for asthma to become uncontrolled in the immediate postpartum period
- Generally there are no changes in therapy requirements

Midwifery Management and Care
- Breast-feeding should be discussed in the antenatal period for the mother to gain greater awareness of the long-term health benefits of breast-feeding and feel more confident to try breast-feeding
- Advise the mother that food allergy appears less likely if foods are introduced at a later stage
- As outlined for medical care above, standard asthma therapy can be used as normal during breast-feeding[6]

5.3 Pneumonia and Chest Infections

Incidence	Risk for Childbearing
4:1000 per year – higher in older people	Variable Risk – except in the rare circumstances of severe pneumonia or unusual complications

EXPLANATION OF CONDITION

Pneumonia is an acute infection within the lower respiratory tract occurring twice as often in the winter months as in the summer.

COMPLICATIONS

Most cases of pneumonia are not severe and can be easily managed at home with appropriate rest and, if necessary, antibiotics. Complications are unusual but include:

- Severe respiratory failure requiring ventilatory support and admission to intensive care
- Parapneumonic pleural effusion and empyema which may require pleural intubation and drainage and sometimes surgery for decortication
- Abscess formation and embolic abscesses
- Generalised septicaemia

NON-PREGNANCY TREATMENT AND CARE

British Thoracic Society guidelines for the management of community-acquired pneumonia[1] have been in existence since the 1990s. These are now living guidelines and can be accessed through the BTS website (www.brit-thoracic.org.uk).

The treatment of pneumonia is guided by an assessment of the severity of the pneumonia and knowledge of the likely causative pathogens[1]. This is often influenced by host factors, epidemiological or circumstantial factors and geographical variations.

In adults, 70% of community-acquired pneumonia cases are caused by bacteria; atypical bacteria cause 20% of cases, and 10% of cases are viral. *Streptococcus pneumoniae* is the commonest pathogen found in around half of identified cases. Other pathogens will vary in importance in relation to host or environmental factors.

Hospital-acquired pneumonia is unusual in pregnancy and mostly affects the elderly in hospital with multiple medical problems. Hospital-acquired pneumonia is often due to the aspiration of bacteria which then colonises the upper respiratory tract, often in association with impaired immunological and mechanical host defences[2].

Assessment

Severity of pneumonia is assessed by scoring one point for each of these factors that are present[1]:

- Confusion
- Urea >7 mmol/l
- Respiratory rate $\geq$30/min
- Blood pressure (systolic <90 mmHg or diastolic $\leq$60 mmHg)
- Age $\geq$65 years

Interpretation of score:

- 0–1: likely suitable for home treatment
- 2: consider supervised hospital treatment
  - short stay in-patient
  - hospital supervised out-patient
- >3: manage in hospital as severe pneumonia
- 4–5: assess for intensive care unit admission

Treatment

Treatment includes supportive care such as bed-rest, analgesia, anti-pyretics, fluids and oxygen if required. In addition, antibiotics are usually given empirically, guided by the severity of the pneumonia, but if there is microbiological confirmation of the causative organism and sensitivities the antibiotic therapy needs to be adjusted accordingly.

The empirical antibiotics of choice, based on severity, are as outlined below[1]:

- **Home-treated, not severe**: oral amoxicillin or, if penicillin allergic, oral erythromycin or clarithromycin
- **Hospital-treated, not severe** (admitted for non-clinical reasons or previously untreated in the community): as for home-treated, not severe
- **Hospital-treated, not severe**:
  - **either** oral amoxicillin plus erythromycin or clarithromycin 500 mg bd
  - **or**, if intravenous therapy is needed, use ampicillin plus erythromycin/clarithromycin
  - in cases of penicillin allergy, or where penicillin has already been given, treat with either levofloxacin or moxifloxacin
- **Hospital-treated, severe**: intravenous co-amoxiclav or cefuroxime plus erythromycin or clarithromycin
  - in cases of penicillin allergy use levofloxacin

PRE-CONCEPTION ISSUES AND CARE

Pneumonia is an acute infection and not a chronic condition and therefore does not have significant pre-conception effects. However, antibiotics do reduce the efficacy of the oral contraceptive pill and women need to be advised about alternative contraception whilst treated with antibiotics.

Pregnancy Issues

Pneumonia is no more common in pregnancy than at other times, but requires prompt attention and, if severe, may have serious complications compromising the woman and baby[3].

The selection of antibiotics needs to be made while remaining cognisant of potential teratogenic effects.

Medical Management and Care
- The management of pneumonia in pregnancy is essentially the same as for the non-pregnant woman
- Care needs to be taken in the selection of antibiotics:
  - penicillin, cephalosporin and macrolides safe in pregnancy
  - quinolones, tetracycline and trimethoprim contraindicated
- Careful consideration required to consider the benefit to the woman with severe pneumonia of using contraindicated antibiotics against the risk to the fetus

Midwifery Management and Care
- If the midwife suspects that the woman may have a chest infection, initiate a plan of care:
  - send a sputum sample
  - make an urgent referral to a doctor
- If the woman is being managed at home, antenatal home visits need to be increased to monitor progress, and adherence to medication should be encouraged
- A further referral may need to be made if, after a course of treatment, symptoms have not improved
- Once the infection has cleared and the woman is back to her usual state of good health she can be transferred back into low risk care

Labour Issues

Sufficient oxygenation of the woman and baby need to be maintained.

Unless maternal oxygen saturations are low, the woman should not need additional oxygen therapy.

There is a risk of pre-term labour, possibly related to pyrexia[2].

Medical Management and Care
- Severe pneumonia in late pregnancy is unusual and in the setting of acute respiratory failure caesarean section and respiratory support may need to be considered

Midwifery Management and Care
- Support and monitoring of baby and woman need to be increased, including continuous EFM
- The woman should have regular BP, temperature, pulse, respiratory rate and oxygen saturations measured and documented appropriately
- With any findings outside normal parameters refer on to appropriate medical staff
- In certain cases the midwife may need to prepare for a pre-term delivery

Postpartum Issues

Potential complications of antibiotic therapy need to be considered.

Medical Management and Care
- Pneumonia in the postpartum period needs to be managed as for pregnancy
- Quinolones, tetracycline and trimethoprim are contraindicated for a breast-feeding woman

Midwifery Management and Care
- In the case of severe pneumonia the woman needs to be adequately monitored in hospital
- If treated at home adherence to medication needs to be encouraged and advice given about potential antibiotic-related side effects, such as diarrhoea, vomiting and reduced feeding, in the breast-feeding child
- With good support from community midwives and other agencies (for example breast-feeding support groups) there should be no reason why the women should not be successful in breast-feeding
- Reassurance should be given that any side effects will be temporary and that the benefit of long-term feeding outweighs the short-term inconvenience

81

5.4 Tuberculosis

Incidence	Risk for Childbearing
1.7 billion affected and 3 million deaths worldwide per annum 6000 cases in England and Wales per annum, TB being prevalent in cities with a high ethnic minority population	High Risk

EXPLANATION OF CONDITION

Tuberculosis (TB) is a bacterial infection, caused by *Mycobacterium tuberculosis*, which is spread by direct contact with an infected individual.

Initial infection with TB often occurs without symptoms, although a positive tuberculin test may show that it has occurred. Only 10–15% of those infected will develop clinical disease over their lifetime, with the highest risk being in the first year after infection. Tuberculosis can affect most parts of the body, but most commonly presents as pulmonary TB[1].

COMPLICATIONS

- TB is associated with significant morbidity and mortality worldwide but in the UK due to careful management and access to appropriate treatment death due to TB is unusual
- The symptoms, signs and complications of TB relate to the sites in the body that are affected. Importantly, TB medication may cause considerable morbidity and in rare cases death so carers need to be mindful of potential complications of treatment as outlined in the section below
- 85% of post-primary TB affects the lungs and sufferers may present with respiratory symptoms such as cough, haemoptysis and breathlessness together with constitutional symptoms like fever, night sweats and weight loss
- Other sites of infection include:
  - peripheral lymph nodes – usually presents with constitutional symptoms alone
  - bones and joints – may present in any joint but most importantly can affect the spine and may lead to cord compression
  - pericardium – may cause a large pericardial effusion, which may compromise the function of the heart and require drainage
  - meninges – TB meningitis is rare in the UK but is associated with significant mortality
  - miliary TB – TB may become generally disseminated, particularly in immunocompromised subjects, and lead to miliary TB, which has a significant mortality

NON-PREGNANCY TREATMENT AND CARE

British Thoracic Society guidelines for the management of TB have been in existence for many years[2]. These are now living guidelines and can be accessed through the BTS website (www.brit-thoracic.org.uk). Current NICE guidance can be accessed through the same website. Due to the potential complications associated with treatment for TB, it is important that the diagnosis should only be made in the presence of a strong clinical suspicion together, where possible, with microbiological confirmation of TB, histological evidence of TB in tissue samples and a positive interferon-gamma test.

Patients diagnosed with active TB should be referred to an appropriate physician trained in treating patients with TB.

The standard treatment regimen for TB is:

- Six months of isoniazid and rifampicin initially, plus pyrazinamide and ethambutol for the first 2 months
- This regimen is appropriate for all types of TB except CNS infection, when treatment is for 12 months in combination with corticosteroid therapy
- Multi-drug-resistant TB and atypical mycobacterial infections particularly associated with an immunocompromised host (e.g. a mother with HIV/AIDS), remain unusual in the UK but pose a considerable challenge to management and require close supervision by appropriate specialists

Side effects from TB treatment are common, although serious complications are rare.

Common side effects include:

- Mild nausea
- Rashes
- Pruritus
- Arthralgia
- Orange discolouration of urine
- Sweat (due to rifampicin)

Serious Side Effects

All of the first-line drugs except ethambutol can cause liver toxicity. This is idiosyncratic and not dose-related. Therefore, liver function is monitored with tests before and throughout the treatment period.

Ethambutol can cause retro-bulbar neuritis, and acuity needs to be tested before treatment. Patients and carers need to be mindful of potential problems with vision and consider stopping treatment and referring to an eye specialist should problems arise.

Isoniazid can cause a neuropathy due to its effect on vitamin B_6 metabolism. Therefore, in patients where dietary intake of this vitamin is a concern, vitamin supplementation with pyridoxine should be given.

PRE-CONCEPTION ISSUES AND CARE

Due to the pressing need to treat TB, the medication is not contraindicated during pregnancy. However, women are advised not to consider pregnancy when undergoing treatment.

TB medication reduces the efficacy of the oral contraceptive pill and therefore women need to be advised about the use of alternative contraception.

Pregnancy Issues

It is well recognised that treatment for pulmonary TB is safe in pregnancy.

There is better neonatal and perinatal survival if treatment is adhered to[3,4].

Even in multi-drug-resistant TB the benefits of treatment outweigh the risks. Of the small number of studies there seem to be few if any teratogenic effects on newborns.

Transmission of pulmonary TB from mother to baby is rare; there has only been a single case report of a mother with endometrial TB who transmitted TB to her unborn baby.

Medical Management and Care

Medical management in pregnancy is the same as for a non-pregnant patient[3,4]:

- Six months of isoniazid and rifampicin initially, plus pyrazinamide and ethambutol for the first 2 months

Midwifery Management and Care

- It is now recommended that all new UK entrant pregnant women and children under 11 have a Mantoux test; midwife should ascertain at the booking visit that this has been done
- A pregnant woman with TB should have shared care with a TB specialist, obstetrician (preferably in a joint clinic), midwife and GP
- Ensure adherence to treatment through regular antenatal visits
- If admitted to antenatal ward will need to be in a single room
- If multi-drug-resistant TB then should be in a specialist centre offering a negative pressure room

Labour Issues

Issues in labour relate to the site and severity of infection.

Epidural anaesthesia will be contraindicated.

Medical Management and Care

- Women established on anti-TB therapy are likely to have an uncomplicated labour
- If the woman has multi-drug-resistant TB or has a new diagnosis and has not been established on TB treatment for at least 2 days then she should be managed in a negative pressure room and precautions taken to prevent infection
- General anaesthetic may be required for operative delivery, so the anaesthetist should review this mother early in the labour

Midwifery Management and Care

- Most women can have a normal labour with delivery conducted by the midwife
- Particular care is required if the woman has a new diagnosis of TB or has multi-drug-resistant TB as the woman will need a negative pressure room
- Women with extra-pulmonary TB may require specific management, e.g. women with spinal TB will need to be assessed as to their suitability for normal delivery and may require particular attention during labour
- Discuss options for pain relief

Postpartum Issues

Treatment needs to be continued.

Breast-feeding is *not* contraindicated.

Medical Management and Care

- Women should be maintained on their current therapy

Midwifery Management and Care

- Encourage continued adherence to anti-TB treatment
- Reassure the woman that there are no contraindications for breast-feeding on standard TB therapy
- Ensure newborn has BCG vaccination[3]
- Baby should have isoniazid or isoniazid and rifampicin combination chemoprophylaxis as per NICE guidelines (www.brit-thoracic.org.uk)
- Paediatric review prior to discharge
- Liaison with community midwife and health visitor for further childhood and family surveillance

5.5 Cystic Fibrosis

Incidence	Risk for Childbearing
1:2500 UK live births	High Risk – maternal mortality ≥12%, related to the risk of maternal hypoxia and pulmonary hypertension[2]

EXPLANATION OF CONDITION

Cystic fibrosis (CF) is the most common life-threatening genetic disorder in Caucasian people. It is an autosomal recessive disorder and the carrier frequency is 1 in 25[1].

The CF gene sits on the long arm of chromosome 7 and encodes for a protein known as the CF transmembrane conducting regulator (CFTR). This protein acts as a chloride channel and also services regulatory functions over membrane chloride channels. Essentially, CF is a disorder in which there are abnormalities in the sodium chloride concentrations in the secretory epithelia occurring throughout the body. This may affect:

- Respiratory tract
- Male reproductive system
- Pancreas
- Hepato-biliary system
- Gastrointestinal tract

Cystic fibrosis often presents in early childhood with cough, loose stools and failure to thrive. Other symptoms include meconium ileus, prolonged neonatal jaundice and rectal prolapse. Heel prick (Guthrie) tests are routinely made in the newborn and additional neonatal screening can be made at 6–9 weeks where a screening policy exists.

COMPLICATIONS

Symptoms and morbidity in general relate to the effects of CF on the respiratory system. However, due to the multisystemic effects of the disease other symptoms and complications can occur.

Complications include[1]:

- Nasal polyps
- Recurrent sinusitis
- Bronchiectasis
- Haemoptysis
- Allergic bronchopulmonary aspergillosis
- Recurrent pneumothoraces
- Intestinal obstruction
- Pancreatic insufficiency
- Malnutrition
- Portal hypertension
- Cirrhosis
- Gallstones
- Male infertility
- Insulin-dependent diabetes
- Osteoporosis
- Vitamin and salt deficiency
- Delayed puberty
- CF associated arthritis

The median survival age of CF sufferers is currently the mid-thirties, but this has increased from a median age of survival of 10 years old some 30 years ago. Therefore it is only recently that women with CF have been able to conceive.

NON-PREGNANCY TREATMENT AND CARE

Diagnosis is critical and is usually made in early childhood, although late presentations have been reported.

Goals of management are to:

- Maintain lung function
- Maintain quality of life

There is a need to ensure treatment regimens are negotiated with patients, so that adherence to therapy is achieved and longer-term effects are minimised.

The patient should undertake daily physiotherapy to clear the lungs, but this, combined with the many medication regimens that patients have to undertake, can be problematic. Hence, it is important to assess compliance with treatment.

Regular assessment, with measurement of lung function, is important, as is early aggressive management of infection. Pulmonary exacerbations, in particular colonisation of the respiratory tract with *Pseudomonas aeruginosa, Staphylococcus aureus, Stenotrophomonas maltophilia* and particularly *Burkholderia cepacia*, need prompt and aggressive treatment. *Burkholderia cepacia*, in particular, causes rapid decline in patients. Often intravenous antibiotics to which the particular organism is sensitive are the treatments of choice and care and management may include teaching patients to manage their own intravenous regimens.

Dietary supplementation is important and patients are often prescribed treatments such as Creon to allow them to absorb their food.

Patients appear to do better under specialised centres and this should always be an option. Often, secondary centres are attached to tertiary centres but care is shared due to the logistical problems of travel. Clearly multidisciplinary input helps address the many problems these patients have.

PRE-CONCEPTION ISSUES AND CARE

There is significant maternal morbidity and mortality, and most women with CF are unlikely to live to see their children reach adulthood. Therefore pre-conception advice and counselling needs to be offered to women with CF and management of the disease optimised.

- Management of women with CF requires specialist multidisciplinary care and needs to be individualised[2]
- Women should be screened for diabetes and advised that a prospective child will be a carrier of cystic fibrosis[3]

Pregnancy Issues

The issues in pregnancy are the same as in the non-pregnant woman, but are more exaggerated.

- Adequate dietary supplementation
- Recurrent infections
- Respiratory failure
- Pulmonary hypertension

Pre-natal diagnosis, with careful consideration of termination of pregnancy, becomes an issue.

Medical Management and Care

- The most serious complications are related to the further compromise of a woman with respiratory failure and pulmonary hypertension. It is important to remember that this can lead to maternal mortality
- Antibiotic therapy may be complicated in CF, and in some circumstances antibiotics that are not recommended in pregnancy (such as quinolones) may need to be given after careful consideration of the benefits versus risks
- Growth scans for prompt identification of IUGR[3]

Midwifery Management and Care

- The management of women with CF is complex and requires a multidisciplinary approach from midwives, physiotherapists, dieticians and clinicians
- Booking at a consultant-led unit
- Role of midwife is to support the woman during pregnancy, to reinforce adherence to treatment and ensure engagement with other health care professionals
- Promote a healthy lifestyle with emphasis on a nutritious diet
- CF does not only affect the respiratory system and pancreatic insufficiency occurs; dietary supplementation is standard treatment
- Monitor closely noting any signs such as increasing breathlessness which will assist in the early recognition of complications; these should be reported promptly to the relevant doctor

Labour Issues

Respiratory failure may compromise the oxygenation of the woman and baby.
Delivery may well be pre-term[3].

Medical Management and Care

- Most women with CF can have a normal labour, but in those with respiratory failure and/or pulmonary hypertension an elective caesarean section needs to be considered
- General anaesthesia may be contraindicated[3], so early review by the anaesthetist is recommended

Midwifery Management and Care

- The midwife needs to be particularly mindful of the potential risk to the woman and baby with respect to respiratory failure and monitoring requirements
- Ensure that oxygen is available in the delivery room, and maternal oxygen saturations should be measured at intervals
- Continuous electronic fetal monitoring[3]
- Avoid prolonged pushing and the Valsalva manoeuvre[3]
- If necessary, prepare for a pre-term delivery and make the paediatricians aware that the mother is in labour

Postpartum Issues

Respiratory infections are common, and whether antibiotics are contraindicated in the breast-feeding woman needs to be considered.

Medical Management and Care

- With most women the postpartum period is uncomplicated, but again be mindful of all of the potential complications of CF

Midwifery Management and Care

- It is important that the woman continues her regular management regimen and additional support may be required in the immediate postpartum period
- Be alert for signs of respiratory infection
- Infant feeding may be an issue if the woman is prescribed quinolones (see Section 5.3); apart from this promote breast-feeding
- Nutritional supplements are still required, especially if breast-feeding
- If paternal genetic screening was negative for the CF gene there should be no neonatal issues for disease inheritance

5.6 Sarcoidosis

Incidence	Risk for Childbearing
Sarcoidosis is rare. The prevalence of active disease is approximately 0.2% and the incidence is 0.1%	Variable Risk – most patients High Risk – small minority of patients with significant disease

EXPLANATION OF CONDITION

Sarcoidosis is a systemic granulomatous condition of unknown cause characterised by frequent pulmonary involvement, although any part of the body may be affected[1].

There are no specific tests to diagnose sarcoidosis. The diagnosis is made by the presence of typical radiological features together with supporting evidence of raised serum levels of angiotensin converting enzyme (ACE), immunoglobulin and calcium[2].

Sarcoidosis is a rare condition and is unlikely to complicate pregnancy.

COMPLICATIONS

Pulmonary sarcoidosis is radiologically staged:

- **Stage I:** bilateral hilar lymphadenopathy
- **Stage II:** as for stage I plus interstitial infiltrates
- **Stage III:** infiltrates without hilar lymphadenopathy
- **Stage IV:** dense fibrosis

Most patients present incidentally with hilar lymphadenopathy, identified when a chest radiograph is performed for another reason. Therefore, in most subjects, the condition is asymptomatic. Even in those with pulmonary involvement the disease is usually self-limiting within two years, although the changes in lung function and lung damage are permanent. It is unusual for the disease to become active again after a period of quiescence.

A minority of patients develop progressive lung disease, with increasing symptoms of breathlessness and lethargy, together with respiratory failure. In extreme circumstances sarcoidosis may cause death due to respiratory failure.

The other organs affected by sarcoidosis include:

- Skin
  - non-specific maculopapular rash
  - erythema nodosum
  - lupus pernio
- Heart – may cause heart block
- Eyes
  - scleritis
  - iritis
  - uveitis
- Joints and muscles
  - arthritis
  - myopathy
- Nervous system
  - peripheral neuropathy
  - spinal sarcoid
  - psychiatric symptoms
- Kidneys
  - renal failure secondary to interstitial nephritis
  - glomerulonephritis
  - IgA nephropathy
  - nephrocalcinosis and nephrolithiasis secondary to hypercalcaemia

NON-PREGNANCY TREATMENT AND CARE

In the presence of symptomatic progressive lung disease and/or significant hypercalcaemia patients should be treated with oral corticosteroids. Vitamin D supplementation can exacerbate the hypercalcaemia and should be avoided in those with active disease. This treatment improves symptoms, reduces progression of disease and hastens resolution. The dose of corticosteroids is high for the first few months and then can be reduced to low dose maintenance therapy.

Treatment for involvement of other organs is also systemic corticosteroids (topical for skin disease), occasionally in combination with corticosteroid-sparing agents.

A respiratory specialist usually manages sarcoidosis, but the management of other organs involved will require specialist care with each relevant organ-based specialist.

In addition to the complications of the condition noted above treatment with oral corticosteroids is also associated with significant side effects. These include corticosteroid-induced myopathy, osteoporosis, diabetes mellitus and hypertension. This list is not exhaustive and highlights the potential issues of systemic corticosteroid therapy.

PRE-CONCEPTION ISSUES AND CARE

Sarcoidosis is not usually a contraindication to pregnancy[3]. In the vast majority of women with sarcoidosis there are no pre-conception issues. Women with significant active disease need to be managed in a specialist clinic.

Particular care is needed with patients treated with systemic corticosteroids due to the increased risk of diabetes mellitus and hypertension. In the rare circumstance of patients with significant respiratory failure women should be advised against pregnancy.

Pregnancy Issues

In most cases there are no pregnancy issues. Rarely respiratory failure and other severe complications may need to be considered.

Medical Management and Care

- The medical management of sarcoidosis is the same in the pregnant and non-pregnant woman
- In most women there are no specific issues, except for those with significant disease and on systemic corticosteroids where particular care is required with respect to complications secondary to the disease and treatment

Midwifery Management and Care

- This is a rare condition in pregnancy and severe sarcoidosis in pregnant women is very unusual[3]
- The woman should be booked into a joint specialist clinic with obstetrician and respiratory consultant care
- Acute breathlessness in a pregnant woman with sarcoidosis is more likely to be due to an alternative cause, e.g. chest infection or pulmonary embolism
- In rare circumstances a woman with sarcoidosis may develop respiratory failure; presents as progressive decline in exercise capacity and development of excessive breathlessness and requires prompt review by a respiratory specialist
- In those women requiring drug therapy the midwife needs to encourage adherence to treatment, but needs to be aware of the potential problems related to corticosteroid therapy
- Advise the mother not to take vitamin D supplements, which may precipitate hypercalcaemia[4]

Labour Issues

Labour is rarely complicated by sarcoidosis except in severe disease.

Medical Management and Care

- Women treated with corticosteroids will require corticosteroid cover during labour[4]
- In the rare circumstance of a woman with significant respiratory failure an elective caesarean section may be required

Midwifery Management and Care

- Only in the exceptional circumstance of respiratory failure does sarcoidosis require any additional midwifery management
- In this setting, as with any woman with respiratory failure, increased monitoring is required to assess whether the woman and baby are adequately oxygenated
- Continuous electronic fetal monitoring

Postpartum Issues

There are no specific postpartum issues with sarcoidosis.

Medical Management and Care

- The woman needs to continue with current therapy and have follow-up arrangements made as appropriate

Midwifery Management and Care

- Breast-feeding is not contraindicated and should be encouraged and supported
- Follow-up with a respiratory specialist is indicated for women with sarcoidosis diagnosed in pregnancy or for those women already under review

S. E. Robson and J. Waugh

5 Respiratory Disorders

PATIENT ORGANISATIONS

British Lung Foundation
73–75 Goswell Road
London
EC1V 7ER
www.lunguk.org

Asthma UK
Summit House
70 Wilson Street
London
EC2A 2DB
Email: info@asthma.org.uk
www.asthma.org.uk

TB Alert
22 Tiverton Road
London
NW10 3HL
www.tbalert.org

Cystic Fibrosis Trust
11 London Road
Bromley
Kent
BR1 1BY
www.cftrust.org.uk

Sarcoidosis and Interstitial Lung Association
www.sarcoidosis.org.uk
info@sarcoidosis.org.uk

ESSENTIAL READING

BTS/SIGN British Guideline on the Management of Asthma 2008 **Thorax**, 63 (Supplement 4), 2009 Update www.brit-thoracic.org.uk

Dilworth JP and Baldwin DR 2002 **Respiratory Medicine Specialist Handbook**. London; Martin Dunitz

Guidelines for the Management of Community Acquired Pneumonia in Adults (2001) **Thorax**, 56 (Supplement IV), 2009 Update www.brit-thoracic.org.uk

NICE 2006 **Clinical Diagnosis And Management Of Tuberculosis, And Measures For Its Prevention And Control**. Guideline **CG033**. London; National Institute for Health and Clinical Excellence. www.nice.org.uk

Price D, Foster J, Scullion J and Freeman D 2004 **Asthma and COPD**. London; Churchill Livingstone

Sarcoidosis European Respiratory Monograph 2005 32:1–339

Scullion JE 2007 **Fundamental Aspects of Nursing Respiratory Disorders**. London; Quay Books

Wells AU, Hirani N on behalf of the British Thoracic Society Interstitial Lung Disease Group in collaboration with the Thoracic Society of Australia and New Zealand and the Irish Thoracic Society Interstitial Lung Disease Guideline (2008) **Thorax**, 63 (Supplement 5) www.brit-thoracic.org.uk

References

5.1 The Breathless Pregnant Woman

1. Dilworth JP and Baldwin DR 2002 **Respiratory Medicine Specialist Handbook**. London; Martin Dunitz
2. Hytten FE and Leitch I 1971 Respiration in **The Physiology of Human Pregnancy**. Oxford; Blackwell Publishing Ltd.
3. Henley-Einon A 2008 Respiratory Disorders in Pregnancy. **Practising Midwife**, 11:48–53

5.2 Asthma

1. Nelson-Piercy C 2001 Asthma in pregnancy. **Thorax**, 56:325
2. Rey E and Boulet L-P 2007 Asthma in pregnancy. **British Medical Journal**, 334:582–585
3. British Thoracic Society/Scottish Intercollegiate Guidelines 2008 Network British guideline on the management of asthma. **Thorax**, 63 (Suppl. 4):i1–i121 update 2009 www.brit–thoracic.org.uk
4. Price D, Foster J, Scullion J and Freeman D 2004 **Asthma and COPD**. London; Churchill Livingstone
5. Scullion JE 2007 **Fundamental Aspects of Nursing – Respiratory Disorders**. London; Quay Books
6. Tan KS and Thompson NC 2000 Asthma in pregnancy. **American Journal of Medicine**, 109:727
7. WHO 2002 **Infant and Young Child Nutrition – Global Strategy in Infancy And Young Child Feeding**. 55th World Assembly. Geneva; World Health Organization
8. Henley-Einon A 2008 Respiratory disorders in pregnancy. **Practising Midwife**, 11:48–53

5.3 Pneumonia and Chest Infections

1. Guidelines for the Management of Community Acquired Pneumonia in Adults 2001 **Thorax**, 56 (Suppl. IV) v1-121 2009 update www.brit–thoracic.org.uk
2. Berkowitz K and Lasala A 1990 Risk factors associated with the increasing prevalence of pneumonia in pregnancy. **American Journal of Obstetrics and Gynecology**, 163:981–985
3. Metlay JP, Kapoor WN and Fine MJ 1997 Does this patient have community-acquired pneumonia? Diagnosing pneumonia by history and physical examination. **Journal of the American Medical Association**, 278:1440

5.4 Tuberculosis

1. NICE 2006 **Guideline CG033: Clinical Diagnosis and Management of Tuberculosis, and Measures for Its Prevention and Control**. London; National Institute for Health and Clinical Excellence. www.nice.org.uk
2. **Guidelines for the Management of Tuberculosis** www.brit–thoracic.org.uk [Accessed March 2011]
3. Omerod P 2001 Tuberculosis in pregnancy and the puerperium. **Thorax**, 56:494
4. de March P 1975 Tuberculosis in pregnancy: five-in-ten year review of 215 patients in their fertile age. **Chest**, 68:800–880

5.5 Cystic Fibrosis

1. Dilworth JP and Baldwin DR 2002 **Respiratory Medicine Specialist Handbook**. London; Martin Dunitz
2. Gilljam M, Antoniou M, Shin J, Dupuis A, Corey M and Tullis DE 2000 Pregnancy in cystic fibrosis. Fetal and maternal outcome. **Chest**, 118:85–91
3. Edenborough FP, Stableforth DE, Webb AK *et al*. 2000 The outcome of 72 pregnancies in 55 women with cystic fibrosis in the UK 1977–1996. **British Journal of Obstetrics and Gynaecology**, 107:254–261

5.6 Sarcoidosis

1. Wells AU, Hirani N on behalf of the British Thoracic Society Interstitial Lung Disease Group in collaboration with the Thoracic Society of Australia and New Zealand and the Irish Thoracic Society Interstital Lung Disease Guideline (2008) **Thorax**, 63 (Supplement 5) v1–58 www.brit-thoracic.org.uk
2. European Respiratory Monograph 2005. **Sarcoidosis** 32:1–339
3. Baughman RP, Lower EE and du Bois RM 2003 Sarcoidosis. **Lancet**, 361:1111–1118
4. Selroos O 1990 Sarcoidosis and pregnancy: a review with results of a retrospective survey. **Journal of Internal Medicine**, 227:221

Appendix 5.2.1 Asthma in Pregnancy:
An Information Leaflet for Pregnant Women

Congratulations on your pregnancy!
The maternal medicine clinic aims to make your pregnancy as problem-free as possible. We try to ensure that you receive the best possible care for your pregnancy and asthma in one location, and to reduce the stress of appointments in several different places. Occasionally we may need to refer you to see a chest consultant.

Naturally you may be a little worried about how your asthma may affect your unborn baby. We hope to dispel some of your common concerns with this leaflet. If this leaflet does not answer all your questions, please ask us and we will try to find out for you.

Asthma is a common condition. Approximately 5% of pregnant women suffer from asthma. We know that approximately one third will see no change in their condition during pregnancy, one third will improve and one third may get worse. It is difficult to predict which category you will fall into.

Will my asthma affect my unborn baby?
It is important that your asthma is well controlled. As you will know, your baby relies on you for his/her supply of oxygen. You are 'breathing for two'. If you are unwell with asthma, your baby may not receive sufficient oxygen and your baby's growth may be affected.

Is it safe to take my asthma medications during pregnancy?
Yes. One of the common concerns of pregnant women with asthma is whether the medication they take for their asthma will affect their baby. There are no known harmful effects from inhaled relievers (e.g. Ventolin, Serevent and Bricanyl) or inhaled steroids (Becotide, Pulmicort or Flixotide). It is therefore safe to take them.

If you need oral steroids (prednisolone) regularly to control your asthma, then you should take them. The benefits of well-controlled asthma outweigh any risk. There is known to be minimal effect with using them. Some of the newer drugs, such as Singular, are untested in pregnancy. However, it is far more harmful to have poorly controlled asthma. Your medications are designed to help you. By keeping you well, they help your baby to develop normally.

What can I safely use for pain relief in labour?
Most drugs are safe to use in labour for most women, but discuss what is on offer and make an informed decision.

You may like to talk to one of our consultant anaesthetists, particularly if your asthma is difficult to control. They will discuss the options with you. They will also discuss your options should the need for a caesarean section arise. An epidural or spinal anaesthetic is generally the safest option for all women, but especially for women with breathing problems.

Will my asthma become worse in labour?
This is rare, but please do not forget to bring **all** your normal medication in with you when you come to hospital. It may help to keep a reliever (blue inhaler) packed in your suitcase ready for coming in.

Can I labour in a *Home from Home* room?
This will depend upon how bad your asthma is. It also depends on how well controlled it is during your pregnancy and at time of labour. Discuss this with your midwife, but remember, nothing is *written in stone* and circumstances or decisions can change. Obviously if you are unwell at the time of labour we will need to monitor the condition of you and your baby closely – and then Home from Home would not be an option.

Will it be safe to breastfeed my baby?
Breastfeeding is the recommended method of feeding for all women, particularly if you suffer from allergies. Recent research shows that children who are breastfed for the first four months of life are less likely to wheeze at six years of age. The amounts of inhaled drugs and even oral steroids that enter breast milk are extremely small. If you are taking **theophylline** it may be better if you take it **after** feeding your baby, to minimise side effects.

What advice should I seek from a professional?
We aim to see all women with moderate or severe asthma in the maternal medicine clinic at booking, then at 28 and 36 weeks of pregnancy. We would also see any asthmatic woman whose condition worsened during pregnancy. Examples of circumstances when you should seek advice include any **one** of the following:

- **Worsening symptoms where you use your reliever more than four times a day**
- **Your reliever is not working, or it works for less than four hours**
- **Being awakened at night by asthma symptoms**
- **Shortness of breath on exertion**
- **Persistent cough**
- **Peak flow below 60% of your normal best**

Who should I contact?
Speak to your community midwife, practice nurse or GP. Ask them to refer you to the maternal medicine clinic, or telephone the clinic directly and ask to speak to a midwife.
Important telephone numbers are . . . .

Finally
Don't forget that smoking is harmful to you and your unborn baby, so we advise you to stop. For advice please telephone . . . .

On the whole your pregnancy should be uneventful. We will work together to make sure it stays that way, but please contact us if you have any concerns.
The Maternal Medicine Team

RENAL DISORDERS

Nigel J. Brunskill and Andrea Goodlife

University Hospitals of Leicester NHS Trust, Leicester UK

6.1 Urinary Tract Infections
6.2 Chronic Kidney Disease
6.3 Dialysis in Pregnancy
6.4 Renal Transplantation
6.5 Nephrotic Syndrome

Medical Disorders in Pregnancy: A Manual for Midwives, Second Edition. Edited by S. Elizabeth Robson and Jason Waugh.
© 2013 John Wiley & Sons, Ltd. Published 2013 by John Wiley & Sons, Ltd.

6.1 Urinary Tract Infections

Incidence	Risk for Childbearing
1–3% of pregnancies are complicated by urinary tract infection, 2–10% by asymptomatic bacteriuria[1]	Moderate Risk

EXPLANATION OF CONDITION

Urinary tract infection (UTI) is caused by bacteria in the urinary tract. Bacteria usually originate from the bowel and the most common causative organism is *Escherichia coli*, which accounts for 80–90% of all acute UTI. In pregnancy UTI may be manifest as the urethral syndrome, acute cystitis (2% of all pregnancies) or acute pyelonephritis (1–3% of pregnancies).

Features of the **urethral syndrome** are frequency and dysuria, whereas those of **acute cystitis** include frequency, urgency and dysuria, offensive smelling urine, haematuria and suprapubic discomfort. Urethral syndrome may be caused by sexually transmitted genital infections such as *Chlamydia trachomatis*. **Acute pyelonephritis** may present with pyrexia, rigors, abdominal/flank pain, nausea and vomiting[1–4].

The presence of $>10^5$/ml of the same bacterial species in a midstream specimen of urine (MSU) in the absence of symptoms is called *asymptomatic bacteriuria* (ABU). This is of greatest significance in pregnancy, and in non-pregnant individuals with structurally abnormal urinary tracts, renal stones or diabetes mellitus[2,5,6].

COMPLICATIONS

- **Acute symptomatic urinary tract infection**
  - developed by ≥30% of women with asymptomatic bacteriuria
  - can lead to pyelonephritis
  - untreated infection may cause kidney damage[2,5,6]
- **Acute cystitis**
  - not usually dangerous but may cause significant discomfort and inconvenience
  - usually an isolated event but can be recurrent and may follow sexual intercourse
  - if untreated may progress to acute pyelonephritis
- **Pre-term labour**
  - in many non-pregnant women uncomplicated asymptomatic bacteriuria resolves spontaneously
  - in pregnancy ABU is associated with premature delivery and low birth weight and is therefore treated with antibiotics
  - ABU occurs in 2–10% of all pregnancies[1]
- **Acute pyelonephritis**
  - a more serious infection
  - if very severe, or inadequately treated, septicaemia may result in acute renal failure, multiple organ failure and death
  - repeated episodes of acute pyelonephritis may be associated with the development of renal scars[4]

NON-PREGNANCY TREATMENT AND CARE

- Identify causative organism by testing an MSU, and treat with appropriate antibiotics
- On completion of antibiotic therapy, an MSU is retested to ensure that the urine is now free of infection
- Treatment is not required in non-pregnant women with uncomplicated asymptomatic bacteriuria
- Affected individuals should be warned to be alert for symptoms suggestive of active urinary infection

Advise on ways to reduce the risk of recurrent UTI:

- Drink 2l of fluid daily, with frequent voiding of urine
- Wipe from 'front to back' after passing urine
- Void to empty the bladder after intercourse
- Drinking cranberry juice may reduce the risk; the dosage is unclear, but approximately 200–300ml (or by capsule), daily appears to be potentially effective[7–9]
- Consider prophylactic antibiotics if recurrent UTI

If UTI is recurrent, consider investigation of underlying cause, such as renal stones or ureteric reflux, with:

- Renal ultrasound
- Abdominal X-ray
- Cystoscopy

Acute pyelonephritis may require:

- Hospitalisation
- Intravenous hydration, monitor fluid balance
- Intravenous antibiotics, changing to oral antibiotics when infection is controlled
- Monitor U&E, urine and blood cultures
- Four-hourly observation of temperature

PRE-CONCEPTION ISSUES AND CARE

- Investigate renal function, and possible underlying causes, prior to pregnancy if recurrent infections have occurred
- Treat and eliminate infections
- Women at risk should be counselled regarding the need for regular urine culture, and the possible requirement for antibiotic therapy during pregnancy
- Advise that there is an increased risk of UTI in pregnancy. This is as a result of relaxation and dilation of the ureters due to hormonal changes and compression at the pelvic brim by the enlarging uterus and ovarian vein[2]. As the pregnancy advances, upward displacement of the bladder into the abdomen results in elongation of the urethra. Under these circumstances, incomplete bladder emptying allows urinary stasis, which in turn encourages infection. If this is accompanied by vesicoureteral reflux ascending bacterial migration and infection is facilitated[2]

Pregnancy Issues

All pregnant women should be offered routine screening for asymptomatic bacteriuria by an MSU culture in early pregnancy, followed by prompt treatment. UTI in pregnancy has been shown to be associated with pre-term birth and low birth weight, although this is controversial[1,3,4].

Generally, if adequately treated, there are no significant effects on the fetus. If the mother has reflux nephropathy as a predisposing cause for UTI there is an increased risk that the baby may also suffer from this condition.

If the organism responsible for the UTI is Group B *Streptococcus* (GBS), this will need to be treated with antibiotics at the time of diagnosis. Intrapartum antibiotics will also be advised. GBS bacteriuria is associated with an increased risk of early onset neonatal sepsis; although the risk is increased, it is not quantified[10].

Medical Management and Care

- Treat confirmed UTI including asymptomatic bacteriuria, promptly[11]
- Ensure antibiotic chosen is safe in pregnancy
- Avoid trimethoprim in the first trimester, as it is a folate antagonist[12]
- Augmentin increases the risk of neonatal necrotising enterocolitis if taken around the time of a premature delivery[13]
- Consider prophylactic antibiotics to prevent recurrent UTI
- In the case of acute pyelonephritis, hospitalise, commence iv antibiotics, converting to oral when tolerated, iv hydration and adequate analgesia
- Monitor renal function and consider renal ultrasound

Midwifery Management and Care

Monthly MSU – more frequently if clinically indicated by:
- Dysuria
- Increased frequency of micturition
- Urine dipstick positive for haematuria/proteinuria or nitrates
- Lower abdominal pain or renal tenderness
- Pyrexia

Always do a *test of cure* MSU after any treatment of UTI and encourage compliance with prescribed antibiotic regime.

Advise:
- Drinking 2l of fluid daily
- Empty bladder after intercourse
- Always wipe from front to back after urinating
- Drinking 200–300 ml cranberry juice (or capsule) daily may reduce the risk of recurrent UTI[7–9]

If GBS is the causative organism, inform the woman, placing an alert note on the case notes for antibiotic cover in labour[10].

Pyelonephritis:
- Refer to hospital if acute pyelonephritis suspected
- Administer analgesia and antibiotics as prescribed
- Observations: hourly temperature, BP, pulse
- Record fluid balance accurately

Labour Issues

If the mother has a UTI in labour, and is pyrexic and tachycardic, this may result in fetal tachycardia. In this case electronic monitoring of the fetal heart rate in labour is indicated.

Urinary catheterisation increases the risk of UTI, so avoid if possible, but if this is required utilise a strict aseptic technique.

Medical Management and Care

- Commence antibiotics and monitor fetal wellbeing especially if the mother is pyrexic in labour. Otherwise manage as normal.

Midwifery Management and Care

- Encourage regular emptying of the bladder
- Good hygiene practices such as offering the mother soap and water for hand washing after using a bedpan
- Avoid urinary catheterisation as this increases the risk of UTI
- Administer any prescribed treatment
- Ensure adequate hydration, if pyrexic iv fluid may be required

Postpartum Issues

If mother has recurrent UTI due to reflux nephropathy, then there is a risk that the baby could also have this condition.

Early detection and prompt treatment of urinary infections in the newborn can help prevent renal scarring and chronic kidney disease later in life.

Medical Management and Care

- Liaise with the GP if there have been recurrent UTIs in pregnancy
- If UTI persists postpartum further investigation is warranted
- A renal ultrasound scan, for reflux nephropathy, should be arranged for the baby

Midwifery Management and Care

- Postnatal care can usually be managed from a normal perspective by the midwife
- Enquires about the occurrence and symptoms of micturition should form part of routine postnatal care, and be acted upon if the mother reports symptoms such as dysuria.
- Encourage the mother to drink regular fluids, especially if breast-feeding
- The mother may need reassurance that antibiotics are safe to be taken when breast-feeding

6.2 Chronic Kidney Disease

Incidence	**Risk for Childbearing**
11% of UK adult population may have CKD[1]	High Risk

EXPLANATION OF CONDITION

Chronic kidney disease (CKD) implies longstanding kidney problems often, but not always, associated with loss of excretory function. CKD is classified according to estimated glomerular filtration rate (eGFR). Five stages are recognised:

1. **Normal:** GFR >90 ml/min/1.73 m² with other evidence of chronic kidney damage*
2. **Mild impairment:** GFR 60–89 ml/min/1.73 m² with other evidence of chronic kidney damage*
3. **Moderate impairment:** GFR 30–59 ml/min/1.73 m²
4. **Severe impairment:** GFR 15–29 ml/min/1.73 m²
5. **Established renal failure:** GFR <15 ml/min/1.73 m² or on dialysis

Other evidence may be urinary dipstick abnormalities or structural abnormalities detected by ultrasound scanning

Estimated GFR is automatically reported by chemical pathology laboratories using a formulaic calculation based on serum creatinine[2], but it is not validated in pregnancy.

Proteinuria in the first trimester of pregnancy may be the first indication of CKD, as this is often the first time a woman's urine has been tested.

COMPLICATIONS

- **Hypertension** – common with CKD
- **Fluid retention** – may cause ankle oedema and contribute to hypertension
- **Anaemia** – increased risk as the kidney produces erythropoietin which stimulates the bone marrow to produce red blood cells; erythropoietin is often deficient
- **Heavy proteinuria** – in the nephrotic range (>3 g per 24 hours); can cause hypoalbuminaemia and oedema
- **Metabolic acidosis** – can develop
- **Renal bone disease** – may occur
- **UTI** – increased risk of infection
- **Impaired renal function** – this may relentlessly and predictably deteriorate over time
- Patients may be given dietary restrictions to help control BP and potassium levels within safe limits

NON-PREGNANCY TREATMENT AND CARE

- Investigations into the cause of CKD may include renal ultrasound scanning or occasionally renal biopsy
- Some causes of CKD may require specific treatments, such as immunosuppression with steroids
- Regular monitoring of renal function in nephrology clinic or primary care
- Antihypertensive medication
- Diuretics to treat fluid retention
- Subcutaneous erythropoietin for anaemia

- Referral to a dietician if dietary restrictions are required to maintain safe blood chemistry levels
- Patient education about disease and treatment
- Dialysis or transplantation is required for stage 5 CKD

PRE-CONCEPTION ISSUES AND CARE

- Referral to a renal/obstetric or maternal medicine clinic for personalised specialised advice and counselling
- The predicted outcome of a pregnancy depends on, and is directly proportional to:
  - how well controlled the BP is at booking
  - the level of renal impairment
  - magnitude of proteinuria
  - the underlying disorder responsible for CKD[3–6]
- Ascertain cause of CKD; if actively under investigation it is prudent to await results before conception
- Always consider previous obstetric history and underlying medical conditions, e.g. patients with lupus nephritis could also have antiphospholipid syndrome[7]
- With progressively worsening CKD, decreasing fertility and need for early conception is balanced against the risk of deteriorating renal function in a pregnancy
- Optimal BP control is essential, and alteration to medications may be required
  - ACE inhibitors are commonly used for patients in CRF because of their protective effect on the kidneys, but they are contraindicated in pregnancy as they cause fetal anuria and subsequent oligohydramnios[8]
- Heavily proteinuric patients are at increased risk of thrombo-embolism in pregnancy
  - prophylactic daily injections of low-molecular-weight heparin might be considered if they become pregnant; must be balanced against the increased risk of bleeding[9]
- Some individuals have familial renal disease and may require referral to clinical genetics for counselling
- Pre-eclampsia risk increases with CKD, being difficult to differentiate from deterioration of underlying CKD
- Increased risk of UTI, so regular MSU testing required with early treatment of symptoms
- If there is significant proteinuria, it may be difficult to measure accurately the alpha-feta protein (AFP) level
  - meaningful interpretation of Down's syndrome screening blood test, usually offered around the 15th week of pregnancy, may not be possible
  - if the kidney is leaking protein, AFP may also, theoretically, be lost in the urine
- Once pregnant, the woman will need to have regular hospital appointments, at a specialised centre

Pregnancy Issues

If the woman did not receive pre-conceptual counselling she should be made fully aware of the effect and risks of pregnancy upon herself, her renal function and her fetus.

The woman should be managed at a maternal medicine or renal/obstetric clinic.

In pregnancy, CKD is associated with:

- IUGR
- Pre-eclampsia
- Premature delivery
- Fetal loss
- UTI
- Deteriorating renal function[3-6]

The predicted outcome of the pregnancy is directly proportional to BP control at booking, the degree of hypertension, the level of renal impairment, magnitude of proteinuria and the underlying disorder responsible for CKD[3-6].

Close supervision of renal function, BP and proteinuria are required.

Although eGFR is now reported as a measure of renal function with all requests for serum creatinine, eGFR is not validated as an accurate measure of renal function in pregnancy[2].

Medical Management and Care

- Specific treatment for underlying renal disease should continue
- Commence 75 mg daily of aspirin, to reduce the risks of pre-eclampsia[10]
- Monitoring renal function necessitates regular blood testing
- Careful BP monitoring is required (see Chapter 3.1)
- Current medications should be reviewed; some agents may need to be omitted or changed to those which are safe for pregnancy
- Administration of erythropoietin may be required to treat anaemia
- Monitor urine for increasing protein excretion
- If heavily proteinuric and/or there is a low serum albumin, it may be necessary for the mother to commence anticoagulant therapy[9]
- Monitor renal function carefully by serum creatinine
- Declining renal function may occasionally necessitate institution of dialysis during pregnancy
- Regular fetal growth scans

Midwifery Management and Care

- Early referral to a renal/obstetric or maternal medicine clinic
- Baseline U&E and LFT with booking blood tests
- Advise about alternative screening methods for Down's syndrome if the serum test was unreliable due to heavy proteinuria; an alternative is nuchal translucency scanning
- Monthly MSU
- Advise the woman about the signs and symptoms of pre-eclampsia
- Encourage compliance with prescribed medications and reassure regarding the safety of the drugs for the fetus, and whilst breast-feeding
- Refer to the pharmacist if further information is required
- Teach administration of anticoagulant injections, if prescribed, and give information about the symptoms of DVT and PE; reinforce with general advice about reducing the risk of thrombosis[9]

Labour Issues

There is no reason why the patient should not have a normal vaginal delivery. However, the woman will be at increased risk of an emergency LSCS, or induction of labour for either maternal or fetal complications.

The ergometrine component of Syntometrine is associated with hypertensive episodes.

Medical Management and Care

- Monitor renal function and BP carefully
- Strict fluid balance
- Monitor fetal wellbeing, being vigilant for fetal distress

Midwifery Management and Care

- If the fetus is premature or growth restricted then continuous fetal monitoring will be indicated
- If the woman is hypertensive, oxytocin will be required for active third-stage management instead of Syntometrine

Postpartum Issues

There is still potential in the immediate post-natal period for instability in the maternal renal function and BP control.

The baby will require a renal ultrasound if the mother has ureteric reflux, because of the familial nature of these conditions.

If the woman suffers from uncontrolled hypertension, or is breast-feeding, the combined oestrogen and progesterone oral contraceptive will be contraindicated.

Medical Management and Care

- Monitor renal function carefully in immediate postpartum period
- BP should be well controlled
- Recommence and change to pre-pregnancy medication if required (avoiding nephrotoxic medications). However, this may be delayed if the mother wishes to breast-feed, dependent upon any contraindications
- Ensure adequate hydration
- Send notification to the woman's lead nephrologist and GP detailing care and pregnancy outcome
- Arrange a renal ultrasound for the baby if required

Midwifery Management and Care

- Follow-up appointment should be arranged in the mother's routine nephrology department
- If alterations are made to hypertensive treatment, more frequent BP monitoring should be arranged
- The woman will not be suitable for an early discharge
- Discuss the alternative methods of contraception available

6.3 Dialysis in Pregnancy

Incidence	Risk for Childbearing
Uncommon – less than 1% of women of childbearing age on dialysis become pregnant each year.	High Risk

EXPLANATION OF CONDITION

Dialysis is a means of removing waste products and water from the body of patients whose kidneys have failed and have lost their ability to excrete water and dissolved waste products as urine (Appendix 6.3.1). These patients would otherwise die.

Two types of dialysis are available.

Haemodialysis

In haemodialysis (HD) blood is circulated through a machine where it is purified before being returned to the patient. This type of dialysis is usually performed on three occasions per week in hospital. HD patients require access to their circulation, usually in the form of an arteriovenous fistula or a semi-permanent plastic catheter inserted into a large vein.

Peritoneal Dialysis

In peritoneal dialysis (PD) the patient has a soft tube inserted into the peritoneal cavity. This is used to drain up to 2.5l of fluid *in and out* of the peritoneal cavity, typically four times a day, by patients in their own home.

Each patient has an individual dialysis prescription and a target 'dry' weight to ensure that the correct amounts of waste products and fluid are removed by their dialysis.

Women of childbearing age receiving dialysis either have reduced fertility or are infertile.

COMPLICATIONS

- Dialysis is an imperfect substitute for normally functioning kidneys and dialysis patients have a reduced life expectancy
- Nearly all dialysis patients are hypertensive and anaemic due to the failure of damaged kidneys to produce erythropoietin
- Dialysis patients suffer from secondary hyperparathyroidism and renal osteodystrophy
- Dialysis patients have greatly increased morbidity and mortality, predominantly as a result of infection and especially cardiovascular disease, including heart disease, cerebrovascular disease and peripheral vascular disease
- Arteriovenous fistulae can clot off and become blocked, and permcaths can become blocked or infected; an urgent alternative has to be arranged
- Patients receiving peritoneal dialysis can develop peritonitis as a result of bacteria entering the peritoneal cavity through the dialysis tube; treatable with antibiotics but a potentially very serious complication

NON-PREGNANCY TREATMENT AND CARE

The patient needs close supervision and care from a multidisciplinary team including doctors, nurses, dieticians, pharmacists and dialysis technicians.

Treatment

- Dialysis – to be performed regularly
- Nearly all patients need antihypertensive medication and erythropoietin injections to prevent severe anaemia
- Strict dietary restrictions to limit intake of fluid, potassium and phosphate
- Regular review clinics are required to assess adequacy of dialysis treatment and to prevent dialysis complications

PRE-CONCEPTION ISSUES AND CARE

Because of the low likelihood of pregnancy occurring in women receiving dialysis, very few actually seek preconceptual advice. However, conception is possible and those of childbearing age should take appropriate contraception precautions to avoid an unwanted pregnancy.

Psychosexual problems are common in dialysis patients and may limit the ability to conceive.

Refer to a joint renal/obstetric or maternal medicine clinic, where they can be seen jointly by a consultant nephrologist and obstetrician and specialised midwife. In some cases this may involve considerable travelling to the appropriate unit.

Advise that pregnancy is at high risk of problems such as:

- Anaemia
- Hypertension
- Pre-eclampsia
- IUGR
- Polyhydramnios
- Premature labour
- **Haemodialysis** – HD requirements will increase, and to help stabilise the blood values dialysis would be performed approximately 6 days a week (compared with three occasions per week as described above)
- **Peritoneal dialysis** – As the pregnancy advances, then smaller, more frequent fluid exchanges may need to be performed; changing to haemodialysis may have to be considered
- If renal transplantation is imminent it may be sensible to wait until after transplantation before trying for a pregnancy
- Down's screening tests will not be interpretable in dialysis patients; nuchal translucency screening or diagnostic tests would have to be considered if requested
- The underlying renal disorder may have an impact on the pregnancy, and this will need to be considered
- Current medications will need review, and probable alteration, by the renal team

Pregnancy Issues

A high-risk pregnancy[1-4] with the risk of:

- IUGR and pre-term labour
- Severe pre-eclampsia (difficult to diagnose in renal patients)
- Polyhydramnios – as the fetus is exposed to high urea levels which increase the diuresis
- Peritonitis with continuous ambulatory peritoneal dialysis
- Dietary restrictions will require modification to accommodate any change in the dialysis prescription
- Anaemia, because the kidney is responsible for erythropoietin which stimulates red cell production

The aim is to minimise the effect of the uraemic maternal environment on fetal development and to prevent large fluctuations in maternal blood chemistry, fluid status and BP.

Target weights need frequent reassessment as weight increases throughout pregnancy. Excellent teamwork and communication between the different members of multidisciplinary team will be essential.

Peritoneal Dialysis (PD)

- More frequent smaller exchanges as the pregnancy advances
- Good exchange technique to avoid peritonitis

Haemodialysis (HD)

- Increase dialysis frequency to 6 days per week
- Avoid hypotensive episodes as dialysis can reduce placental blood flow

Medical Management and Care

- Ensure the woman *understands* risks of proceeding with a pregnancy
- Aim to deliver in a unit with both obstetric and nephrology support
- Consider if the underlying disease has any impact on the pregnancy
- Assess current medications for their compatibility with pregnancy
- Commence 75 mg daily of aspirin, to reduce the risks of pre-eclampsia[5]
- Increase the frequency and duration of dialysis through pregnancy
- Frequent monitoring of:
  - serum biochemistry
  - haemoglobin
  - bacteriuria
  - fluid balance
  - maternal weight
- Close input from specialised renal dietician
- Regular ultrasound scans for fetal growth
- Conventional Down's syndrome screening investigations will be difficult to interpret as a result of the dialysis so discuss alternatives such as nuchal translucency screening or amniocentesis
- Aim to maintain haemoglobin >10 g/dl, which may require increasing erythropoietin, iron supplementation, or having a blood transfusion

Midwifery Management and Care

- Refer to renal/obstetric or maternal medicine clinic
- No phlebotomy or taking of BP on the arm if there is an arteriovenous fistula as this increases the risk of damaging the access for dialysis
- Monthly MSU
- Advice on prevention of urinary tract infection
- Educate about the symptoms of pre-eclampsia; ensure the mother has appropriate contact numbers if there is concern
- Plan regular antenatal appointments
- Encourage compliance with dietary advice, medication and treatment
- Liaise closely with the renal unit, coordinate care and try to avoid repetition of blood tests which could be taken whilst on haemodialysis
- Due to increasing hospitalisation and visits, consider referral to social services or support group to offer financial or practical support, such as assistance with transport problems
- If a pre-term delivery is likely arrange a tour of the relevant neonatal unit for the mother and significant others

Labour Issues

The dialysis mother could in principle have a normal delivery, but there is an increased likelihood that they will need to be delivered early because of pre-eclampsia, concerns about IUGR or for maternal reasons. Hence, the majority of pregnant dialysis women will be delivered by caesarean section.

Medical Management and Care

- Dialysis prior to elective delivery with close monitoring of blood biochemistry
- Strict BP control and fluid balance
- If caesarean section performed PD should be discontinued, and all PD fluid drained out pre-operatively; PD can be restarted immediately post-delivery if there are no complications

Midwifery Management and Care

- Continuous electronic fetal monitoring, being alert for fetal distress
- Strict control of any iv fluids and record fluid balance
- Liaise with renal team/nurses regarding prescribed dialysis
- Clearly document and report up-to-date blood results

Postpartum Issues

The mother can now return to pre pregnancy medications (if not breast-feeding) and dialysis prescription.

Caesarean section should not preclude continuation of PD, however if unable to do PD following abdominal surgery, temporary HD may be required until wounds healed.

Medical Management and Care

- Review medications and dialysis prescriptions
- The Mirena intrauterine system (IUS) would be the contraceptive of choice; reduces menstrual blood loss, therefore reduces anaemia, and is very effective in preventing unplanned pregnancies

Midwifery Management and Care

- Ensure specific dietary requirements are met whilst an in-patient
- Liaise with renal unit regarding dialysis requirements
- Breast-feeding is possible, although awkward whilst actually on HD

6.4 Renal Transplantation

Incidence	Risk for Childbearing
Over 14 000 pregnancies have been documented in renal transplant recipients	High Risk

EXPLANATION OF CONDITION

The patient will have developed end-stage renal failure as a consequence of either acute or chronic kidney disease. At this stage renal replacement therapy is required. The options are haemodialysis, peritoneal dialysis or renal transplantation. Most patients spend some time receiving dialysis before receiving a kidney transplant. Kidneys for transplantation may be obtained from a cadaver donor or be donated by a living relative. Although non-functional, the patient's own kidneys do not cause a significant problem and are not removed.

The transplanted kidney is placed superficially in the lower part of the abdomen in the left or right iliac fossa. To avoid rejection the patient requires lifelong immunosuppressive therapy.

The success of the transplant may vary. Most transplanted kidneys function well for many years, whereas others function less well or not at all. Commonly, however, kidney transplants work well initially, but their function declines slowly over time.

COMPLICATIONS

- Risk of rejection and loss of renal function
- Immunosuppressive treatment increases the risk of infection and malignancy
- The patient may experience side effects from the immunosuppressive medications
- Transplant patients are commonly hypertensive, and are at particular risk of cardiovascular disease
- Progressive decline in transplant kidney function may occur, until the transplant fails and dialysis is needed

NON-PREGNANCY TREATMENT AND CARE

Regular hospital appointments are needed to address:

- Blood and urine analysis to monitor kidney function and immunosuppressive treatment
- Annual review for long-term stable transplant patients
- Ensure well-controlled BP
- Advice on general good healthy lifestyle, no smoking, good weight control, dietary intake and good hygiene
- Importance of seeking prompt treatment if unwell or if infection is suspected

For women of childbearing age, transplantation improves libido, and restores fertility[1], therefore discussions need to take place around family planning, and contraceptive advice.

PRE-CONCEPTION ISSUES AND CARE

- If the underlying disease is an inherited condition, the patient may require a clinical genetics referral to discuss potential implications for the fetus, and the possibility of pre-natal testing
- Referral to renal/obstetric or maternal medicine clinic for specific individual advice and counselling is very important
- Prospective mothers with transplanted kidneys, and their partners, should be informed that pregnancy in renal transplant recipients is associated with an increased risk of pre-eclampsia, IUGR, premature delivery and fetal loss
- Risks increase as kidney transplant function declines or if BP is poorly controlled[2]
- Regardless of the level of transplant function all patients should be regarded as having renal insufficiency
- Advise the woman to wait for at least 1 year after transplant, with no evidence of rejection in past year, before attempting pregnancy[3]
- Aim for stable and adequate kidney function
- Achieve good BP control
- The woman should be taking maintenance doses of immunosuppressive drugs at stable dosages. Some newer immunosuppressive drugs are not safe for the fetus in pregnancy (see Appendix 11.1.1) and will require changing before conception; this process is associated with an increased risk of rejection
- Women may be taking other medications that are not safe in pregnancy, e.g. ACE inhibitors or statins, which need to be changed for safer drugs, or discontinued pre-conception[2]
- Outcome of pregnancy may be influenced by other co-existing morbidity:
  - diabetes
  - cardiovascular status
  - level of transplant function
  - hypertension
  - aetiology of the original kidney disease
- Generally, pregnancy outcomes in kidney transplant recipients are good

Pregnancy Issues

It is essential that the pregnancy is managed jointly by nephrologists, obstetricians and midwives who are experienced in renal disease and pregnancy[1-4].

Pregnancy outcome is highly dependent on stable transplant with good function, well-controlled BP and minimal co-morbidity. If these factors are optimised then this will improve the outcome of the pregnancy[1-4].

The woman is at risk of pre-eclampsia, hence she requires careful BP monitoring.

Kidney transplant rejection can occur in pregnancy and may require transplant biopsy.

Signs of infection may be less obvious or unusual with immunosuppressant therapy and must not be overlooked.

Medical Management and Care

- Review medications, and change or omit drugs which are contraindicated in pregnancy
- Commence 75 mg daily of aspirin, to reduce the risks of pre-eclampsia[5]
- Regular renal function checks with serum investigations, and urinalysis for proteinuria
- Monitor immunosuppressive drug levels, altering dosages as required
- Regular MSU to check for urinary infection
- Regular fetal growth scans
- Be alert for pre-eclampsia
- Remain aware that transplant rejection may occur, or that underlying renal disease may have an impact on transplant function during the pregnancy[3,4]
- Maintain a good haemoglobin level

Midwifery Management and Care

- Refer early to a specific joint renal/obstetric or maternal medicine clinic for high-risk care
- Regular antenatal appointments and prompt referral if there are any concerns, ensuring the midwifery team and the mother have appropriate contact telephone numbers
- If the mother has an arteriovenous fistula used for previous dialysis, avoid that arm for phlebotomy or BP measurement
- Minimise risk of UTI (see Section 6.1)
- Reassure the woman that the baby will not 'squash' the new kidney, and the baby will have room to grow
- Ensure compliance with medications and emphasise their importance in optimising pregnancy outcome
- Be alert for signs of infection, referring if problems are suspected
- Breast-feeding may not be contraindicated, dependent on the drugs used; refer to a pharmacist for specialised advice if required

Labour Issues

A normal vaginal delivery is not contraindicated because of the presence of a transplanted kidney. Caesarean section is reserved for standard obstetric indications.

If the labour is protracted or complicated by pre-eclampsia, there must be good fluid balance control, particular avoidance of dehydration and hypotensive episodes, which would reduce renal blood flow and increase the risk of acute renal failure.

Medical Management and Care

- Increase steroid cover during labour
- Monitor BP regularly in labour
- Strict input/output fluid balance
- Prompt fluid replacement if there is significant haemorrhage
- Inform and involve the renal team of the woman's admission, updating them if there are any medical concerns in labour

Midwifery Management and Care

- Administer any prescribed (including regular) medications
- Maintain an accurate fluid balance record
- Encourage regular micturition, but avoid bladder catheterisation
- Report any hyper- or hypotensive episodes

Postpartum Issues

Ensure renal function is stable, and BP well controlled (therefore the mother is not suitable for early discharge).

The baby will require a renal ultrasound if the mother has scarring nephropathy or ureteric reflux, due to the familial nature of these conditions.

For non-rubella immune mothers, the live rubella vaccine should be avoided as it is contraindicated with immunosuppressants[1].

If the woman has uncontrolled hypertension the combined oral contraceptive will not be advised.

Medical Management and Care

- Monitor renal function and immunosuppressive drug levels in the immediate postpartum period
- Aim for well-controlled BP
- Re-commencement of pre-pregnancy drugs may be required, but ensure there are no contraindications if the patient is breast-feeding
- Arrange a renal ultrasound of the baby if required
- Arrange an appointment at the routine transplant clinic

Midwifery Management and Care

- Good hygiene, being alert for early signs of sepsis, as the woman is immunosuppressed, with prompt medical referral if concerned
- Administer medications as prescribed
- Regular BP monitoring, reporting hypo- or hypertensive episodes
- Advise on contraception available to the woman

6.5 Nephrotic Syndrome

Incidence	Risk for Childbearing
Uncommon	High Risk

EXPLANATION OF CONDITION

Nephrotic syndrome is a classical clinical syndrome of renal disease compromising a triad of features:

1. Proteinuria (usually >3.5 g/24 h)
2. Low plasma albumin
3. Oedema

Most patients also have high cholesterol and high triglyceride levels. The loss of protein into the urine results in a fall in plasma albumin concentration, but other circulating proteins are also lost. Falling plasma oncotic pressure encourages fluid to leave the circulation, and this results in oedema.

The development of nephrotic syndrome indicates that the patient has renal disease affecting the glomerulus, i.e. glomerulonephritis. Many different types of glomerular disease may cause nephrotic syndrome (e.g. membranous nephropathy, diabetic nephropathy) and a renal biopsy is usually required to make a precise histological diagnosis.

COMPLICATIONS

- Oedema
- Hypertension
- Infection
- Hyperlipidaemia – may result in atherosclerosis over time
- Thrombo-embolism – loss of protein in the urine results in an imbalance in blood clotting systems with increased risk of thrombo-embolic disease
- Kidney failure – for some patients with nephrotic syndrome

NON-PREGNANCY TREATMENT AND CARE

- Fluid retention and oedema are treated with diuretics, often in high dosages, and dietary restriction of salt
- Hypertension may require treatment; ACE inhibitors and angiotensin receptor blockers (ARB) are the agents of first choice
- Even if nephrotic patients are normotensive, they will receive either an ACE inhibitor or an ARB since these agents reduce protein leakage into the urine and protect kidney function
- Some patients may receive a statin
- Some patients may be anticoagulated
- Some patients may receive treatment aimed specifically at the cause of the nephrotic syndrome, usually some form of immunosuppression

PRE-CONCEPTION ISSUES AND CARE

The woman requires referral to a renal/obstetric or maternal medicine clinic for specialised advice. This encompasses:

- Ascertain the underlying cause of nephrotic syndrome by renal biopsy prior to pregnancy if possible
- Determine the level of renal functional impairment if present
- Ensure hypertension is controlled prior to conception
- The combination of pregnancy (a hypercoagulable state), and nephrotic syndrome, will put the woman at a markedly increased risk of thrombo-embolism[1]; prospective mothers should be advised to:
  - reduce their weight if obese
  - stop smoking
  - wait, if possible, until the protein loss is minimal and stable
- Be aware that during pregnancy daily subcutaneous (sc) injections of low-molecular-weight heparin may be prescribed; this is balanced against the risk of causing bleeding problems
- Consider cessation of ACE inhibitors and angiotensin receptor blockers as they are contraindicated in pregnancy; if used as an antihypertensive they can be changed to methyldopa[2]
- Consider cessation of other drugs (e.g. diuretics, statins)
- The Down's screening test may not be reliable in pregnancy (as yet unproven), but if serum protein is lower because of increased excretion, then serum levels of alpha-feta protein could also be lower; nuchal translucency scanning or diagnostic tests (amniocentesis) are to be considered if required
- Advise the prospective mother that pregnancy entails increased risk of:
  - Pre-eclampsia, although this is difficult to distinguish from deteriorating renal function, therefore regular monitoring and frequent blood and urine testing would be required
  - IUGR
  - Premature delivery

Pregnancy Issues

There is increased risk of:

- Pre-eclampsia
- IUGR
- Deteriorating renal function
- Thrombo-embolism

Because of the high risk and complex nature of nephrotic syndrome in pregnancy[3], the woman will need to be referred to a specialist renal/obstetric or maternal medicine clinic.

The woman must be made aware that pregnancy itself is a hypercoagulable state, and she will be at an increased risk of thrombosis if the pregnancy continues.

There is no clear evidence as to what level of proteinuria, and/or lowered serum albumin, requires commencement of prophylactic anticoagulation. This is usually given as daily sc injection of low-molecular-weight heparin. A careful balance of the risk of thrombosis versus the concern about haemorrhage must be made in discussion with the mother.

Developing pre-eclampsia may be difficult to distinguish from deterioration of the underlying renal condition. Regular assessment of all signs and symptoms of pre-eclampsia must be evaluated carefully.

Although there is heavy urine protein loss, increasing dietary intake of protein is not indicated as this simply results in increased urinary protein leakage.

Urinary tract infection is more common.

Medical Management and Care

- Aim to deliver in a unit with obstetric and nephrology support
- Outline risks of thrombosis with continuing pregnancy
- Commence 75 mg daily of aspirin, to reduce the risks of pre-eclampsia[5]
- Monitor: U&E and LFT (specifically plasma albumin levels), urine protein, creatinine ratios and 24-h urinary protein excretion
- Consider investigation of underlying cause of nephrotic syndrome by renal biopsy, if not already identified
- Assessment of thrombosis risk factors:
  - overweight
  - limited mobility
  - previous thrombotic episodes
  - low plasma albumin <30 g/l
  - 24-hour urinary protein loss >3 g/24 hours
  - smoking
- Consider prescribing low-molecular-weight heparin anticoagulant therapy, by daily sc injection[1]
- Consider referral to haemostasis clinic for monitoring of heparin assay levels if low-molecular-weight heparin is prescribed (see Chapter 15)
- Careful monitoring and good control of BP
- Down's risk screening test will be difficult to interpret; consider nuchal translucency screening or diagnostic tests (amniocentesis) if required
- Fetal growth surveillance by regular ultrasound scans
- Monthly MSU

Midwifery Management and Care

- Refer to a renal/obstetric or maternal medicine clinic
- Investigations for U&E and LFT simultaneous with 'booking bloods'
- Teach self-administration of low-molecular-weight heparin injections
- To reduce the risk of thrombosis, advise the mother:
  - do not sit with legs crossed
  - at rest, raise legs on footstool, make circle movements with feet
  - wear support stockings, evenly applied (no creases)
- Advise on the signs and symptoms of thrombosis or embolism (and to seek immediate help if occur) (see Chapter 15)
  - acutely painful swollen calf
  - pleuritic pain, cough or breathlessness
- Weigh regularly (helps to monitor for fluid retention)
- Be alert for signs and symptoms of pre-eclampsia
- Fortnightly antenatal appointments

Labour Issues

Whilst there is an increased risk of labour being induced if the pregnancy is complicated, there are no reasons for the woman not to have a normal delivery.

In order to reduce the risk of postpartum haemorrhage, low-molecular-weight heparin is omitted on the day of delivery.

Medical Management and Care

- Omit low-molecular-weight heparin on the day of delivery
- If receiving steroids an increase in 'cover' will be required for labour

Midwifery Management and Care

- Mobilise the mother as much as possible throughout the labour
- Strict fluid balance
- If Fragmin has been given, be aware of the increased risk of PPH
- Apart from the above, labour can usually be managed normally by the midwife

Postpartum Issues

The increased risk of thrombosis continues into the postpartum period. Six weeks appears to be the acceptable time frame to continue with anticoagulant therapy[4].

Serum albumin and total protein urine excretion will need to be assessed along with the patient's risk factors for thrombosis, in order to individualise care.

Avoid the combined oral contraceptive pill, because of the increased risk of DVT.

Medical Management and Care

- Continue with anticoagulants for approximately 6 weeks, dependent upon serum albumin and proteinuria levels[1]
- Monitor for signs of infection
- Arrange follow-up appointment in a general nephrology clinic

Midwifery Management and Care

- TED stockings to be worn whilst in hospital
- Reassurance that it is safe to breast-feed whilst on anticoagulants
- Give advice on alternative contraception

6 Renal Disorders

PATIENT ORGANISATIONS

National Kidney Federation
6 Stanley Street
Worksop
Nottinghamshire S81 7HX
www.kidney.org.uk/main/nkf_work.html

British Kidney Patient Association
Bordon
Hampshire GU35 9JZ
www.britishkidney-pa.co.uk

Kidney Alliance
26 Oriental Road
Woking
Surrey GU22 7AW
www.kidneyalliance.org.uk

Kidney Research UK
Kings Chambers
Priestgate
Peterborough PE1 1FG
www.kidneyresearchuk.org

Kidney Patient Guide
www.kidneypatientguide.org.uk

American Association of Kidney Patients
www.aakp.org

Edinburgh Royal Infirmary Patient Information
www.renux.dmed.ed.ac.uk/edren/EdRenINFOhome.html

Group B Strep Support
PO Box 203
Haywards Heath
West Sussex RH16 1GF
www.gbss.org.uk

Action on Pre-eclampsia – APEC
84–88 Pinner Road
Harrow
Middlesex HA1 4HZ
www.apec.org.uk

ESSENTIAL READING

Barcelo P, Lopez-Lilo J, Cabero L and Del Rio G 1986 Successful pregnancy in primary glomerular disease. **Kidney International**, 30:914–919

Davison JM 2001 Renal disorders in pregnancy. **Current Opinion in Obstetrics and Gynaecology**, 13:109–114

Hou S 1999 Pregnancy in chronic renal insufficiency and end stage renal disease. **American Journal of Kidney Disease**, 33:235–252

James DK, Steer PJ, Weiner CP and Gonik B (Eds) 2006 *Thromboembolic disorders*, pp. 938–948; *Autoimmune disease*, pp. 949–985; *Renal disorders*, pp 1098–1124; *Pregnancy after renal transplantation*, pp. 1174–1186. In: **High Risk Pregnancy: Management Options**. Philadelphia; W.B. Saunders

Jepson RG, Milhaljevic L and Craig J (2004) Cranberries for preventing urinary tract infections. **The Cochrane Database of Systematic Reviews**, Issue 2.Art.No.CD001321. DOI:10.1002/14651858.CD001321

Lewis G (Ed) 2011 **Saving Mothers Lives: Reviewing maternal deaths to make motherhood safer: 2006–08**; Supplement to British Journal of Obstetrics and Gynaecology, vol.118; London; Centre for Maternal and Child Enquiries

McKay DB and Josephson MA 2006 Pregnancy in recipients of solid organs – effects on mother and child. **New England Journal of Medicine**, 354:1281–1293

Queenan JT (Ed.) 1999 *Renal disease* in **Management of High Risk Pregnancy**. Oxford; Blackwell Publishing Ltd. 236–245.

RCOG 2003 **Prevention of early onset neonatal group B streptococcal disease. Guideline No 36**, p. 6

Smaill F 2002 Antibiotics for asymptomatic bacteriuria in pregnancy. **The Cochrane Database of Systematic Reviews**, Issue 2. Art. No.: CD000490. DOI: 10.1002/14651858. CD000490

Thorsen MS and Poole JH (2002) Renal disease in pregnancy. **Journal of Perinatal Neonatal Nursing**, 15:13–26

Williams DJ 2001 Renal disease and fluid balance in pregnancy. **Current Obstetrics and Gynaecology**, 11:146–152

Williams D and Lightstone L 2007 Chapt. 4 *Renal disorders* in Greer I, Nelson-Piercy C and Walters B (eds) **Maternal Medicine: Medical Problems in Pregnancy**. Edinburgh: Churchill Livingstone 53–69

References

6.1 Urinary Tract Infections

1. NICE 2008 **Clinical Guideline: Antenatal care**. London; National Institute for Health and Clinical Excellence http://www.nice.org.uk/nicemedia/live/11947/40115/40115.pdf
2. Williams D 2006 Renal disorders in James DK, Steer PJ, Weiner CP, Gonik B (Eds) **High Risk Pregnancy: Management Options**, 3rd Edn. Philadelphia; W.B. Saunders 1098–1124
3. Lindheimer MD, Grunfeld JP and Davison JM 2000 *Renal disorders* in Baron WM and Lindheimer MD (Eds) **Medical Disorders During Pregnancy**. Chicago; Mosby Inc. 39–70
4. Davison JM 2001 Renal disorders in pregnancy. **Current Opinion in Obstetrics and Gynaecology**, 13:109–114
5. Kincaid-Smith P and Bullen M 1965 Bacteriuria in pregnancy. **Lancet**, 1:1382–1387
6. Brumfitt W 1975 The effects of bacteriuria in pregnancy on maternal and fetal health. **Kidney International**, 8(Suppl.): S113–119
7. Avorn J, Monane M, Gurwitz JH, Glynn RJ, Choodnovskiy I and Lipsitz LA 1994 Reduction of bacteriuria and pyuria after ingestion of cranberry juice. **Journal of the American Medical Association**, 271:751–754
8. Griffiths P 2003 The role of cranberry juice in the treatment of urinary tract infections (mini-review). **British Journal of Community Nursing**, 8:557–561
9. Jepson RG, Milhaljevic L and Craig J 2004 Cranberries for preventing urinary tract infections. **The Cochrane Database of Systematic Reviews** Issue 2. Art. No: CD001321.DOI: 10.1002/14651858.CD001321
10. RCOG 2003 **Clinical Guideline 36 Prevention of Early Onset Neonatal Group B Streptococcal Disease**. London; Royal College of Obstetricians and Gynaecologists 6
11. Smaill F 2001 Antibiotics for asymptomatic bacteriuria in pregnancy. **The Cochrane Database of Systematic Reviews**. 2. Art. No.: CD000490. DOI: 10.1002/14651858.CD000490
12. British National Formulary 2006 **Issue 51** http: www.bnf.org/bnf/bnf/current/127074.htm [Accessed 08-05-2006]
13. Hass DM 2005 Antibiotic treatment for preterm rupture of the membranes. http://www.clinicalevidence.co/ceweb/conditions/pac/1404/1404_13.jsp [Accessed 04-05-2006]

6.2 Chronic Kidney Disease

1. www.dh.gov.uk/assetRoot/04/10/26/80/04102680.pdf [Accessed 14-09-2006]
2. The Short CKD eGuide, derived from UK CKD Guidelines. 2005 http://www.renal.org/eGFR/eGFR/eguide.html [Accessed 18-05-06]
3. Jones DC and Hayslett JP 1996 Outcome of pregnancy in women with moderate or severe renal insufficiency. **New England Journal of Medicine**, 335:226–226
4. Jungers P and Chaveau D 1997 Pregnancy in renal disease. **Kidney International**, 52:871–885
5. Hou S 1999 Pregnancy in chronic renal insufficiency and end stage renal disease. **American Journal of Kidney Disease**, 33:235–252
6. Davison JM 2001 Renal disorders in pregnancy. **Current Opinion in Obstetrics and Gynaecology**, 13:109–114
7. Branch DW and Porter FF 2006 Chapt. 44 *Autoimmune disease* in James DK, Steer PJ, Weiner CP and Gonik B (Eds) **High Risk Pregnancy: Management Options**, 3rd Edn. Philadelphia; W.B. Saunders 949–985
8. Cooper WD, Hernandez Dias S, *et al.* 2006 Major congenital malformations after exposure to ACE inhibitors. **New England Journal of Medicine**, 344:2443

9. RCOG 2009 **Clinical Guideline No.37a – Thrombosis and embolism during pregnancy and the puerperium, reducing the risk**. London; Royal College of Obstetricians and Gynaecologists
10. NICE 2010 **Clinical Guideline: Hypertension in Pregnancy**. London; National Institute for Clinical Excellence http://www.nice.org.uk/guidance/CG107

6.3 Dialysis in Pregnancy

1. Hou SH 1994 Pregnancy in women on haemodialysis and peritoneal dialysis. **Baillière's Clinical Obstetrics and Gynaecology**, 8:481–500
2. Jungers P and Chaveau D 1997 Pregnancy in renal disease. **Kidney International**, 52:871–885
3. Hussey MJ and Pombar X 1998 Obstetric care for renal allograft recipients or for women treated with haemodialysis or peritoneal dialysis during pregnancy. **Advanced Renal Replacement Therapy**, 5:3–13
4. Hou S 1999 Pregnancy in chronic renal insufficiency and end stage renal disease. **American Journal of Kidney Disease**, 33:235–252
5. NICE 2010 **Clinical Guideline: Hypertension in Pregnancy**. London; National Institute for Clinical Excellence http://www.nice.org.uk/guidance/CG107

6.4 Renal Transplantation

1. Eardley KS and Lipkin GW 2000 Pregnancy in the renal transplant recipient. **Transplant Topics**, 7:1–6
2. Davison JM 2001 Renal disorders in pregnancy. **Current Opinion in Obstetrics and Gynaecology**, 13:109–114
3. McKay DB and Josephson MA 2006 Pregnancy in recipients of solid organs – effects on mother and child. **New England Journal of Medicine**, 354:1281–1293
4. Hussey MJ and Pombar X 1998 Obstetric care for renal allograft recipients or for women treated with haemodialysis or peritoneal dialysis during pregnancy. **Advanced Renal Replacement Therapy**, 5:3–13
5. NICE 2010 **Clinical Guideline: Hypertension in Pregnancy**. London; National Institute for Clinical Excellence http://www.nice.org.uk/guidance/CG107

6.5 Nephrotic Syndrome

1. RCOG 2007 **Clinical Guideline No.37b – Thromboembolic Disease in Pregnancy and the Puerperium: Acute Management**. London; Royal College of Obstetricians and Gynaecologists
2. Cooper WD, Hernandez Dias S, *et al.* 2006 Major congenital malformations after exposure to ACE inhibitors. **New England Journal of Medicine**, 344:2443
3. Barcelo P, Lopez-Lilo J, Cabero L and Del Rio G 1986 Successful pregnancy in primary glomerular disease. **Kidney International**, 30:914–919
4. Farquharson RG and Grieves M 2006 Chapt. 43 *Thromboembolic disease* in James DK, Steer PJ, Weiner CP and Gonik B (Eds) **High Risk Pregnancy: Management Options**, 3rd Edn. Philadelphia; W.B. Saunders 938–948
5. NICE 2010 **Clinical Guideline: Hypertension in Pregnancy**. London; National Institute for Clinical Excellence http://www.nice.org.uk/guidance/CG107

Appendix 6.3.1 Replacement of Renal Function by Dialysis

In medicine, dialysis is a method of replacing renal function that has been lost due to either acute or chronic renal failure. Dialysis works on the principle of diffusion of low molecular weight solutes down a concentration gradient across a semi-permeable membrane. Fluid can be removed by exerting a hydrostatic or osmotic gradient across the membrane. Blood is present on one side of the semi-permeable membrane and dialysis fluid on the other.

The concentration of undesired solutes, such as potassium, in the dialysis fluid is low and a buffer is also present to facilitate the removal of metabolic acid. There are two types of dialysis.

HAEMODIALYSIS (HD)

During haemodialysis the patient's blood is pumped by machine through a filter (dialyser) containing a semi-permeable membrane with a large surface area. A physiological dialysis fluid (dialysate), is pumped on the other side of the semi-permeable membrane in the opposite direction. Excess water and metabolic waste products are cleared from the blood by the processes of diffusion, convection and ultrafiltration.

To prevent the blood from clotting whilst circulating through the machine, a low dose of heparin is infused into the blood tubing.

Normally a patient will receive haemodialysis three times per week, for approximately four hours at a time. Some dialysis patients pass no urine at all, and fluid intake is usually restricted to only 500 ml per day (equivalent to daily insensible losses through breathing, sweating, etc.), plus the amount of the previous day's urinary output. Otherwise, in between dialyses this fluid will accumulate in the body causing 'overload', hypertension and pulmonary oedema.

There are other dietary restrictions such as potassium, which if elevated will cause cardiac arrhythmias, and phosphate which can accumulate and lead to renal bone disease and extravascular calcification.

Access to the vascular system is required for haemodialysis by:

- Insertion of a dual lumen catheter (VasCath) into a major vein
- Arterio-venous fistula: surgical procedure to join together an artery and a vein, usually at the wrist; blood from the artery then flows directly into the vein, the increased pressure causes the vein to thicken and dilate
- Arterio-venous graft (synthetic such as Gore-Tex), again between the artery and a vein, just beneath the skin

It is very important not to cannulate, or take blood, or blood pressure on the arm with the graft or the fistula, as this may cause unnecessary damage to it.

PERITONEAL DIALYSIS (PD)

With PD, the peritoneal membrane serves as a semi-permeable membrane and its blood supply provides blood flow. After the insertion of a soft plastic tube into the peritoneal cavity, dialysis fluid (usually ~2l), is infused. The fluid is left to dwell in the peritoneal cavity, dialysis occurs and the fluid is then drained out and discarded. Fresh fluid is instilled back into the peritoneal cavity and the cycle is repeated.

Most commonly patients perform four exchanges per day, at breakfast, lunch, teatime, and bedtime, and the fluid remains in the abdomen for approximately four hours between exchanges. This is called continuous ambulatory peritoneal dialysis (CAPD). Another alternative is to use a machine that automatically cycles the fluid exchanges in and out of the peritoneal cavity continuously overnight whilst the patient sleeps. This is called automated peritoneal dialysis (APD).

The composition of the dialysis fluid is similar to that used for haemodialysis. The major difference is that PD fluid contains high concentrations of glucose to enable the removal of fluid from the patient by osmosis. Therefore, for example, a patient may instil in 2l of fluid and then later drain out 2.5l of fluid.

The PD fluid is prepared with different glucose concentrations so that the amount of fluid removal can, to some degree, be tailored to individual patient requirements. Because this fluid is warm and sugary, there is a high chance of infection. This may result in PD peritonitis, a painful and potentially serious complication of treatment. Scrupulous hygiene is therefore required when changing the bags.

Dietary restrictions are less rigorous for PD patients because dialysis is occurring constantly. Patients must avoid constipation, as this will restrict the draining out of the dialysis fluid.

7 ENDOCRINE DISORDERS

Robert Gregory and Diane Todd

University Hospitals of Leicester NHS Trust, Leicester, UK

7.1 Hypothyroidism
7.2 Thyrotoxicosis
7.3 Type 1 Diabetes Mellitus
7.4 Type 2 Diabetes Mellitus
7.5 Gestational Diabetes Mellitus
7.6 Addison's Disease (Adrenal Insufficiency)
7.7 Prolactinoma

7.1 Hypothyroidism

Incidence	**Risk for Childbearing**
0.3–0.7% Hypothyroidism	Variable Risk
2.2–2.5% Subclinical hypothyroidism	

EXPLANATION OF CONDITION

Hypothyroidism comprises a lack of thyroid hormones, thyroxine (T4) and tri-iodothyronine (T3). This may be primary (impaired functioning of thyroid tissue) or central (due to pituitary or hypothalamic disease).

T4 circulates in the blood in two forms:

1. T4 which is protein-bound, and
2. Free T4 (fT4) which is unbound and may enter target tissues to exert its effect. Free T4 is a more accurate indicator of thyroid function, fT4 is used for laboratory testing of thyroid function.

Causes

The commonest causes encountered in pregnancy are autoimmune thyroiditis, with or without goitre (Hashimoto's or atrophic thyroiditis), and a history of thyroidectomy or radioiodine treatment.

Autoimmune thyroid disease occurs in families; sometimes in association with other organ-specific autoimmune diseases, e.g. type 1 diabetes, reflecting a genetic predisposition to organ-specific autoimmunity. Auto-antibodies to thyroid peroxidase (TPO) are usually present in serum.

Symptoms

The symptoms are independent of the cause and may affect multiple systems. They include:

- Weight gain
- Constipation
- Cold intolerance
- Alopecia
- Dry skin
- Hoarseness
- Lethargy
- Ataxia
- Cognitive impairment
- Normochromic normocytic anaemia
- Menorrhagia
- Bradycardia[1]

However, the majority of cases have few or no symptoms at diagnosis.

Signs

Slow-relaxing ankle reflexes, coarse skin, cool skin, periorbital puffiness.

Subclinical hypothyroidism is defined biochemically as a raised TSH concentration with normal free T4 (fT4) and free T3 (fT3) concentrations[2]. This condition can resolve spontaneously, but 2.6% of antibody negative and 4.3% of antibody positive subjects become hypothyroid per year.

Investigations

Investigation consists of the measurement of circulating thyroid hormones with thyroid function tests. In primary hypothyroidism thyroid stimulating hormone (TSH) will be raised, free thyroxine (fT4) will be reduced, as will fT3, although this is not always measured. In central hypothyroidism the TSH will also be low.

TPO antibodies are usually positive in autoimmune thyroiditis. Up to 5% of women have positive antibodies in early pregnancy.

COMPLICATIONS

Myxoedema coma is a rare complication that occurs in undiagnosed or chronically untreated hypothyroidism. There is loss of consciousness with hypothermia, hypoventilation and bradycardia.

There are pregnancy associated complications:

- To mother:
  - Reduced fertility
  - Pregnancy induced hypertension
- To baby:
  - Low birth weight
  - Psychomotor retardation

NON-PREGNANCY TREATMENT AND CARE

The standard treatment is thyroid hormone replacement with oral L-thyroxine at a dose sufficient to restore TSH to the normal range – usually 50–150 micrograms once daily.

In central hypothyroidism the dose is adjusted to keep the fT4 in the normal range.

PRE-CONCEPTION ISSUES AND CARE

Women with hypothyroidism may have anovulation and may present with infertility.

Pre-conception care is especially important, as the prospective mother and future child are at risk of:

- **Pregnancy induced hypertension** – this is two–three times as common in overt or subclinical hypothyroidism
- **Low birth weight** – but there is no excess of congenital malformations
- **Reduced psychomotor development** – associated with hypothyroidism in early pregnancy
- **Lower IQ in children at age 8 years** – associated with untreated maternal hypothyroidism; fetal thyroid starts to produce hormones at 10–12 weeks and early fetal brain development depends on small amounts of maternal thyroid hormone that cross the placenta[3,4]

Women who are known to have hypothyroidism should be informed of the above issues, but can be reassured that adequate treatment with thyroxine will reduce the risks to a minimum. They should be reminded to take their thyroxine regularly throughout the pregnancy.

A measurement of fT4 and TSH should be taken as baseline and the dose of thyroxine adjusted if necessary to ensure the woman is euthyroid at the time of conception.

Women with recently-diagnosed hypothyroidism should be advised to delay conceiving until their TSH is restored to a normal level.

Women with subclinical hypothyroidism, who are contemplating pregnancy, should be treated with thyroxine to correct the TSH concentration. As weight gain and lethargy are common problems, the BMI should be estimated (see Appendix 13.1.1) and if overweight a reducing diet advised and an exercise plan recommended.

Pregnancy Issues

Women may be diagnosed with hypothyroidism at any stage of pregnancy and should be treated promptly.

In pregnancies complicated by hypothyroidism the TSH rises, indicating a rising demand for thyroxine. The usual increase in dose is 25–50%.

Medical Management and Care

- Check fT4 and TSH at booking and 4–6 weekly throughout the pregnancy
- Adjust the dose of thyroxine to maintain TSH in the lower half of the reference range[2]
- Encourage compliance with thyroxine supplementation
- If previous IUGR associated with hypothyroidism has occurred, then serial fetal growth scans are indicated

Midwifery Management and Care

- Mother is suitable for routine, shared antenatal care, unless there are any other medical or obstetric issues
- Any concerns regarding restricted fetal growth, refer immediately to the obstetric unit
- Ensure that regular fT4 and TSH blood tests are performed and acted upon
- Be alert for pregnancy-induced hypertension

Labour Issues

- As for normal pregnancy

Medical Management and Care

- No specific medical issues

Midwifery Management and Care[5]

- As for low-risk pregnancy – unless there are any other underlying medical or obstetric issues
- All infants are checked for congenital hypothyroidism at 6 days old, in conjunction with other neonatal screening tests, therefore a placental clotted sample is no longer required

Postpartum Issues

- Reduced demand for thyroxine to pre-pregnancy level
- Neonatal screening is of paramount importance
- The parents are likely to be anxious that the baby could have inherited the maternal condition

Medical Management and Care

- Reduce dose of thyroxine to pre-pregnancy dose (assuming the woman was euthyroid then) in order to avoid overtreatment postpartum
- Check fT4 and TSH 6 weeks after delivery

Midwifery Management and Care

- Routine care for type of delivery
- Breast-feeding should be encouraged
- Arrange paediatric review of baby[6]
- Emphasise to the mother the importance of attending any outpatient appointments arranged, especially for the baby
- It is important that the neonatal screening blood test (formally the Guthrie test) is performed promptly and well, and mention made of the maternal condition on the request form[6]
- Support and reassure the mother who may have been alarmed over indiscreet mention of 'cretinism' and fearful for long-term prospects for the baby

7.2 Thyrotoxicosis

Incidence	Risk for Childbearing
Graves' disease approximately 1:1000	High Risk
Other causes are rare	

EXPLANATION OF CONDITION

Thyrotoxicosis is the clinical syndrome caused by high serum concentrations of thyroid hormones. Symptoms and signs include:

- Heat intolerance
- Weight loss (despite good appetite)
- Insomnia
- Agitation
- Tremor
- Retraction of the upper eyelid
- Sweating
- Tachycardia and bounding pulse
- Diarrhoea
- Oligo- or amenorrhoea

Since several of these features occur in normal pregnancy, the clinical diagnosis of thyrotoxicosis can be difficult to make in this context. The combination of raised serum free thyroxine (fT4), and low thyroid stimulating hormone (TSH) confirms the diagnosis. Occasionally the fT4 is in the normal range, but if the fT3 is raised T3 toxicosis occurs[1].

Causes

Graves' disease: Most women with primary hyperthyroidism in pregnancy will have Graves' disease (GD), an autoimmune condition in which thyrotoxicosis is caused by autoantibodies to the thyroid stimulating hormone receptor (TSHR). These thyroid stimulating immunoglobulins (TSIg) mimic the effects of TSH on its receptor, but in an unregulated way. Endogenous TSH falls in response to high levels of fT3 and fT4, but production and release of these hormones continues to be stimulated by TSIgs. A smooth, symmetrical goitre (enlarged thyroid gland) is often present, over which a *bruit* may be heard. In some cases Graves' disease is associated with other organ-specific autoimmune conditions, e.g. type 1 diabetes and pernicious anaemia.

Excess thyroid hormone ingestion: This may be iatrogenic (overtreatment of hypothyroidism) or factitious (taking thyroid hormone surreptitiously, perhaps to aid weight loss).

HCG-dependent hyperthyroidism: Human chorionic gonadotrophin (HCG) shows a degree of homology with TSH, and can act as a weak TSHR agonist. Conditions characterised by raised concentrations of HCG may cause hyperthyroidism. The commonest is hyperemesis gravidarum which results in transient hyperthyroidism in one-third of cases. Trophoblastic tumours such as hydatidiform mole may rarely cause thyrotoxicosis[1].

COMPLICATIONS

- **Graves' ophthalmopathy** (GO) describes the range of eye symptoms and signs seen in up to 50% of patients with GD. These range from a stare due to retraction of the upper eyelid to exophthalmos of one or both eyes that may result in diplopia and even blindness due to optic nerve compression. Corneal damage can occur when the patient cannot close her eyes properly. Smoking is a risk factor for GO. The disease is thought to be due to an immune response directed against orbital antigens resembling TSHR[2]
- **Graves' dermopathy** is an uncommon feature characterised by localised, usually pre-tibial, myxoedema

- **Thyrotoxic storm** is severe life-threatening thyrotoxicosis, usually precipitated by the withdrawal of antithyroid drug treatment or intercurrent illness. Features include high fever, tachycardia, drowsiness and coma[3]

NON-PREGNANCY TREATMENT AND CARE

Antithyroid Drugs

Carbimazole (CBZ) (methimazole in the US) and propylthiouracil (PTU) block the organification of iodine – an essential step in the manufacture of thyroid hormones. They are also weakly immunosuppressive and may induce long-term remission of GD.

Treatment is usually started at a high dose, which reduces fT4 and fT3 to normal in approximately 4 weeks. Propranolol, a non-selective beta-blocker, may be prescribed to relieve symptoms during this phase, but is not required long term. In order to avoid iatrogenic hypothyroidism it is necessary either to reduce the dose of CBZ or PTU to that required to keep the concentration of fT4 in the normal range (*dose titration*) or to continue with high dose CBZ or PTU in combination with L-thyroxine (*block and replace*). After treatment for 12–18 months with dose titration, or 6–12 months with block and replace, medication is stopped.

Remission is induced in 60% of cases. Some who relapse opt for long-term CBZ or PTU (titrated dose), others choose radioiodine treatment or surgery. Side effects include urticaria and arthralgia. Agranulocytosis (incidence 0.2–0.5%) is potentially life threatening and patients must be counselled when starting treatment[1].

Radioiodine (^{131}I)

The thyroid gland in GD is avid for iodine and will take up ^{131}I given orally. This radioactive isotope causes a thyroiditis that eventually destroys sufficient thyroid tissue to lower thyroid hormone levels to normal, or subnormal. Women are counselled not to conceive for 6 months following ^{131}I treatment.

Thyroidectomy

Subtotal thyroidectomy is usually reserved for cases of GD uncontrolled by large doses of antithyroid drugs, or where there is a large goitre.

PRE-CONCEPTION ISSUES AND CARE

The woman is at risk of oligo-/amenorrhoea and consequently reduced fertility.

There are additional risks of fetal and neonatal transfer of the thyroid antibodies causing neonatal thyroid dysfunction.

Women on block and replace treatment are switched to a titrated dose of CBZ or PTU. The woman should be euthyroid by fT4 before conception. If uncontrolled by drug therapy, surgery is considered prior to cessation of contraception[2]. Women should continue with contraception for 6 months following ^{131}I treatment.

Aplasia cutis is a rare defect of the skin of the scalp. It has only been reported in babies born to mothers who took CBZ and not PTU in pregnancy. Some endocrinologists recommend using PTU rather than CBZ in pregnancy[4].

Pregnancy Issues

Thyrotoxicosis increases the risk of miscarriage. Diagnosis of thyrotoxicosis may be difficult because some of the symptoms and signs are mimicked by normal pregnancy. Serum investigations are necessary.

Graves' disease (GD) tends to improve in pregnancy, and may remit completely during the second half of pregnancy.

Fetal or neonatal thyrotoxicosis affects 2–10% of Graves' disease pregnancies. This can cause a small for dates baby, premature labour and intrauterine or neonatal death. It is also associated with craniostenosis.

Overtreatment of maternal thyrotoxicosis will cause fetal hypothyroidism and goitre.

If ultrasound scans show a fetal goitre the differential diagnosis is fetal hypothyroidism or fetal thyrotoxicosis. This is an indication for cordocentesis to measure fetal TSH and fT4[2].

Medical Management and Care

- The aim of treatment is to achieve maternal euthyroidism (normal thyroid function) and maintain this for the entire pregnancy
- fT4 should ideally be in the upper half of the reference range
- Block and replace regimens are contraindicated in pregnancy because, while CBZ and PTU cross the placenta, relatively little thyroxine does and this would cause fetal hypothyroidism
- The lowest dose of CBZ or PTU that achieves target fT4 levels is used
- Serial measurements of fT4 and TSH every 4 weeks will usually allow withdrawal of antithyroid drugs in the third trimester
- If large doses of CBZ or PTU appear to be required to treat maternal thyrotoxicosis, it is worth considering referral for subtotal thyroidectomy after the first trimester to avoid fetal hypothyroidism
- The risk of fetal/neonatal thyrotoxicosis is highest in women with uncontrolled thyrotoxicosis in later pregnancy, those who have had this complication before, and those who have had radioiodine or surgical treatment
- Measurement of TSIg in the third trimester in such cases may help those at highest risk, but this assay is not readily available in the UK and many centres rely on careful obstetric monitoring of fetal thyroid status

Midwifery Management and Care

- Accurate booking history and early referral to specialist obstetric unit
- Ensure regular fT4 and TSH tests are performed and acted upon
- Serial ultrasound growth scans should be organised
- Regular assessment of fetal heart rate to detect fetal tachycardia (>160/min is suggestive) is essential

Labour Issues

- Detection of previously undiagnosed fetal thyrotoxicosis.

Medical Management and Care

- To manage as high risk[2]

Midwifery Management and Care

- Manage as high-risk labour
- Continuous fetal monitoring to detect fetal tachycardia
- Alert the paediatrician when labour is established

Postpartum Issues

Management of Neonatal Thyrotoxicosis
Neonatal thyrotoxicosis, caused by placental transfer of maternal TSIgs, is self-limiting, but gets worse transiently when the maternally transferred antithyroid drugs disappear.

Relapse
Graves' disease can 'flare' postpartum.

Antithyroid Drugs and Breast-feeding
PTU is preferred to carbimazole if the mother wishes to breast-feed, as it is transferred to breast milk less readily. However carbimazole in low dose (<15 mg daily) does not affect infant thyroid function.

Medical Management and Care

- The baby may require temporary treatment with antithyroid drugs and propranolol
- Maternal thyroid hormone levels must be checked 6 weeks postpartum to identify relapse of GD and treatment reintroduced or increased as necessary[5]

Midwifery Management and Care

- Extend the period of postnatal observations, with emphasis on pulse
- Promote breast-feeding and reassure the mother that low dose carbimazole does not affect infant thyroid function
- When examining the baby, be vigilant for signs of goitre (swollen neck) and if suspected report this immediately
- Be alert for signs of neonatal thyrotoxicosis, which may be delayed for a week[6], and include: weight loss, jitteriness, tachycardia, irritability and poor feeding
- The baby may be transferred to a neonatal unit, in which case the mother requires support and measures to promote infant 'bonding'

7.3 Type 1 Diabetes Mellitus

Incidence	**Risk for Childbearing**
2–4:1000 pregnancies	High Risk

EXPLANATION OF CONDITION

Type 1 diabetes mellitus (T1DM) accounts for 15–20% of all diabetes mellitus. Since it usually presents in childhood or early adulthood, it accounts for the majority of cases of pregestational diabetes. It is caused by autoimmune destruction of the insulin-producing β-cells of the pancreatic islets leading to insulin dependency, and there is a genetic predisposition to the condition.

The symptoms are of hyperglycaemia and include thirst, polydipsia, weight loss, fatigue and blurred vision. If not diagnosed at this stage, diabetic ketoacidosis may develop – a medical emergency, characterised by dehydration, and metabolic acidosis, that can lead to coma and death. Diagnostic criteria are included in Appendix 7.3.1. Most patients with T1DM would have had symptoms at presentation and a raised fasting or random venous plasma glucose..

COMPLICATIONS[1]

Microvascular Complications

These are caused by chronic hyperglycaemia and are preventable if patients can achieve near normal blood glucose concentrations for much of the time.

Retinopathy

The early stages are asymptomatic, so annual photographic screening is essential. The stages progress from background (requiring no specific treatment) through pre-proliferative to proliferative retinopathy in which retinal ischaemia has stimulated new vessel formation on the optic disc or in the periphery of the retina. New vessels are prone to tear leading to vitreous haemorrhage. The fibrous stalk carrying the new vessels can cause traction retinal detachment. Each scenario can cause blindness. Laser photocoagulation is an effective treatment for pre-proliferative and proliferative retinopathy.

Nephropathy

The earliest sign is microalbuminuria (albumin:creatinine ratio >3.5 mg/mmol). Angiotensin converting enzyme inhibitors (ACEI) are indicated at this stage to reduce the risk of progression. The next stage is overt proteinuria (Albustix® positive). Renal function deteriorates and blood pressure increases. Renal failure progresses to chronic kidney disease (CKD). Some may require dialysis or transplantation.

Neuropathy

The commonest presentation is with a symmetrical sensory polyneuropathy of the feet and legs; this confers a risk of foot ulceration. Less commonly there may be diabetic mononeuropathies and autonomic neuropathy that can cause postural hypotension, gastroparesis, diarrhoea and bladder dysfunction.

Cataract Formation

Three to four times more likely in those under the age of 60 years.

NON-PREGNANCY TREATMENT AND CARE

The aims of treatment are to prevent symptomatic hyper- and hypoglycaemia, and the development of complications. Treatment is with subcutaneous insulin injections. Although insulin preparations are of standard strength, they differ considerably in the rate of onset and duration of action. Patients may take 2–5 injections per day. Injections are given with disposable syringes and needles or with pen-injectors. Some patients use a continuous subcutaneous insulin infusion (CSII) (insulin pump).

The diabetic diet is designed to achieve and maintain a healthy weight. It is high in unrefined carbohydrate (60%) and low in fat (<30%).

Patients are encouraged to monitor their own capillary glucose concentrations to help them to achieve target values. Carbohydrate counting and appropriate adjustment of the insulin dose is the cornerstone of modern diabetes management. However, not all patients achieve ideal control. Routine care includes assessment of diabetic control by measuring HbA1c, physical examination for complications, retinal photography, screening urine for microalbumin and measurement of serum creatinine.

PRE-CONCEPTION ISSUES AND CARE

Pre-pregnancy counselling is essential because of the risks of miscarriage, congenital anomalies, IUGR, pre-eclampsia, macrosomia, polyhydramnios and IUFD. This should be part of routine diabetes care wherever this is provided, but women who are considering pregnancy should have access to a multidisciplinary pregnancy preparation service.

The aim is a planned pregnancy with the woman taking high-dose folic acid (5 mg daily)[2] and having the best possible diabetic control at the time of conception[3]. Women with suboptimal diabetic control (HbA1c >53 mmol/mol) should be encouraged to use contraception while efforts are made to improve control[4,5]. There should be a thorough assessment of complications, as retinopathy and nephropathy can deteriorate as a result of pregnancy, placing both mother and baby at risk.

Medication should be reviewed and where possible changed to agents that are safer in pregnancy. In particular ACE inhibitors should be stopped, and, where treatment for hypertension is required, methyldopa substituted. Insulin regimens may be intensified – twice daily injections with biphasic preparations are unlikely to allow sufficient flexibility of dose adjustment. Only *insulin aspart* (NovoRapid) is licensed for use in pregnancy. Theoretical concerns about insulin glargine (Lantus ®) and animal insulins mean that human isophane insulins or *insulin detemir* (Levemir ®) are preferred as basal insulins[4] (though increasing evidence now supports insulin glargine use in pregnancy).

Pregnancy Issues

Booking:
- Dating/viability scan
- HbA1c
- Complication check and retinal examination
- Medication review
- Blood glucose monitoring strategy
- Dietetic review
- *Potential issues*
  - miscarriage*
  - hypoglycaemia
  - hyperemesis gravidarum
  - Down's risk assessment (nuchal thickness and amniocentesis)

Week 20:
- Detailed ultrasound scan
- *Potential issues*
  - congenital malformation*

Weeks 28, 32, 36:
- Growth scans
- *Potential issues*
  - IUGR*
  - macrosomia*
  - polyhydramnios*
  - premature labour
  - pre-eclampsia

Week 35 onwards:
- Plan mode and timing of delivery
- Plan insulin management during labour and postpartum
- *Potential issues*
  - – unexplained fetal death *
  - *Outcomes influenced by diabetic control*

Medical Management and Care (Figure 7.3.1)
- Planned pregnancy – check if pre-pregnancy actions were carried out
- Unplanned pregnancy – start folic acid 5 mg daily[2], review insulin regimen and alter if necessary, and undertake pre-pregnancy actions
- Arrange retinal screening and, if retinopathy detected, arrange regular ophthalmological monitoring
- Advise about risk of hypoglycaemia (especially if vomiting is a problem); ensure the woman and her partner are equipped to treat hypoglycaemia – glucose tablets or drinks (GlucoGel) and glucagon injection (GlucaGen)
- Advise and assist the woman to achieve target blood glucose levels (<5 mmol/l pre-meals and <7 mmol/l 2 hours after meals)
- Advise on aspirin treatment from 12 weeks gestation[1]
- From 20–36 weeks of gestation maternal insulin resistance increases due to placental production of counter regulatory hormones, especially human placental lactogen; insulin dose will need to be increased to deal with this
- Delivery should be at term unless there is any concern about fetal growth or wellbeing or if the diabetic control has been suboptimal, in which case earlier delivery may be recommended

Midwifery Management and Care
- Immediate referral to combined diabetes–obstetric antenatal clinic
- Maintain regular contact with specialist team either by clinic attendance or telephone every 1–2 weeks
- Ensure that all screening procedures concerning maternal and neonatal complications of diabetes are performed in a timely manner
- Advise on weight management as appropriate[6]
- Discuss plans for infant feeding and provide information on colostrum harvesting where appropriate
- Ensure plan for delivery has been made in partnership with the woman and is clearly and accurately documented in the notes
- Advise woman to come to the unit if she becomes unwell or has concerns about fetal movements
- Offer parentcraft education including advice on the management of diabetes during delivery and postpartum

Labour Issues
- High-risk labour (not suitable for home delivery or birthing pool)
- Management of diabetes
- Monitoring fetal wellbeing – there is a risk of fetal distress
- Paediatrician should be available for delivery

Medical Management and Care
- Managed as per high-risk pregnancy
- Optimise blood glucose control at 4–7 mmol/l using intravenous insulin and D-glucose as per local guidelines (for suggested insulin regimen for labour see Appendix 7.3.1)
- Prevent maternal hyperglycaemia and neonatal hypoglycaemia
- Avoid maternal hypoglycaemia
- Prophylactic antibiotics for operative or instrumental delivery

Midwifery Management and Care
- Hourly measurement of maternal blood glucose
- Continuous EFM is indicated
- Anticipate shoulder dystocia (awareness of local obstetric protocols)
- Notify paediatricians once labour is established, and call for delivery

Postpartum Issues
- Neonatal hypoglycaemia
- Insulin regimen
- Breast-feeding
- Contraception advice

Medical Management and Care
- Insulin sensitivity increases promptly after delivery
- Stop insulin infusion once the woman has re-commenced eating
- Optimise maternal blood glucose levels, avoiding hypoglycaemia
- Adjust postpartum insulin doses according to blood glucose levels
- Breast-feeding typically reduces insulin requirements by 30%

Midwifery Management and Care
- Routine postnatal care appropriate for the type of delivery and observe for maternal hypoglycaemia
- Infants should be offered early feeding, observe baby closely for signs of hypoglycaemia (jitteriness)
- Neonatal blood glucose levels should be monitored as per local policy
- Breast-feeding should be actively encouraged[7]
- Not appropriate to have early 6-hour discharge
- Information should be offered regarding future pregnancies, and pre-pregnancy care
- A follow-up appointment should be made with the diabetes team

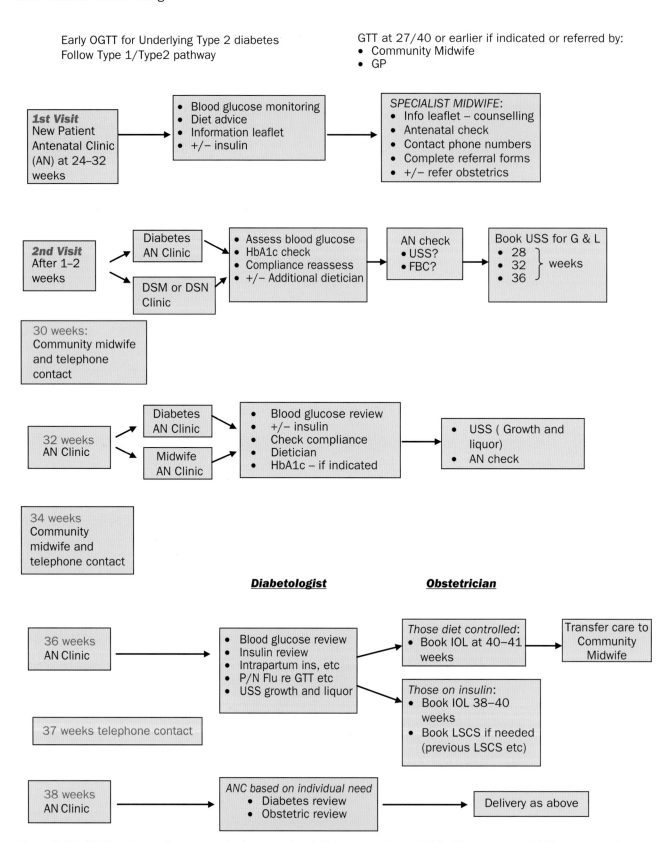

Figure 7.3.1 NICE guidance for antenatal care gestational diabetes mellitus (GDM). AN, antenatal. LSCS, lower section caesarean section. DSN, Diabetes Specialist Nurse. DSM, Diabetes Specialist Midwife. FBC, full blood count. G&L, growth and liquor. GP, General Practitioner. IOL, induction of labour. OGTT, oral glucose tolerance test. GTT, glucose tolerance test. ANC, antenatal clinic. USS, ultrasound scan. This figure is downloadable from the book companion website at www.wiley.com/go/robson

7.4 Type 2 Diabetes Mellitus

Incidence	**Risk for Childbearing**
Approximately 1:1000 pregnancies, but depends on ethnicity of the clinic population	High Risk

EXPLANATION OF CONDITION

Type 2 diabetes (T2DM) accounts for 80–85% of all diabetes mellitus. The prevalence of T2DM is rising worldwide, but the rate of rise is fastest in developing countries. It usually presents in middle age or later life, but along with the global epidemic there is a trend for earlier presentation, particularly in minority ethnic populations, so women with T2DM are becoming pregnant. Some of these women will have had gestational diabetes previously.

T2DM is characterised by two metabolic defects – insulin resistance and impaired insulin secretion. There is an inherited predisposition (polygenic) that can be unmasked by obesity and physical inactivity. Besides raised blood glucose, non-esterified fatty acid (NEFA) concentrations are raised. NEFA reduce the uptake of glucose by muscle, and stimulate gluconeogenesis in the liver.

Early in the disease patients respond to diet or oral hypoglycaemic agents, but many ultimately require insulin treatment. T2DM was commonly regarded as 'mild diabetes' because patients did not need to be treated with insulin to keep them alive. However, the adjective is inappropriate because patients are at increased risk of cardiovascular mortality and morbidity.

COMPLICATIONS[1]

Microvascular Complications

Microvascular complications are caused by chronic hyperglycaemia and are preventable if patients can achieve near normal blood glucose concentrations for much of the time.

Macrovascular Disease

Macrovascular disease occurs because insulin resistance is part of the 'metabolic syndrome' (see Appendix 7.3.1), each component of which is a risk factor for cardiovascular disease. Consequently the management of T2DM is not just about controlling blood glucose concentrations: it encompasses the management of as many of these risk factors as possible.

Pregnancy Complications

* Miscarriage
* Congenital malformations
* IUGR
* Macrosomia
* Polyhydramnios
* Intrauterine fetal death (IUFD)

NON-PREGNANCY TREATMENT AND CARE

The aims of treatment are to prevent symptomatic hyper- and hypoglycaemia and the development of micro- and macrovascular complications.

Initially, lifestyle modification (increasing physical activity and reducing dietary energy consumption) that leads to weight reduction may improve glucose tolerance and control diabetes adequately.

With time it is often necessary to use oral antidiabetic agents. Metformin is the drug of choice for overweight patients and is increasingly used in polycystic ovarian syndrome (PCOS) to augment ovulation induction. Other agents include sulfonylureas (e.g. glibenclamide, gliclazide, glipizide), the thiazolidinedione pioglitazone, gliptins (saxagliptin, sitagliptin and vildagliptin). GLP-1 mimetics (exenatide and liraglutide) are injectable therapies indicated for obese patients with T2DM. If oral agents alone or in combination are ineffective then insulin injections are added or substituted, and management of this is as for T1DM.

Patients are often prescribed antihypertensives (especially ACE inhibitors), statins to lower cholesterol concentrations and aspirin as primary prophylaxis against cardiovascular events.

Routine care is as for T1DM (see Section 7.3).

PRE-CONCEPTION ISSUES AND CARE

Pre-pregnancy counselling is essential for all women of childbearing age with T2DM. This should be part of routine diabetes care wherever this is provided, but women who are considering pregnancy should have access to a multidisciplinary pregnancy preparation service. There is evidence to suggest that women with T2DM are more likely to be cared for in primary care and are less likely to receive pregnancy advice than women with T1DM. This is associated with worse outcomes[2,3].

The aim is the same as for women with T1DM.

Pre-pregnancy assessment is as for women with T1DM. Women with T2DM are likely to be overweight or obese and they should be actively encouraged to lose weight before conceiving if possible.

Pre-pregnancy medication review is very important. Women are likely to be taking potentially teratogenic drugs including statins and ACE inhibitors, which must be discontinued.

Oral antidiabetic/hypoglycaemic agents should be discontinued and treatment with insulin started as for T1DM. Increasing evidence indicates metformin is not teratogenic, and some clinicians advise women with PCOS who conceive whilst receiving it to continue to take it at ≥32 weeks to prevent deterioration in glucose tolerance.

Women with suboptimal diabetic control (HbA1c >5 mmol/mol should be encouraged to use contraception while efforts are made to improve control[2,4].

Pregnancy Issues

Booking:
- Dating/viability scan
- HbA1c
- Complication check and retinal examination
- Medication review
- Blood glucose monitoring strategy
- Dietetic review
- *Potential issues*
  - miscarriage*
  - hypoglycaemia
  - hyperemesis gravidarum
  - Down's risk assessment (nuchal thickness and amniocentesis)

Week 20:
- Detailed ultrasound scan or fetal echocardiogram
- *Potential issues*
  - congenital malformation*

Weeks 28, 32, 36:
- Growth scans
- *Potential issues*
  - IUGR*, macrosomia*
  - polyhydramnios*
  - premature labour
  - pre-eclampsia[2,5]

Week 35 onwards:
- Plan mode and timing of delivery
- Plan insulin management during labour and postpartum
- *Potential issues*
  - unexplained fetal death*
  - *Outcomes influenced by diabetic control*

Medical Management and Care
- Planned pregnancy – check if pre-pregnancy actions were carried out
- Unplanned pregnancy – start folic acid 5 mg daily[5], review insulin regimen and alter if necessary, and undertake pre-pregnancy actions
- Arrange retinal screening and, if retinopathy detected, arrange regular ophthalmological monitoring
- Advise about risk of hypoglycaemia (especially if vomiting is a problem); ensure the woman and her partner are equipped to treat hypoglycaemia – glucose tablets or drinks (Glucogel) and glucagon injection (Glucagen)
- Advise and assist the woman to achieve target blood glucose levels (<5 mmol/l pre-meals and <7 mmol/l 2 hours after meals)
- Advise on aspirin treatment from 12 weeks gestation[6]
- From 20–36 weeks gestation maternal insulin resistance increases due to placental production of counter-regulatory hormones, especially human placental lactogen; insulin may be required to compensate for this
- Delivery should be at term unless there is any concern about fetal growth or wellbeing or if the diabetic control has been suboptimal, in which case earlier delivery may be recommended

Midwifery Management and Care
- Immediate referral to combined diabetes–obstetric antenatal clinic
- Maintain regular contact with specialist team either by clinic attendance or telephone every 1–2 weeks
- Ensure that all screening procedures concerning maternal and neonatal complications of diabetes are performed in a timely manner
- Advise on weight management as appropriate[7]
- Discuss plans for infant feeding and provide information on colostrum harvesting where appropriate
- Ensure plan for delivery has been made in partnership with the woman and is clearly and accurately documented in the notes
- Advise woman to come to the unit if she becomes unwell or has concerns about fetal movements
- Offer parentcraft education including advice on the management of diabetes during delivery and postpartum

Labour Issues
- High-risk labour (not suitable for home delivery or birthing pool)
- Management of diabetes
- Monitoring fetal wellbeing – there is a risk of fetal distress
- Paediatrician should be available for delivery

Medical Management and Care
- Managed as per high-risk pregnancy
- Optimise blood glucose control at 4–7 mmol/l using intravenous insulin and D-glucose as per local guidelines (for suggested insulin regimen for labour see Appendix 7.3.1)
- Prevent maternal hyperglycaemia and neonatal hypoglycaemia
- Avoid maternal hypoglycaemia
- Prophylactic antibiotics for operative or instrumental delivery

Midwifery Management and Care
- Hourly measurement of maternal blood glucose
- Continuous EFM is indicated
- Anticipate shoulder dystocia (awareness of local obstetric protocols)[1]
- Notify paediatricians once labour is established, and call for delivery

Postpartum Issues
- Neonatal hypoglycaemia
- Insulin regimen
- Breast-feeding
- Contraception advice

Medical Management and Care
- Insulin sensitivity increases promptly after delivery
- Generally women require c.25% reduction in pre-pregnancy insulin doses
- Stop insulin infusion once the woman has re-commenced eating
- Optimise maternal blood glucose levels, avoiding hypoglycaemia
- Adjust postpartum insulin doses according to blood glucose results
- Breast-feeding typically necessitates a further reduction insulin requirements

Midwifery Management and Care
- Routine care as appropriate for the type of delivery
- Observe baby closely for signs of hypoglycaemia (jitteriness)
- Monitor neonatal blood glucose levels as per local policy
- Breast-feeding should be actively encouraged[8]
- Some oral antidiabetic agents should not be used until weaning
- Insulin treatment is preferred
- Information should be offered regarding contraception (suitable for oral contraceptives), future pregnancies and pre-pregnancy care[2]
- A follow-up appointment should be made with the diabetes team or local GP

7.5 Gestational Diabetes Mellitus

Incidence	Risk for Childbearing
3–18% of pregnancies (depending on definition used and on population studied – however, this figure is known to be increasing)	High Risk[4]

EXPLANATION OF CONDITION

Gestational diabetes mellitus (GDM) is glucose intolerance that is diagnosed during pregnancy. This may represent previously undiagnosed type 1 or type 2 diabetes, but the majority of cases are due to transient, pregnancy-induced glucose intolerance.

Pathophysiology

Glucose tolerance changes during normal pregnancy: fasting blood glucose concentration falls and postprandial glucose concentration rises up to 36 weeks gestation. From week 20 increasing levels of placental hormones, including human placental lactogen, are responsible for increasing maternal insulin resistance. If the woman has sufficient insulin secretory reserve, then the rise in plasma glucose is minor: if she has limited reserve, then glucose intolerance or diabetes may result.

Definition

There has recently been progress towards adopting a universal definition of GDM. The International Association of Diabetes and Pregnancy Study Groups (IADPSG)[1] has based its recommendation on detailed analysis of the epidemiological data from the Hyperglycemia and Adverse Pregnancy Outcome (HAPO) study[2]. These confirmed a continuum of risk to mother and fetus from increasing maternal glycaemia detected by a 75 g oral glucose tolerance test (OGTT) at 24–28 weeks gestation. The IADPSG recommend a diagnostic threshold of fasting plasma glucose ≥5.1 mmol/l, 1-hour glucose ≥10 mmol/l, 2-hour glucose ≥8.5 mmol/l. The fasting glucose is significantly lower than the NICE-endorsed WHO definition, ≥7 mmol/l, while the 2-hour value is ≥7.8 mmol/l. The consequence of changing from the NICE/WHO to the IADPSG criteria will be an increase in the number of women diagnosed with GDM, but there will be some women who would have been diagnosed on the basis of a 2-hour glucose in the range 7.8–8.4 mmol/l who will no longer be considered to have GDM.

Screening

Since nearly all women with GDM will be asymptomatic, it will be necessary to screen.

NICE recommends that selective screening of high-risk groups is cost-effective[3]. Groups at high risk include women with:

- BMI above 30 kg/m^2
- First degree relative with diabetes
- Previous macrosomic baby weighing 4.5 kg or above
- Previous GDM
- Family origin with high prevalence of diabetes (South Asian, Black Caribbean and Middle Eastern)

To these may be added previous stillbirth and polycystic ovarian syndrome.

Glycosuria is a poor predictor of GDM and usually reflects hyperfiltration of pregnancy. However, glycosuria before 20 weeks is unusual and should not be ignored as it may indicate pre-existing undiagnosed diabetes.

The IADPSG recommends universal screening rather than selective screening. This was rejected as not cost-effective by NICE. To date there have been two randomised controlled trials investigating the effect of treating glucose intolerance in pregnancy, neither of which defined GDM as proposed by IADPSG. The Australian Carbohydrate Intolerance Study in Pregnant Women (ACHOIS)[2] showed that treatment was associated with a significant reduction of composite outcomes (death, shoulder dystocia, fractures, nerve palsies) from 4% to 1%. The Maternal Fetal Medicines Unit Network multicentre, randomised trial of treatment for mild GDM showed no difference in these outcomes, but there were significant reductions in birth weight, %LGA babies, and caesarean section rate.

COMPLICATIONS

Increased maternal glucose concentration leads to increased delivery of nutrients to the fetus, which stimulates fetal insulin production. The potential effects of diabetes on the fetus include:

- Polyhydramnios
- Macrosomia (risk of shoulder dystocia)
- Hepatomegaly
- Polycythaemia
- IUFD
- Hyaline membrane disease
- Neonatal hypoglycaemia

Since the onset of GDM is after 12 weeks, it does not confer an increased risk of congenital malformation or miscarriage.

TREATMENT AND CARE

Unless the woman has symptomatic hyperglycaemia it is usual to start by offering lifestyle advice and home blood glucose monitoring. Most women (80%) will be adequately controlled by diet and exercise. A dietetic assessment is essential. Women should be advised to eat regular meals, and to take 50% of their diet as unrefined carbohydrate. If they are overweight/obese it is safe to aim for limited weight gain during the pregnancy, by modest energy restriction[4].

The memory of the blood glucose meter should be interrogated at each clinic visit. Consistent failure to meet target blood glucose concentrations is an indication to start insulin treatment. Oral antidiabetic agents are not generally used, although glibenclamide (glyburide) and Metformin (Glucophage) are safe, effective and becoming a popular choice of treatment.

Raised post-meal glucose values are best treated by short-acting analogues *insulin aspart* (NovoRapid®), which has a licence for use in pregnancy, *insulin lispro* (Humalog®) or insulin glulisine (Apidra®) while raised pre-meal values are treated with human isophane insulin, or, where nocturnal hypoglycaemia is a problem, *insulin detemir* (Levemi).

Pregnancy Issues
- Explanation of condition
- Dietetic advice
- Blood glucose monitoring instruction
- Dietetic review
- Review maternal blood glucose results: if consistently above target, commence insulin treatment and titrate dose until targets achieved

Weeks 28, 32, 36:
- Growth scans
- *Potential issues*
  - macrosomia*
  - polyhydramnios*
  - premature labour
  - pre-eclampsia
  - IUGR

Week 35 onwards:
- Plan mode and timing of delivery
- Plan insulin management during labour and postpartum
- *Potential issues*
  - – unexplained fetal death*
  - **Outcomes influenced by diabetic control*

Medical Management and Care (Figure 7.5.1)
- Advise and assist woman to achieve target blood glucose levels (<5 mmol/l before meals and <7 mmol/l 2 hours after meals)
- From 20–36 weeks gestation maternal insulin resistance increases, due to placental production of counter-regulatory hormones, especially human placental lactogen; insulin may be required to compensate for this
- Delivery should be at term unless there is any concern about fetal growth or wellbeing or if the diabetic control has been suboptimal, in which case earlier delivery may be recommended

Midwifery Management and Care
- Full explanation of GDM and the implications for pregnancy should be given
- Maintain regular contact with specialist team either by clinic attendance or telephone every 1–2 weeks to permit adjustment of treatment where necessary and to arrange regular ultrasound scans
- Ensure plan for delivery has been made in partnership with the woman and is clearly and accurately documented in the notes
- Advise the woman to come to the unit if she becomes unwell or has concerns about fetal movements
- Offer parentcraft education including advice on the management of diabetes during labour and postpartum

Labour Issues
- High-risk labour (not suitable for home delivery or birthing pool)
- Management of diabetes
- Monitoring fetal wellbeing – there is a risk of fetal distress
- Paediatrician should be available for delivery

Medical Management and Care
- If insulin-treated, manage as per type 1 DM high-risk pregnancy
- Optimise blood glucose control using intravenous insulin and D glucose as per local guidelines – as for type 1 and type 2 diabetes
- If on diet treatment alone, monitor blood glucose levels as per local guidance, no requirement for insulin therapy in labour if blood glucose levels are normal
- Prophylactic antibiotics for operative or instrumental delivery

Midwifery Management and Care
- In addition to routine labour care, take hourly measurements of maternal blood glucose, and adjust insulin as appropriate
- Continuous EFM is indicated
- Anticipate shoulder dystocia (consult local obstetric protocols)
- Notify paediatricians once labour is established, and call for delivery

Postpartum Issues
- Neonatal hypoglycaemia
- Assess glucose intolerance
- Encourage breast-feeding
- Lifestyle advice
- Contraceptive advice

Medical Management and Care
- Stop insulin immediately after delivery and monitor maternal blood glucose concentrations before meals for 24 hours
- If blood glucose >7 mmol/l seek advice from diabetes team
- Arrange repeat glucose tolerance test at 6 weeks postpartum
- Classify glucose tolerance according to result and manage accordingly

Midwifery Management and Care
- Observe baby closely for signs of hypoglycaemia (jitteriness)
- Neonatal blood glucose levels should be monitored as per local policy
- Breast-feeding should be actively encouraged
- Ensure understanding of increased risk of type 2 diabetes and advise about lifestyle modifications to minimise that risk. Educate about symptoms of diabetes and recommend an annual test of glucose tolerance
- Advise that the woman should have an oral GTT before she conceives again, and during every subsequent pregnancy to screen for type 2 diabetes mellitus

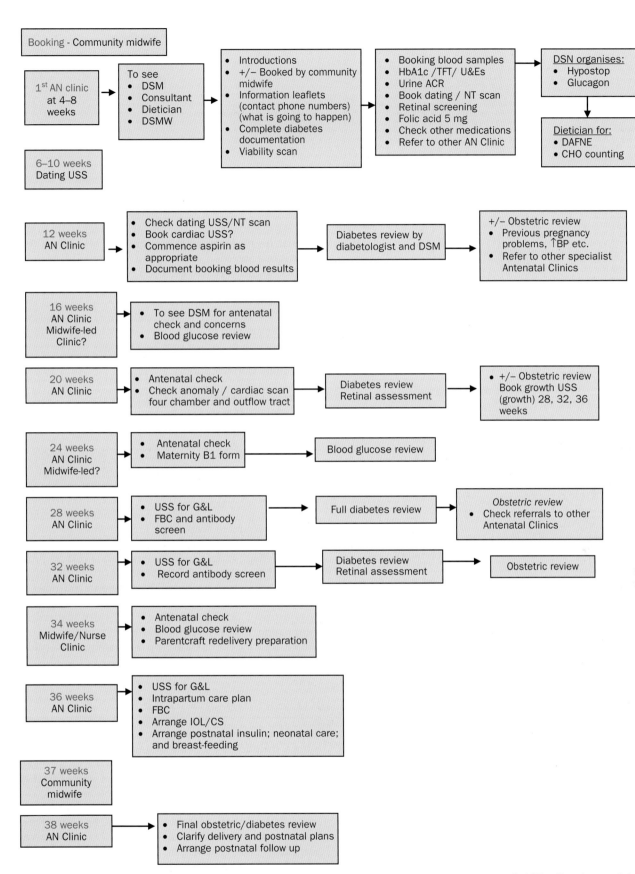

Figure 7.5.1 NICE guidance for antenatal care type 1 and type 2 diabetes mellitus. AN, antenatal. ACR, albumin-creatinine ratio. CHO, carbohydrate. CS, caesarean section. DSN, Diabetes Specialist Nurse. DSM, Diabetes Specialist Midwife. DAFNE, dose adjustment for normal eating. FBC, full blood count. G&L, growth and liquor. GP, General Practitioner. IOL, induction of labour. OGTT, oral glucose tolerance test. TFT, thyroid function test. NT, nuchal translucency screening (11^{+2} to 14^{+1} weeks). USS, ultrasound scan. This figure is downloadable from the book companion website at www.wiley.com/go/robson

7.6 Addison's Disease (Adrenal Insufficiency)

Incidence	Risk for Childbearing
Rare <1:1000	High Risk

EXPLANATION OF CONDITION

Adrenal insufficiency is the deficiency of gluco- and miner-alocorticosteroids produced by the cortex of the adrenal glands[1]. This may be primary (damage to the glands) or secondary, due to the lack of pituitary adrenocorticotrophic hormone (ACTH).

Addison's disease refers to primary adrenal insufficiency. Of all cases, 70–90% are due to autoimmune destruction of the adrenal cortex (either alone or associated with other organ-specific autoimmune conditions, e.g. type 1 diabetes, autoimmune thyroid disease). Of the remainder, most cases are due to tuberculosis. Autoantibodies to the enzyme 21-hydroxylase are often present in autoimmune Addison's disease.

Symptoms

Symptoms include:

- Anorexia
- Nausea
- Vomiting
- Weight loss
- Weakness
- Lassitude
- Syncope
- Hyperpigmentation (not in secondary adrenal insufficiency)
- The patient may be hypotensive or have postural hypotension

Diagnosis

Biochemical changes include:

- Low serum sodium
- Raised serum potassium
- Hypoglycaemia

but they may be absent. A low plasma cortisol concentration at 9 a.m. supports the diagnosis.

A paired ACTH measurement is needed to differentiate primary (ACTH raised) from secondary (ACTH low) cases. If the morning plasma cortisol is borderline, the ability of the adrenal cortex to respond to synthetic ACTH (tetracosactrin) is tested by measuring plasma cortisol before and 30 minutes after an intramuscular injection of synthetic ACTH – the 'short Synacthen test'. The incremental rise in plasma cortisol is subnormal in Addison's disease[1].

COMPLICATIONS

Acute Adrenal Crisis (Addisonian Crisis)

This is a medical emergency in which a patient with primary adrenal insufficiency suffers a stressful event such as an intercurrent infection or trauma. The normal physiological increase in corticosteroid secretion cannot occur. The patient presents in hypovolaemic shock with features of the precipitating event.

The stress of elective or emergency surgery is covered by the administration of intramuscular hydrocortisone in high doses tapering to normal over several days.

Pregnancy Complications

- IUGR – if undiagnosed
- Hypovolaemic shock – following labour

NON-PREGNANCY TREATMENT AND CARE

Patients are treated with oral corticosteroids for life. Typically glucocorticoid replacement is with hydrocortisone 20–30 mg daily, given as 2–3 doses. The adequacy of the dose is assessed by patient wellbeing, supplemented by measurement of 24-h urinary free cortisol excretion (which should be in the reference range) and possibly plasma cortisol profiles measured as a day case. It is important to avoid chronic over replacement in order to avoid osteoporosis and other features of Cushing's syndrome. Patients should increase their dose to cover intercurrent illness, and carry medical alert information about their diagnosis and treatment. They should seek urgent medical help if vomiting and unable to absorb oral steroids.

PRE-CONCEPTION ISSUES AND CARE

There should be no adverse effects on pregnancy of treated adrenal insufficiency. It is important to check that the woman is adequately but not excessively replaced with steroids as above. She should be advised to carry a steroid card and medical alert bracelet or tag with her at all times.

Although there is no need to increase the steroid doses routinely in pregnancy, the woman should be aware that she should seek medical advice in the event of vomiting in early pregnancy that prevents her absorbing oral steroids[2]. She should also be counselled about the need to cover labour and the puerperium with higher doses of steroids[2].

Pregnancy Issues
No changes in regular treatment required

Special Circumstances:
- Hyperemesis
- Intercurrent illness
- Risk of Addisonian crisis

Medical Management and Care
- Hyperemesis may result in insufficient oral steroid being absorbed by women with treated adrenal insufficiency
- Admission for parenteral steroid administration may be necessary
- Undiagnosed Addison's disease should be suspected in women with persistent nausea and vomiting beyond 20 weeks gestation, especially if this is associated with fatigue and weight loss

Midwifery Management and Care
- High-risk pregnancy – shared care with community and obstetric teams
- Women with intercurrent illness during pregnancy should be reminded to increase their corticosteroid dose exactly as they would do normally
- Promote correct administration of medication
- Immediate admission for signs of adrenal crisis, e.g. nausea and vomiting, profound epigastric pain or hypotension

Labour Issues
- Increased corticosteroid requirement for labour and delivery
- Intravenous fluids to prevent hypovolaemia

Medical Management and Care

Suggested Labour Regimen:
- Hydrocortisone: 100 mg 6-hourly im

Midwifery Management and Care
- This is a high-risk labour, managed by the obstetricians although the midwife should be able to deliver the baby if the labour itself progresses normally
- Continuous EFM is required
- Hourly blood pressure monitoring
- Care of the IVI and strict recording of fluid balance
- Send for immediate medical assistance for signs of adrenal crisis, e.g. nausea, vomiting, profound epigastric pain or hypotension
- Be aware that epidural anaesthesia may mask epigastric pain
- Promote correct administration of steroids
- Ensure that appropriate pharmacological therapy is available for an adrenal crisis[2]

Postpartum Issues
The physiological diuresis of the puerperium may cause significant hypotension.

Medical Management and Care
- Steroid dose should be tapered gradually over 6 days to cover the physiological diuresis in the puerperium
- *Suggested labour regimen:*
  - Day 1: Hydrocortisone 100 mg 6-hourly intramuscularly
  - Day 2: Hydrocortisone 50 mg 6-hourly intramuscularly
  - Day 3: Hydrocortisone 40 mg morning, 20 mg evening orally
  - Days 4 and 5: Hydrocortisone 30 mg morning, 15 mg evening orally
  - Day 6: Usual maintenance dose
- Ensure the woman is taking her maintenance dose of steroids on discharge

Midwifery Management and Care
- Routine care appropriate for type of delivery
- This mother is not suitable for early discharge from hospital
- Continue to monitor blood pressure and observe for signs of adrenal crisis
- Breast-feeding is considered safe and should be actively encouraged[2]

7.7 Prolactinoma

Incidence	Risk for Childbearing
Rare <1:1000	High Risk

EXPLANATION OF CONDITION

Prolactinomas are the commonest hormone-secreting pituitary adenomas and the only ones likely to be encountered in routine obstetric practice. They arise from the monoclonal proliferation of a lactotroph cell in the anterior pituitary gland. These cells synthesise and secrete prolactin (PRL), the hormone that promotes lactation. Of these adenomas, 90% are microadenomas (<10mm diameter) and 10% are macroadenomas (≥10mm). Microadenomas may regress spontaneously and do not usually grow significantly, with very few enlarging to become macroadenomas. Macroadenomas are more likely to expand[1].

The clinical features are due to hyperprolactinaemia and the space-occupying effects of the tumour. Hyperprolactinaemia causes secondary amenorrhoea and infertility; it inhibits pulsatile gonadotropin releasing hormone (GnRH) release which results in anovulation and low oestrogen levels. Raised PRL levels can also cause galactorrhoea.

Serum prolactin is always raised: in general higher levels are seen with macroprolactinomas. It is important to exclude other causes of hyperprolactinaemia (pregnancy, untreated hypothyroidism, antipsychotic and antiemetic drugs) before imaging the pituitary with MRI.

COMPLICATIONS

If the prolactinoma is large enough, it may compress the surrounding normal pituitary cells, causing partial or complete hypopituitarism, with deficiencies of growth hormone, ACTH, leading to hypocortisolaemia, and TSH, leading to hypothyroidism.

Large macroadenomas may cause pressure symptoms with headache, and, if optic chiasmal compression occurs, visual field defects, usually bitemporal hemianopia. Further expansion beyond the pituitary fossa may cause diplopia due to involvement of cranial nerves III, IV and VI.

NON-PREGNANCY TREATMENT AND CARE

Microprolactinoma

Medical treatment with a dopamine (DA) agonist is almost always successful in restoring normal prolactin concentration and stopping galactorrhoea. Bromocriptine was the first drug to be used. Cabergoline and quinagolide are alternatives. Bromocriptine is cheapest, but has to be taken 2–3 times daily, is less well tolerated and marginally less effective than cabergoline. Cabergoline is taken once or twice a week and is the preferred agent outside pregnancy.

All have side effects:

- Nausea
- Vomiting
- Constipation
- Postural hypotension
- Nasal congestion
- Raynaud's phenomenon

Women must be warned about these effects. Compliance is helped by starting with a low dose and slowly increasing.

Long-term use has been associated with pulmonary, pericardial and retroperitoneal fibrosis.

Since 10–20% microprolactinomas remit after medical treatment, it is reasonable to withdraw medication every 2–3 years to see whether it is still required.

Trans-sphenoidal surgery to remove the adenoma is reserved for women who cannot tolerate, or who do not respond to, DA agonists. It is as effective as medical treatment, but carries greater risks, including a degree of hypopituitarism.

MACROPROLACTINOMA

First-line treatment, even with the largest adenomas, is with DA agonists. These induce falls in prolactin concentrations within 24h and tumour shrinkage within weeks. These improvements continue with duration of treatment. The visual field defects usually recede, and PRL concentrations return to normal in 58% of cases. Rapid shrinkage may result in a leak of cerebrospinal fluid from the nose (CSF rhinorrhoea).

If tumours do not shrink as expected, trans-sphenoidal surgery to debulk the tumour mass in the sella followed by radiotherapy is recommended.

PRE-CONCEPTION ISSUES AND CARE

There is a risk of amenorrhoea and infertility.

Safety of DA Agonists

There is no evidence of increased rates of spontaneous abortion, ectopic pregnancy or teratogenicity with bromocriptine therapy. There is less experience with cabergoline, which is therefore not the first choice agent for women wishing to conceive, but may have to be used for those women with tumours that are unresponsive to bromocriptine. Women receiving DA agonists should be advised to use barrier methods of contraception for the first few menstrual cycles, which may be irregular, to facilitate accurate dating of pregnancy.

Risk of tumour expansion

As oestrogen levels rise in pregnancy they stimulate the growth of lactotrophs that, in normal women, cause the pituitary gradually to double its size: prolactinomas may also grow. The risk of clinically significant expansion of micro prolactinomas is low (1.6–4.7%) compared with 27–46% of macroprolactinomas. Women with microprolactinomas should be advised to stop taking the DA agonist as soon as pregnancy is confirmed. Macroprolactinomas are less likely to expand during pregnancy in women who have been treated for more than a year before conceiving.

The management of macroprolactinoma depends on the size of the tumour. If it is confined to the sella, the DA agonist can be stopped after conception. In women with larger macroadenomas, options to be considered before making an individualised plan include:

- Trial withdrawal of DA agonist
- Continuing bromocriptine throughout pregnancy
- Pre-pregnancy trans-sphenoidal surgery to debulk the tumour

Pregnancy Issues

Monitor for symptoms and signs of tumour expansion

Medical Management and Care

Since normal pregnancy is associated with increasing PRL concentrations, it is not possible to use PRL measurements to indicate prolactinoma enlargement.

Microprolactinomas
- Discontinue DA agonist
- Monitor clinically for symptoms and signs of tumour expansion
  - headache
  - visual symptoms
- Check visual fields clinically by direct confrontation

Macroprolactinomas
Decide whether to continue with DA agonist. Monitor clinically for symptoms and signs of tumour expansion as for microprolactinoma. In addition perform monthly visual perimetry to detect early signs of optic chiasmal compression. Serial MRI scanning is not recommended in view of a lack of proof of its safety in pregnancy.

If there is a suggestion of tumour expansion, this should be confirmed with an urgent MRI scan and bromocriptine started immediately. The subsequent management involves endocrinologist, obstetrician and neurosurgeon. Lack of response to bromocriptine is a neurosurgical emergency.

Early delivery may be indicated according to the gestational age.

Midwifery Management and Care

- Accurate booking history, noting any past treatments/surgery and current medication
- Care shared with community midwife and medical obstetric team
- Routinely ask about headaches and visual symptoms
- Refer to specialist unit if indicated

Labour Issues

No particular issues except if a woman is known to have an expanding macroprolactinoma.

Medical Management and Care

If the woman has an expanding tumour, she will need to be prepared for elective forceps delivery to avoid a rise in intracranial pressure during labour.

Midwifery Management and Care

- Routine shared care, unless expanding tumour as above or any other underlying obstetric or medical complications
- Be prepared for induction of labour before 38 weeks and prepare for a pre-term delivery

Postpartum Issues

Breast-feeding
Suckling has no effect on PRL concentrations and there is no evidence that it causes tumour expansion. DA agonists should not be given while breast-feeding.

Contraception
Oestrogens in combined oral contraceptives might stimulate growth of prolactinomas.

Restarting Medical Treatment
In most cases there should be no immediate need to restart DA agonist treatment after delivery. It is reasonable to wait and see whether the original symptoms return and to measure serum PRL if they do.

Medical Management and Care

- Advise the woman to report a recurrence of her original symptoms
- Confirm hyperprolactinaemia before restarting medical treatment
- Note that PRL concentrations return to normal by 3 weeks postpartum in normal women
- Women with macroprolactinomas should have an MRI scan postpartum to estimate tumour size

Midwifery Management and Care

- Routine postnatal care appropriate for type of delivery
- Encourage breast-feeding provided the woman does not need to restart DA agonists
- Discuss contraceptive options; theoretical risk of oestrogen-containing oral contraceptives should be discussed

7 Endocrine Disorders

PATIENT ORGANISATIONS

British Thyroid Foundation
PO Box 97
Clifford
Wetherby
West Yorkshire LS23 6XD
www.btf-thyroid.org

Diabetes UK
10 Parkway
London NW1 7AA
www.diabetes.org.uk

The Addison's Disease Self Help Group
21 George Road
Guildford
Surrey GU1 4NP
www.adshg.org.uk

The Pituitary Foundation
PO Box 1944
Bristol BS99 2UB
www.pituitary.org.uk

ESSENTIAL READING

Billington M and Stevenson M 2007 **Critical Care in Childbearing for Midwives**. Oxford; Blackwell Publishing Ltd. 55–62

Bronstein MD, Paraiba DB and Jallad RS 2011 Management of pituitary tumors in pregnancy. **Nature Review Endocrinology**, 7: 301–310

Girling JC 2006 Thyroid disorders in pregnancy. **Current Obstetrics and Gynaecology**, 16:47–53

Holt RIG, Coleman MA and McCance DR 2011 The implications of the new International Association of Diabetes and Pregnancy Study Groups (IADSPG) diagnostic criteria for gestational diabetes. **Diabetic Medicine**, 28:382–385

Lindsay RS and Catalano PM 2011 Diagnosis and Treatment of Gestational Diabetes. Royal College of Obstetricians and Gynaecologists Scientific Advisory Committee Opinion Paper 23

Powerie R, Greene M and Camann W (2010) *Chapt. 11 Diabetes mellitus in pregnancy* 293–321. *Chapt. 12 Thyroid disease in pregnancy* 322–334. *Chapt. 13 Pituitary & renal disease in pregnancy* 335–35 in **de Swiet's Medical Disorders in Obstetric Practice**, 5th Edn, Oxford; Wiley-Blackwell

Taylor R and Davison JM 2007 Type 1 diabetes and pregnancy. **British Medical Journal**, 334:742–745

Turner HE and Wass JAH (Eds) (2009) **Oxford Handbook of Endocrinology and Diabetes**, 2nd Edn. Oxford; Oxford University Press

Wier FA 2006 Clinical controversies in screening women for thyroid disease during pregnancy. **Journal of Midwifery and Women's Health**, 51:152–158

References

7.1 Hypothyroidism

1. Tonacchera M, Chiovato L and Pinchera A 2002 *Clinical assessment and systemic manifestations of hypothyroidism* in Wass JAM and Shalet SM (Eds) **Oxford Textbook of Endocrinology and Diabetes**. Oxford; Oxford University Press 491–502
2. Girling JC and DeSwiet M 1992 Thyroxine dosage during pregnancy in women with primary hypothyroidism. **British Journal of Obstetrics and Gynaecology**, 99:368–370
3. Girling JC 2003 Thyroid disorders in pregnancy. **Current Obstetrics and Gynaecology**, 13:45–51
4. Franklyn J 2002 *Subclinical hypothyroidism* in Wass JAM and Shalet SM (Eds) **Oxford Textbook of Endocrinology and Diabetes**. Oxford; Oxford University Press 518–522
5. Hershman JM 2002 *Thyroid disease during pregnancy* in Wass JAM and Shalet SM (Eds) **Oxford Textbook of Endocrinology and Diabetes**. Oxford; Oxford University Press 522–524
6. Rennie JM and Roberton NRC 2002 **A Manual Of Neonatal Intensive Care**, 4th Edn. London; Arnold 281–282

7.2 Thyrotoxicosis

1. Orgiazzi J. *Management of Graves' hyperthyroidism* in Wass JAM and Shalet SM (Eds) **Oxford Textbook of Endocrinology and Diabetes**. Oxford; Oxford University Press 453–458
2. Girling JC 2003 Thyroid disorders in pregnancy. **Current Obstetrics and Gynaecology**, 13:45–51
3. Davis LE, Lucas MJ, Hankins GDV, *et al.* 1989 Thyrotoxicosis complicating pregnancy. **American Journal of Obstetrics and Gynecology**, 160:63–70
4. Hershman JM 2002 *Thyroid disease during pregnancy* in Wass JAM and Shalet SM (Eds) **Oxford Textbook of Endocrinology and Diabetes**. Oxford; Oxford University Press 522–524
5. Rennie JM and Roberton NRC 2002 **A Manual of Neonatal Intensive Care**, 4th Edn. London; Arnold 281–282
6. Nelson-Piercy C 2002 **Handbook of Obstetric Medicine**. London; Martin Dunitz 100–105

7.3 Type 1 Diabetes Mellitus

1. NICE 2010. **The Management of Hypertensive Disorders During Pregnancy**. London; National Institute for Health and Clinical Excellence. www.nice.org
2. Lumley J, Watson L, Watson M and Bower C 2006 Periconceptional supplementation with folate and/or multivitamins for preventing neural tube defects. **Cochrane Pregnancy and Childbirth Group, Cochrane Database of Systematic Reviews**, 3
3. Casson IF, Clarke CA, Howard CV, *et al.* 1997 Outcomes of pregnancy in insulin dependent diabetic women: results of a five year population cohort study. **British Medical Journal**, 315(7103):275–278
4. CEMACH 2007 **Findings of a National Enquiry: Diabetes in Pregnancy: Are we providing the best care? England, Wales and Northern Ireland**. London; Confidential Enquiry into Maternal and Child Health
5. CEMACH 2005 **Findings of a National Enquiry: Pregnancy In Women With Type 1 And Type 2 Diabetes, England, Wales and Northern Ireland**. London; Confidential Enquiry into Maternal and Child Health
6. NICE 2010.**Weight Management Before, During and After Pregnancy**. London; National Institute for Health and Clinical Excellence. www.nice.org.uk
7. Jackson W 2004 Breast-feeding and Type 1 diabetes mellitus. **British Journal of Midwifery**, 12:158–165

7.4 Type 2 Diabetes Mellitus

1. Casson IF, Clarke CA, Howard CV, *et al.* 1997 Outcomes of pregnancy in insulin dependent diabetic women: results of a five year population cohort study. **British Medical Journal** 315(7103):275–278
2. CEMACH 2007 **Findings of a National Enquiry: Diabetes in Pregnancy: Are we providing the best care? England, Wales and Northern Ireland**. London; Confidential Enquiry into Maternal and Child Health
3. CEMACH 2005 **Findings of a National Enquiry: Pregnancy In Women With Type 1 And Type 2 Diabetes, England, Wales and Northern Ireland**. London; Confidential Enquiry into Maternal and Child Health
4. Dunne FP, Brydon P, Smith T, Essex M, Nicholson H and Dunne J 1999 Pre-conception diabetes care in insulin-dependent diabetes mellitus. **Quarterly Journal of Medicine**, 92:175–176
5. Lumley J, Watson L, Watson M and Bower C 2006 Periconceptional supplementation with folate and/or multivitamins for preventing neural tube defects. **Cochrane Pregnancy and Childbirth Group, Cochrane Database of Systematic Reviews**, 3
6. NICE 2010. **The Management of Hypertensive Disorders During Pregnancy**. London; National Institute for Health And Clinical Excellence. www.nice.org.uk
7. NICE 2010. **Weigh Management Before, During and after Pregnancy**. London; National Institute for Health and Clinical Excellence. www.nice.org.uk
8. Jackson W 2004 Breast-feeding and Type 1 Diabetes Mellitus. **British Journal of Midwifery**, 12:158–165

7.5 Gestational Diabetes Mellitus

1. International Association of Diabetes and Pregnancy Study Groups Consensus Panel 2010 International Association of Diabetes and Pregnancy Study Groups.:Recommendatioans on the Diagnosis and Classification of hyperglycaemia in Pregnancy. **Diabetes Care**, 33, 676–682
2. Crowther CA, Hille JE, Moss JR, *et al.* 2005 The Australian carbohydrate intolerance study in pregnant women (ACHOIS): Trial group – effect of treatment of gestational diabetes mellitus on pregnancy outcomes. **New England Journal of Medicine**, 352:2477–2486
3. NICE 2008 **Diabetes in Pregnancy**. London; National Institute for Health and Clinical Excellence. www.nice.org.uk
4. NICE 2010.**Weight management before, during and after Pregnancy**. London; National Institute for Health and Clinical Excellence. www.nice.org.uk

7.6 Addison's Disease

1. Parker KL and Kovacs WJ 2002 *Addison's disease (adrenal insufficiency)* in Wass JAM and Shalet SM (Eds) **Oxford Textbook of Endocrinology and Diabetes**. Oxford; Oxford University Press 837–844.
2. Molitch ME 1998 Pituitary disease in pregnancy. **Seminars in Perinatology**, 22:157–170

7.7 Prolactinoma

1. Bevan JS 2002 *Prolactinomas* in Wass JAM and Shalet SM (Eds) **Oxford Textbook of Endocrinology and Diabetes**. Oxford; Oxford University Press 172–181

Appendix Reference

1. World Health Organization. **Definition, Diagnosis and Classification of Diabetes Mellitus and its Complications: Report of a WHO Consultation. Part 1: Diagnosis and Classification of Diabetes Mellitus**. Geneva; World Health Organisation 1999

Appendix 7.3.1 Diabetes Mellitus

CRITERIA FOR THE DIAGNOSIS OF DIABETES MELLITUS

The 1999 WHO Revised Criteria for Glucose Intolerance:

- Diabetes mellitus requires symptoms of hyperglycaemia and a fasting venous plasma glucose concentration ≥7.0 mmol/l and/or random venous plasma glucose ≥11.1 mmol/l
- Otherwise an oral glucose tolerance test is required:

75 g Oral Glucose Tolerance Test		Venous Plasma Glucose Concentration (mmol/l)
Diabetes mellitus	Fasting 2 h	>7.0 ≥11.1
Impaired glucose tolerance	Fasting 2 h	<7.0 >7.8 and <11.1
Increased fasting glucose	Fasting 2 h	≥6.1 and <7.0 <7.8

SUGGESTED REGIMEN FOR MANAGEMENT OF DIABETES DURING LABOUR

The target capillary blood glucose should be within the range of 4–8 mol/l.
Once the woman is in established labour insert an intravenous cannula and infuse:

- Line 1: 5% D-glucose + 10 mmol potassium chloride 500 ml at 100 ml/h
- Line 2: 0.9% sodium chloride 49.5 ml + human soluble insulin (50 units) via a syringe driver
- Titrate the rate of infusion against capillary blood glucose level according to the scale below
- Give parallel infusions through a Y-connector; avoid three-way taps
- Monitor glucose hourly during labour
- All results to be charted by the midwife
- After delivery continue infusion until woman is able to eat and drink
- Subcutaneous insulin must be given 30 min before the infusion is stopped

Capillary Blood Glucose Concentration (mmol/l)	Insulin Infusion Rate (IU/h)
<3.5	• Stop infusion and recheck blood glucose in 20 min • Inform doctor
3.5–4	0.5
4.1–7	1.0
7.1–11	2.0
11.1–14	3.0
14.1–17	4.0
>17	8.0 • Check urine for ketones and inform doctor

FEATURES OF THE METABOLIC SYNDROME

Abnormal glucose tolerance (type 2 diabetes or IGT) plus two or more of the following:

- Insulin resistance
- Central obesity
  - body mass index >30 kg/m^2
  - waist:hip ratio >0.85 (females)
- Hypertension: BP >160/90 mmHg
- Dyslipidaemia
  - fasting triglycerides >1.7 mmol/l
  - HDL-cholesterol <1.0 mmol/l (females)
- Microalbuminuria
- Albumin:creatinine ratio >3.5 (females)

NEUROLOGICAL DISORDERS

8

Fionnuala McAuliffe[1], Eleanor Burns-Kent[2], Deborah Frost[3] and Edmund S. Howarth[2][†]

[1]University College Dublin and National Maternity Hospital, Dublin, Ireland
[2]University Hospitals of Leicester NHS Trust, Leicester, UK
[3]University of Leicester, Leicester, UK
[†]Deceased

8.1 Migraine and Headaches
8.2 Epilepsy
8.3 Cerebrovascular Disease and Stroke
8.4 Bell's Palsy
8.5 Carpal Tunnel Syndrome
8.6 Myasthenia Gravis
8.7 Multiple Sclerosis

Medical Disorders in Pregnancy: A Manual for Midwives, Second Edition. Edited by S. Elizabeth Robson and Jason Waugh.
© 2013 John Wiley & Sons, Ltd. Published 2013 by John Wiley & Sons, Ltd.

8.1 Migraine and Headaches

Incidence
Most common neurological disease[3]
Migraine affects 1 in 4 women and 1 in 12 men[1-3]

Risk for Childbearing
Variable Risk – dependent on cause

EXPLANATION OF CONDITION

Headache

Headache is an extremely common neurological disorder, the most common being 'tension' type headaches, accounting for nearly 90% of all headaches which affect approximately 3% of the population[4]. Tension headaches last from 30 minutes to 7 days and are mild to moderate in intensity, not accompanied by nausea or any other symptoms affecting the nervous system. They are thought to occur due to scalp muscle contraction resulting in a sensation of bilateral tightness in the head and pressure behind the eyes[5]. Often related to stress, such headaches may be precipitated by noise, depression, fatigue and concentrated visual work. The diagnosis is made by careful history taking and performing a neurological examination to exclude differential diagnosis[5,6].

Cluster Headaches

Cluster headaches are rare in women and more common in men[7,8], usually appear rapidly, peak within 10 minutes, last 15–180 minutes and occur from once every other day to eight times a day. Pain is severe, usually non-pulsatile, unilateral and may be centred on one eye. Symptoms include lacrimation (tear formation), eyelid oedema, nasal congestion and rhinorrhoea (runny nose) with 60% of cases causing ptosis and miosis[5].

Migraine

Migraine is a genetically influenced chronic brain condition marked by paroxysmal attacks of moderate to severe throbbing headache[5] influenced by fluctuating oestrogen levels.[9-11] There are two main types:

Migraine without aura (common migraine) is the commonest type of migraine with recurrent headaches manifesting in attacks lasting 4–72 hours. Typical characteristics of the headache are unilateral location, pulsating quality, moderate or severe intensity, aggravation by routine physical activity and association with nausea and/or photophobia and phonophobia (sensitivity to sound)[12].

Migraine with aura (classical migraine) occurs when patients experience premonitory symptoms up to 48 hours before a migraine attack. Symptoms include depression, irritability and yawning, difficulty concentrating, stiff neck and food cravings. Other symptoms may include visual disturbances affecting one side of the visual field (scintillating scotoma, geometric patterns) and unilateral paraesthesia or numbness. Each aura symptom develops gradually over 5–20 minutes and lasts no longer than 60 minutes. Headache begins during the aura period or within an hour of the aura ceasing and manifests in the same way as migraine without aura[12].

Migraine headache is thought to be due to vasodilation of cerebral blood vessels and stimulation of cerebral nerves. The release of 5-hydroxytryptamine, a vasoactive substance, is known to rise at the onset of prodromal symptoms and fall during the headache.

Migraines may be induced in a minority of patients by[1]:

- *Emotional triggers*: stress, anxiety, tension, excitement, shock
- *Physical triggers*: tiredness, poor posture, shift work, neck or shoulder tension, poor quality sleep, travelling long distances
- *Dietary triggers*: lack of food, dehydration, alcohol, food additives, caffeine, specific foods like cheese, chocolate and citrus fruits
- *Environmental triggers*: bright/flickering lights, smoking, loud noises, strong smells and a change in climate
- *Medicinal triggers*: oral contraceptives, hormone replacement therapy (HRT), some sleeping tablets and vasodilators

COMPLICATIONS

Migraine with aura has been consistently linked with an increased risk of ischaemic stroke and might also be a marker of increased risk for other ischaemic events[12,13]. Severe headache with rapid deterioration was a key presenting feature in eight of the 15 neurological indirect maternal deaths in the latest CMACE report[14].

NON-PREGNANCY TREATMENT AND CARE

Headache

- Investigation to confirm the benign nature of the headaches
- Simple analgesia: paracetamol and/or a NSAID
- Avoid agents which may exacerbate headache, e.g. alcohol, nicotine
- Cluster headaches are primarily treated as migraine

Migraine

A detailed neurological examination should be performed to ensure accurate diagnosis. Hemiplegic, visual and hemisensory symptoms must be distinguished from thrombo-embolic transient ischaemic attacks (TIA). In addition:

- Patient to complete a diary to ascertain any triggers[1]
- Discontinue oral contraceptives if appropriate
- Simple analgesia as a first-line treatment, with or without an anti-emetic[1]
- Vasoconstrictors such as ergotamine tartrate can be used during an attack administered orally, rectally or by subcutaneous injection
- Triptan medicines like sumatriptan (a $5HT_1$ agonist) are commonly used for acute attacks either orally, as a nasal spray or by injection[1]
- Beta-blockers, antidepressants, serotonin agonists and anticonvulsants can be used as prophylaxis[1]
- Feverfew, a herbal remedy, is a preventative treatment for migraine and may reduce the frequency of migraines[15]

PRE-CONCEPTION ISSUES AND CARE

Women should be accurately counselled regarding the risks and benefits of continuing any prescribed or *over the counter* medication.[14,16]

Pregnancy Issues

Headaches and migraine during pregnancy are the most common neurological disorders seen in obstetrics[14,17–19]. Tension headaches do not usually improve in pregnancy[19].

Of women with pre-existing classical migraine, 50–80% will improve during pregnancy, particularly in the third trimester[3,19–22] and only 4–8% experience worsening[1,16,21].

Women aged over 40 are twice as likely to have pregnancy related migraine compared with women less than 20 years old.[3]

New onset migraine with aura is not common in pregnancy[1,20,23]. Therefore, it is paramount to consider differential diagnosis, including:

- Subarachnoid haemorrhage
- Meningitis
- Encephalitis
- Cerebral vein thrombosis
- Benign intracranial hypertension
- Pre-eclampsia
- Intracranial mass lesions

Women with peripartum migraine have an increased risk of hypertensive disorder[24], a twofold increased risk of developing pre-eclampsia[25,26] and an increase risk of stroke and vascular disease[25].

Ergotamine and feverfew (which contain ergot alkaloids) should be avoided throughout pregnancy[15,27].

Preventative treatment of migraines includes: trigger avoidance, stopping smoking, sleep deprivation and eating regular meals[3].

Medical Management and Care[3,19]

- Careful diagnosis, history taking and neurological examination
- Prolonged neurological signs and symptoms for >12 hours require further investigation. Consider pre-eclampsia at all times
- Consider non-pharmacological measures first: ice, massage, sleep and biofeedback
- Paracetamol and low dose caffeine are first line agents in drug therapy[28]
- NSAIDs should be used with caution in the first and second trimester only; extended use should be avoided
- Consider prophylaxis if attacks are frequent or long lasting; aspirin 75 mg once daily is safe and effective
- Consider beta-blockers; note that use of these in pregnancy has been associated with IUGR (see Appendix 4.3.1)
- If beta-blockers and aspirin are ineffective consider tricyclic antidepressants (25–50 mg amitriptyline)
- Consider anti-emetics if presentation of nausea and vomiting; metoclopramide decreases gastric atony and increases absorption of other administered medications[29]
- Narcotics (morphine) can be used if severity warrants (avoid in third trimester)
- Avoid ergotamine and benzodiazepines[28]
- Sumatriptan is safe to use in the first trimester of pregnancy with no increased risk of teratogenicity[30]. Newer triptans: more evidence is needed to support these in pregnancy[30]
- Prenatal obstetric anesthetic assessment should be sought in significant neurologic disease

Midwifery Management and Care

- Neurological disorders fall outside the midwives normal sphere of practice. Referral to a consultant-led unit for obstetric, specialist advice for ongoing care should be sought following a detailed booking history[31]
- Advice to avoid triggers
- Advocate regular meals, adequate hydration, moderate exercise and relaxation, plenty of sleep and restriction of smoking and alcohol[32]
- Ensure physical observations are noted to exclude other diagnosis
- Women who present with headaches in late second and third trimester should be screened for pre-eclampsia (blood pressure measurement and urinalysis) and referred for urgent medical assessment if necessary (see Section 3.2)

Labour Issues

Triggers such as stress, pain and starvation can induce headache or a migraine attack[1].

Emerging evidence[33] indicates a possible increased risk of LBW, preterm babies and caesarean delivery although this is disputed[21,26].

Medical Management and Care[3,19]

- As above

Midwifery Management and Care

- Condition may cause anxiety about labour and analgesia; discuss and refer to anaesthetic team if necessary
- Encourage adequate nutritional intake and hydration
- Tranquil delivery room environment; avoid triggers such as flickering lights
- Utilise relaxation techniques

Postpartum Issues

Postnatal headache can worsen in 40% of cases[19].

Differential diagnosis includes[34]:

- Migraine
- Meningitis
- Subarachnoid haemorrhage
- Cardiovascular attack
- Puerperal psychosis
- Imminent eclampsia
- Dural puncture headache
- Diabetic hypoglcaemia
- Raised intracranial pressure
- Encephalopathy

Migraine often recurs postpartum[29] as oestrogen levels fall[3] and may present for the first time[29] in 4.5% patients[19].

No adverse fetal outcome is associated with maternal migraines[19].

Medical Management and Care

- Careful examination and history taking are essential[19]; post-dural headache will usually improve when the mother is lying prone
- Women with classical migraine should not take oestrogen-containing oral contraceptives[6]
- Post-delivery consider pre-pregnancy treatment, ensuring no contraindications if breast-feeding
- Avoid aspirin and chlorpromazine[16,19,35]
- Sumatriptan: withhold breast-feeding for 12 hours after last dose[30,35]
- Other triptans; withhold breast-feeding for 24 hours after last dose[16,35]

Midwifery Management and Care

- Carefully history taking
- Referral to medical team if necessary
- Encourage rest, hydration and relaxation[16]

8.2 Epilepsy

Incidence	Risk for Childbearing
50/100 000[1]	Variable Risk – depending on nature of epilepsy and seizure control
Prevalence rate of 6.2:1000[2]	
1 in 131 people[3]	
Affects 0.5% pregnancies[4]	

EXPLANATION OF CONDITION

Epilepsy is a common neurological condition with a tendency to have recurrent (two or more) seizures[5]. A seizure is caused by a sudden burst of excess electrical activity in the brain, causing a temporary disruption in the normal message passing between cortical neurons (brain cells). This disruption results in the brain's messages becoming halted or mixed up depending on the site and extent of activity within the brain. Seizures can occur at any time and the severity differs from person to person but can be broadly classified into two categories: *partial and generalised seizures*[5,6] (see Table 8.2.1 and 8.2.2).

Seizure triggers are circumstances or substances that could trigger an epilepsy seizure. These triggers include[7,8]:

- Stress, anxiety
- Lack of sleep
- Lack of food
- Excess alcohol, particularly binge drinking
- Illegal drugs: cocaine, ecstasy, heroin, codeine, methadone, amphetamines.
- Missing a dose of anti-epileptic drugs (AEDs)
- Flickering lights (rare, affects 5% of people with epilepsy known as photosensitive epilepsy)
- Illness and health conditions that cause a high temperature
- Certain medications and supplements: antidepressants, antihistamines, evening primrose oil
- Hormonal changes with menstrual cycle: known as catamenial epilepsy

COMPLICATIONS

- **Status epilepticus:** a seizure that lasts >30 min or longer or a series of seizures without regaining consciousness in between. In rare cases it can be fatal[9]
- **Sudden unexpected death in epilepsy (SUDEP):** phenomenon whereby person with epilepsy dies suddenly and no anatomical or toxicological cause of death can be found. SUDEP causes 500 deaths a year with the single most important risk factor being chronic epilepsy with uncontrolled generalised tonic clonic seizures[8,10]
- **Trauma** occurring at the time of the convulsion, including tongue biting, head trauma, hot water burns, etc.; patients with epilepsy should be counselled regarding precautions and how to minimise harm
- **Maternal mortality, indirect deaths in pregnant women:** epilepsy attributed to 14 deaths in the latest CMACE report. SUDEP was categorised in 11 of the 14 deaths[11]

Table 8.2.1 Two Types of Partial Seizures[5,6]. Commonly affects the temporal lobe

Simple Partial	· Remain conscious
	· Experience an aura; change in the way things look, smell, taste or sound
	· Déjà vu – experienced something before
	· Pins and needles in arms/legs
	· Muscles in arms/legs may become stiff with twitching on one side of body.
	· Flushed face or goes pale
	· Sweating
Complex Partial	· Change in awareness; looses memory of the event
	· Rubbing of hands
	· Smacking of lips; chewing
	· Picking at clothes
	· Fiddling with objects
	· Making random noises
	· Adopting unusual posture

Secondary Generalised
Partial seizures begin in one part of the brain and spread to the whole brain and tonic clonic seizures occur. An aura may be experienced warning of imminent full seizure activity.

Table 8.2.2 Generalised Seizures[5,6]. The whole brain is affected straight away without warning and in most cases the person is completely unconscious

Absence	Staring and blinking, daydreaming, mainly affect children and lose awareness for 5–20 seconds
Myoclonic	Brief muscle jerking of one or both arms, legs. Last a fraction of a second and remain conscious
Tonic	All muscles of the body contract causing falling but without convulsions. Lasts <20 seconds
Tonic Clonic	Most common seizure (60%) with two stages: whole body contracts and then arms and legs convulse/twitch. Lasts 1–2 minutes with possible incontinence. Very sleepy after
Atonic	All muscle tone lost very briefly; fall limply to ground. Head injury likely. No confusion and gets up straight away

NON-PREGNANCY TREATMENT AND CARE

The aim of treatment in both pregnancy and non-pregnancy is to achieve optimum, seizure-free status without adverse effects. Epilepsy is the most common neurological disorder of pregnancy[4,12,13].

Anti-epileptic drugs (AEDs) are commonly used to treat epilepsy either with a single drug (monotherapy) or if epilepsy is difficult to treat then with two or more AEDs (polytherapy)[6,14] (see Appendix 8.2.1 for current UK AED therapy). Seizure control occurs in 52% of people with epilepsy. It is estimated 70% could be seizure free with the right treatment[15]. Neurological surgery, vagus nerve stimulation, and a ketogenic diet (for children only) are other proven methods of treatment[6,14,15].

PRE-CONCEPTION ISSUES AND CARE

Women considering pregnancy should seek pre-conceptual advice from an appropriately experienced health care professional. Figure 8.2.1 provides advice on the management of epilepsy pre-pregnancy through to postpartum.

Counselling should review current medications, explain risk of fetal defects and formulate a plan for the pregnancy to optimise both maternal and fetal outcome[11,16–19].

- **Review of epilepsy**: previous medical and obstetric history. Defer pregnancy until seizure control is optimal. If seizure free for a minimum of 2 years may consider withdrawing AEDs altogether or until the end of first trimester when organogenesis is complete. This should be planned well before conception and implications for driving and risk of seizure recurrence should be explored[17]
- **AEDs**: increase the risk of folate deficiency, neural tube defect (NTD) and major congenital malformations (MCMs). Monotherapy, at the lowest dose to control seizures (if needed at all) is preferable to polytherapy[16,17,20,21], as this increases the risk of congenital malformations[17,22] and can reduce cognitive developmental outcomes in the baby[23]. Changing AED therapy should be completed *before* conception with effective contraception to avoid pregnancy whilst possibly receiving polytherapy[17,19]
- **Folic acid**: supplementation of 5 mg daily 12 weeks before pregnancy continuing until the end of the first trimester[14,16,17,21,24]. Women with epilepsy and particularly those taking AEDs have an increased risk of folate deficiency and NTD[21,25–27]
- **Antenatal screening**: options discussed and due to an increased risk of malformations, a detailed fetal anatomic survey at 18–22 weeks gestation is recommended along with serum AFP[16, 17, 21]
- **Vitamin K:** oral supplementation needed at the end of pregnancy if AEDs are enzyme inducing[14,17] (see Table 8.2.3)
- **Labour advice:** regarding pain relief, continuation of AEDs in labour and seizure risk[17]
- **Breast-feeding:** is encouraged in all women with epilepsy[16,17,21]
- **Care of the newborn baby**: and safety advice in the postnatal period[17,18]. See postpartum issues.
- **General health promotion and well being:** including lifestyle, dental care, exercise, healthy eating, alcohol consumption, smoking and reliable contraception, etc.[17, 28]

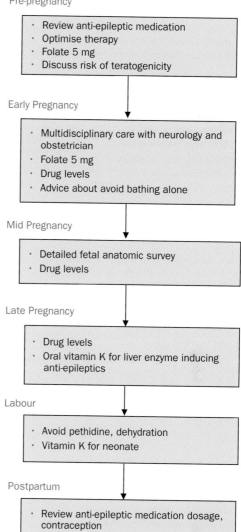

Pre-pregnancy

- Review anti-epileptic medication
- Optimise therapy
- Folate 5 mg
- Discuss risk of teratogenicity

Early Pregnancy

- Multidisciplinary care with neurology and obstetrician
- Folate 5 mg
- Drug levels
- Advice about avoid bathing alone

Mid Pregnancy

- Detailed fetal anatomic survey
- Drug levels

Late Pregnancy

- Drug levels
- Oral vitamin K for liver enzyme inducing anti-epileptics

Labour

- Avoid pethidine, dehydration
- Vitamin K for neonate

Postpartum

- Review anti-epileptic medication dosage, contraception
- Safety precautions when caring for baby

Figure 8.2.1 Management of epilepsy algorithm. This figure is downloadable from the book companion website at www.wiley.com/go/robson

Table 8.2.3 Anti-epileptic Drugs

Enzyme-inducing AEDs	Non-enzyme-inducing AEDs
Phenobarbital	Clonazepam
Phenytoin	Clobazam
Primidone	Ethosuximide
Carbamazepine	Gabapentin
Topiramate	Lamotrigine*
Oxcarbazepine	Levetiracetam
Rufinamide	Sodium valproate
	Tiagabine
	Vigabatrin
	Zonisamide

*Lamotrigine is not an enzyme inducer but interacts with the efficacy of hormonal contraception[6]. Lamotrigine levels are lowered by the combined oral contraceptive pill (COCP)[17]

Pregnancy Issues

Women with epilepsy are likely to have healthy pregnancies with over 95% having a baby without an abnormality[22].

Seizure Control

* 15–37% of women will see an increase in the frequency of seizures in pregnancy[14] with the majority seeing no change or a decrease in seizure frequency[17,29–31]
* If seizure free for 9 months prior to pregnancy 84–92% remain seizure free during pregnancy[32]
* Simple partial, complex partial, absence and myoclonic seizures are thought not to affect the pregnancy or developing fetus unless a fall or injury is sustained[14]
* Tonic clonic seizures have a relatively low risk to the fetus[14] but could influence future cognitive development[33]

AEDs

* All AEDs cross the placenta with varying rates of teratogenicity
* Fetal malformation risk[22]:
  ○ in general population: 1–2%
  ○ epilepsy but not taking AEDs: 3.5%
  ○ one AEDs: 3.7%
  ○ two AEDs: 6%
  ○ three or more AEDs: 15% plus

Major Congenital Malformation (MCM)

* MCM occur in <5% of fetuses of women taking AEDs during pregnancy.
* Polytherapy regimes increase MCM risk[22]. MCM are structural defects requiring medical or surgical intervention including heart, neural tube, urogenital defects and orofacial clefts[21].
* Fetal anticonvulsant syndrome with distinctive facial features is common with AEDs exposure [17, 34]
* Sodium valproate is associated with an increased risk of MCM (dose related)[22,23,35–37], long-term developmental delay, cognitive impairment in children[33,35,38–41] and more distinct facial features[17,34]
* Carbamazepine is associated with the lowest MCM risk[22,23]
* Lamotrigine drug levels fall in all three trimesters of pregnancy. An increase in dosage is required in the majority of women[11,29,42]

Folic Acid

Increased risk of folate deficiency and NTD particularly those taking AEDs [21,25–27].

Antenatal Screening

Increased risk of fetal malformations[14,17,21].

Vitamin K

Enzyme-inducing AEDs affect vitamin K production and synthesis in the maternal intestines reducing fetal uptake[16,17].

Medical Management and Care

* Care of women with epilepsy should be shared between the obstetrician, midwife and a neurology specialist[14,17]
* All women with epilepsy are encouraged to register with the UK Epilepsy and Pregnancy Register to contribute to greater understanding of epilepsy and AEDs use in pregnancy[14,17] (www.epilepsyand pregnancy.co.uk)

Seizure Control

* Achieving seizure freedom is important for successful pregnancies and highly predictive of seizure freedom during pregnancy[17,43]
* If seizures increase, ensure AEDs compliance first and foremost, alleviate concerns and advocate AEDs continuation throughout pregnancy[14,22,44]
* Seizures may increase as a result of[14]:
  ○ poor or non-compliance with AEDs medication
  ○ decreased drug levels due to nausea and vomiting
  ○ decreased gastrointestinal absorption
  ○ sleep deprivation
  ○ raised hepatic and renal clearance leads to insufficient drug levels
* New onset seizures in pregnancy require investigation to rule out other causes; eclampsia should always be considered until proven otherwise[4]

AEDs (see Appendix 8.2.1 for review of AEDs)

* Continue all monotherapy at the lowest dose considering slow-release preparation to achieve seizure freedom[17]
* If seizure control is inefficient, consider alternative monotherapy first
* Consider polytherapy if monotherapy is unsuccessful[14,17,20,21,45]
* Emerging evidence[11,27,37,46–49] suggests clinicians therapeutically monitor drug AED levels during each trimester as the haemodilution effects of pregnancy can reduce drug availability and serum levels[4,29,31,42,50,51]
* Avoid sodium valproate where possible or use in slow release form as monotherapy[17, 35, 36, 48, 52, 53] ideally <1000 mg/day[17,54]

Folic Acid

* Prescribe 5 mg per day early in first trimester if not commenced pre-conceptually and continue until 12 weeks gestation[14,21,54,55]
* Women taking sodium valproate should continue folic acid 5 mg per day for the remainder of the pregnancy[54,56]

Antenatal Screening

* Detailed fetal ultrasound performed at 18–22 weeks for structural anomalies[4,14,17,21,43]

Vitamin K

Women taking enzyme inducing AEDs (see Table 8.2.3) should receive oral vitamin K 20 mg per day from 36 weeks gestation until delivery or for 4 weeks prior to delivery[17,21,57].

Midwifery Management and Care

* Epilepsy is outside the normal sphere of midwifery practice[58]
* Detailed booking history with emphasis on current drug therapy
* Refer to a consultant-led unit with shared care by multi-disciplinary team consisting of obstetrician, neurologist and midwife[11,14]
* Advocate importance and compliance with AEDs therapy and refer to medical staff if increase, or onset, of seizures occurs
* Advise against unattended bathing and steamy environments. Showers are preferable and the bathroom door should remain unlocked[11]
* Ascertain expectations; discuss a realistic birth plan and options available. Discourage from unrealistic schemes, such as water-birth[14]
* Encourage breast-feeding and discuss post-delivery safety issues[17,21]

Labour Issues

- The risk of a tonic clonic seizure during labour is low: 1–2%[14,16,17,59]
- Hyperventilation, exhaustion, dehydration, emotional stress and pain can induce a seizure[16,17]
- Prolonged or repeated seizures can cause fetal hypoxia leading to transient bradycardia, reduced beat to beat heart rate variability and decelerations for about 30 minutes after a seizure[16]
- *Status epilepticus* is a medical emergency and necessitates input from obstetric and anaesthetic teams
- Pethidine is metabolised to norpethidine and may induce a seizure; its use should be avoided in labour[55,60]
- Women with epilepsy taking AEDs show no substantially increased risk of caesarean section, late pregnancy bleeding, premature labour or delivery[30,36]

Medical Management and Care

- Continue normal AED regime[4,16,17]

Management of Status Epilepticus- a Medical Emergency[14]
- Senior obstetric and anaesthetic staff to be present
- Secure the airway, give oxygen therapy
- Intravenous access in large vein
- Assess cardiac and respiratory function
- Ensure safe environment to maintain safety of patient
- First line treatment of prolonged seizures is iv lorazepam 4 mg, which is less sedative and longer acting than diazepam.
- Investigations – FBC, U&E and consider AED levels
- Consider alternative causes
- Seek advice from neurologist if lorazepam is not effective
- Consider iv phenytoin with continuous EEG monitoring
- If phenytoin unsuccessful, paralyse, sedate and ventilate mechanically
- Consider delivery of the fetus at this point

Midwifery Management and Care

- Delivery should be in a consultant-led obstetric unit equipped with facilities for maternal and neonatal resuscitation[14,16,17]
- Do not leave alone in labour[59]
- Use of the birthing pool is contraindicated on safety grounds[14,59]
- Ensure compliance and continuation of prescribed AEDs[16,17]
- If seizure free during labour, treat as for any other laboring woman[54]
- Limit stress and anxiety and ensure adequate hydration[16,17]
- Avoid exhaustion and hyperventilation[16,17]
- Consider appropriate pain relief which includes: TENS, epidural anaesthesia and entonox[16,17]
- Adhere to unit policy for the management of epilepsy

Postpartum Issues

- During the first 24 hours postpartum there is an additional 1–2% risk of tonic clonic seizures[14,16,17,59]
- Enzyme inducing AEDs have been shown to interfere with vitamin K metabolism in the newborn and may lead to haemorrhagic disease[14,16,17,21]
- Physiological changes that occurred in pregnancy are reversed, which may lead to an increase in AED levels[61]
- AEDs are secreted in breast milk but the dose received is less than the therapeutic level for neonates and less than that received *in utero*[4,17,55]
- Infants that are breast fed whose mothers take AEDs have no additional problems at the age of 3[62]
- Lamotrigine is eliminated slowly in breast fed infants but no adverse neonatal effects have been reported caused by lactation[51,55]
- There are no contraindications to the use of non-hormonal forms of contraception or the Mirena coil[17]
- Hormonal forms of contraception are affected by enzyme-inducing AEDs and lamotrigine[16,17,19,63]
- Lamotrigine levels are lowered by the combined oral contraceptive pill[17]

Medical Management and Care

- Review AEDs regime and levels; consider return to pre-pregnancy dosage if increased in pregnancy[4,16,17]
- Prescribers should consult the British National Formulary (BNF) for guidance on prescribing AEDs whilst breast-feeding[14]
- New onset seizures require investigation to rule out other causes (e.g. eclampsia, infection, intracerebral haemorrhage)[4]
- Ensure appropriate contraception prescribed; enzyme-inducing AEDs decrease the efficacy of combined oral contraceptive pill and progestogen-only contraceptive pill[16,17]
- Advocate pre-conceptual counselling prior to next pregnancy[17]

Midwifery Management and Care

- Vitamin K 1 mg intramuscular to babies at birth whose mothers are taking enzyme inducing AEDs[14,16,17,21]
- Breast-feeding should be encouraged[14,16,17,50]
- Observe neonate closely; report concerns promptly to paediatrician
- Advise parents about simple safety precautions (Box 8.2.1)[4,14,17,60]

Box 8.2.1 Safety Precautions For Mothers Caring for the Baby

√ Share care of baby at night to avoid exhaustion
√ When feeding the baby, sit safely with a back rest
√ Consider feeding on the floor
√ Dress and change baby on floor to prevent falling
√ Carry baby up or down stairs using a carrycot or car seat
√ Bath the baby when support is available and in shallow water
√ Use high chair in lowest setting in safe surroundings, making sure it cannot be knocked over
√ Use a buggy/pram with brakes preferably that initiate when you release the handle
√ Use safety gates at all times.

8.3 Cerebrovascular Disease and Stroke

Incidence	Risk for Childbearing
Pregnancy-related stroke: 11–26:100 000 deliveries[1]	High Risk

EXPLANATION OF CONDITION

Cerebrovascular accidents (CVA), also known as **strokes**, result from cerebral infarction and are the most common brain disorder in the general population[2]. They occur when the flow of blood carrying essential oxygen to the brain is disrupted, causing brain cells to die[3].

Stroke is divided into three categories:

1. **Ischaemic:** from decreased blood flow as a result of vascular occlusion by embolism or atherosclerosis[2] within an artery
2. **Thrombotic:** a venous event
3. **Haemorrhagic** (subarachnoid haemorrhage [SAH]) due to a ruptured blood vessel in the brain

With CVA there can be an abrupt onset of neurological symptoms that vary in severity due to the location and extent of the damage caused. They range from mild strokes, where recovery occurs within 24 hours, to severe brain damage or death[3]. In the case of a small CVA neurons near to the damaged area may sprout new dendrites, make new synaptic connections and take over some of the functions of the lost neurons[2], thereby reducing the patient's physical neurological symptoms.

Risk Factors

- **Ischaemic stroke:**
  - hypertension
  - hypercholesterolaemia
  - heart disease
  - previous transient ischaemic attacks
  - diabetes
  - vasculitis
  - smoking
  - obesity
  - excessive alcohol intake[2]
  - over 35 years old[4]
  - black ethnicity[4]
- **Thrombotic stroke:**
  - thrombophilia
  - dehydration
  - infection[5,6]
  - smoking
  - operative delivery
- **Haemorrhagic stroke**
  - hypertension
  - vasoactive drugs (amphetamine, cocaine)

Strokes usually appear in healthy women, with only one-third of cases having a risk factor[4]. Whilst history and risk factors may give guidance as to which type of CVA has occurred, there is considerable symptom overlap and appropriate imaging is essential. For example, cerebral vein thrombosis (CVT) may have an insidious symptom onset with headache followed by impairment of consciousness, and SAH classically presents with a 'thunderclap' headache,

vomiting, hypertension and progressive loss of consciousness[6,7], but neither history is conclusive.

COMPLICATIONS

Ischaemia resulting from a CVA is a major cause of death or permanent disability which may be experienced as:

- Dizziness
- Weakness
- Numbness
- Paralysis in a limb or a side of the body
- Headache
- Slurred speech or difficulty understanding speech
- Partial loss of vision
- Nausea and vomiting[2] (Figure 8.3.1)

NON-PREGNANCY TREATMENT AND CARE

The principal aim of management is the prevention of neurological complications and death. It is essential to establish as quickly as possible if the stroke is due to cerebral ischaemia or haemorrhage[1]. Appropriate brain imaging by CT or MRI should be carried out urgently after symptom onset to determine the type of CVA (Figure 8.3.2).

Thrombophilia screening is essential[1]. Cerebrospinal fluid (CSF) examination is beneficial if an infection is suspected[5], and for the presence of blood if a SAH is suspected. If cardiac origin is suspected, an ECG and echocardiogram should be performed. Blood/urine toxicology would be beneficial to rule out substance misuse.

Management is ultimately dependent upon the precise type of CVA.

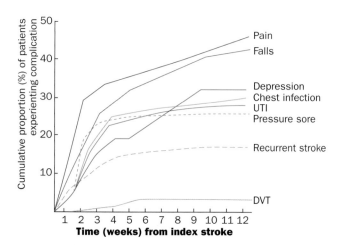

Figure 8.3.1 Problems experienced following stroke (Mant and Walker, 2011). This figure is downloadable from the book companion website at www.wiley.com/go/robson

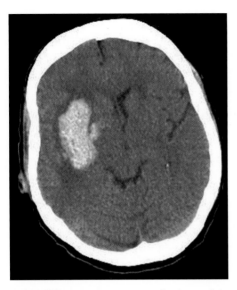

Figure 8.3.2 A CT scan appearance of primary intracerebral haemorrhage (Donnelly, 2001). This figure is downloadable from the book companion website at www.wiley.com/go/robson

The presence of significant haemorrhage is a contraindication to anticoagulation[7], whereas therapeutic anticoagulation is essential to prevent further episodes if thrombotic stroke is diagnosed.

Surgery may be necessary to remove the blood clot, or to repair a ruptured aneurysm, if there is a SAH.

PRE-CONCEPTION ISSUES AND CARE

Women who have had a stroke are unlikely to have a recurrence in pregnancy unless there is an underlying risk factor[8]. However, the majority of women who experience stroke in pregnancy have underlying risk factors[9]. Women who have had six or more pregnancies have an increased risk of all types of stroke[10].

- **Previous CVA** – these women require review prior to pregnancy, including assessment of medication
- **Previous ischaemic stroke** – these women will be receiving anti-platelet medication, most commonly aspirin, dipyridamole or clopidrogel. If receiving either of the latter two, then conversion to aspirin 75–300 mg per day prior to pregnancy would be recommended. Discontinuation of all anti-platelet medication would be unwise during pregnancy and the puerperium
- **Previous thrombotic stroke** – if the woman is taking warfarin, consideration should be given to changing this to subcutaneous heparin prior to conception to reduce the risk of warfarin embryopathy[1,11]

Pregnancy Issues

Previous CVA

- Warfarin embryopathy may occur with exposure of the fetus to warfarin from 6 to12 weeks gestation
- Close consultation with haematology required for a patient requiring anticoagulation during pregnancy
- Thrombophilia screen may be performed during pregnancy but the results should be interpreted with caution as some of the factors are altered in pregnancy (e.g. protein S may fall in pregnancy)

At risk of CVA

- Underlying risk factors of poorly controlled hypertension, obesity, thrombophilia, vasculitis need to be identified
- Antenatal thromboprophylaxis may be required if more than three risk factors are present for thrombosis

Development of CVA during Pregnancy

- For patient with a history of haemorrhagic stroke brain imaging may be required to assess for presence of residual vascular malformations

Subarachnoid Haemorrhage

- Pregnancy does not appear to increase the incidence of SAH, although the physiological changes occurring during pregnancy such as increased blood volume, stroke volume and cardiac output, as well as increased oestrogen levels resulting in vasodilatation of an already abnormal vessel, can precipitate this.
- SAH is often associated with pre-eclampsia and eclampsia[4]. In fact, nine women died from intracranial haemorrhaging secondary to pre-eclampsia or eclampsia between 2006 and 2008[12]

Medical Management and Care

- The nature of previous CVA, persisting neurological disability and current treatment dictate care during pregnancy
- If previous **ischaemic** stroke, then anti-platelet therapy in the form of aspirin 75–300 mg per day should be continued
- If previous **thrombotic** stroke, commence anticoagulation in the form of subcutaneous heparin as prophylaxis continued for at least 6 weeks postnatally
- If currently receiving warfarin, risk of warfarin embryopathy (15%) should be acknowledged, and request for termination of pregnancy respected
- If wishing to continue with pregnancy, subcutaneous heparin should be substituted for warfarin ideally prior to 6 weeks gestation
- If no persisting vascular malformations, then pregnancy carries no specific care needs for women who have previously had a **SAH**, although if this was in relation to substance misuse, then a urine toxicology screen to exclude persistent use of these recreational drugs should be considered
- The existence of pre-existing risk factors should alert clinicians to appropriate investigations should a woman present with relevant symptoms and signs
- Careful clinical assessment and documentation of neurological findings and relevant history and risk factors
  - early imaging is essential, with MRI the investigation of choice
  - CT scans may be performed with appropriate abdominal shielding[7]
- Full anticoagulation is of benefit in the presence of cerebral vein thrombosis, but may cause bleeding into an ischaemic stroke and lead to its extension
- Once the acute treatment has been initiated, early physiotherapy and speech therapy are essential in maximising recovery

Midwifery Management and Care

- Appropriate referral for care is essential and should be prioritised as urgent[11]. Care of such women should be centralised in units with a multidisciplinary team, including a neurologist, obstetrician, haematologist and rehabilitation services[1]
- Women should be advised to continue their medications until medical review
- Persisting neurological disability should be recognised and appropriate arrangements for care should be in place and may include:
  - ensuring the availability of disabled parking at the maternity unit for appointments
  - advice regarding childcare
  - alerting the maternity unit to any special needs when admitted
- The existence of pre-existing risk factors should alert clinicians to appropriate investigations should a woman present with relevant symptoms and signs
- The risk of SAH with poorly controlled hypertension should be a particular concern
- Support, reassurance and basic nursing care are essential; these women may require help with toileting and pressure-area care
- Contribution to physiotherapy in the form of guided exercises under the direction of the physiotherapy services will aid recovery

Labour Issues

1. Labour and delivery after SAH

2. Labour and delivery after CVT

3. Labour and delivery after ischaemic stroke

Medical Management and Care (Figure 8.3.3)

1. Treatment of SAH by surgical or neuroradiological intervention should be undertaken initially; fetal outcome is dependent on maternal outcome. After successful treatment and in the absence of persisting arterial malformation, labour and vaginal delivery pose no additional risk to mother and baby. Elective instrumental delivery can be employed if valsalva manoeuvre is to be avoided

2. If receiving low-molecular-weight subcutaneous heparin prophylactically, then this should be discontinued on the day of delivery to permit use of regional anaesthesia if required. Prophylactic heparin does not contribute to excessive blood loss at delivery. Adequate hydration and mobilisation, along with TED stockings are important

3. Should be treated as normal. If taking clopidogrel, then this needs to be discontinued at least a week before labour if regional anaesthesia is anticipated

Midwifery Management and Care

General DVT prevention is essential, therefore ensure:

- TED stockings are worn
- The mother is well hydrated and well mobilised
- Regular maternal observations are taken
- Supportive care related to any neurological disability is undertaken
- Commonly used forms of analgesia (including epidural) may be used after review and discussion by the obstetrician, neurologist and anaesthetist[13]
- Do not administer Syntometrine in the presence of hypertension (three women died between 2006 and 2008 from cerebral haemorrhage after developing very high blood pressure shortly after giving birth and receiving Syntometrine for the third stage[12]). Use Syntocinon im instead (see also Section 15.2)

Postpartum Issues

Thrombo-embolic Risk
- Thrombotic and ischaemic stroke is most commonly identified in the puerperium but not in pregnancy itself[1,11]
- Although the exact cause is unknown, it is thought the profound coagulation changes occurring during a pregnancy and the puerperium may be a factor

Persisting Disability
- Disability affects parenting skills and childcare
- Social isolation may become an issue
- Continued involvement with physiotherapy, occupational therapy and speech therapy services may be required to assist the woman in providing care for her baby

Medical Management and Care

- An assessment of risk should be made on all women undergoing LSCS and thromboprophylaxis instituted as appropriate
- Women who have had a CVT and/or persisting limited mobility require thromboprophylaxis for at least 6 weeks postpartum
- Liaison with haematologist, and other relevant specialists, for ongoing care
- Refer to physiotherapy and speech therapy, occupational therapy as indicated
- Discuss contraceptive options

Midwifery Management and Care

- Encourage and assist with breast-feeding
- Aspirin[1], warfarin[14] and heparin[15] are safe during breast-feeding
- Women with persisting disability requires additional help with breast-feeding
- Make relevant outpatient appointments
- Collaborative working with other services to ensure a safe, supportive setting in which the mother can care for her children as independently as possible
- Advice on contact with voluntary agencies (p.147) for ongoing support and to encourage socialisation

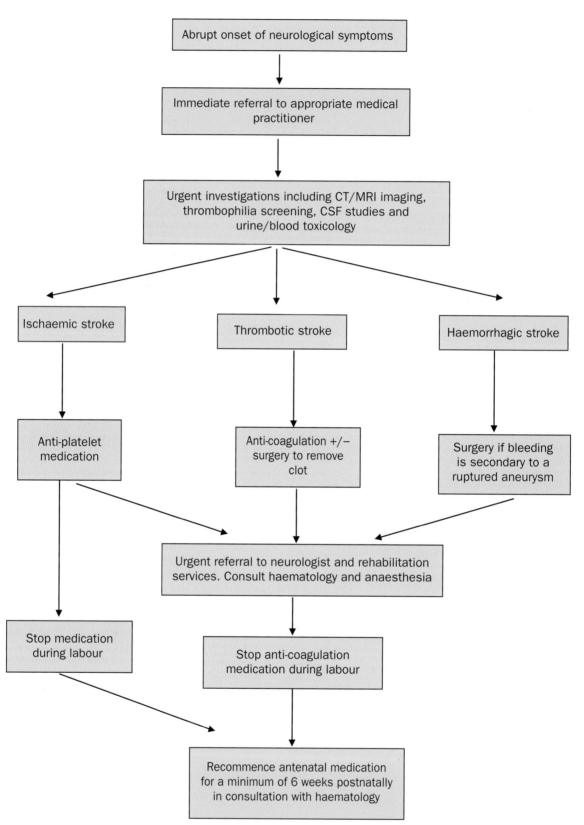

Figure 8.3.3 Stroke management algorithm. This figure is downloadable from the book companion website at www.wiley.com/go/robson

8.4 Bell's Palsy

Incidence	Risk for Childbearing
45:100 000 pregnancies[1,2] 17: 100 000 general population[1-3]	Low Risk

EXPLANATION OF CONDITION

Bell's palsy is an idiopathic peripheral facial paralysis, resulting from inflammation or compression of the VIIth cranial nerve within the temporal bone. It is the most common acute facial paralysis[4]. It usually develops over hours to days and is often discovered in the morning. Bell's palsy manifests as drooping of the brow and corner of the mouth, as well as an inability to close the eye on the affected side, even during sleep (Figure 8.4.1). A diminished sense of taste over the anterior two-thirds of the tongue is experienced and whistling is usually impossible[5]. Hyperacusis is common as is pain in and around the ear. Bell's phenomenon – upward diversion of the eye on attempted closure of the lid – is seen when eye closure is incomplete.

The underlying cause is not known, although occurrence in late pregnancy and puerperium may be caused by oedema, hypertension, pre-eclampsia[6] or secondary to infection[7-9]. The paralysis is usually temporary even when untreated[10]. In one large study 85% of patients recovered within 3 weeks and the remaining 15% after 3–5 months. Sequelae were slight in 12% of patients, mild in 13% and severe in 4%. Contracture and associated movements were found in 17% and 16% of patients, respectively[11]. However, the prognosis for a recovery of a pregnant woman with **complete** facial paralysis is significantly worse compared with the general population[11].

COMPLICATIONS

Due to an inability to close the eyelid as well as a reduction in the production of tears, damage and infection to the eye can occur. For similar reasons, it is cosmetically disfiguring.

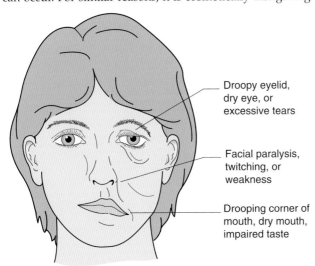

Droopy eyelid, dry eye, or excessive tears

Facial paralysis, twitching, or weakness

Drooping corner of mouth, dry mouth, impaired taste

Figure 8.4.1 Possible symptoms of Bell's palsy. This figure is downloadable from the book companion website at www.wiley.com/go/robson

Pain is common in and around the ear. Frequently, a misdiagnosis of Ramsay Hunt syndrome (facial palsy due to *Herpes zoster* of the geniculate ganglion) is made.

NON-PREGNANCY TREATMENT AND CARE

The diagnosis of Bell's palsy is made clinically:

- An MRI should be performed if there is any possibility of a stroke or a brain tumour, particularly if there is hearing loss or a slow onset of paralysis
- An examination of the external auditory meatus, soft palate and tongue for herpetic vesicles is necessary to prevent being mistreated as Ramsay Hunt syndrome
- If the herpes virus is evident, treat with aciclovir in combination with steroids[4]
- Commencement on high-dose corticosteroids within 24 hours of onset is evidence-based and considered safe and effective in the treatment of Bell's palsy[4,12]
- If there is a history of a tick bite, a thorough physical examination of the limbs or trunk for erythemamigrans should be undertaken to rule out Lyme disease (which may cause facial palsy)[13]
- Eye care is essential to prevent morbidity and should include artificial tears. Eye patches are often counterproductive because the eyelid easily gets dislodged from the patch, allowing the eye to brush against the patch, causing discomfort and potential damage[5]
- Physiotherapy including massage and facial exercises may be of some benefit
- Because of the cosmetically disfiguring nature of Bell's palsy, psychological support is essential[1]

PRE-CONCEPTION ISSUES AND CARE

Bell's Palsy

- Pregnancy is not contraindicated if a woman is being treated for Bell's palsy
- Aciclovir and steroids are safe in pregnancy[14,15]
- If a woman has experienced Bell's palsy outside of pregnancy, it may recur during pregnancy, particularly during the third trimester and the early puerperium. Among these women, a higher rate of gestational hypertension and pre-eclampsia was reported[6]

Pregnancy Issues

- Acute onset with an increased frequency during the third trimester and immediate postpartum period[7,8]
- Pain
- Disfiguring and embarrassing
- Bell's palsy can be associated with hypertensive disorders of pregnancy[6]
- Complete recovery of Bell's palsy during pregnancy is less when compared with Bell's palsy outside pregnancy[11,16]

Medical Management and Care (Figure 8.4.2)

- Thorough examination for the exclusion of Ramsay Hunt syndrome and commencement of corticosteroids
- Prednisolone is usually effective for treatment in pregnancy[15], but needs to be commenced as soon as possible following diagnosis
- Close monitoring for hypertension and pre-eclampsia, and manage accordingly[6]

Midwifery Management and Care

- At the onset of symptoms, referral to the appropriate medical practitioner
- Reassurance of the short-term nature of Bell's palsy, and that it does not affect the course of pregnancy
- Referral to physiotherapy may be of benefit
- Paracetamol for analgesia if painful
- Ensure adequate eye care is given
- Psychological support and information provision

Labour Issues

- If the mother had prolonged antenatal corticosteriod use, she will require hydrocortisone cover during labour
- Be aware that the mother may feel embarrassed by her facial appearance and speech may be impaired when she becomes tired

Medical Management and Care

- Consider the necessity of intravenous hydrocortisone cover
- Intravenous access is required for hydrocortisone during labour

Midwifery Management and Care

- Labour and birth in an obstetric unit, because iv drugs may be needed
- Basic care in labour to include eye and mouth care
- Assistance with administering oral medication, as she may 'dribble'
- There may be difficulty in using a mouthpiece with inhalational analgesia, such as Entonox, so a face mask may be preferred

Postpartum Issues

- As for antenatal issues

Medical Management and Care

- Prednisolone is safe for breast-feeding[15]

Midwifery Management and Care

- Provide reassurance of a good prognosis and potentially a swift recovery

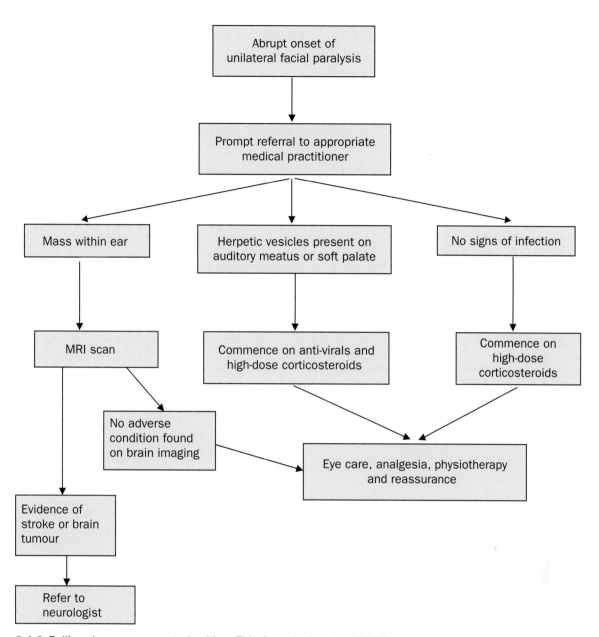

Figure 8.4.2 Bell's palsy management algorithm. This figure is downloadable from the book companion website at www.wiley.com/go/robson

8.5 Carpal Tunnel Syndrome

Incidence	Risk for Childbearing
Estimated incidence of 21–62% of pregnancies[1]	Low Risk

EXPLANATION OF CONDITION

Carpal tunnel syndrome (CTS) results from compression of the median nerve as it passes from the forearm into the hand via the carpal tunnel at the wrist[2] (Figure 8.5.1). It results in pain, pins and needles, weakness and numbness of the thumb and fingers (forefinger, middle finger and half of the ring finger) supplied by the median nerve. In severe cases, wasting of the muscle at the base of the thumb (*thenar eminence*) can occur[2].

A decrease in the size of the carpal tunnel or an increase in the volume within the tunnel results in compression of the median nerve, as with trauma, oedema and repetitive flexion of the wrist[3] as occurs with long-term use of crutches and walking sticks. Symptoms are worse at night and often disrupt sleep. It tends to occur in the dominant hand but can be present simultaneously in both hands.

CTS is associated with a wide variety of clinical conditions including obesity, rheumatoid arthritis, diabetes, thyroid dysfunction, renal dialysis, trauma and pregnancy[4].

COMPLICATIONS

There is a loss of manual dexterity and weakness in grip resulting in dropping things. Injuries to numb fingers are common. Sleep is often disturbed by pain or the pins and needles sensation. If severe, it can be disabling and cause muscle wasting.

NON-PREGNANCY TREATMENT AND CARE

- The diagnosis is made clinically from the history given and if positive to Phalen's test (wrist flexion provoking tingling in the median innervated fingers within 60 seconds) and Tinel's sign (percussion of the median nerve at the wrist creating tingling in the median innervated fingers)[2,4]. Electrophysiological tests will also show a decreased conduction in the median nerve but are rarely required

- Physiotherapy referral is a treatment option; splinting of the wrists into a neutral position opens the carpal tunnel and thus minimises pressure on the median nerve. Most hand therapists prefer the use of splints at night only[4]
- Occupational therapists can offer workers and their employer's advice on task modification which can often control mild of moderate symtoms[4]
- Anti-inflammatory analgesics to reduce pain and swelling are often necessary[5]
- Diuretics to reduce fluid retention[5] are of uncertain benefit
- Injections of steroids (sometimes combined with a local anaesthetic[6]) into the radial or ulnar side of the median nerve reduces the inflammation and can provide temporary relief[2,5], but in severe cases surgical decompression and release of the trapped nerve will be required

PRE-CONCEPTION ISSUES AND CARE

- Pregnancy is not contraindicated
- CTS is the most frequent mononeuropathy in pregnancy[7]
- Women should be advised that the fluid retention brought about by hormonal changes of pregnancy can result in further swelling within the carpal tunnel, and the pregnancy hormone relaxin may result in further narrowing of the carpal tunnel thus increasing compression of the median nerve[2] and worsening the symptoms
- Symptoms should resolve spontaneously after birth[8]
- If a woman has suffered with carpal tunnel syndrome in a prior pregnancy it may recur in subsequent pregnancies[9]
- If a woman requires walking aids, she may benefit from wrist splinting prior to developing symptoms
- Excessive weight gain is a predisposing factor[10] so ideal weight management should be emphasised
- Symptoms may also begin during lactation and resolve after weaning[8]

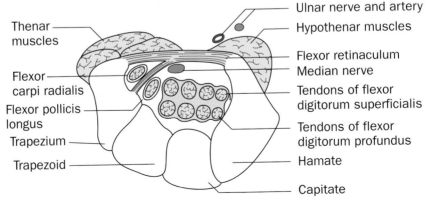

Figure 8.5.1 Cross-section of a wrist (Faiz *et al.* 2011). This figure is downloadable from the book companion website at www.wiley.com/go/robson

Pregnancy Issues
- Usually presents in the second and third trimesters[8]
- Pain
- Disturbed sleep
- Disabling

Medical Management and Care
- Corticosteroid injection into the carpal tunnel may be indicated, and is safe during pregnancy[1,11]
- Nerve decompression under local anaesthesia is safe during pregnancy, but is best avoided since symptoms resolve or are significantly reduced soon after birth

Midwifery Management and Care
- Conservative management aimed at the relief of symptoms is preferred
  - referral to a physiotherapist for splinting may be of benefit
  - paracetamol for analgesia
- Give a thorough explanation of CTS and reassurance that it almost always settles after birth

Labour Issues
- Digital numbness and weak wrists
- Writing, such as signing consent forms, may be difficult as the dominant hand is the one most likely to be affected
- Hydrotherapy for labour and/or birth will allow ease of movement

Medical Management and Care
- Avoid cannulation in the affected hand or hands

Midwifery Management and Care
- Avoidance of birth positions that involve flexion of the wrists for prolonged periods, e.g. kneeling on all fours
- Risk assessment if hydrotherapy is to be used in labour as there may be difficulty in getting out of the pool with the weakened arm; hence hoist might be required
- Support and patience if consent forms are to be signed
- Assistance with basic tasks such as holding a beaker of water
- Assistance with holding the baby immediately after delivery

Postpartum Issues
- May present for the first time during the puerperium
- Weakness of hands
- Loss of manual dexterity, making caring for baby difficult
- Difficulty positioning baby for breast-feeding
- Oral contraceptives tend to cause fluid retention and may provoke CTS[4]
- Risk of developing CTS again in later life if experienced during pregnancy

Medical Management and Care
- Surgical decompression if symptoms persist or are significantly troublesome
- Discuss contraception options

Midwifery Management and Care
- Advise that domestic help is available to assist the mother with the 'trickier' tasks of changing and nursing a newborn
- Extra help and support whilst establishing breast-feeding
- Encourage feeding positions that result in little pressure on the wrists, e.g. using pillows for support
- If wrists are weak and gripping is an issue, advise the mother against holding the baby whilst standing and walking with the baby in her arms, until some strength has returned

8.6 Myasthenia Gravis

Incidence
2–10:100 000[1]
Female to male ratio 2:1[2]

Risk for Childbearing
High Risk – both maternal and fetal

EXPLANATION OF CONDITION

Myasthenia gravis (MG) is a chronic autoimmune disease. Its name translated from Latin means grave muscle weakness. First reported in 1672, MG is characterised by fatigue on exertion and skeletal muscle weakness[3]. This occurs as a result of breakdown in the communication between the nerve and muscle at the neuromuscular junction, due to the presence of autoantibodies which block the acetylcholine receptors.

It is suggested that an abnormal thymus gland induces the developing immune cells to produce autoantibodies. Of patients with MG, 50–60% exhibit lymphofollicular hyperplasia and 10–20% have a thymoma[4].

Patients with MG will present with erratic muscle weakness that worsens with sustained or repeated exertion and recovers with rest[5]. MG may affect any voluntary muscle although in many cases it is limited to the ocular muscles. The degree of muscle weakness may vary greatly, ranging from the localised ocular form to a generalised form affecting swallowing, walking and breathing. Symptoms may include:

- Ptosis (drooping eyelid)
- Diplopia (double vision)
- Unstable gait
- Limb weakness
- Dysphagia (impaired swallowing)
- Dysarthria (impaired speech)
- Dyspnoea (impaired breathing)

COMPLICATIONS

- Respiratory arrest
- **Myasthenic crisis** as a result of exacerbation of MG characterised by acute bulbar or respiratory paralysis which may necessitate mechanical ventilation; death may occur as a result of severe respiratory muscle fatigue[1]
- **Cholinergic crisis** caused by overdosage of anticholinesterase drugs, resulting in:
  - severe muscle weakness
  - hypersalivation
  - constriction of pupils
  - sweating
  - vomiting
  - lacrimation
- Adverse drug response

NON-PREGNANCY TREATMENT AND CARE

MG is one of the most treatable neurological disorders[3], with several therapies available to improve muscle weakness.

- Therapeutic anticholinesterase agents used include neostigmine and pyridostigmine

- Pyridostigmine is currently the most utilised long-acting medication for the treatment of MG: oral pyridostigmine 240–1500 mg per day[1]
- Immunosuppressive drugs include:
  - prednisone (60–80 mg per day)
  - ciclosporin
  - azathioprine
  - significant side effects may occur
  - use with caution (see Appendix 11.1.1)
- Plasmapheresis – plasma exchange involving the removal of abnormal antibodies from blood
- Intravenous immunoglobulin (IVIG), high dosages of which temporarily modify the immune system, provides the recipient with normal donated antibodies
- Thymectomy reduces symptoms in >70% of patients without thymoma; usually performed in patients under 45 years of age[6]

PRE-CONCEPTION ISSUES AND CARE

Onset of MG can occur at any age. Female incidence peaks in the third decade therefore during peak childbearing age. Evidence suggests there is a greater risk of death from MG during a pregnancy in the first year of the disease, with a marked decrease in risk after this time. It is therefore suggested that pregnancy be postponed in women with newly-diagnosed MG. However, therapeutic abortion is not generally advocated[7].

- Ensure medical advice is sought pre-pregnancy to ensure maximum clinical improvement prior to conception. Input is required from neurology in planning a pregnancy
- Advise of the slight increased risk of spontaneous abortion[7]
- Adjustment of medication to establish good control of symptoms may be required, although generally the usual drug therapy may be maintained
- If disease severity is minimal consider discontinuing medication
- Educate women with regard to the need for close supervision, potential for increased fatigue and respiratory compromise and the risk of pre-term birth and neonatal myasthenia gravis

Pregnancy Issues

The effect of myasthenia gravis on pregnancy is variable and unpredictable:

- Disease may remain stable, result in partial or complete remission or deteriorate and may differ in each pregnancy
- Pregnancy does not worsen the long-term outcome of myasthenia gravis[8]
- Relapses or remissions tend to occur in the first trimester[7]
- Effect of nausea and vomiting on gastric emptying may influence medication levels
- Exacerbated by stress, physical exertion, minor infections and fatigue
- Exacerbation in pregnancy less likely if patient has undergone previous thymectomy
- Hypermagnesaemia inhibits release of acetylcholine
- Acetylcholinesterase receptor antibodies in the mother may cross to the fetus and cause arthrogryposis (limb contracture)
- There is no significant increase in preterm labour and growth restriction[9]

Medical Management and Care

- Specialist multidisciplinary team approach; input required from neurology and anaesthetic teams, to ensure medications that may precipitate a crisis are avoided
- Delivery should be planned for tertiary level maternity unit with access to anaesthesia, high risk obstetrics and neonatology[10]
- Assess extent of muscle weakness
- Regular monitoring of maternal disease and fetal health (including regular USS)
- Treat if necessary with acetylcholinesterase inhibitor therapy: drug of choice is pyridostigmine 240–1500 mg orally, in divided doses 3–8 hourly[1]
- Thymectomy is not recommended in pregnancy
- Magnesium sulfate for treatment of pre-eclampsia, should *not* be used in patients with MG, as it may precipitate a crisis
- The following drugs should be avoided: non-depolarising muscle relaxants such as suxamethonium, halothane, ether

Midwifery Management and Care

- Encourage rest
- Ensure women are referred to appropriate medical staff
- Frequent antenatal appointments for maternal and fetal assessment
- Advise regarding fetal movement
- Advise to avoid stress, limit exercise and to ensure prompt treatment of infections
- Referral to anaesthetic team to explore possible maternal concerns regarding possible effects of regional analgesia on disease

Labour Issues

- Increased risk of respiratory insufficiency and aspiration of gastric contents in severe disease[11]
- Expulsive efforts in second stage may be reduced
- Acetylcholinesterase inhibitor requirements may be difficult to estimate, due to reduced gastric absorption and worsening weakness
- Insufficient dosage may lead to severe weakness (myasthenic crisis); excessive dosage may induce a cholinergic crisis (muscle weakness, sweating and abdominal colic)

Medical Management and Care

- Prophylactic antacids in labour
- Consider the need for elective instrumental delivery if mother unable to push effectively in the second stage of labour
- Caesarean section is indicated for usual obstetric reasons
- Consider need for anticholinesterase medications to be administered parentally to avoid erratic absorption
- Consider iv hydrocortisone if mother is taking regular prednisolone
- Avoid gentamicin, ritodrine, salbutamol and narcotics, which may exacerbate muscle fatigue[2]

Midwifery Management and Care

- Careful observation and monitoring of excessive fatigue
- Avoid stress and prolonged second stage of labour
- Regional analgesia may minimise stress of labour and prevent sedative effects of Entonox (nitrous oxide and oxygen) and opioids

Postpartum Issues

- Decreasing circulating volume post delivery may require rapid adjustment of medication
- A worsening of symptoms occurs in one third of women postpartum
- Myasthenia gravis is exacerbated by stress and infection
- Acetylcholine receptor antibodies may enter fetal circulation via the placenta; 12% of babies born to mothers with MG may display transient muscle weakness (this usually resolves within 8 weeks)

Medical Management and Care

- Close observation in short-term postnatal period in order to adjust drug therapy
- In the longer term it is necessary to re-establish pre-pregnancy treatment regime
- Paediatric review to assess for presence of transient neonatal muscle weakness
- Review contraception

Midwifery Management and Care

- Ensure support for women at home and advise regarding rest
- Assistance with baby care is needed following birth
- Advise and observe for signs of uterine and wound infection; refer for treatment promptly if appropriate
- Observe neonate for signs of muscle weakness, e.g. floppiness, feeble cry, poor feeding and respiratory distress; refer to the paediatrician if identified
- Liaison with specialist public health nurse (health visitor) who may wish to be involved at an early stage
- Advise that pyridostigmine is not contraindicated if breast-feeding

8.7 Multiple Sclerosis

Incidence	Risk for Childbearing
100–120:100 000[1]	Variable Risk
Twice as many women as men have MS[2,3]	

EXPLANATION OF CONDITION

Multiple sclerosis (MS) is an unpredictable, progressive demyelinating disease that affects the central nervous system at different levels and at varying times[4]. It is a chronic, disabling, autoimmune neurological condition[5,6] (Table 8.7.1). The white matter within the brain or spinal cord becomes inflamed then destroyed by the person's own immune system. The inflamed areas of myelin sheaths on neurons deteriorate. This destruction of the myelin sheath slows and short-circuits the conduction of nerve impulses, resulting in neurological symptoms. Often there is an acute onset of symptoms, including:

- Diplopia
- Vertigo
- Bladder incontinence
- Loss of vision
- Fatigue
- Muscular weakness[7]

The autoimmune response that causes multiple sclerosis has an unknown aetiology[6,8,9]. Increasingly there is thought to be an interaction of a genetic tendency with environmental factors[10,11]. It typically presents during child-bearing years and is more common in women.

There are several clinical types of MS, but the most common types are:

- **Relapsing–remitting**: clearly defined disease relapses with good recovery between relapses. There are variations in severity and frequency of relapses; 85% of patients have this form of MS. Some are normal for years between attacks
- **Secondary progressive**: initially relapsing–remitting course followed by progression with or without an occasional relapse; 50% of people with relapsing–remitting MS develop secondary progressive MS during the first 10 years of their illness[1]
- **Primary progressive**: disease progresses from its onset, with temporary minor improvements; 10–15% have this form from the onset[1]

COMPLICATIONS

- **Optic neuritis** (inflammation of the optic nerve): often acute in onset and painful, resulting in a reduction or loss of vision in an eye[1]
- **Transverse myelitis**: impairment of motor control, sensory function and control over bladder, bowel and sexual functions[1]

NON-PREGNANCY TREATMENT AND CARE

Diagnosis

There is no single test that can confirm an MS diagnosis. It is diagnosed clinically by accumulating evidence from history, examinations and investigations. Clinical manifestations indicate the involvement of motor, sensory, visual and autonomic systems, but many other symptoms and signs can occur[11].

Common investigations are:

- Brain imaging via an MRI to identify lesions
- CSF studies for the presence of oligoclonal bands

Treatment

In MS the majority of interventions are targeted at masking the individual symptoms, and improving everyday life rather than the disease itself. Pharmacological treatment for MS patients with relapsing–remitting disease or with secondary progressive MS may involve using beta interferon or glatiramer acetate, although neither is recommended by NICE because of their clinical and cost effectiveness[12].

Acute episodes are treated with a course of high-dose corticosteroids and should be started as soon as possible after onset of relapse.

Further pharmacological therapies are dependent on the severity of the relapse and the specific problem (Appendix 8.2.1 and 11.1.1). They generally include antispasmodics, analgesics and medications for bladder urgency.

Referral to a specialist neurological rehabilitation service, which involves occupational therapists, speech therapists and physiotherapists, is essential for every person with MS.

PRE-CONCEPTION ISSUES AND CARE

- MS does not affect fertility, but sometimes MS sufferers experience difficulties with intercourse[2], from severe spasticity of the legs or the presence of indwelling catheters, and may require assisted conception
- It is ideal to plan a pregnancy during a remission period when the woman may be off her medication
- The teratogenic effects of MS medication are uncertain, and many therapies are for symptomatic relief only. Review of medication prior to pregnancy and discontinuation where appropriate is important. Waiting for 3 months prior to conception is advocated[2]
- The woman contemplating pregnancy can be advised that MS has no apparent adverse effects on pregnancy, labour and delivery. There does not appear to be an increased risk of spontaneous abortion, congenital malformation or stillbirth
- Pregnancy does not affect the overall rate of disease progression[13]. There can be improvement of MS during the pregnancy with fewer relapses occurring[14]. There is a marked increase in relapses during the initial postpartum period with 20–40% of patient's affected[13]. This is attributed to immune activation following delivery
- Feelings of fatigue and an increased rate of depression may be heightened when pregnancy and parenthood are contemplated[6]
- Children of MS mothers have a 1:50 risk of acquiring the disease, compared with a population risk of 1:800[15]

Pregnancy Issues

- Having MS has no effect on pregnancy, labour and birth
- Women with MS are no more likely to experience complications than other women[13]
- Half of all people with MS experience cognitive losses[1] and may have impaired ability to learn and remember, to plan, to concentrate and to handle information quickly
- If there is urinary tract involvement, screen regularly for asymptomatic bacteriuria[7]
- Any physical therapy and stretching exercises required prior to pregnancy should be continued[7]
- Relapses during pregnancy tend to be mild and leave no or minimal residual deficits[13]

Medical Management and Care

- Multidisciplinary care including neurology
- Mild relapses may only need supportive treatment
- Severe relapses are usually treated with high-dose corticosteriods[16]

Midwifery Management and Care

- Continuity of midwifery care would be beneficial
- The midwife should check the woman has understood all issues and provide written material where available
- Good communication between health care professionals is essential in the management of these women
- Refer to an obstetrician who has the knowledge of supporting women with disabilities
- Referral to anaesthetists so a plan of labour analgesia can be drawn up and documented[9]
- Refer to local services and support groups for mothers with disabilities
- Parentcraft groups are beneficial for the support element from other pregnant women
- To conserve energy, provide antenatal care at the woman's home[17]

Labour Issues

- If the mother has had prolonged antenatal corticosteroid use, she will require hydrocortisone cover during labour[7]
- More likely to become exhausted quickly
- Many women suffer with urinary retention outside of pregnancy, and this can be a particular problem during labour
- Those mothers who are immobile are at an increased risk of pressure ulcers and DVT
- For those with restricted mobility, the use of a birthing pool may be beneficial
- Epidural analgesia is safe and does not increase the rate of relapse[18,13]
- Relapse may occur after a stressful event, such as delivery of a baby[9]

Medical Management and Care

- Obstetric care as usual

Midwifery Management and Care

- Bladder care is essential
  - palpation for a bladder and attention to urinary output is needed
  - catheterisation may be required
- For those who are immobile, use pressure-relieving procedures
- Inspect the skin areas at risk, and record a pressure-ulcer risk score; use of an appropriate specialist mattress may be needed
- DVT prevention (TED stockings, leg exercises and adequate hydration) is essential (see Section 15.2)
- Access to a birthing pool will provide analgesia as well as aiding mobility. However, a hoist must be available
- Provide reassurance to those mothers who have epidural analgesia regarding the temporary loss of sensation
- Careful documentation of pre-existing neurological deficit in legs to avoid any postpartum exacerbation of MS being inappropriately attributed to a regional block[18]
- Adequate analgesia for the benefit of reducing stress in labour[9]

Postpartum Issues

- Exacerbation of MS is reported to increase 20–40% during first 6 months after delivery[13]
- Nearly all new mothers are fatigued; this can be exacerbated in MS sufferers, and therefore it is important that extra help and support is made available
- Longer maternity leave may be required to cover the period of highest risk of relapse[2]
- Breast-feeding should be encouraged, unless prescribed medication precludes it
- Infections have been associated with worsening of disability and can trigger a relapse[1]
- Since MS does not affect fertility, the usual decisions about contraception need to be made[2]

Medical Management and Care

- Re-starting MS therapy shortly after delivery may decrease the frequency of postpartum relapse[13]
- If mobility is affected or if a severe relapse occurs following the birth, the mother may require thromboprophylaxis for the initial 6 weeks postpartum (see Section 15.2)

Midwifery Management and Care

- Those with disability will require extra help with infant care[18]
- Breast-feeding has no adverse effect on the rate of relapse[2,13,18]
- If manual dexterity is reduced the mother will require extra help and support with feeding
- Be vigilant for the signs and symptoms of infections and act promptly
- The type of contraception will be dependent on the areas affected by the MS and the other medications that are being taken. If manual dexterity is reduced, barrier methods are impractical. If bladder problems are experienced, diaphragms may increase the likelihood of UTI. If mobility is an issue or if the mother is on medication and oral contraceptives are used, the mother may be susceptible to DVT or to reduced efficacy of the 'pill'
- Discussion of appropriate contraception

Table 8.7.1 Symptoms, Signs and Non-Pregnancy Treatment of Multiple Sclerosis by Site (modified from Compston and Coles, 2008)

	Symptoms	Signs	Treatment (Established Efficacy)
Cerebrum	Cognitive impairment	Deficits in attention, reasoning, and executive function; dementia	
	Hemisensory and motor	Upper motor neuron signs	Antidepressant drugs
	Affective (mainly depressive)		
	Epilepsy (rare)		Anticonvulsant drugs
	Focal cortical deficits (rare)		
Optic nerve	Unilateral painful loss of vision	Scotoma, reduced visual activity, colour vision, and relative afferent papillary defect	Low vision aids
Cerebellum and cerebellar pathways	Tremor	Postural and action tremor, dysarthria	
	Clumsiness and poor balance	Limb incoordination and gait ataxia	
Brainstem	Diplopia, oscillopsia	Nystagmus, internuclear and other complex opthalmoplegias	
	Vertigo		
	Impaired swallowing	Dysarthria	Anticholinergic drugs
	Impaired speech and emotional liability	Pseudobulbar palsy	Tricyclic antidepressant drugs
	Paroxysmal symptoms		Carbamazepine, gabapentin
Spinal cord	Weakness	Upper motor neuron signs	
	Stiffness and painful spasms	Spasticity	Tizanidine, baclofen, dantrolene, benzodiazepines, intrathecal baclofen
	Bladder dysfunction		Anticholinergic drugs and/or intermittent self-catherisation, suprapubic catherisation
	Constipation		Bulk laxatives, enemas
Other	Pain		Carbamazepine, gabapentin
	Fatigue		Amantadine

8 Neurological Disorders

PATIENT ORGANISATIONS

Migraine Action Association
4th Floor
27 East Street
Leicester LE1 6NB
www.migraine.org.uk

The Migraine Trust
52–53 Russell Square
London WC1B 4HP
www.migrainetrust.org

Epilepsy Action (British Epilepsy Association)
New Anstey House
Gate Way Drive
Yeadon
Leeds LS19 7XY
www.epilepsy.org.uk

National Society for Epilepsy
Chesham Lane
Chalfont St Peter
Buckinghamshire SL9 0RJ
www.epilepsynse.org.uk

Multiple Sclerosis Society
MS National Centre
372 Edgware Road
London NW2 6ND
www.mssociety.org.uk

Stroke Association
Stroke House
240 City Road
London EC1V 2PR
www.stroke.org.uk

Bell's Palsy Association
www.bellspalsy.org.uk

Myasthenia Gravis Association
The College Business Centre
Uttoxeter New Road
Derby
DE22 3WZ
www.mgauk.org

ESSENTIAL READING

Adab N and Chadwick DW 2006 Management of women with epilepsy during pregnancy. **The Obstetrician and Gynaecologist**, 8:20–25

Briggs GG, Freeman RK and Yaffe SJ 2005 **Drugs in Pregnancy and Lactation**, 7th Edn. Philadelphia, USA: Lippincott

Carhuapoma J, Tomlinson M and Levine S 2011 *Neurologic complications* in James D (Ed.) **High Risk Pregnancy: Management Options**, 4th Edn. Oxford: Elsevier Saunders

Centre for Maternal and Child Enquiries (CMACE) 2011 Saving Mothers' Lives: Reviewing Maternal Deaths to Make Motherhood Safer: 2006–2008. 8th Report of the Confidential Enquiries into Maternal Deaths in the United Kingdom. **BJOG: An International Journal of Obstetrics & Gynaecology**, 118:1–203

Crawford P 2005 Best practice guidelines for the management of women with epilepsy. **Epilepsia**, 46(Suppl 9):117–124

Epilepsy Action booklets:
Epilepsy, Facts, Figures and Terminology
Mothers in Mind
Epilepsy, Diagnosis, Treatment and Healthcare
Seizures Explained
From: www.epilepsy.org.uk

Heaney DC, Williams DJ, O'Brien P and Elton C 2010 *Neurologic disorders In Obstetric Practice* in Powrie R, Greene M, and Camman W (Eds) **de Swiet's Medical Disorders in Obstetric Practice**, 5th Edn. Oxford: Wiley-Blackwell

MS Essentials Booklet 15 – Multiple Sclerosis Society
From: www.mssociety.org.uk

NICE Clinical Guidelines:
20: 2004 The Epilepsies – The Diagnosis and Management of the Epilepsies in Adults and Children in Primary and Secondary Care.
8: Multiple Sclerosis; Management of Multiple Sclerosis in Primary and Secondary Care
From: www.nice.org.uk

Rozette C and Houghton-Clemmey R 2003 A review of carpal tunnel syndrome in pregnancy. **British Journal of Midwifery**, 11:136–139.

References

8.1 Migraine and Headaches

1. NHS Institute for Innovation and Improvement 2008 **Migraine – NHS Clinical Knowledge Summaries** http://www.cks.nhs.uk/migraine/management/scenario_adults#-463689 [Accessed 16-03-2011]

2. The Neurological Alliance 2003 **Neuro numbers** http://www.neural.org.uk/store/assets/files/20/original/NeuroNumbers.pdf [Accessed 16-03-2011]

3. Heaney DC, Williams DJ, O'Brien P and Elton C 2010 *Neurologic disorders in obstetric practice* in Powrie R, Greene M and Camman W (Eds) **de Swiet's Medical Disorders in Obstetric Practice**, 5th Edn. Oxford: Wiley-Blackwell

4. Rasmussen BK, Jensen R, Schroll M and Olesen J 1991 Epidemiology of headache in a general population; a prevalence study. **J Clin Epidemiol**, 44:1147–1157

5. Institute for Clinical Systems Improvement 2011 **Diagnosis and Treatment of Headache** 10th Edn. http://www.icsi.org/headache/headache__diagnosis_and_treatment_of_2609.html [Accessed 16-03-2011]

6. Nelson-Piercy C 2002 **Handbook of Obstetric Medicine**, 2nd Edn. London: Martin Dunitz

7. Juergens TP, Schaefer C and May A 2009 Treatment of cluster headache in pregnancy and lactation. **Cephalalgia**, 29:391–400

8. Calhoun AH and Peterlin BL 2010 Treatment of cluster headache in pregnancy and lactation. **Current Pain and Headache Reports**, 14:164–173

9. Zacur HA 2006 Hormonal changes throughout life in women. **Headache**, 46(Suppl 2):S49–54

10. Lay CL and Broner SW 2009 Migraine in women. **Neurologic Clinics**, 27:503–511

11. Allais G, Gabellari IC, Borgogno P, De Lorenzo C and Benedetto C 2010 The risks of women with migraine during pregnancy. **Neurological Sciences: Official journal of the Italian Neurological Society and of the Italian Society of Clinical Neurophysiology**, 31 Suppl 1

12. Olesen J 2004 The International Classification of Headache Disorders 2nd Edn. **Cephalalgia**; 24(Suppl 1):23–136

13. Kurth T, Kase CS, Schürks M, Tzourio C and Buring JE 2010 **Migraine and risk of haemorrhagic stroke in women: prospective cohort study** http://www.bmj.com/content/341/bmj.c3659.full#cited-by [Accessed 16-05-2011]

14. Centre for Maternal and Child Enquiries (CMACE) 2011 Saving Mothers' Lives: Reviewing Maternal Deaths to Make Motherhood Safer: 2006–2008. 8th Report of the Confidential Enquiries into Maternal Deaths in the United Kingdom. **BJOG: An International Journal of Obstetrics & Gynaecology**, 118:1–203

15. The Migraine Trust 2010 **Feverfew and Migraine.** http://www.migrainetrust.org/factsheet-feverfew-and-migraine-10904 [Accessed 16-05-2011]

16. The Migraine Trust 2009 **Pregnancy, Breast-feeding and Migraine.** http://www.migrainetrust.org/factsheet-pregnancy-breast-feeding-and-migraine-10901 [Accessed 16-05-2011]

17. Das S, Muhasseb MK and Loughney AD 2005 Migraine in pregnancy. **Fetal and Maternal Medicine Review**, 16:179–193

18. Loder E 2007 Migraine in pregnancy. **Semin Neurol**, 27: 425–433

19. Carhuapoma J, Tomlinson M and Levine S 2011 *Neurologic complications* in James D (Ed.) **High Risk Pregnancy: Management Options**, 4th Edn. Oxford: Elsevier Saunders

20. Pfaffenrath Rehm M 1998 Migraine in pregnancy: what are the safest treatment options? **Drug Safety**, 19:383–388

21. Aube M 1999 Migraine in pregnancy. **Neurology**, 53:S26–S28

22. Aegidius K, Zwart J, Hagen K and Stovner L 2009 The Effect of Pregnancy and Parity on Headache Prevalence: The Head-HUNT Study. **Headache**, 49:851–859

23. Torelli P, Allais G and Manzoni GC 2010 Clinical review of headache in pregnancy. **Neurological Sciences: Official Journal of the Italian Neurological Society and of the Italian Society of Clinical Neurophysiology**, 31 Suppl 1

24. Facchinetti F, Allais G, Nappi RE, *et al.* 2009 Migraine is a risk factor for hypertensive disorders in pregnancy: a prospective cohort study. **Cephalalgia**, 29:286–292

25. Bushnell CD, Jamison M and James AH 2009 Migraines during pregnancy linked to stroke and vascular diseases: US population based case-control study. **BMJ**, 10; 338:b664–b664

26. Banhidy F, Acs N, Horvath-Puho E and Czeizel AE 2007 Pregnancy complications and delivery outcomes in pregnant women with severe migraine. **European Journal of Obstetrics Gynecology and Reproductive Biology**, 134:157–163

27. Goadsby PJ, Goldberg J and Silberstein SD 2008 Migraine in pregnancy. **BMJ**, 336(7659):1502–1504

28. Fox AW, Diamond ML and Spierings EL 2005 Migraine during pregnancy: options for therapy. **CNS Drugs**, 19:465–481

29. Silberstein SD 2005 Headaches in pregnancy. **Journal of Headache and Pain**, 6:172–174

30. Duong S, Bozzo P, Nordeng H and Einarson A 2010 Safety of triptans for migraine headaches during pregnancy and breast-feeding. **Canadian Family Physician**, 56:537–539

31. Nursing and Midwifery Council 2004 **Midwives Rules and Standards.** http://www.nmc-uk.org/Documents/Standards/nmcMidwivesRulesandStandards.pdf [Accessed 14-04-2011]

32. Airola G, Allais G, Castagnoli Gabellari I, Rolando S, Mana O and Benedetto C 2010 Non-pharmacological management of migraine during pregnancy. **Neurological Sciences: Official journal of the Italian Neurological Society and of the Italian Society of Clinical Neurophysiology**, 31 Suppl 1

33. Chen H, Chen S, Chen Y and Lin H 2010 Increased risk of adverse pregnancy outcomes for women with migraines: a nationwide population-based study. **Cephalalgia**, 30:433–438

34. Warren R and Arulkumaran S 2009 **Best Practice in Labour and Delivery**. Cambridge: Cambridge University Press

35. BNF 2011 **British National Formulary** Issue 61. http://bnf.org/bnf/. [Accessed 14-05-2011]

8.2 Epilepsy

1. Sander JW 2003 The epidemiology of epilepsy revisited. **Curr Opin Neurol**, 16:165–170

2. Booth L and Thompson G 2010 **Epilepsy Statistics.** http://www.parliament.uk/briefingpapers/commons/lib/research/briefings/SNSG-05691.pdf [Accessed 16-03-2011]

3. The Joint Epilepsy Council of the UK & Ireland 2005 **Epilepsy Prevalence, Incidence and Other Statistics.** http://www.jointepilepsycouncil.org.uk/downloads/Epilepsy%20Prevalence,%20Incidence%20and%20Other%20Statistics.pdf [Accessed 14-04-2011]

4. Heaney DC, Williams DJ, O'Brien P and Elton C 2010 *Neurologic disorders in obstetric practice* in Powrie R, Greene M and Camman W (Eds) **de Swiet's Medical Disorders in Obstetric Practice**, 5th Edn. Oxford: Wiley-Blackwell

5. Epilepsy Action 2008 **Epileptic Seizures Explained** http://www.epilepsy.org.uk/info/education/professionals/seizures-explained [Accessed 16-03-2011]

6. Epilepsy Action 2008 **Epilepsy: Diagnosis, Treatment and Healthcare.** http://www.epilepsy.org.uk/info/treatment [Accessed 24-03-2011]

7. Epilepsy Action 2010 **Possible Seizure Triggers.** http://www.epilepsy.org.uk/info/triggers [Accessed 24-03-2011]

8. NHS Institute for Innovation and Improvement 2008 **Epilepsy –NHS Clinical Knowledge Summaries** http://www.cks.nhs.uk/patient_information_leaflet/epilepsy [Accessed 14-03 2011]

9. Epilepsy Action 2010 **Status Epilepticus.** http://www.epilepsy.org.uk/info/seizures/status-epilepticus [Accessed 14-03-2011]

10. Epilepsy Action 2011 **SUDEP** http://www.epilepsy.org.uk/info/sudep-sudden-unexpected-death-in-epilepsy [Accessed 14-03-2011]

11. Centre for Maternal and Child Enquiries (CMACE) 2011 Saving Mothers' Lives: Reviewing Maternal Deaths to Make Motherhood Safer: 2006–2008. 8th Report of the Confidential Enquiries into Maternal Deaths in the United Kingdom. **BJOG: An International Journal of Obstetrics & Gynaecology**, 118:1–203

12. Nelson-Piercy C 2002 **Handbook of Obstetric Medicine**, 2nd Edn. London: Martin Dunitz

13. Adab N 2006 Birth defects and epilepsy medication. **Expert Review of Neurotherapeutics**, 6:833–845

14. NICE 2004 **Clinical Guideline 20 The Epilepsies – The Diagnosis and Management of the Epilepsies in Adults and Children in Primary and Secondary Care.** London: National Institute for Health and Clinical Excellence. www.nice.org.uk

15. Epilepsy Action 2011 **Epilepsy facts, figures and terminology.** http://www.epilepsy.org.uk/press/facts-figures-terminology. [Accessed 14-03 2011]

16. Betts T and Crawford P 1998 **Women and Epilepsy**, 1st Edn. London: Martin Dunitz

17. Crawford P 2005 Best practice guidelines for the management of women with epilepsy. **Epilepsia**, 46(Suppl 9):117–124

18. Tatum WO 2006 Use of antiepileptic drugs in pregnancy. **Expert Review of Neurotherapeutics**, 6:1077–1086

19. Thomas SV 2006 Management of epilepsy and pregnancy. **Journal of Postgraduate Medicine**, 52:57–64

20. Adab N, Tudur SC, Vinten J, Williamson P and Winterbottom J 2004 Common antiepileptic drugs in pregnancy in women with epilepsy. **Cochrane Database of Systematic Reviews**, 3:CD004848

21. Adab N and Chadwick DW 2006 Management of women with epilepsy during pregnancy. **The Obstetrician and Gynaecologist**, 8:20–25

22. Morrow J, Russell A, Guthrie E, et al. 2006 Malformation risks of antiepileptic drugs in pregnancy: a prospective study from the UK Epilepsy and Pregnancy Register. **Journal of Neurology, Neurosurgery and Psychiatry**, 77:193–198

23. Harden CL, Meador KJ, Pennell PB, et al. 2009 Practice parameter update: management issues for women with epilepsy–focus on pregnancy (an evidence-based review): teratogenesis and perinatal outcomes: report of the Quality Standards Subcommittee and Therapeutics and Technology Assessment Subcommittee of the American Academy of Neurology and American Epilepsy Society. **Neurology**, 73:133–141

24. Harden CL, Pennell PB, Koppel BS, et al. 2009 Practice parameter update: management issues for women with epilepsy – focus on pregnancy (an evidence-based review): vitamin K, folic acid, blood levels, and breast-feeding: report of the Quality Standards Subcommittee and Therapeutics and Technology Assessment Subcommittee of the American Academy of Neurology and American Epilepsy Society. **Neurology**, 73:142–149

25. Rosa FW 1991 Spina bifida in infants of women treated with carbamazepine during pregnancy. **New England Journal of Medicine**, 324:674–677

26. Lindhout D, Omtzigt JG and Cornel MC 1992 Spectrum of neural-tube defects in 34 infants prenatally exposed to antiepileptic drugs. **Neurology**, 42(Suppl 5):111–118

27. Morrow JI, Hunt SJ, Russell AJ, et al. 2009 Folic acid use and major congenital malformations in offspring of women with epilepsy: a prospective study from the UK Epilepsy and Pregnancy Register. **Journal of Neurology, Neurosurgery and Psychiatry**, 80:506–511

28. Walker SP, Permezel M and Berkovic SF 2009 The management of epilepsy in pregnancy. **BJOG: An International Journal of Obstetrics & Gynaecology**, 116:758–767

29. Brodtkorb E and Reimers A 2008 Seizure control and pharmacokinetics of antiepileptic drugs in pregnant women with epilepsy. **Seizure**, 17:160–165

30. Harden CL, Hopp J, Ting TY, et al. 2009 Practice parameter update: management issues for women with epilepsy – focus on pregnancy (an evidence-based review): obstetrical complications and change in seizure frequency: report of the Quality Standards Subcommittee and Therapeutics and Technology Assessment Subcommittee of the American Academy of Neurology and American Epilepsy Society. **Neurology**, 73: 126–132

31. Tomson T and Battino D 2009 Pregnancy and epilepsy: what should we tell our patients? **Journal of Neurology**, 256: 856–862

32. Harden CL, Hopp J, Ting TY, et al. 2009 Management issues for women with epilepsy – focus on pregnancy (an evidence-based review): I. Obstetrical complications and change in seizure frequency: Report of the Quality Standards Subcommittee and Therapeutics and Technology Assessment Subcommittee of the American Academy of Neurology and the American Epilepsy Society. **Epilepsia**, 50:1229–1236

33. Adab N, Kini U, Vinten J, et al. 2004 The longer term outcome of children born to mothers with epilepsy. **Journal of Neurology, Neurosurgery and Psychiatry**, 75:1575–1583

34. Kini U, Adab N, Vinten J, Fryer A and Clayton-Smith J 2006 Liverpool and Manchester Neurodevelopmental Study Group. Dysmorphic features: an important clue to the diagnosis and severity of fetal anticonvulsant syndromes. **Archives of Disease in Childhood Fetal & Neonatal Edition**, 91:F90-5

35. Meador KJ, Baker GA, Finnell RH, et al. 2006 In utero antiepileptic drug exposure: fetal death and malformations. **Neurology**, 67:407–412

36. Battino D and Tomson T 2007 Management of epilepsy during pregnancy. **Drugs**, 67:2727–2746

37. Pennell PB 2008 Antiepileptic drugs during pregnancy: what is known and which AEDs seem to be safest? **Epilepsia**, 49 (Suppl 9):43–55

38. Adab N, Jacoby A, Smith D, Chadwick D 2001 Additional educational needs in children born to mothers with epilepsy. **Journal of Neurology, Neurosurgery & Psychiatry**, 70:15–21

39. Meador K, Reynolds MW, Crean S, Fahrbach K and Probst C 2008 Pregnancy outcomes in women with epilepsy: a systematic review and meta-analysis of published pregnancy registries and cohorts. **Epilepsy Research**, 81:1–13

40. Vinten J, Bromley RL, Taylor J, et al. 2009 The behavioral consequences of exposure to antiepileptic drugs in utero. **Epilepsy & Behavior**, 14(1):197–201

41. Banach R, Boskovic R, Einarson T and Koren G 2010 Long-term developmental outcome of children of women with epilepsy unexposed or exposed prenatally to antiepileptic drugs: a meta-analysis of cohort studies. **Drug Safety**, 33:73–79

42. Adab N 2006 Therapeutic monitoring of antiepileptic drugs during pregnancy and in the postpartum period: is it useful? **CNS Drugs**, 20:791–800

43. Robinson JN and Cleary-Goldman J 2008 Management of epilepsy and pregnancy: an obstetrical perspective. **International Review of Neurobiology**, 83:273–282

44. DeToledo J 2008 Pregnancy in epilepsy: issues of concern. **International Review of Neurobiology**, 83:169–180

45. NICE 2004 **Newer Drugs for Epilepsy in Adults: Quick Reference Guide**. London: National Institute for Health and Clinical Excellence. www.nice.org.uk

46. Harden CL, Pennell PB, Koppel BS, et al. 2009 Management issues for women with epilepsy – focus on pregnancy (an evidence-based review): III. Vitamin K, folic acid, blood levels, and breast-feeding: Report of the Quality Standards Subcommittee and Therapeutics and Technology Assessment Subcommittee of the American Academy of Neurology and the American Epilepsy Society. **Epilepsia**, 50:1247–1255

47. Harden CL 2007 Pregnancy and epilepsy. **Seminars in Neurobiology**, 27:453–459

48. Harden CL and Sethi NK 2008 Epileptic disorders in pregnancy: an overview. **Current Opinion in Obstetrics and Gynecology**, 20:557–562

49. Longo B, Forinash AB and Murphy JA 2009 Levetiracetam use in pregnancy. **Annals of Pharmacotherapy**, 43:1692–1695

50. Pack AM 2006 Therapy insight: clinical management of pregnant women with epilepsy. **Nature Clinical Practice Neurology**, 2:190–200

51. Sabers A and Tomson T 2009 Managing antiepileptic drugs during pregnancy and lactation. **Current Opinion in Neurology**, 22:157–161

52. Genton P, Semah F and Trinka E 2006 Valproic acid in epilepsy: pregnancy-related issues. **Drug Safety**, 29:1–21

53. Kalviainen R and Tomson T 2006 Optimizing treatment of epilepsy during pregnancy. **Neurology**, 67(Suppl 4):S59–63

54. University Hospitals of Leicester NHS Trust 2001 Maternal Medicine Clinic/Department of Neurology. **Epilepsy and Pregnancy Guideline**. Reviewed 2006

55. British National Formulary 2011 (61). http://bnf.org/bnf/ [Accessed 16-03-2011]

56. Koch S, Jäger-Roman E, Lösche G, Nau H, Rating D and Helge H 1996 Antiepileptic drug treatment in pregnancy: drug side effects in the neonate and neurological outcome. **Acta Pædiatrica** 85:739–746

57. Cornelissen M, Steegers-Theunissen R, Kollee L, et al. 1993 Increased incidence of neonatal vitamin K deficiency resulting from maternal anticonvulsant therapy. **American Journal of Obstetrics & Gynecology**, 168(3 Pt 1):923–928

58. Nursing and Midwifery Council 2004 **Midwives Rules and Standards** http://www.nmc-uk.org/Documents/Standards/nmcMidwivesRulesandStandards.pdf [Accessed 12-04-2011]

59. Warren R and Arulkumaran S 2009 **Best Practice in Labour and Delivery**. Cambridge: Cambridge University Press

60. Epilepsy Action 2008 Mothers in Mind http://www.epilepsy.org.uk/sites/epilepsy/files/images/about/epilepsyaction_mothersinmind.pdf [Accessed 04-03-2011]

61. Carhuapoma J, Tomlinson M and Levine S 2011 *Neurologic complications* in James D (Ed.) **High Risk Pregnancy: Management Options**, 4th Edn. Oxford: Elsevier Saunders

62. Karceski S and Pack A 2010 Seizure medications, pregnancy, and breast-feeding. **Neurology**, 75:E90–E91

63. Doggett-Jones S 2007 Contraception for women with epilepsy. **Practice Nurse**, 33(4)

8.3 Cerebrovascular Disease and Stroke

1. Davie CA and O'Brien P 2008 *Stroke and pregnancy*. **Journal of Neurology, Neurosurgery and Psychiatry**, 79;240–245

2. Tortora GJ and Grabowski SR 1996 **Principles of Anatomy and Physiology**, 8th Edn. New York; Harper Collins 424–425

3. NHS Choices 2010 **Stroke.** http://www.nhs.uk/conditions/Stroke/Pages/Introduction.aspx?WT.mc_id=110901 [Accessed 26-03-2011]

4. Parlakgumus HA and Haydardedeoglu B 2010 A review of cardiovascular complications of pregnancy. **Ginekologia Polska**, 81 292–297

5. Lowe SA and Sen R 2005 Neurological disease in pregnancy. **Current Obstetrics and Gynaecology**, 15:166–173

6. Carbuapoma JR, Tomlinson MW and Levine SR 2006 *Neurologic disorders* in James DK, Steer PJ, Weiner CP and Gonik B (Eds) **High Risk Pregnancy: Management Options**, 3rd Edn. London: Saunders/Elsevier 1067–1074

7. Barron W and Lindheimer M 2000 **Medical Disorders during Pregnancy**. London: Mosby 517–520

8. Nelson-Piercy C 2002 **Handbook of Obstetric Medicine**, 2nd Edn. London: Martin Dunitz 174–178

9. Walsh J, Murphy C, Murray C, O'Laoide R, McAuliffe FM 2010. Maternal cerebrovascular accidents in pregnancy: incidence and outcomes. **Obstetric Medicine**, 3:152–155

10. Qureshi AI, Giles WH, Croft JB, et al. 1997 Number of pregnancies and risk for stroke and stroke subtypes. **Archives of Neurology**, 54:203–206

11. Cheng SJ, Chen PH, Chen LA and Chen CP 2010 Stroke during pregnancy and puerperium: clinical perspectives. **Taiwan Journal of Obstetrics and Gynecology**, 49:395–399

12. Centre for Maternal and Child Enquiries (CMACE). 2011 Saving Mothers' Lives: Reviewing Maternal Deaths to Make Motherhood Safer: 2006–2008. The Eighth Report on Confidential Enquiries into Maternal Deaths in the United Kingdom. **BJOG**, 118(Suppl 1):1–203

13. Kuczkowski KM 2006 Labour analgesia for the parturient with neurological disease: what does an obstetrician need to know? **Archives of Gynecology and Obstetrics**, 274:41–46

14. British National Formulary 2011 **Warfarin.** http://www.bnf.org/bnf/bnf/current/201052.htm [Accessed 26-03-11]

15. British National Formulary 2011 **Heparin.** http://www.bnf.org/bnf/bnf/current/2762.htm [Accessed 26-03-11]

8.4 Bell's Palsy

1. Holland NJ and Weiner G 2004 Recent developments in Bell's palsy. **British Medical Journal**, 329:553–557

2. Mylonas I, Kastner R, Sattler C, Kainer F and Friese K 2005 Idiopathic facial paralysis (Bell's palsy) in the immediate puerperium in a patient with mild preeclampsia: a case report. **Archives of Gynaecology and Obstetrics**, 272:241–243

3. Falco NA and Eriksson E 1989 Idiopathic facial palsy in pregnancy and puerperium. **Surgery Gynaecology and Obstetrics**, 169: 337–340

4. Hato N, Murakami S and Gyo K 2008 Steroid and antiviral treatment for Bell's palsy. **Lancet**, 371:1818–1820

5. Hain TC **Bell's Palsy – What Is It?** http://www.bellspalsy.org.uk/phprint.php [Accessed 04-01-11]

6. Shmorgun D, Chan WS and Ray JG 2002 Association between Bell's palsy in pregnancy and pre-eclampsia. **QJM – Monthly Journal of the Association of Physicians**, 95:359–362

7. Carbuapoma JR, Tomlinson MW and Levine SR 2006 *Neurologic disorders* in James DK, Steer PJ, Weiner CP and Gonik B (Eds) **High Risk Pregnancy: Management Options**, 3rd Edn. London: Saunders Elsevier 1081

8. Barron W and Lindheimer M 2000 **Medical Disorders During Pregnancy**. London: Mosby 520–521

9. Lowe SA and Sen R 2005 Neurological disease in pregnancy. **Current Obstetrics and Gynaecology**, 15:170–171

10. Lockhart P, Daly F, Pitkethly M, Comerford N and Sullivan F 2009 Antiviral treatment for Bell's palsy (idiopathic facial paralysis). **Cochrane Database of Sytstematic Reviews**. Issue 4. Art. No.:CD001869. DOI:10.1002/14651858.CD001869.pub4

11. Peitersen E 2002 Bell's palsy: the spontaneous course of 2500 peripheral facial nerve palsies of different etiologies. **Acta Oto-Laryngologica**, 122:4–30

12. Davenport RJ, Sullivan F, Smith B, Morrison J and McKinstry B 2008 Treatment for Bell's palsy. **Lancet**, 372(9645):1219–1220

13. Stanek G and Strle F 2003 Lyme borreliosis. **Lancet**, 362(9396):1639–1647

14. British National Formulary 2011 **Aciclovir.** http://www.bnf.org/bnf/bnf/current/3994.htm [Accessed 36-03–2011]

15. British National Formulary 2011 **Prednisolone.** http://www.bnf.org/bnf/current/200132.htm [Accessed 26-03-2011]

16. Gillman GS, Schaitkin BM, May M and Klein SR 2002 Bell's palsy in pregnancy – a study of recovery outcomes. **Otolaryngology – Head and Neck Surgery**, 126:26–30

8.5 Carpal Tunnel Syndrome

1. NHS Evidence – women's health 2009 **Annual Evidence Update on Antenatal and Pregnancy Care – Backache, Symphysis Pubis Dysfunction and Carpal Tunnel Syndrome during Pregnancy.** http://www.library.nhs.uk/womenhealth/viewResource.aspx?resID=324406 [Accessed 15-02-2011]

2. Rozette C and Houghton-Clemmey R 2003 A review of carpal tunnel syndrome in pregnancy. **British Journal of Midwifery**, 11:136-139

3. Tortora GJ and Grabowski SR 1996 **Principles of Anatomy and Physiology**, 8th Edn. New York: HarperCollins 380

4. Burke FD, Ellis J, McKenna H and Bradley MJ 2003 Primary care management of carpal tunnel syndrome. **Postgraduate Medical Journal**, 79:433–437

5. Medinfo 2011 **Carpal Tunnel Syndrome.** http://www.medinfo.co.uk/conditions/carpaltunnel.html [Accessed 26–03–2011]

6. Lowe SA and Sen R 2005 Neurological disease in pregnancy. **Current Obstetrics and Gynaecology**, 15:170–171

7. Padua L, Di Pasquale A, Pazzaglia C, Liotta GA, Librante A and Mondelli M 2010 Systematic review of pregnancy-related carpal tunnel syndrome. **Muscle & Nerve**, 42:697–702

8. Williams Sax T and Rosenbaum RB 2006 Neuromuscular disorders in pregnancy. **Muscle & Nerve**, 34:559–571

9. Sweet BR (Ed.) 1997 **Mayes' Midwifery: A Textbook for Midwives**, 12th Edn. London: Baillière Tindall 241–242

10. Carbuapoma JR, Tomlinson MW and Levine SR 2006 *Neurologic disorders* in James DK, Steer PJ, Weiner CP and Gonik B (Eds) **High Risk Pregnancy: Management Options**, 3rd Edn. London: Saunders Elsevier 1081

11. British National Formulary 2011 **Corticosteroids** http://www.bnf.org/bnf/current/200132.htm [Accessed 26–03–2011]

8.6 Multiple Sclerosis

1. The National Collaborating Centre for Chronic Conditions 2004 **Multiple Sclerosis: National Clinical Guidelines ror Diagnosis and Management in Primary and Secondary Care**. London: Royal College of Physicians of London

2. Neild C 2008 **MS Essentials: Women's issues – Pregnancy, Menstruation, Contraception and Menopause**. London: Multiple Sclerosis Society http://www.mssociety.org.uk/downloads/MS_Essentials_15_Women's_Health_-_web.6662A342.pdf [Accessed 26-03-2011]

3. Borchers AT, Naguwa SM, Keen CL and Gershwin ME 2010 The implications of autoimmunity and pregnancy. **Journal of Autoimmunity**, 34 287–299

4. Poser CM, Paty DW, Scheinberg L, *et al.* 1983 New diagnostic criteria for multiple sclerosis: guidelines for research protocols. **Annals of Neurology**, 13:227–231

5. Tortora GJ and Grabowski SR 1996 **Principles of Anatomy and Physiology**, 8th Edn. New York: HarperCollins 336

6. Bothamley J and Boyle M 2009 **Medical Conditions Affecting Pregnancy and Childbirth**. Oxford: Radcliffe Publishing 192–193

7. Carbuapoma JR, Tomlinson MW and Levine SR 2006 *Neurologic disorders* in James DK, Steer PJ, Weiner CP and Gonik B (Eds) **High Risk Pregnancy: Management Options**, 3rd Edn. London: Saunders Elsevier 1085

8. Barron W and Lindheimer M 2000 **Medical Disorders during Pregnancy**. London: Mosby 527–528

9. Yentis S, Brighouse P, May A, Bogod D and Elton C 2001 **Analgesia, Anaesthesia and Pregnancy – A Practical Guide**. London: Saunders 278

10. Wylie L and Bryce H 2008 **The Midwives' Guide to Key Medical Conditions: Pregnancy and Childbirth**. London: Churchill Livingstone Elsevier 116

11. Compston A and Coles A 2008 Multiple sclerosis. **Lancet**, 372 1502–1517

12. NICE 2002 **Technology Appraisal Guidance 32 – Beta Interferon and Glatiramer Acetate for the Treatment of Multiple Sclerosis**. London: National Institute for Health and Clinical Excellence. www.nice.org.uk

13. Bennett KA 2005 Pregnancy and multiple sclerosis. **Clinical Obstetrics and Gynecology**, 48:38–47

14. Hughes M 2004 Multiple sclerosis and pregnancy. **Neurologic Clinics**, 22:757–769

15. Compston A and Coles A 2002 Multiple sclerosis. **Lancet**, 359:1221–1231

16. Lowe SA and Sen R 2005 Neurological disease in pregnancy. **Current Obstetrics and Gynaecology**, 15:166–173

17. Payne D and Mcpherson KM 2010 Becoming mothers. Multiple sclerosis and motherhood: a qualitative study. **Disability and Rehabilitation**, 32:629–638

18. Nelson-Piercy C 2002 **Handbook of Obstetric Medicine**, 2nd Edn. London: Martin Dunitz 167–168

8.7 Myasthenia Gravis

1. Flint Porter T and Ware Branch D 2006 *Autoimmune disease* in James DK Steer PJ Weiner CP and Gonik B (Eds) **High Risk Pregnancy: Management Options**, 3rd Edn. London: Saunders Elsevier 949–985

2. Nelson-Piercy C 2002 **Handbook of Obstetric Medicine**, 2nd Edn. London: Martin Dunitz 169–173

3. Shah A 2006 **Myasthenia Gravis**. http://www.emedicine.com/neuro

4. Idan S 2005 **Myasthenia Gravis and Pregnancy**. http://www.emedicine.com/neuro

5. Ciafaloni E and Massey J 2004 *Myasthenia Gravis and Pregnancy* in Washington J (Ed.) **Neurologic Disorders in Pregnancy**. London; Parthenon

6. Buckley C and Newsom-Davis J 2007 **Myasthenia Gravis**. http://www.netdoctor.co.uk/diseases/facts/myastheniagravis.htm

7. Barron W and Lindheimer M 2000 **Medical Disorders During Pregnancy**. London: Mosby 523–524

8. Batocchi AP, Majolini L, Evoli A, Lino MM, Minisci C, Tonali P 1999 Course and treatment of myasthenia gravis during pregnancy. **Neurology**, 52:447–52

9. Wen JC, Liu TC, Chen YH, Chen SF, Lin HC, Tsai WC 2009 No increased risk of adverse pregnancy outcomes for women with myasthenia gravis: a nationwide population-based study. **European Journal of Neurology**, 16:889–894. Epub 2009 May 22

10. Gveric-Ahmetasevic S, Coliæ A, Elvedji-Gasparoviæ V, Gveriæ T and Vukeliæ V 2008 Can neonatal myasthenia gravis be predicted? **Journal of Perinatal Medicine**, 36:503–506

11. Yentis S, Brighouse D, May A, Bogod D and Elton C 2001 **Analgesia, Anaesthesia and Pregnancy: A Practical Guide**. London: W.B. Saunders

Figure References

Donnelly R, London NJM 2009 **ABC of Arterial and Venous Disease**, 2nd Edn. Oxford: BMJ Books, Wiley-Blackwell

Faiz O, Blackburn S and Moffat D 2011 **Anatomy at a Glance**, 3rd Edn. Oxford: Wiley-Blackwell

Mant J and Walker MF 2011 **ABC of Stroke**. Oxford: BMJ Books, Wiley-Blackwell

Appendix Reference

1. Morrow J, Russell A, Guthrie E, *et al.* 2006 Malformation risks of epileptic drugs in pregnancy: a prospective study from the UK Epilepsy and Pregnancy Register. **Journal of Neurology, Neurosurgery and Psychiatry**, 77:193–198

151

Appendix 8.2.1 Drugs Used for Neurological Conditions

Drug Name	Possible Side Effects	Potential Effects on Fetus	Rate of Major Congenital Malformation (MCM) (%)
Carbamazepine	Acne, hirsutism, dizziness, double vision, headaches, decreased appetite, aplastic anaemia, thrombocytopenia, erythrocytopenia, leucocytopenia, hypotension, vitamin K deficiency and folate deficiency	• Neural tube defects • Craniofacial defects • Digital defects • Cardiac malformations • Developmental delay	2.2[1]
Phenytoin	Slurred speech, ataxia, insomnia, twitching, nausea, vomiting, constipation, rash with fever, gingival hyperplasia, megaloblastic anaemia, vitamin K deficiency, hypocalcaemia, folate deficiency and systemic lupus erythematosus	• Craniofacial, limb and digital abnormalities • Hernias • IUGR • Development delay • Congenital heart defects • Orofacial clefts	3.7[1]
Sodium valproate	Ataxia, tremors, sedation, increased weight gain, gastric irritation, liver dysfunction, pancreatitis, rash, hair loss, thrombocytopenia, folate deficiency, and vitamin K deficiency	• Fetal valproate syndrome, facial dysmorphia, impaired psychomotor development • Neural tube defects • Digital defects • Urogenital defects	6.2[1]
Lamotrigine	Rashes, fever, malaise, drowsiness, hepatic dysfunction, dizziness		3.2[1]
Benzodiazepine	–	–	
Topiramate	–	–	7.1[1]
Gabapentin	–	–	3.2[1]
Levetiracetam	Drowsiness, asthenia, dizziness	–	Insufficient data
Primidone	Extreme sedation, vitamins D and K deficiencies	• Dysmorphic face • Digital abnormalities • Hypoplastic fingernails	Insufficient data

Midwives: Mothers should be advised to continue with existing medication until a doctor with experience of prescribing such medications in pregnancy has been consulted, because sudden cessation of any medication without careful thought for substitution can be associated with a poor pregnancy outcome.

Doctors: This simple table cannot address factors for prescribing, and a more authoritative source **must** be used, e.g. Briggs GG, Freeman RK and Yaffe SJ 2005 **Drugs in Pregnancy and Lactation**, 7th Edn. USA; Lippincott. Morrow J, Russell A, Guthrie E *et al.* 2006 Malformation risks of epileptic drugs in pregnancy: a prospective study from the UK Epilepsy and Pregnancy Register. **Journal of Neurology, Neurosurgery and Psychiatry** 77, 193–198.

MUSCULOSKELETAL DISORDERS

9

S. Elizabeth Robson[1], Marie C. Smith[2],
Edmund S. Howarth[3][†] and Javed Iqbal[3][†]

[1]De Montfort University, Leicester, UK
[2]Royal Victoria Infirmary and Newcastle University,
Newcastle upon Tyne, UK
[3]University Hospitals of Leicester NHS Trust,
Leicester, UK
[†]Deceased

9.1 Back and Pelvic Pain
9.2 Diastasis Recti Abdominis
9.3 Pregnancy Related Pelvic Girdle Pain
9.4 Hypovitaminosis D
9.5 Osteoporosis

Medical Disorders in Pregnancy: A Manual for Midwives, Second Edition. Edited by S. Elizabeth Robson and Jason Waugh.
© 2013 John Wiley & Sons, Ltd. Published 2013 by John Wiley & Sons, Ltd.

9.1 Back and Pelvic Pain

Incidence	**Risk for Childbearing**
Back pain – 60–78% of pregnant women[1]	Variable Risk
Pelvic pain – 16–20% of pregnant women[1]	

EXPLANATION OF CONDITION

Back pain is a common disorder, accounting for significant use of health service resources and sick leave[2]. A childbearing woman may either have a previous history of medical or 'alternative' treatments. Alternatively, they may present for the first time in pregnancy. 'Backache' is so common in pregnancy that it is described as one of the adaptations to pregnancy[3] with symptoms usually presenting between 4 and 7 months of gestation[4]. A variety of classifications are in use and there is a lack of consensus about the manifestations and treatments[5].

Common presentations comprise:

- Low back pain
- Pelvic girdle pain
- Sacroiliac dysfunction
- Sciatica

Diagnosis is complex. Backache is often referred pain, in particular from the pelvic organs. This needs consideration prior to assuming that the pain is orthopaedic in nature. There is a psychological impact, and this can influence the perception of pain and disability[6].

COMPLICATIONS

- Worsening mobility
- Impaired driving ability
- Difficulty continuing with everyday tasks, work commitments, or caring for other children
- Insomnia leading to tiredness and irritability
- Fear avoidance behaviour[2] leading to physical deconditioning, further pain and employment difficulties[6]

NON-PREGNANCY TREATMENT AND CARE

Careful assessment and treatment are required for any back or pelvic joint dysfunction, including orthopedic or physiotherapy referral.

Modern management encourages mobility and an early return to work[6] with reasonable adjustment to prevent recurrence of the injury. Treatment is specific to the cause.

Low Back Pain

Pain is usually low in the back, sometimes radiating into the buttocks and thighs, and occasionally down the legs as sciatica. There is also a great variation in the severity of symptoms between individuals. Some women have transitory stiffness or discomfort, whilst others are severely affected[4]. Pain is exacerbated by prolonged standing or sitting, forward bending and lifting. Some women experience pain over the symphysis pubis or thoracic spine at the same time.

Associated factors include[7]:

- Increased parity
- Back pain in a previous pregnancy
- Increased weight and tiredness
- Postural changes and adaptations
- Joint and ligamentous laxity

Treatment includes:

- Individual education can reduce symptoms[8] by empowering women to understand their condition[9]
- Back care and postural advice[4]
- Management of activities of daily living to keep pain level as low as possible[4]
- Maintain a comfortable level of activity and exercise[10]
- Analgesia may be prescribed on a gradient, or 'pain ladder' (see Appendix 9.1.1) and adjusted accordingly[11]

Sacroiliac Dysfunction

Pregnancy can affect the sacroiliac joints in several ways:

- Joint laxity may allow enough repetitive new movement at one or both joints to cause pain (a hypermobile joint)
- Alternatively, the newly permitted movement could result in the uneven joint surfaces moving on one another and then becoming 'stuck' (a hypomobile joint)[12]

Treatment includes:

- Appropriate exercise and advice
- It is sometimes appropriate for *gentle* manipulative or self-manipulative techniques to be tried by a physiotherapist[4]

Sciatica

Pain in the distribution of the sciatic nerve occurs, which may accompany backache and sacroiliac dysfunction and rarely occurs alone. The sciatic nerve runs immediately in front of the sacroiliac joint and could become involved in any dysfunction or inflammatory process that is occurring there. The most common cause is a prolapsed intervertebral disc. An exaggerated lumbar curve could also affect the nerve, especially in lying and standing.

Treatment includes:

- Assessment by a physiotherapist or doctor to exclude other back problems and assess the sacroiliac joints[13]
- Pelvic support might be fitted to assist with a co-existing problem such as pelvic instability[10,13]
- Advise sleeping on her side with a pillow between her knees[13]
- Advise the woman to roll over in bed keeping knees and shoulders in line to avoid twisting[13]

PRE-CONCEPTION ISSUES AND CARE

- Women who have had back problems in previous pregnancies are more susceptible in subsequent pregnancies, and may benefit from referral for stability exercises pre-conceptually
- Women with current back symptoms need a medical review of current drug treatments, especially for fetal risk, and substitutions made where indicated (see Appendices 9.1.1 and 11.1.1)
- Measures to reduce obesity
- Encourage physical activity to increase muscular strength

Pregnancy Issues

Previous back pain can be exacerbated by the release of progesterone and relaxin, which relaxes the pelvic ligaments. Alternatively, respite from discomfort may arise if the pain is ligamentous in origin.

Back pain can present for the first time in pregnancy, influenced by the above hormones and postural changes due to the gravid uterus altering the woman's centre of gravity. This condition gets progressively worse as the pregnancy continues.

Associated factors specific to pregnancy include:

- Multiple pregnancy
- Fetal position, especially malposition

Vitamin D deficiency/osteoporosis can present in pregnancy. Here initial symptoms may be symmetrical lower back pain spreading to the pelvis and upper legs and ribs[14].

Back pain can impede mobility, driving, child caring ability and employment. If her job cannot be adapted she might have to take sick leave or take maternity leave sooner than anticipated.

Physiotherapy[15] and planned exercise programmes can reduce pain[16]. Water exercise has reduced pain enabling women to remain at work[1]. Acupuncture[1] and TENS[1,11] can be beneficial for chronic back pain.

Regular use of a pelvic belt decreases mobility of the sacroiliac joints[17] and may be beneficial for some[18] but the evidence is conflicting. Women of short stature have difficulty with fitting a pelvic belt effectively[18] and 60% discontinue use due to excessive heat and other discomforts[19].

Medical Management and Care

- Take a pain history with attention to pain on standing and sitting
- Physical examination. European guidelines recommend[24]:
  - *For pelvis function*: active straight leg raising test
  - *For sacro-iliac (SIJ) pain*: posterior pelvic pain provocation test; Patrick's faber test; palpation of the long dorsal SIJ ligament
  - *For symphisis pain*: palpation of symphysis pubis; Trendelenburg's test of the pelvic girdle
- Investigations of any neurological symptoms
- Be aware that backache can be musculoskeletal or can be associated with other pelvic conditions such as infection
- Analgesia with regular review; augment as per symptoms (see Appendix 9.1.1)
- Early maternity leave may be needed, and 'sick note' required

Midwifery and Physiotherapy Care

- Accurate booking history to identify previous 'backache' and treatment
- Be aware that increasing lower back pain in dark-skinned or veiled women may indicate vitamin D deficiency requiring medical referral
- The care and advice of non-pregnancy (previous page) should be reinforced
- Advise to wear low-heeled shoes and *bend at the knees* when lifting
- Monitor the progression of symptoms to determine if referral is necessary
- Specific exercise advice and encouragement for[25]:
  - Strengthening exercises
  - Pelvic floor exercises
  - Sitting pelvic tilt exercises
  - Aquarobics (water gymnastics)
- Encourage good posture and to avoid 'slumping' when sitting[25]
- Ascertain if a pelvic support belt would be suitable for the mother, and assist with fitting. A simple belt is most likely to increase compliance[19]
- Physiotherapist can advise the most suitable positions for labour and delivery
- Maternal concerns should be taken seriously
- Antenatal pilates and yoga exercises are beneficial; the mother should be advised to check that the instructor is qualified to teach ante/postnatal women[25]
- If a mother asks about acupuncture she must be advised to only consult a practitioner experienced and trained in using acupuncture in pregnancy[25]

Labour Issues

- Some women are best remaining comfortably supported in labour rather than moving around, which could exacerbate symptoms[20]
- Epidurals are not harmful per se, but the relief they give allows positions to be adopted which may further exacerbate the pre-existing condition. There is no evidence to link use of epidurals with subsequent back pain[21]
- Mothers may request water immersion in the first stage; note there is a theoretical chance of difficulty in getting out of a bath/pool

Medical Management and Care

- Review analgesia options
- Avoid, or take care with lithotomy position which may cause nerve root compression from disc protrusion

Midwifery Management and Care

- Agree a birth plan which allows for flexibility with choice of mobility or rest during labour, and position for delivery
- For water immersion confer with obstetrician; ensure a hoist is available
- Suitable delivery positions may include side-lying, kneeling on all fours or semi-reclining with the legs well supported[14]
- If the woman requires assistance to move her legs, they must be moved together at the same time

Postpartum Issues

- The ligamentous changes of pregnancy can take up to 6 months to reverse[10]
- Many women who have back pain during pregnancy find that it persists, or recurs, after the birth[15,22]
- Persistent postpartum backache requires accurate investigation and a diagnosis made before further pregnancies are planned, as the pain may result from an underlying condition such as osteoporosis, which could be exacerbated by subsequent childbearing[23]

Medical Management and Care

- As for antenatal care
- Women who continue to have poor postpartum mobility may require venous thrombo-embolism prophylaxis

Midwifery and Physiotherapy Care

- Re-refer to a physiotherapist if pain persists
- Arrange any necessary outpatient appointments
- Midwife and physiotherapist to give consistent advice on:
  - good posture when feeding, nappy changing, etc.
  - wearing flat-heeled shoes
  - appropriate postnatal exercises
  - the best time to resume pre-pregnancy exercise regimes
  - seeking medical advice if the back pain persists beyond the postnatal period

9.2 Diastasis Recti Abdominis

Incidence	Risk for Childbearing
66% of third trimester mothers[1]	Low Risk – unless there is a pendulous abdomen

EXPLANATION OF CONDITION

Diastasis of recti abdominis, aka divarication of recti abdominis is known colloquially as 'abdominal separation'. It is a separation of the recti abdominis muscles, often appearing in the second or third trimester, or as a result of bearing down during delivery[1].

The abdominal muscles are stretched and elongated during pregnancy, and can become separated along the linea alba, which has become softer and more elastic. The hormonal and mechanical stresses placed on the abdominal wall are believed to facilitate this separation[2].

The diastasis can vary from a small vertical gap 2–3 cm wide and 12–15 cm long, above or below the umbilicus, to a gap measuring 12–20 cm wide and extending almost the whole length of the recti muscles[3]. This weakens the abdominal support, which potentially could increase the vulnerability of the back to injury.

Women Most at Risk

- Multiple pregnancy
- Polyhydramnios
- Multiparae
- Women with a narrow pelvis and large baby
- Women with weak abdominal muscles pre-pregnancy

COMPLICATIONS

If left untreated, diastasis recti abdominis can lead to long-term problems, in particular:

- Abnormal posture
- Back pain
- Pendulous abdomen (with sequelae of fetal malpresentation and malposition in subsequent pregnancies)

Rupture of the rectus abdominus muscles is very rare, mainly occurs in multigravid women, presenting in late pregnancy and is often precipitated by expulsive coughing[4].

NON-PREGNANCY TREATMENT AND CARE

All newly-delivered women with the condition should ideally be referred to an obstetric physiotherapist, who is likely to first check the width of the gap.

With the woman in crook lying, supported on one pillow, she raises her head to reach with her hands towards her feet. With the fingertips of one hand placed widthways across the abdomen in the midline, just below the umbilicus, the medial edges of the two recti muscles can be palpated as the woman raises her head. The degree of separation is measurable in fingertip widths[5].

The physiotherapist will then:

- Teach appropriate abdominal exercise[6]
- Advise regarding activities of daily living

- Encourage constant awareness of the abdomen, so that the woman retracts her abdominal muscles frequently[7]
- Encourage the woman to roll onto her side to get into and out of bed, reducing the amount of strain placed on the muscles and the back
- Determine if the woman would benefit from wearing an abdominal support such as Tubigrip, in the interim period, to provide some abdominal support
- Review the woman regularly until the diastasis has improved

In extreme cases, where the condition persists after physiotherapy and abdominal musculature is severely impaired, corrective surgery by abdominoplasty may be considered. This entails suturing the rectus bellies together and removing the distended pendulous fat and skin[7].

PRE-CONCEPTION ISSUES AND CARE

It is thought that women who take regular exercise before pregnancy have a reduced risk of developing diastasis recti abdominis because their muscle tissue is healthier as a result[8]. Hence all women should be encouraged to exercise, and this especially applies to women with a past history of diastasis as well as women generally in the pre-conception period.

The woman with a past history of the condition should be encouraged to:

- Use effective contraception until the diastasis has improved, and effective muscle tone has been achieved
- Exercise regularly, especially swimming
- Have a well-balanced diet to reduce obesity
- Adopt a positive body image
- Avoid, or take care, with lifting – especially lifting her own children[6]

If a woman has had surgical treatment by abdominoplasty, further pregnancies are not usually recommended, as the repaired abdominal muscles may not stretch adequately in pregnancy. If a woman still wishes for a pregnancy she would benefit from advice and counselling, because she is likely to experience increasing discomfort as the pregnancy progresses.

Pregnancy Issues

- Healthy pregnant women should be encouraged to remain active. Mild to moderate exercise is beneficial, provided that overheating or exhaustion does not occur[5]
- Swimming provides a toning and strengthening activity which increases physical fitness as well as promoting a sense of wellbeing
- A mild diastasis, with inter-recti distance of two finger widths is considered normal, and should not prevent the mother from having low-risk midwifery care, unless further complications occur
- An inter-recti distance of four or more finger widths is considered abnormal
- Fetal parts are readily identifiable on abdominal palpation, and the fetus is theoretically more vulnerable to trauma under the diastasis gap. Skin over the gap may be inflamed or itchy
- There is a theoretical risk of pendulous abdomen developing in grand multiparae, which can pre-dispose to fetal malpresentation or malposition
- Women with previous abdominoplasty will experience significant pain and discomfort. It is difficult to palpate the abdomen, and it is misleading to measure fundal height against the umbilicus, necessitating ultrasonic scans

Medical Management and Care

- Examine the mother and monitor the condition if referred
- No specific medical interventions are proven
- Skin treatment may have to be prescribed if moisturisers have failed
- Refer to the obstetric physiotherapist for treatment as below

Midwifery and Physiotherapy Management and Care

- Be aware that a mother with a previous diastasis may have a recurrence in the current pregnancy, and that diastasis can also present for the first time in the second/third trimester[1]
- Take care when performing abdominal palpation, as a mother with diastasis may feel especially sensitive in the midline
- Advise the use of moisturiser cream for itchy/flaky abdominal skin
- If a pendulous abdomen develops refer to the obstetrician, and be alert for fetal malpresentation or malposition
- Ascertain if the mother has an occupational risk of contact pressure on her abdomen, which may necessitate adaptation of occupation
- Refer the mother to the obstetric physiotherapist if the diastasis presents (or re-occurs) with an inter-recti distance ≥4 finger widths
- The physiotherapist might fit a Tubigrip abdominal support in late pregnancy or in readiness for labour[11]

Midwife and Physiotherapist Should Advise the Mother

- To roll onto her side to get in and out of bed, to reduce excessive strain on the abdominal muscles
- To avoid strenuous abdominal exercises (sit-ups) and contact sports which might worsen the condition.
- To attend aquanatal classes, informing the instructor of her condition
- That labour is likely to be normal, unless other problems develop

Labour Issues

- A woman with a significant diastasis may benefit from wearing a piece of size 'L' Tubigrip (xiphisternum to symphysis pubis) during labour to help to support the abdomen, if tolerated

Medical Management and Care

- This is dictated by fetal malposition, otherwise labour can be managed normally by the midwife

Midwifery Management and Care

- Gentle, but accurate, abdominal examination in labour as it is important to identify fetal malposition or malpresentation
- Assist the mother with significant diastasis to put on the Tubigrip belt, and be aware that the mother may feel 'hot and sweaty' under the belt and require assistance with washing
- Labour should otherwise be managed normally

Postpartum Issues

- Whilst the inter-recti distance should reduce after delivery, some degree of diastasis may persist for 30–60% of postpartum women[1] and non-resolution postpartum is associated with chronic lower back pain[9]
- Advice and treatment in the puerperium remains the same as for non-pregnancy
- The inter-recti distance should reduce naturally, but some degree of the gap is likely to persist for up to 12 weeks postpartum[10]. The gap is larger when measured in a resting posture postpartum[10]

Medical Management and Care

- Be aware of the risk of bowel incarceration, which can result when muscle tone improves and the gap narrows

Midwifery Management and Care

- Assess the inter-recti distance as part of the routine postnatal examination, measuring in both active and resting positions[10]
- Re-refer the mother to the obstetric physiotherapist, who is likely to assess the width of the diastasis gap, and advise on abdominal exercise (see previous page)
- Reinforce the advice of the obstetric physiotherapist
- Give practical advice to the mother on posture and picking up her baby, and returning to pre-pregnancy fitness; in particular, to 'draw-in' her abdomen when walking and prior to picking up the baby
- Advise the mother that this condition could recur with future pregnancies, and she should wear abdominal support promptly[11]

9.3 Pregnancy Related Pelvic Girdle Pain

Incidence	Risk for Childbearing
Symphysis pubis dysfunction (SPD)[1] 1:36	Variable Risk
Diastasis of the symphysis pubis (DSP)[2] 1:569	

EXPLANATION OF CONDITION

The symphysis pubis forms the strong midline union between the pubic bones of the pelvis. It is a unique joint comprising a fibrocartilaginous disc sandwiched between the articular surfaces of the pubic bones and is capable of a 2 mm amount of movement and 1° rotation[3]. The hormones of pregnancy, especially relaxin, induce resorption of the symphyseal margins and structural changes in the fibrocartilaginous disc thus increasing the symphyseal width and mobility during pregnancy[3].

Pain and varying degrees of dysfunction of the symphysis pubis can present in some pregnant women and a plethora of classifications exist. European guidelines now advocate the use of the 'umbrella' term *pregnancy related pelvis girdle pain* (PRPGP)[4] which encompasses more specific conditions as described below.

Symphysis Pubis Dysfunction (SPD)

Symphysis pubis malfunction results in varying immobility or disability. It is associated with obesity especially when the BMI >30[5], and is also more common in those with joint hypermobility problems and connective tissue diseases especially Marfan's and Ehlers–Danlos syndromes[6]. There are no definitive tests that prove or disprove its presence, the diagnosis being made on the basis of symptoms alone.

Signs and symptoms of SPD include:

- Mild to severe pain in the symphysis pubis joint, hips, groin, lower abdomen, inner thighs and back
- Exacerbated by all weight-bearing activities, especially walking, stairs, sitting to standing, standing on one leg, abducting the legs (e.g. getting in and out of a car)
- Painful to roll over in bed
- Clicking or grinding noises from the symphysis pubis
- Women often walk in a 'waddling' fashion

NB, Palpation of the symphysis pubis should be performed cautiously as it can be extremely tender.

The pelvic girdle is responsible for the transference of large forces from the upper body onto the legs during walking. It is therefore essential that the three joints of the pelvis are strongly supported and stable. Stability of the pelvic ring is provided by close fitting joint surfaces, strong pelvic ligaments and support from pelvic and trunk muscles. This means that any dysfunction (stiffness or hypermobility) at one joint could have an effect on the others. Women presenting with SPD often complain of low back pain and vice versa.

During pregnancy, pelvic stability can be compromised by ligamentous laxity that occurs as a result of the hormonal changes. The normal gap between the pubic bones in pregnancy varies from 4.5 to 9 mm. However, separation can exceed 10 mm. In some cases, severe dysfunction and pain can occur as a result of these changes.

Symphysiolysis

Symphysiolysis is the name given to pain in the symphysis pubis only. This group of patients tend to hormonally-mediated changes alone[7,8] (the other groups have additional biomechanical and articular changes) and the best outcome with full postpartum recovery[7].

Diastasis of the Symphysis Pubis (DSP)

Diastasis (separation) of the symphysis pubis (DSP) may develop from chronic SPD, or present acutely with the same symptoms. Definitive diagnosis can, however, only be made radiologically. The definition is separation of the symphysis pubis of 10 mm or more, and a vertical shift of 5 mm or more[9]. There is often no association between the severity of symptoms and the degree of separation at the symphysis pubis[10]. Traumatic separation can occur as a result of:

- Precipitous delivery
- Cephalo-pelvic disproportion
- Excessive abduction of the thighs during delivery[3]
- Pelvic girdle pain in a previous pregnancy
- Previous pelvic damage

COMPLICATIONS

- Long-term morbidity can be experienced by some women, who may ultimately require internal fixation
- Adverse impact on daily life, parenting skills, housekeeping
- Mechanical difficulty with sexual relationship
- Feeling of frustration, helplessness and loss of control[11]
- Increased risk of recurrence in subsequent pregnancy

NON-PREGNANCY TREATMENT AND CARE

Symptoms may persist postpartum and women may require physiotherapy for several months with an emphasis on:

- Advice on adapting to daily living and employment
- Promoting good posture
- Teaching core stability exercises
- Hydrotherapy enhances movement whilst causing less joint pain

Most cases resolve by 6 months postpartum. In non-resolving cases orthopaedic referral may be necessary, and, on occasion, surgery for internal fixation of the symphysis pubis may be necessary.

PRE-CONCEPTION ISSUES AND CARE

- SPD often starts earlier in subsequent pregnancies, and symptoms can be more pronounced
- It is best to recover from previous pregnancy effects before embarking on another, hence effective contraception is required
- Calculate the BMI and consider weight reduction measures
- Identification of women with hypermobility or connective tissue disorders, especially Marfan's syndrome, who may need referral for that condition and also exercise advice as below
- Pelvic stability exercises can assist future pregnancies
- Once pregnant early referral to a physiotherapist is advisable for assessment and prompt symptom control

Pregnancy Issues

- PRPGP can present at any stage in pregnancy.
- The mother may experience a range of severity with symptoms and complications, which include:
  - pain
  - instability
  - immobility
  - inability or difficulty with weight-bearing
- Symptoms worsens with multiple pregnancy
- The disabling nature of the condition is under-appreciated[11]
- Women experience practical difficulties caring for themselves and their children, and become increasingly dependent upon others[12]
- Disabling situations and pain can influence[12]:
  - domestic and driving mobility
  - employment situation
  - social isolation
  - psychological wellbeing
  - family relationships
  - sexual function
  - enthusiasm for the pregnancy
- Hydrotherapy is popular, and the buoyancy encourages pain-free movement allowing exercise to improve muscle tone[6]. The mother should make the instructor aware of her condition and the pool should permit easy entrance and exit

Medical Management and Care

- Analgesia amended on a gradient as symptoms alter (see Appendix 9.1.1)
- Antenatal epidural has been described in extreme situations[14], necessitating hospital admission
- Women with limited mobility will require VTE prophylaxis

Midwifery and Physiotherapy Management and Care

- Midwife should liaise with an obstetric physiotherapist for assistance in managing the condition. This would include:
  - advice on back care and exercises
  - management of joint dysfunction
  - correction of muscle imbalance
  - assess effectiveness of a pelvic support belt if used, as there is conflicting evidence as to its effectiveness[15,16]
  - provision of elbow crutches
- Check pain-free range of hip abduction prior to labour[17] and liaise management of labour with the named midwife
- Assess for suitability of TENS for pregnancy use if symptoms persist[17]
- Advise[17] the mother to:
  - reduce non-essential weight-bearing activities, e.g. lifting, shopping
  - rest – in short doses, as long periods usually aggravate symptoms when starting to walk again
  - avoid straddle movements
  - sit to get dressed
  - wear flat-heeled shoes
- Referral to the multi-disciplinary team may be required as follows:
  - occupational therapist for appropriate aids and wheelchair
  - home assessment if symptoms are severe
  - medical social worker if assistance with benefits, home help or childcare assistance is required

Labour Issues

- Mothers may request water immersion in the first stage; note there is a theoretical chance of difficulty in getting out of a bath/pool
- If the woman 'pushes' with her feet on the midwife's hips, this can lead to SPD worsening to become diastasis
- This can be 'masked' if a mother has an epidural or spinal analgesia[12]
- Acute presentation of diastasis in the second stage, with audible 'popping' noise has been associated with McRoberts manoeuvre for shoulder dystocia[13]

Medical Management and Care

- Epidural can be used, but care is needed with lithotomy position
- Keep lithotomy position to the shortest time period possible, and legs should be moved into position at the same time

Midwifery Management and Care

- Enable woman to adopt the most comfortable position in all stages of labour, e.g. side lying, kneeling[17], but avoid squatting position[18]
- Keep hip abduction to a minimum[12]
- Vaginal examinations in the most comfortable position, often lateral
- The woman should **not** rest her feet on the attendant's hips[17]
- Labour can be managed normally
- For water immersion, confer with obstetrician; ensure a hoist is available

Postpartum Issues

- The disability of the antenatal period is likely to continue into the puerperium, although some level of pain might abate[7]
- The mother with mobility problems is at risk of VTE and postnatal depression
- Whilst diastasis might have occurred acutely in labour, it might be recognised first in the puerperium, possibly after the mother has been discharged home, hence all cases of postpartum suprapubic pain should be taken seriously.

Medical Management and Care

- Analgesic/anti-inflammatory medication if possible
- Anticoagulants if bed-rest exceeds 24 hours
- If symptoms persist, imaging may be required (flamingo posture by standing on one leg) and an orthopaedic referral arranged[19]

Midwifery and Physiotherapy Management and Care

- Bed-rest until acute pain subsides, usually 24–48 hours
- TED stockings and leg exercises if on bed-rest[18]
- Basic nursing care of mother and baby while on bed-rest
- Daily postnatal examination to assess if condition improving or worsening
- Wheelchair to toilet, and gradual mobilisation as pain allows
- Ascertain status of social services support
- Community midwife to extend period of postnatal visiting
- Promote maternal–infant attachment
- Be alert for signs of depression
- Counselling – 68–85% risk of recurrence in future pregnancies[19]

9.4 Hypovitaminosis D

Incidence	Risk for Childbearing
Up to 90% of certain migrant women to North West Europe; 3% indigenous women in North West Europe	Variable

EXPLANATION OF CONDITION

Vitamin D

Vitamin D is essential for calcium and phosphorus absorption for skeletal mineralisation[1]. The major source of vitamin D for most women in the UK is exposure of skin to sunlight[2,3]. Smaller amounts of vitamin D are obtained in certain foods (e.g. oily fish, eggs). The supply of vitamin D from standard European diets is inadequate[2,4].

Vitamin D is transported to the liver to produce the main circulating form, calcidiol, which is further metabolised in the kidney to produce the active hormonal form of vitamin D, calcitriol (see Figure 9.4.1). Maternal vitamin D status is particularly important because the fetus is entirely dependent on vitamin D supply from the mother[5].

Hypovitaminosis D

Serum calcidiol level of <50 nM/l indicates vitamin D insufficiency; <25 nM/l indicates deficiency[6,7]. Other characteristic biochemical changes occur. Serum calcium and phosphorus may become low, but parathyroid hormone (PTH) and later the serum bone alkaline phosphatase rise[8]. These changes are diagnostic in any age group. Although mild hypovitaminosis D seems to be prevalent in many populations worldwide, resurgence of severe vitamin D deficiency, first described in the 1960s in migrants from the Indian subcontinent to the UK[9], seems to be a continuing issue in several migrant groups and particularly in women of reproductive age[10–15].

Risk Factors for Hypovitaminosis D

* Migrant women from the Southeast Asian Indian subcontinent, Middle East, Afro-Caribbean countries coming to the UK and Europe or Australia
* Women with a predominantly indoor lifestyle
* Women with a body mass index >30 kg/m²

COMPLICATIONS

Osteomalacia

With severe vitamin D deficiency, calcium and phosphorus supply to bone are diminished and an excess of new collagen, osteoid, is formed. This is diagnostic of osteomalacia (bone softening) and is diagnosed on bone biopsy[16,17]. Clinically there may be:

* Bone pain
* Pseudofractures, partial linear stress lines in the cortex of bone, can progress to complete fractures of:
    ◦ pelvis
    ◦ upper femora
    ◦ ribs
* With hypocalcaemia there is risk of paraesthesia and seizures
* Mild muscular pains, which are not uncommon, can progress to severe proximal myopathy with paresis[16,17]

Rickets

Bone softening results in bowing of the legs, knock knees in older children, swollen wrists, dental hypoplasia, frontal bossing and/or rickety rosaries (swollen costochondral joints)[18]. This typically presents at age 1–2 years when walking begins.

Pregnancy and Neonatal Complications

Women with established osteomalacia may experience severe skeletal complications including fractures of the femur and pelvic deformity and fracture[19–21] in pregnancy. Rarely, intrauterine rickets may be diagnosed in fetuses of mothers with severe vitamin D deficiency[22,23].

Vitamin D deficiency is particularly common in breast-fed infants[24] of at risk mothers who have *not* been taking supplements[25,26]. Neonates of mothers with severe vitamin D deficiency, are prone to hypocalcaemia[27]. This can cause serious complications including seizures which are resistant to treatment leading to brain injury[28] or neonatal heart failure[29].

NON-PREGNANCY TREATMENT AND CARE

* Women from at risk migrant populations, particularly those who cover themselves, are advised to take regular vitamin D supplements
* A treatment regime of im cholecalciferol (300 000 IU) twice monthly with an oral course of calcium (1000 mg) and cholecalciferol (20 micrograms daily) should resolve vitamin D deficiency within 3 months[30]
* 'Sensible sunlight' exposure should be encouraged

AREAS FOR FUTURE RESEARCH

* The optimal dose of vitamin D supplementation in pregnancy needs to be determined. The current recommended daily dose of 10 micrograms (400 IU) prevents the major complications of severe deficiency but higher doses may be required to achieve neonatal vitamin D repletion
* Further studies are needed to clarify the association between hypovitaminosis D and other complications of pregnancy, e.g. preeclampsia

PRE-CONCEPTION ISSUES AND CARE

* All at risk prospective mothers should be routinely supplemented with vitamin D
* Those with severe deficiency should avoid pregnancy until this has been corrected
* Vitamin and mineral deficiencies may be precipitated by repeated pregnancies at short intervals – appropriate family spacing is a way of minimising this risk

Pregnancy Issues

Ideally, as the population most at risk from vitamin D deficiency is well defined, routine supplementation with vitamin D, 10 micrograms (400 IU) should be given daily. This should avoid any of the rare cases of advanced osteomalacia presenting in pregnancy with possible skeletal complications.

The Committee on Medical Aspects of Food and Nutritional Policy (COMA) has recommended vitamin D supplementation of 10 μg (400 IU) daily to all pregnant women, especially women with a cultural background predisposed to vitamin D deficiency. This has subsequently been endorsed by NICE[31] and the RCOG[32].

Medical Management and Care

- Prescribe vitamin D 10 micrograms (400 IU) daily supplements to *at risk* mothers from onset of pregnancy
- If vitamin D deficiency is encountered later in pregnancy other dosage schedules have been used: from the third trimester onwards 1000 IU of vitamin D daily[33] or a single dose of 100 000–200 000 IU of vitamin D in the sixth or seventh month of pregnancy[34] (the latter should only be used under specialist supervision)
- Generalised musculoskeletal symptoms may be difficult to evaluate and blood biochemistry is diagnostic: raised serum alkaline phosphatase of bone origin indicates more advanced vitamin D deficiency with possible skeletal complications and these women need careful monitoring

Midwifery Management and Care

- Report any musculoskeletal symptoms to the medical team
- Encourage mother to comply with nutritional doses of vitamin D supplements
- Advise women that if they use antacids heavily this could inhibit their vitamin D absorption[35,36]

Labour Issues

- In women with a contracted pelvis from childhood complications and osteomalacia, deformity will need to be carefully assessed

Medical Management and Care

- Careful assessment to see if caesarean section will be required

Midwifery Management and Care

- If pre-pregnancy treatment has been successful with no pelvic anomalies, then labour can be managed normally
- Careful observation of the progress of labour and relate to pelvic shape on vaginal examination
- Be aware that asynclitism can be an indication of a rachitic, contracted pelvis[35]

Postpartum Issues

Mother

- The mother should continue taking calcium and vitamin D supplements in the postpartum period.

Neonate

- There may be some days before neonatal hypocalcaemia develops and mother and baby may already be discharged, so it is important to assess the biochemistry before discharge. Any jitteriness, muscular jerks or twitching should be taken seriously and appropriate treatment considered before full-blown grand mal seizures occur
- Infant biochemistry is diagnostic. Low 25(OH) vitamin D levels lead to low serum calcium and phosphate, raised serum alkaline phosphatase and parathyroid hormone levels (PTH). Some of these tests may take longer to obtain, especially 25[OH] vitamin D and PTH
- Treatment should be instigated in the infant on empirical grounds, but especially if there is hypocalcaemia and/or a raised alkaline phosphatase

Medical Management and Care

- Mothers will need assessment of their vitamin D status with appropriate biochemistry and consider bone densitometry
- Women with severe symptoms plus abnormal biochemistry may need pelvic and femoral X-rays after delivery to exclude pseudo fractures
- If there has been any suspicion of maternal vitamin D deficiency during pregnancy, especially during the third trimester, then very careful assessment of the newborn will be required; close liaison should be kept with a neonatologist
- Bone biochemistry should be checked in high risk neonates and appropriate calcium and calciferol supplements prescribed.
- If neonatal fits occur, urgent paediatric assessment should be sought

Midwifery Management and Care

- If breast-feeding, women will require adequate vitamin D supplementation and advice about avoidance of a further pregnancy until the condition is completely resolved
- Breast-feeding should not be prolonged in the presence of maternal hypovitaminosis D or osteomalacia
- Upon discharge, the parents should be advised about signs of neonatal seizures and the need to seek urgent medical advice

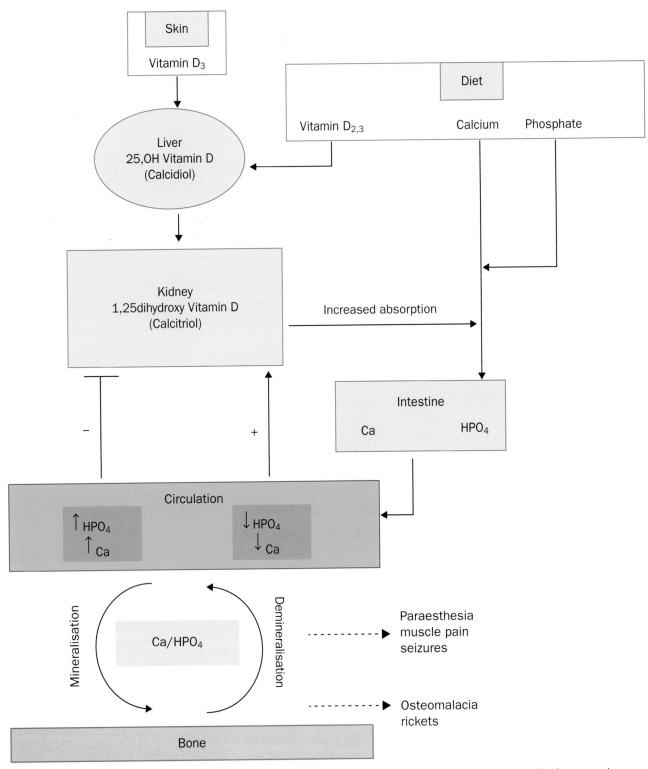

Figure 9.4.1 Schematic representation of calcium homeostasis. This figure is downloadable from the book companion website at www.wiley.com/go/robson

9.5 Osteoporosis

Incidence	Risk for Childbearing
1:3 post-menopausal women[1]	Variable Risk
Rare in pregnancy	

EXPLANATION OF CONDITION[1,2]

Osteoporosis

Osteoporosis is a progressive, systemic skeletal disease characterised by low bone mass and micro-architectural deterioration of bone tissue with a consequent increase in bone fragility and susceptibility to bone fracture.

A more clinically relevant definition of osteoporosis is made on bone mineral density measurement (BMD). BMD is usually measured at the lumbar spine, hip and the radius. Results are expressed in grams per centimetre squared (g/cm^2) as an area density expressed as standard deviations related to the BMD of young adults (T-score). Results can be expressed as standard deviation related to age; this constitutes the Z-score. The WHO diagnostic classification is:

- T-score −1 or better: normal
- T-score between −1 and −2.5: osteopenia
- T-score below −2.5: osteoporosis
- T-score below −2.5 plus one or more osteoporotic fractures: clinical osteoporosis

These criteria strictly apply to women, and at the sites of measurement of hip, spine and forearm.

Osteoporosis Associated with Pregnancy[2,3,4]

This is a rare condition in which women present with severe back pain and height loss due to vertebral collapse, usually in the third trimester of pregnancy. Often the diagnosis is not made until after delivery. Lateral spinal X-rays will show vertebral collapse. The aetiology is not clear but may be related to previous prolonged amenorrhoea, anorexia nervosa or mild forms of **osteogenesis imperfecta**. Osteogenesis imperfecta is an inherited bone disorder due to defective collagen known colloquially as 'brittle bone disease' that results in fractures of varying frequency and severity.

Pregnancy-related Osteoporosis of the Hip (transient)

This is a rare condition characterised by pain in the hip in the late second or third trimester of the pregnancy. There is no associated history of trauma or illness. Physical examination is essentially normal apart from pain in the hip on hip movement. This needs to be differentiated from joint infection or fracture and although X-rays are relatively contraindicated they need to be considered. This condition may be due to neurovascular ischaemia.

COMPLICATIONS[1,2]

Osteoporosis leads to bone fracture, especially lower radius, vertebral and hip fractures. There are estimated to be around 250 000 osteoporotic fractures each year in the UK.

Osteoporosis is common, with up to one in three women over the age of 50 years affected, especially very elderly women. In women of child-bearing age, osteopenia and oste-oporosis are less common, but those with a family history of repeated fractures, prolonged amenorrhoea, and steroid use are at risk of worsening bone density during pregnancy and breast-feeding. This may increase chances of worsening post-menopausal bone health with risk of fractures in later life.

NON-PREGNANCY TREATMENT AND CARE

Women of child-bearing age who have osteopenia or osteoporosis will require appropriate medical attention either in primary and/or secondary care. Advice on diet and exercise are as below. Also see note below regarding bisphosphonate therapy.

PRE-CONCEPTION ISSUES AND CARE

Women with osteoporosis or osteogenesis imperfecta contemplating pregnancy should be encouraged to seek pre-conception care. This should be tailored to the physical condition and personal circumstances, to encompass:

- Re-referral to a physician if an existing treatment is associated with osteoporosis, in particular low molecular weight heparin and certain steroids
- Calculate the body mass index (see Appendix 13.1.1) to determine if weight needs to be gained, as with anorexia nervosa, or lost, as with obesity[4]
- Encourage a well-balanced diet, rich in calcium, vitamin D and other vitamins[4] (daily dietary requirements are to be found in Appendix 1.2)
- Some mothers may require vitamin supplementation
- Smoking and alcohol consumption should be strongly discouraged[4]
- Encourage regular, gentle exercise of which swimming is a good example[4]
- Specific relaxation techniques to help with pain, and exercises to develop muscle strength, are found in the National Osteoporosis Society's booklet (see Essential Reading)
- Advise that breast-feeding may not be possible for some
- Old fractures to femur, hip or spine can cause sexual difficulties, so advice on coital position may be needed[4]
- Women receiving bisphosphonate therapy should be made aware that the safety of these drugs is unproven in pregnancy and lactation[5] and are therefore contraindicated in pregnancy; bisphosphonates remain in bones for a long time, and will continue to be released into the woman's circulation ≥18 months[6]
- Women having had osteoporosis in a previous pregnancy need careful assessment and advice prior to planning a future pregnancy

163

Pregnancy Issues

Osteoporosis Associated with Pregnancy

Vertebral collapse presenting for the first time in pregnancy is rare and making the diagnosis is all important. Characteristically, vertebral collapse occurs in the third trimester but may occur any time until after delivery. Sudden, severe back pain in the thoracic and/or lumbar spinal region, persisting for some weeks or even months, are the main clinical features.

Pregnancy-Related Osteoporosis of the Hip

For cases of sudden onset of pain in the hip, fracture, infection, tendonitis and muscle sprain osteoporosis will need to be considered.

Related Issues

Some medications – steroids, prolonged heparin therapy – are associated with increased risk of osteoporosis.

Identification of fractures in pregnant women raises a possibility of domestic violence. Hence, there is a theoretical risk of misattribution of fractures to domestic violence with the possibility of osteoporosis being overlooked.

Medical Management and Care

Osteoporosis Associated with Pregnancy

- Lateral spinal X-rays showing vertebral collapse would be diagnostic, and careful judgement would be needed about the need to do these as there is a relative contraindication
- Other imaging modalities may be discussed with local radiology services
- Pain management (see Appendix 9.1.1)
- Apart from calcium and vitamin D preparations other specific treatment for osteoporosis can be deferred until after delivery

Pregnancy-Related Osteoporosis of the Hip

- To exclude possible infection of the hip: pulse and temperature, together with FBC including WBC and CRP, will be needed
- To exclude hip fracture X-rays will need to be considered and this will require careful clinical judgement about the need to do this
- Reduced bone density on X-rays is characteristic of this condition

Midwifery Management and Care

- Careful booking history including weight, BMI and dietary history
- Advice on a calcium- and vitamin-D-rich diet with *no* alcohol, referring to a dietician if indicated
- Calcium-based antacids rather than magnesium based (see Section 9.4)
- Confer with medical staff over vitamin supplementation
- Take the mother's concerns seriously and do not dismiss pain as a minor disorder of pregnancy, UTI or even signs of labour
- Observe the mother's gait at every appointment, as anomalies may indicate hip or pelvic pathology
- Be alert for signs of infection (see above)
- Ascertain infant feeding expectations, preparing for the possibility of formula feeding
- Tailor antenatal education (parentcraft) accordingly

Labour Issues

- Labour will be managed according to the clinical circumstances. In the unusual circumstance of collapsed vertebra or fracture of pelvis occurring during labour appropriate management will need to be considered
- The level of vertebral collapse will influence the possibility or otherwise of regional anaesthesia. Anaesthetic review is therefore recommended
- There is increased risk of venous thromboembolism (VTE) if the mother has restricted mobility

Medical Management and Care

Osteoporosis Associated with Pregnancy

- If vertebral collapse is suspected or confirmed the mode of delivery needs review

Midwifery Management and Care

- Care with handling should lithotomy position be required
- TED stockings and gentle passive exercises may be necessary to address the VTE risk

Postpartum Issues

- If the diagnosis has not been confirmed then lateral spinal X-rays and bone mineral density investigations will be needed
- Vertebral fractures may present anytime after delivery up to a few weeks or a month or so; sudden onset of severe and persistent back pain should be therefore considered carefully

Future Pregnancies

If no cause is found, recurrence of spinal osteoporosis is not usual but osteoporosis of the hip can recur. Careful review and advice will need to be given.

Medical Management and Care

Osteoporosis Associated with Pregnancy

- Calcium and vitamin D supplementation will need to be considered
- Specialist advice will need to be sought about starting bisphosphonate or other specific therapy for osteoporosis
- If this problem arises after delivery, then X-rays and other management issues discussed above will need to be considered

Pregnancy-Related Osteoporosis of the Hip

- X-ray bone densitometry
- Specific therapy requires specialist input
- Physiotherapy will normally be helpful

Midwifery Management and Care

- Controlling pain postpartum
- Breast-feeding needs careful assessment and may not be advisable
- Address practical issues, such as picking up the baby and self-care

9 Musculoskeletal Disorders

PATIENT ORGANISATIONS

The Pelvic Partnership
26 Manor Green
Harwell
Oxon OX11 OEL
www.pelvicpartnership.org.uk

Disability, Pregnancy & Parenthood International
National Centre for Disabled Parents
Unit F9, 89-93 Fonthill Road
London N4 3JH
www.dppi.org.uk

Association to aid the Sexual and Personal Relationships of People with a Disability (SPOD)
www.spod-uk.org

National Osteoporosis Foundation USA
www.nof.org

National Osteoporosis Society
Camerton
Bath BA2 OPJ
www.nos.org.uk
Osteoporosis in pregnancy forum http://www.nos.org.uk/forum/Forum17-1.aspx

Brittle Bones Society
Grant Patterson House
30 Guthrie Street
Dundee DD1 5BS
www.brittlebone.org

Strongbones Children's Charitable Trust
www.strongbones.org.uk

Women's Health (UK)
www.womenshealthlondon.org.uk

Food Standards Agency
www.food.gov.uk

The British Pain Society
Churchill House
35 Red Lion Square
London WC1R 4SG
www.britishpainsociety.org

Backcare (National Back Pain Association)
16 Elmtree Road
Teddington
Middlesex TW11 8ST
www.backcare.org.uk

ESSENTIAL READING

Campbell G, Compston J and Crisp A 1993 **The Management of Common Metabolic Bone Disorders**. Cambridge; Cambridge University Press

Compston JE and Rosen CJ 2009 **Fast Facts – Osteoporosis**, 5th Edn. Oxford; Health Press

Fordham J 2004 **Your Questions Answered: Osteoporosis**. London; Churchill Livingstone/Elsevier

Jain S, Eedarapalli P, Jamjute P and Sawdy R 2006 Review – symphysis pubis dysfunction: a practical approach to management. **The Obstetrician and Gynaecologist**, 6:153–156

Kanakaris N, Roberts C and Giannoudis, P 2011 Pregnancy-related pelvic girdle pain: An update **BMC Medicine**, 9, art. no. 15. http://www.ncbi.nlm.nih.gov/pmc/articles/PMC3050758/pdf/1741-7015-9-15.pdf

NOS 2003 **Osteoporosis Associated with Pregnancy**. Bath; National Osteoporosis Society

RCOG **Exercise in Pregnancy** 2006 Statement No. 4 http://www.rcog.org.uk/resources/Public/pdf/exercise_pregnancy_rcog_statement4.pdf

Richens Y, Smith K and Leddington Wright S 2010 Lower back pain during pregnancy: advice and exercises for women. **British Journal of Midwifery**, 18:562–566

Sutcliffe A 2006 **Osteoporosis: A Guide for Health Professionals**. Chichester; Whurr/John Wiley & Sons, Ltd

References

9.1 Back and Pelvic Pain

1. Pennick V, Young G. 2007 Interventions for preventing and treating pelvic and back pain in pregnancy. **Cochrane Database of Systematic Reviews** Issue 2. Art. No.: CD001139. DOI: 10.1002/14651858.CD001139.pub2 [Accessed 9-6-2011]

2. Dawson A, Schluter P, Hodges P, *et al.* 2011 Fear of movement, passive coping, manual handling, and severe or radiating pain increase the likelihood of sick leave due to low back pain. **Pain**; 151 on line http://www.sciencedirect.com/science?_ob=PublicationURL&_tockey=%23TOC%234865%239999%23999 9999999%2399999%23FLA%23&_cdi=4865&_pubType=J&_auth=y&_acct=C000039118&_version=1&_urlVersion=0&_userid=3725461&md5=38047ef035f9e62d830b20d81dafdbfe [Accessed 9-6-2011]

3. Fraser D and Cooper M 2009 **Myles Textbook for Midwives**. London; Elsevier 215

4. Mantle J, Haslam J and Barton S 2003 **Physiotherapy in Obstetrics and Gynaecology**, 2nd Edn. Oxford; Butterworth/Heinemann

5. Kanakaris N, Roberts C and Giannoudis, P 2011 Pregnancy-related pelvic girdle pain: an update. **BMC Medicine**, 9, art. no. 15, http://www.ncbi.nlm.nih.gov/pmc/articles/PMC3050758/pdf/1741-7015-9-15.pdf

6. Wegener S, Castillo R, Haythornthwaite J *et al.* 2011 Psychological distress mediates the effect of pain on function. **Pain**, 151 on line [Accessed 9-6-11]

7. Bastiaanssen JM, Bie RA and Bastiaenen CGH 2005 A historical perspective on pregnancy related low back and/or girdle pain. **European Journal of Obstetrics and Gynaecology**, 120:3–14

8. Ostgaard HC, Zetherstrom G, Roos-Hansson E, *et al.* 1994 Reduction of back and posterior pelvic pain in pregnancy. **Spine**, 19:894–900

9. Ostgaard HC 1996 Assessment and treatment of low back pain in working pregnant women. **Seminars in Perinatology**, 20:61–69

10. Perkins J, Hammer RL and Loubert PV 1998 Identification and management of pregnancy-related low back pain. **Journal of Nurse-Midwifery**, 43:331–340

11. Roche S and Hughes EW 1999 Pain problems associated with pregnancy and their management. **Pain Reviews**, 6:239–261

12. Polden M and Mantle J 1990 **Physiotherapy in Obstetrics and Gynaecology**. Oxford; Butterworth Heinemann

13. Brayshaw E 2003 **Exercises for Pregnancy and Childbirth: A Practical Guide for Educators**. London; Books for Midwives/Elsevier 27–28

14. De Torrente del la Jara G, Pecoud A and Favrat B 2004 Musculoskeletal pain in female asylum seekers and hypovitaminosis D. **British Medical Journal**, 329:156–157

15. Lennard F 2003 Physiotherapy for back and pelvic pain. **British Journal of Midwifery**, 11:97–102

16. Garshasbi A and Zadeh SF 2005 The effect of exercise on the intensity of low back pain in pregnant women. **International Journal of Obstetrics and Gynaecology**, 88; 271–275

17. Carr CA 2003 Use of a maternity support binder for relief of pregnancy related back pain. **Journal of Obstetric, Gynecologic and Neonatal Nursing**, 32:495–502

18. Mens JMA, Damen L and Snijders CJ 2005 The mechanical effect of a pelvic belt in patients with pregnancy-related pelvic pain. **Clinical Biochemics**, 21:122–127

19. Ho S, Yu W, Lao T *et al.* 2009 Garment needs of pregnant women based on content analysis of in-depth interviews. **Journal of Clinical Nursing**, 18:2426–2435

20. Boissonnault JS 2002 Positioning in labour and delivery for women with pre-existing spine or pelvic girdle dysfunction. **Journal of the Association of Chartered Physiotherapists in Women's Health**, 90:3–5

21. Anim-Somuah M, Smyth R and Howell C 2005 Epidural versus non-epidural or no analgesia in labour. **Cochrane Database of Systematic reviews** Issue 4 No: CD000331 DOI

22. Brynhilsden J, Hansson A, Persson A and Hammar M 1998 Follow-up of patients with low back pain during pregnancy. **Obstetrics and Gynaecology**, 91:182–186

23. Brayshaw E 2002 Pregnancy associated osteoporosis. **Journal of the Chartered Physiotherapists in Women's Health**, 91:3–9

24. Vleeming A, Hanne B, Ostgaard H *et al.* 2008 European Guidelines for the diagnosis and treatment of pelvic girdle pain. **European Spine Journal**, 17:789–819 [Accessed 9-6-11]. http://www.backpaineurope.org/web/files/WG4_Guidelines.pdf

25. Richens Y, Smith K and Leddington Wright S 2010 Lower back pain during pregnancy: advice and exercises for women. **British Journal of Midwifery**, 18;562–566

9.2 Diastasis Recti Abdominis

1. Boissonault J and Blaschak M 1988 Incidence of diastasis recti abdominis during the childbearing year. **Physical Therapy**, 68:1082–1086

2. Noble E 1988 **Essential Exercises for the Childbearing Years**, 3rd Edn. USA; Houghton Mifflin

3. Polden M and Mantle J 1990 **Physiotherapy in Obstetrics and Gynaecology**. Oxford; Butterworth Heinnemann

4. Chandraharan E and Arulkumaran S 2008 Acute abdomen and abdominal pain in pregnancy **Obstetrics, Gynaecology and Reproductive Medicine**, 18:205–212

5. Mantle J, Haslam J and Barton S 2004 **Physiotherapy in Obstetrics and Gynaecology**, 2nd Edn. Oxford; Butterworth Heinemann

6. Sheppard S 1996 Part I: Management of postpartum gross divarication recti. **Journal of the Association of Chartered Physiotherapists in Women's Health**, 79:22–24

7. Sheppard S 1996 Part II: The role of transversus abdominus in post-partum correction of gross divarication recti. **Journal of the Association of Chartered Physiotherapists in Women's Health**, 79:24–26

8. Candido G, Lo T and Janssen PA 2005 Risk factors for diastasis of the recti abdominis. **Journal of the Association of Chartered Physiotherapists in Women's Health**, 97:49–54

9. Das S and Jones S 2002 **Abdominal Muscle Performance in Women Who Are 12 To 22 Weeks Post Partum**. www.physiotherapy.curtin.e...onours/99_honours_abstracts.shtm [Accessed 4-6-2006]

10. Hsia M and Jones S 2000 Natural resolution of rectus abdominis diastasis: two single case studies. **Australian Journal of Physiotherapy**, 46:301–307

11. Brayshaw E 2003 **Exercises for Pregnancy and Childbirth: A Practical Guide for Educators**. London; BFM/Elsevier 31–34

9.3 Pregnancy Related Pelvic Girdle Pain

1. Owens K, Pearson A and Mason G 2002 Symphysis pubis dysfunction – a cause of significant obstetric morbidity. **European Journal of Obstetrics, Gynecology and Reproductive Biology**, 105:143–146

2. Snow RE and Neubert AG 1997 Peripartum pubic symphysis separation: a case series and review of the literature. **Obstetrical and Gynecological Survey**, 52:438–443

3. Becker I, Woodley S and Stringer M 2010 The adult symphysis pubis: a systematic review. **Journal of Anatomy** 217:475–487

4. Vleeming A, Hanne B, Ostgaard H *et al.* 2008 European Guidelines for the diagnosis and treatment of pelvic girdle pain. **European Spine Journal**, 17:794–819. [Accessed 9-6-2011]

5. Denison F, Norrie G, Graham B, Lynch J, Harper N and Reynolds R. 2009 Increased maternal BMI is associated with an increased risk of minor complications during pregnancy with consequent cost implications **BJOG**, 116:1467–1472

6. Clarke C 2010 Joint hypermobility syndrome and symphysis pubis dysfunction. **British Journal of Midwifery**, 18:92–97

7. Albert H, Godskegen M and Westergaard J 2001 Prognosis in four syndromes of pregnancy-related pelvic pain. **Acta Obsterica et Gynecologica Scandinavia**, 80:505–510

8. Coldron Y 2005 'Mind the Gap!' Symphysis pubis dysfunction revisited. **Journal of the Association of Chartered Physiotherapists in Women's Health**, 96:3–15

9. Hagen R 1974 Pelvic girdle relaxation from an orthopaedic point of view. **Acta Orthopaedica Scandinavica**, 45:550–563

10. Bjorklund K, Bergstrom S, Nordstrom ML and Ulmsten U 2000 Symphyseal distention in relation to serum relaxin levels and pelvic pain in pregnancy. **Acta Obstetricia et Gynecologica Scandinavica**, 79:269–275

11. Crichton M and Wellock V 2008 Pain, disability and symphysis pubis dysfunction: women talking. **Evidence Based Midwifery**, 6:9–17

12. Shepherd J and Fry D 1996 Symphysis pubis pain. **Midwives**, 109 (1302):199–201

13. Culligan P, Hill S and Heit M 2002 Rupture of the symphysis pubis during vaginal delivery followed by two successful uneventful pregnancies. **Obstetrics and Gynaecology**, 100: 1114–1117

14. Scicluna J, Alderson J, Webster V and Whiting P 2004 Epidural analgesia for acute symphysis pubis dysfunction in the second trimester. **International Journal of Obstetric Anesthesia**, 13: 50–52

15. Depledge J, McNair P, Smith C and Williams M 2005 Management of symphysis pubis dysfunction during pregnancy using exercise and support belts. **Physical Therapy**, 85:1290–1300

16. Ostgaard HC, Zetherstrom GG, Roos–Hansson E and Svanberg B 1994 Reduction of back and posterior pelvic pain in pregnancy. **Spine**, 19:894–900

17. ACPWH 2007 **Guideline for Health Professionals Pregnancy-related Pelvic Girdle Pain**. London; Association of Chartered Physiotherapists in Women's Health. http://www.acpwh.org.uk/docs/ACPWH-PGP_HP.pdf

18. Wellock V 2002 The ever widening gap – symphysis pubis dysfunction. **British Journal of Midwifery**, 10:348–353

19. Jain S, Eedarapalli P, Jamjute P and Sawdy R 2006 Review – symphysis pubis dysfunction: a practical approach to management. **The Obstetrician and Gynaecologist**, 6:153–156

9.4 Hypovitaminosis D

1. Hollick MF 2002 Vitamin D, the under-appreciated D-lightful hormone that is important in skeletal and cellular health. **Current Opinion in Endocrinology, Diabetes and Obesity**, 9:87–98

2. Glerup H, Middelsen K, Poulsen L, *et al*. 2000 Commonly recommended daily intake of vitamin D is not sufficient if sunlight exposure is limited. **Journal of Internal Medicine**, 247:260–268

3. Hollick MF 1998 Vitamin D requirements for humans of all ages; new increased requirements for women and men 50 years and older. **Osteoporosis International**, Suppl. 8:S24–29

4. Henderson L, Gregory J and Swan G 2003 **The nutrition and diet survey adults age 19–64 years. Vitamin and mineral intake and urinary analyses**. www.food.gov.uk/multimedia/pdf/ndnsv3.pdf

5. Clements MR and Fraser DR 1998 Vitamin D supply to the rat fetus and neonate. **Journal of Clinical Investigation**, 81:1768–1773

6. Ford L, Graham V, Wall A and Berg J 2006 Vitamin D concentration in a UK city with multicultural outpatient population. **Annals of Clinical Biochemistry**, 43:468–475

7. Boucher BJ 2006 Evidence of deficiency and insufficiency of vitamin D in the UK; national diet and nutrition data survey 1994–2004 in Gillie O (Ed.) **Sunlight Vitamin D and Health; Health Research Forum Report No. 2**. London; White Hall Park

8. Iqbal SJ, Kaddam IMS, Wassif W, Walls J and Nichol F 1994 Continuing clinically severe vitamin D deficiency in Asians in the UK (Leicester). **Postgraduate Medical Journal**, 70:708

9. Dunnigan MG, Patton JPG, Hass ES, McNichol GW and Smith GM 1962 Late rickets and osteomalacia in the Pakistani community in Glasgow. **Scottish Medical Journal**, 7:159–167

10. Allgrove J 2004 Is nutritional rickets returning? **Archives of Diseases of Childhood**, 89:699–701

11. Lakhani S, Srinivasen L, Buchanan C and Allgrove J 2004 Presentation of vitamin D deficiency. **Archives of Diseases of Childhood**, 89:781–784

12. Sehra E, Newton P, Ali H, *et al*. 1999 Prevalence of hypovitaminosis D in Indo-Asian patients attending a rheumatology clinic. **Bone**, 25:609–611

13. Pal BR, Marshal T, James C and Shaw N 2003 Distribution analysis of vitamin D highlights – differences in population subgroups; preliminary observations from a pilot study in UK adults. **Journal of Endocrinology**, 179:119–129

14. Grover SR and Morely R 2001 Vitamin D deficiency in veiled or dark skinned pregnant women. **Medical Journal of Australia**, 175:251–252

15. Nozza JM and Rozza CP 2001 Vitamin D deficiency in mothers of infants with rickets. **Medical Journal of Australia**, 175: 253–255

16. Smith R and Wordsworth P 2005 **Clinical and Biochemical Disorders of the Skeleton**. Oxford; Oxford University Press 173–200

17. Francis R and Selby P 1997 Osteomalacia. **Baillière's Clinical Endocrinology and Metabolism**, 11:1454–1463

18. Behrman RE, Kliegman R and Jenson HB (Eds) 2000 Rickets of vitamin D deficiency in Nelson, **Textbook of Pediatrics**, 16th Edn. Philadelphia; Saunders (sec 44.10) 184–187

19. Henry A and Bowyer L 2003 Fracture of the neck of femur and osteomalacia in pregnancy. **British Journal of Obstetrics and Gynaecology**, 110:329–330

20. Dane C, Dane B and Kural C 2005 A rare case of severe dyspareunia: post-osteomalacia contracted pelvic outlet. **Acta Obstetrica et Gynecologica Scandinavica**, 84:407–408

21. Hollingworth J, Howley JH, Davidson AC and Iqbal SJ 1994 Severe vitamin D deficiency in pregnancy. **Journal of Obstetrics and Gynaecology**, 14:430–434

22. Innis AM, Seshi MM, Prasad C, El Syeth S, *et al*. 2002 Congenital rickets caused by maternal vitamin D deficiency. **Paediatrics and Child Health**, 7:455–458

23. Blonde MH, Gould F, Pierre F and Burger C 1997 Nutritional foetal rickets: one case report. **Journal de la Gynecologie Obstetrique et Biologie de la Reproduction**, 26:834–836

24. Mughal MZ, Selma H, Greenway T, *et al*. 1999 Florid rickets associated with prolonged breast-feeding without vitamin D supplementation. **British Medical Journal**, 318:39–40

25. Alfaham M, Woodhead S, Pask G and Davies D 1995 Vitamin D deficiency: a concern in pregnant Asian women. **British Journal of Nutrition**, 73:881–887

26. Iqbal SJ, Walker C and Swift PG 2001 The continuing problem of vitamin D deficiency in pregnant Asian women and their offspring, an interface audit as a prelude to action. **Archives of Diseases of Childhood**, 1:84, Suppl. A36

27. Casey M, West J, Shannon R, Iqbal SJ, Madira W and Simpson H. 1994 Persistent vitamin D deficiency in Asian children in the UK (Leicester). **Proceedings of 9th Workshop on Vitamin D**, Orlando, Florida 148

28. Shenoy SD, Cody D, Swift P and Iqbal SJ 2005 Maternal vitamin D deficiency, refractory neonatal hypocalcaemia and nutritional rickets. **Archives of Diseases of Childhood**, 90:437–44330

29. Carlton-Conway D, Tulloh R, Wood L and Kanabar D 2004 Vitamin D deficiency and cardiac failure in infancy. **Journal of the Royal Society of Medicine**, 97:238–239

30. De Torrente del la Jara G, Pecoud A and Favrat B 2004 Musculoskeletal pain in female asylum seekers and hypovitaminosis D. **British Medical Journal**, 329(7458):156–157

31. NICE (National Institute for Health and Clinical Excellence) CG6: Antenatal Care: Routine Care for the Healthy Pregnant Woman. 2008

32. RCOG 2009 **Scientific Advisory Committee Paper 16: Vitamin Supplementation in Pregnancy**. London; Royal College of Obstetricians and Gynaecologists

33. Brooke OG, Brown IR and Bone CD 1980 Vitamin D supplements in pregnant Asian women: effects on calcium status and fetal growth. **British Medical Journal**, 280(6216):751–754

34. Hellouin de Menibus C, Mallet E, Henocq A, *et al.* 1990 Neonatal hypocalcemia. Results of vitamin D supplement in the mother. Study on 13 377 newborn infants. **Bulletin of the Academy of National Medicine**, 174:1051–1060

35. Tytgat GN, Heading RC, Muller-Lissner, *et al.* 2003 Contemporary understanding and management of reflux and constipation in the general population and pregnancy: a consensus meeting. **Alimentary Pharmacology and Therapeutics**, 18:291–301

36. Henderson C and Macdonald S 2004 **Mayes' Midwifery**, 13th Edn. London; Elsevier 74

9.5 Osteoporosis

1. Compston JE and Rosen CJ 2009 **Fast Facts – Osteoporosis**, 6th Edn. Oxford; Health Press

2. Smith R and Wordsworth P 2005 **Clinical and Biochemical Disorders of the Skeleton**. Oxford; Oxford University Press 109–172

3. Smith R, Athenasou NA, Ostlere SJ, *et al.* 1995 Pregnancy associated osteoporosis. **QJM**, 88:865–878

4. NOS 2003 **Osteoporosis Associated With Pregnancy**. Bath; National Osteoporosis Society

5. Briggs GG, Freeman RK and Yaffe SJ 2011 **Drugs in Pregnancy and Lactation**, 8th Edn. Philadelphia, USA; Lippincott

6. Lasseter KC, Porras AG, Denker A, Santhanagopal A and Daifotis A 2005 Pharmacokinetic considerations in determining the terminal elimination half-lives of bisphosphonates. **Clinical Drug Invest igation**, 25:107–114(8): online as www.ingentaconnect.com/content/adis/cdi/2005/00000025/00000002/art00003;jsessionid=u0b26

Appendix References

1. Roche S and Hughes EW 1999 Pain problems associated with pregnancy and their management. **Pain Reviews**, 6:239–261

2. Briggs GG, Freeman RK and Yaffe SJ 2005 **Drugs in Pregnancy and Lactation**, 7th Edn. USA; Lippincott

Appendix 9.1.1 Pain Therapy Ladder for Pregnancy

Step		Step
3	**Methadone**[1] **Use:** Long-term pain management[1] **Risk Factor:** B (or D with prolonged use, or high doses at term)[2] or **Morphine**[1] **Use:** Intravenous patient controlled analgesia or a combination of slow-and rapid-release oral preparations for acute short-term interventions[1] **Risk Factor:** C	3

↑

Step		Step
2	**Orphenadrine**[1] **Dose:** 50 mg, three times daily[1] **Use:** Skeletal muscle spasm **Risk Factor:** C or **Mexiletine**[1] **Dose:** 50–100 mg initially, increasing to 360 mg controlled release once daily, then twice daily[1] **Use:** Neuropathic pain **Risk Factor:** C **Caution:** Nausea (take with food), test blood levels[1] or **Amitriptyline**[1] **Dose:** 10–50 mg *nocte*[1] **Use:** Neuropathic pain, visceral spasm, headache prophylaxis/treatment[1] **Risk Factor:** C or **Diclofenac**[1] **Dose:** 75 mg once daily (second trimester only)[1] **Use:** Musculoskeletal pain and headache **Risk Factor:** B (D in third trimester)[2] **Caution:** Oligohydramnios[1] or **Clonidine Patch Transdermal Therapeutic System TTS-1** **Dose:** = 100 µg per day; one or two patches daily[1] **Use:** Neuropathic pain; place patch over affected nerves/nerve root **Risk Factor:** C **Caution:** If a rash occurs under patch, change to clonidine tablets 150 µg once or twice daily[1]	2

↑

Step		Step
1	**Paracetamol**[1] **Dose:** 1 g 4 hourly[1] **Use:** Mild to moderate pain	1

↑
Local Pharmacotherapy[1]
Local anaesthetics
↑
Non Pharmacological Therapies[1]
e.g. heat, physiotherapy, TENS, acupuncture, hypnotherapy

Risk to Fetus Key: A, little or no risk (human studies)[2]; **B**, little risk (animal studies)[2]; **C**, some adverse effects (animal studies); used if benefit outweighs risk[2]; **D**, positive evidence of risk (human studies); used with serious conditions[2]; **X**, risk outweighs possible benefits, contraindicated in pregnancy[2]

GASTROINTESTINAL DISORDERS

10

Rosemary Lydall[1], Manjiri Khare[1], Caroline Farrar[2] and S. Elizabeth Robson[2]

[1]University Hospitals of Leicester NHS Trust, Leicester, UK
[2]De Montfort University, Leicester, UK

10.1 Gastro-oesophageal Reflux and Hiatus Hernia
10.2 Coeliac Disease
10.3 Ulcerative Colitis
10.4 Crohn's Disease
10.5 Irritable Bowel Syndrome
10.6 Haemorrhoids
10.7 Anal Sphincter Disorders
10.8 Obstetric Cholestasis
10.9 Gall Bladder and Pancreatic Disease

171

Medical Disorders in Pregnancy: A Manual for Midwives, Second Edition. Edited by S. Elizabeth Robson and Jason Waugh.
© 2013 John Wiley & Sons, Ltd. Published 2013 by John Wiley & Sons, Ltd.

10.1 Gastro-oesophageal Reflux and Hiatus Hernia

Incidence	Risk for Childbearing
Heartburn: 20–40% adults[1] and >80% pregnant women[2] Hiatus Hernia: 20% of endoscopy patients[3]	Low Risk

EXPLANATION OF CONDITION

Heartburn

Heartburn is a burning sensation experienced in the region of the heart and in the throat[4] usually resulting from gastro-oesophageal reflux[5].

Gastro-Oesophageal Reflux

Gastro-oesophageal reflux occurs when stomach contents regurgitate into the oesophagus, and is common in health[4]. As the stomach contents contain hydrochloric acid, the mucosa of the oesophagus is easily irritated resulting in the burning sensation of heartburn. **Dyspepsia** may result, entailing pain and discomfort after eating, sometimes accompanied by flatulence or belching, and is commonly known as 'indigestion'.

Reflux and heartburn are a particular problem in pregnancy, where progesterone reduces the muscle tone of the lower oesophageal sphincter, resulting in impaired competence with regards to closure[6]. Intra-abdominal pressure from the growing fetus, and delayed gastric emptying, may exacerbate this problem. The effects are elaborated on the next page.

Gastro-oesophageal Reflux Disease (GORD; GERD in USA)

After repeated reflux episodes **oesophagitis** can result. When combined with the cardinal symptom of heartburn[1], it becomes a disease with significant morbidity. Over time[1] insomnia and disturbed eating patterns may develop. Fortunately the mortality rate is low at 1:100000[1].

Risk of developing GORD increases with age, noticeably once over 40 years of age[1]. It is associated with cigarette smoking, heavy alcohol consumption and increased intra-abdominal pressure[7] often associated with obesity or pregnancy.

Hiatus Hernia

Weakness of the diaphragmatic sphincter enables the lower oesophagus and upper part of the stomach to rise up through the diaphragm into the thorax[8]. This can take up to two years to develop[3] and is associated with obesity[9]. Gastro-oesophageal reflux may, or may not, accompany this[8] and impaired oesophageal emptying may ensue[10]. There are two forms:

1. **Sliding hiatus hernia** (Figure 10.1.1) in which the gastro-oesophageal junction literally 'slides up' through the hiatus (opening in the diaphragm) to lie just above the diaphragm but *below* the oesophagus[11]. It is more common in those aged >50 years, with oesophageal reflux usually the sole symptom[11]

2. **Rolling hiatus hernia** (Figure 10.1.1) in which part of the top of the stomach (fundus) literally 'rolls up' and herniates through the hiatus to lie *alongside* the oesophagus. The gastro-oesophageal junction stays below the diaphragm and remains competent[7,11]. There can be severe pain from volvulus or strangulation, usually necessitating surgery[11]

Investigations comprise barium swallow or endoscopy to identify the hernia and exclude other causes of symptoms[8].

COMPLICATIONS

- Altered weight
  - *weight gain* – as symptoms may be temporarily relieved by eating high carbohydrate or starch-based food
  - *weight loss* – due to dysphagia and dyspepsia[11]
- Dysphagia – difficulty with swallowing
- Oesophageal ulcers – can result with risk of bleeding[12]
- Barrett's oesophagus
  - acid reflux causes the squamous epithelium to be replaced by columnar epithelium
  - this neoplasia is a pre-malignant condition[12]

NON-PREGNANCY TREATMENT AND CARE

About 80% of people with reflux self-medicate with antacids, and only consult their GP once symptoms are prolonged and troublesome[5].

First-line Management (Lifestyle and Diet)

- Measures to reduce obesity[5,7,8]
- Smoking cessation, and reduction of alcohol consumption[5]
- Avoidance of reflux-inducing foods, e.g. greasy, spicy foods, acidic products, carbonated drinks[5] and chocolate[13]
- Postural measures, such as raising the head of the bed by 10–15cm, and avoiding lying down for 3 hours after eating[5,8]
- Antacids for immediate relief, purchased over-the-counter[5]

Second-line Management

- Histamine$_2$-receptor antagonists (H$_2$RA)[5] to treat oesophagitis, e.g. cimetidine or ranitidine[12]
- Proton-pump inhibitors (PPI), e.g. omeprazole or rabeprazole, inhibit gastric secretions and are the mainstay of medical treatment healing 80–85% of oesophageal lesions[14]
- Prokinetic drugs to increase oesophageal sphincter tone and enhance gastric emptying, e.g. metoclopramide

Third-line Management and Surgery

- Surgical repair of hernia in extreme cases[12,15]
- In obese patients hernia repair might be performed on the same occasion as gastric band surgery[16]
- Emergency surgery may be needed for volvulus
- Malignancy investigation of Barrett's oesophagus

PRE-CONCEPTION ISSUES AND CARE

- High dose aluminium-based antacids can cause osteomalacia (rickets) in children[5], so a calcium-based alternative needs consideration for mothers at risk of osteomalacia or osteoporosis (see Sections 9.4 and 9.5)
- H$_2$RAs require review; ranitidine is preferred for pregnancy
- Proton-pump inhibitor drugs are no longer thought to be teratogenic[14]
- If a woman is pending surgery she should be advised to delay conception until a full post-operative recovery has been made

Pregnancy Issues

Heartburn and Reflux

- Pregnancy might be the first time that a woman experiences heartburn and reflux
- Reflux and heartburn are common due to progesterone reducing the muscle tone of the lower oesophageal sphincter[6]
- Traditionally termed *minor disorders of pregnancy* reflux and heartburn are a normal occurrence in a healthy pregnancy
- Symptoms in pregnancy do not differ from the non-pregnant period, although they are exacerbated with multiple pregnancy
- Symptoms may worsen in pregnancy as both the progesterone level and intra-abdominal pressure increase
- Psychological support is necessary as many women feel 'miserable' with the symptoms as they worsen over pregnancy
- Serious reflux complications are rare in pregnancy; invasive tests are used infrequently; and barium studies are contraindicated[13]
- Antacids should not be taken at the same time as other drugs as they may impair absorption or damage enteric coating designed to prevent dissolution in the stomach[17] and PPI should be taken before a meal[13]

Hiatus Hernia

- Pregnancy increases the chance of developing hiatus hernia as the rising progesterone level and mechanical effect of the expanding uterus cause the lower oesophageal sphincter to rise and become intrathoracic[6]; 10–20% of women are affected by late pregnancy[18]
- As hiatus hernia is age-related, more women in the future could potentially present with this as a pre-existing condition if the average maternal age continues to rise

Medical Management and Care

Pre-existing Condition

- Antacids remain the first line treatment in pregnancy (see Figure 10.1.2) and those containing alginate, e.g. Gaviscon, form a raft that floats on the stomach contents to inhibit reflux and protect the oesophageal mucosa
- Avoid antacids containing sodium bicarbonate as they cause maternal or fetal metabolic alkalosis and fluid overload
- If on H_2RA, e.g. cimetidine, switch to ranitidine[5] for theoretical risk of interaction of cimetidine with androgen receptors; metoclopramide is also considered safe[2]
- PPI are more effective in reducing gastric acid secretion and can be used in pregnancy[14]; a meta-analysis of women with first trimester exposure did not show increased risk of teratogenicity[20]

Condition Presenting in Pregnancy

- Advise lifestyle modifications and antacids[13]
- If the above methods fail, PPI or histamine₂ receptor antagonists are tried[13] (see Figure 10.1.2 algorithm for treatment options)
- If there is dysphagia, bleeding, frequent vomiting or excessive weight loss refer for diagnostic evaluation[5]
- Endoscopy for diagnosis in cases with intractable reflux or atypical cases should not be delayed due to pregnancy as this can be performed safely under sedation[15]

Midwifery Management and Care

- Accurate booking history to determine and record previous treatment, and to identify current management and medication. Be aware that surgery to insert a gastric band may have repaired hiatus hernia on the same occasion
- If already taking H_2RA such as cimetidine, or PPI such as omeprazole, re-refer to a doctor
- Heartburn and reflux without any other complications should not preclude a woman from low-risk midwifery care schemes
- Calculate the body mass index (Appendix 13.1.1), and if appetite is poor consider weighing the mother at each antenatal visit
- Reinforce lifestyle advice and use of antacids suitable for pregnancy
- The midwife should take the mother's concerns seriously and not dismiss them because of the 'minor disorders' classification
- Be aware that extreme symptoms of dysphagia or bleeding or frequent vomiting or excessive weight loss are suggestive of hiatus hernia and complications such as 'strangulated hernia'. Such mothers require prompt medical review

Labour Issues

- The mechanical changes to the abdomen and thorax during labour may exacerbate symptoms
- It is preferable to avoid eating in labour as there is a potentially increased chance of reflux, with a theoretical risk of Mendelson's syndrome if general anaesthesia is undertaken

Medical Management and Care

- Avoid prolonged second stage pushing in women with known hiatus hernia
- Prophylactic ranitidine for women at risk, especially caesarean section under general anaesthesia, obese women and those with known GORD

Midwifery Management and Care

- Labour can be managed normally by the midwife
- Prompt administration of ranitidine and allow water or isotonic drinks
- Additional antacids *might* be useful in this circumstance
- Have a vomit bowl discreetly near the mother throughout labour

Postpartum Issues

- In mothers without a prior history of reflux, symptoms usually abate after delivery[13]
- Aluminium- and magnesium-based antacids are not concentrated in breast milk and are considered safe for breast-feeding mothers
- Cimetidine is compatible with breast-feeding[19]
- Limited amounts of ranitidine pass into breast milk with an unknown effect on the infant[19] so it is used with caution
- The PPI omeprazole passes into breast milk in small quantities, and is best avoided until further research has been evaluated[19]

Medical Management and Care

- Gaviscon is the antacid of choice
- H_2RA ranitidine is commonly used as second line management and PPI are used in a select group of women with severe symptoms of GORD not responding to other therapies
- If iron is required postnatally as well as antacids, it is best to advise that they be taken at different times to allow absorption of the iron

Midwifery Management and Care

- Explain that symptoms should improve as placental hormones diminish
- Encourage breast-feeding; the mother should not return to her pre-pregnancy drugs without medical review, especially if breast-feeding; here advice on formula milk feeds may be necessary
- Reinforce the first-line treatment and use of antacids (see previous page)
- Advise the mother to consult her general practitioner if her symptoms persist significantly after the puerperium

Normal stomach

Lower oesophageal (cardiac) sphincter. In non-pregnancy it is closed to prevent reflux of the acidic stomach contents. Hormonal effects of pregnancy relax the sphincter muscle leaving the sphincter partly open

Oesophagus

Hiatus (opening in the diaphragm)

Diaphragm

(a)

Duodenum

Pyloric sphincter

Stomach

Flap valve

Chyme (partly digested food mixed with hydrochloric acid and other gastric juices)

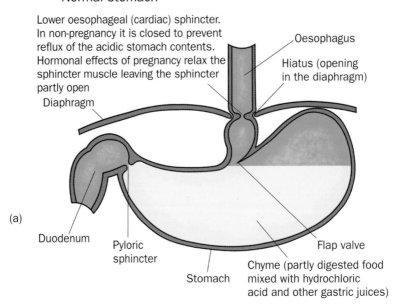

Sliding hiatus hernia
(95% of case)

The "tightening effect" of the diaphragm is compromised, and part of the stomach slides upwards through the hiatus. Acidic stomach contents then reflux into the lower oesophagus.

Hemia

Lower oesophageal (cardiac) sphincter

(b)

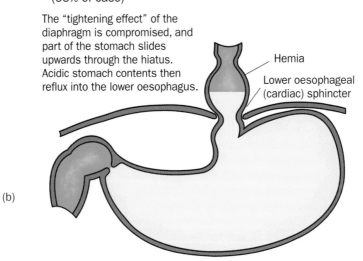

Rolling hiatus hernia
(5% of case)

The "tightening effect" of the diaphragm is severe, and the fundus of the stomach herniates through the hiatus to lie alongside the oesophagus. This can twist causing "strangulation" resulting in intense pain becoming medico-surgical emergency.

Lower oesophageal (cardiac) sphincter

(c)

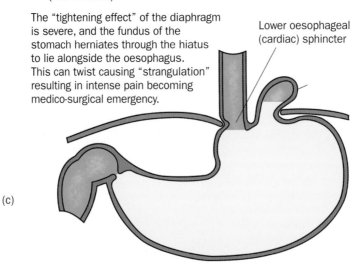

Figure 10.1.1 (a) Normal stomach, (b) sliding and (c) rolling hiatus hernia. This figure is downloadable from the book companion website at www.wiley.com/go/robson

174

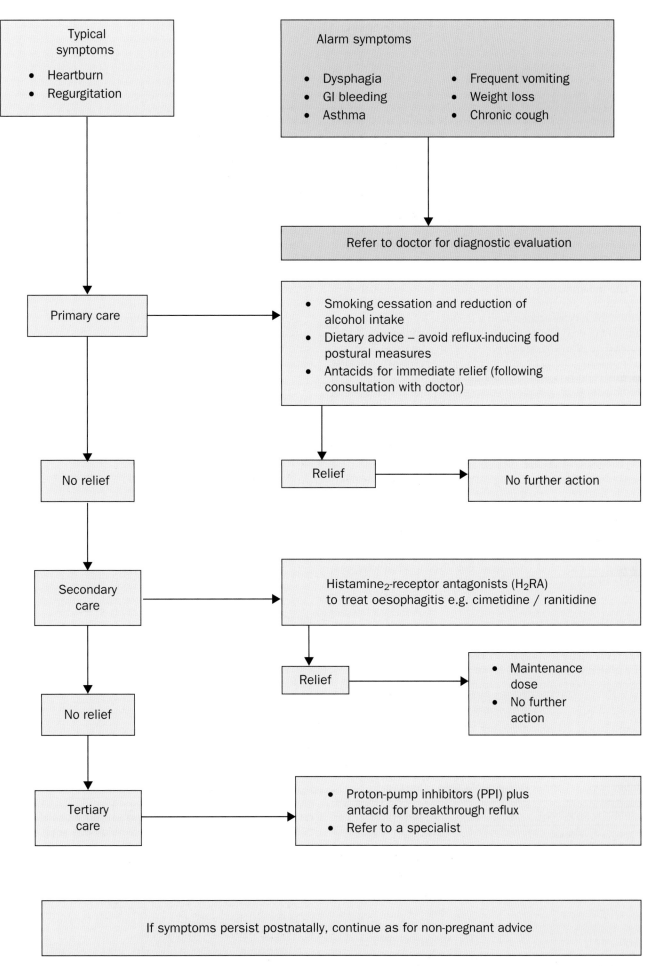

Figure 10.1.2 Treatment algorithm for reflux in pregnancy. This figure is downloadable from the book companion website at www.wiley.com/go/robson

10.2 Coeliac Disease

Incidence	Risk for Childbearing
Active or symptomatic coeliac disease is approximately 1 per 1000 in Europe[1]	Variable Risk

EXPLANATION OF CONDITION

Coeliac disease is a common lifelong, often under diagnosed, inflammatory condition of the mucosa of the small intestine, which has been induced by gluten, a protein in cereals, wheat, rye and barley. The estimated ratio of diagnosed to undiagnosed individuals is 1:8[2]

The inflammation, caused by gluten, leads to malabsorption in the proximal small intestine due to atrophy of the villi, which is associated with a decrease in the activity and amount of enzymes present in the surface epithelium. Injury caused to the intestinal villi is by an abnormal immune response to gliadin, a component of gluten. The precise cause of this condition still remains unknown but is related to a combination of genetic predisposition and environmental factors[3]. Factors such as the amount of gluten ingested, stress of a pregnancy or operation, or a gastrointestinal infection can exacerbate the condition, and if such stress factors are relieved the mucosa may return to normal.

Diagnosis of coeliac disease in more recent years is by sensitive and specific serological markers but the gold standard is made by a small intestine biopsy together with serological tests for antigliadin and endomysial antibodies. It is becoming increasingly diagnosed with the use of serological screening tests that reveal cases of occult enteropathy[4].

Clinical features of this disease may become apparent during infancy and childhood but also in adulthood (see Table 10.2.1).

COMPLICATIONS

There are many complications associated with coeliac disease if a gluten-free diet (GFD) is not adhered to. Anaemia, osteoporosis, short stature and reproductive problems are associations secondary to malabsorption from coeliac disease. Some of the associated autoimmune disorders, cancer and neurological complications are more complex associations and cannot be explained by diet alone[5].

Table 10.2.1 Clinical Features of Coeliac Disease

Infancy/childhood	Adulthood
Failure to thrive	Diarrhoea
Muscle wasting	Malabsorption
Diarrhoea	Anorexia
Abdominal distension	Weight loss
Short stature	Lethargy
Anaemia	Anaemia
	Infertility
	Abdominal pain
	Early menopause
	Recurrent miscarriage

Malignant disease, such as small intestinal lymphoma, is increased as well as carcinoma of the small bowel. Although rare there are some reports related to an increased risk of squamous cell carcinoma of the oesophagus and pharynx[1].

Infertility is another associated complication of coeliac disease, including delayed menarche, relative infertility in men and women and premature menopause. Fertility will improve with treatment which includes a gluten-free diet and correction of nutritional deficiencies.

Other associations include **autoimmune** diseases, such as insulin dependent diabetes, thyroid disease and neurological syndromes. Another complication, which can affect up to 90% of patients, is **dermatitis herpetiformis**[1].

NON-PREGNANCY CARE

It is essential to follow a GFD by avoiding products made from wheat, barley and rye. Some literature suggests oats should be initially avoided, if possibly contaminated by wheat flour[1]. If oats have not been contaminated by wheat flour they can be re-established safely into the diet.

A response is noticeable within at least 3 months in adults, and is clearly evident in children within a few weeks.

To be able to optimise care and ensure correct management, review of nutritional status of each patient is essential, together with regular follow-up appointments. It is important to consider this as a life-long condition that requires a gluten-restricted diet for life. If there is no improvement within 3 months this is usually due to non-compliance either intentional or accidental.

PRE-CONCEPTION ISSUES AND CARE

The disease is unaffected by pregnancy but gastrointestinal symptoms that may have been experienced in childhood may be seen again in pregnancy. This needs to be highlighted to the patient to ensure an awareness of the importance of a gluten-free or gluten-restricted diet and adherence to this as well.

Due to the nutritional requirements of pregnancy, referral to a dietician prior to pregnancy may alleviate any fears or anxieties the patient may have. Consequently, dietary advice can be discussed and monitored and any nutritional deficiencies can be addressed accordingly with dietary supplements if necessary.

As women with this condition have a predisposition to folate malabsorption, they should be advised to take higher doses of folate (5 mg) and iron supplementation pre-conceptually, in order to optimise their levels of folic acid. By restricting to a GFD this will be an effective treatment and therefore can lead to complete remission within weeks.

If the prospective mother has any other associated autoimmune diseases, issues surrounding the management of these conditions should be addressed on an individual basis.

Pregnancy Issues

Women who have been diagnosed with coeliac disease can experience an aggravated response during pregnancy and the puerperium.

Haematological disorders, for example megaloblastic and iron-deficiency anaemia, can present during pregnancy (see Sections 14.1 and 14.2).

Some studies have shown coeliac disease that is left untreated appears to carry an increased risk of miscarriage, fetal growth restriction and lower birth weight babies[6].

A GFD and further vitamin and mineral supplementations need to be given, especially folic acid, to aid protection against neural tube defects.

In the UK people with coeliac disease are able to obtain certain gluten-free dietary products on NHS prescription; however, they usually have to pay prescription charges which can have an influence on dietary adherence.

The association between urinary tract infection in pregnancy and coeliac disease has been debated in the literature[7–9].

Medical Management and Care

- Strict adherence to a GFD should be advised throughout pregnancy
- Anaemia can be associated as a common disorder in coeliac disease, therefore iron, folate and possibly vitamin B_{12} supplementation should be monitored and used appropriately
- Unexplained iron-deficiency or anaemia not responding to oral iron therapy, folate deficiency or vitamin B_{12} deficiency during pregnancy should be investigated to exclude coeliac disease
- Base-line calcium level measurement should be arranged at booking, and appropriate calcium supplementation given if hypocalcaemia is diagnosed
- Serial fetal growth scans should be arranged for pregnant women with coeliac disease

Midwifery Management and Care

- Ascertain if folic acid was initiated peri-conceptually, if not this needs to be implemented promptly in the first trimester
- Consideration should be given to vitamins and minerals within the diet, these include: vitamin B_{12}, folic acid, iron and trace elements such as zinc
- Encourage pregnant women to adhere to a GFD, because pregnancy has additional nutritional demands
- Prompt issuing of certification of pregnancy that entitles a mother to free prescriptions during pregnancy in the UK, which include coeliac dietary products
- If a referral to a dietician is necessary this should be initiated promptly to consider appropriately any nutritional corrections that are required; such referrals are important if diabetes mellitus co-exists
- The consideration of increased folic acid is especially significant, due to the risk factor of neural tube defects; a nutritional assessment is required for both diet and supplements
- Ask about bowel motions as the mother is at risk of constipation, especially if taking iron tablets, and laxatives might be required
- Be alert for risk of urinary tract infections

Labour Issues

Anaemia can be considered an issue in labour and therefore it is important to be aware of the woman's haemoglobin status in view of blood loss at delivery.

Medical Management and Care

- Intrapartum care should reflect the increased awareness of anaemia and consequences in labour
- The medical team should be aware of any related coeliac disease if performing a caesarean section as some sutures contain gluten and can act as an irritant

Midwifery Management and Care

- Discuss with the medical team if a FBC should be taken when the woman is admitted in labour, and if samples should be taken for group and save
- In view of a low haemoglobin status, active management of the third stage may be initiated, reducing the risk of a postpartum haemorrhage

Postpartum Issues

Breast-feeding appears to offer protection and decrease the risk of the development of coeliac disease in the newborn. This is dependent on breast-feeding exclusively[10] and also continuing to breast-feed during the introduction of gluten within the diet[11].

Breast-feeding will provide protective benefits against gastrointestinal and respiratory infections[12].

Medical Management and Care

- Appropriate management of nutritional anaemia and continued emphasis on adherence to a GFD should be an integral part of the care that these women receive from health professionals
- Encourage breast-feeding for its added benefits to the baby

Midwifery Management and Care

- If a woman's choice is to breast-feed exclusively this may act as a protective feature in the delay of onset of coeliac disease for the child, as symptoms usually occur at the time of weaning; hence the midwife should encourage and support breast-feeding
- The mother may worry that the baby could inherit the condition so the mother can be encouraged to seek advice from the specialist public health nurse (health visitor) and attend child wellbeing clinics where weaning and infant feeding advice are given

S. E. Robson and J. Waugh

10.3 Ulcerative Colitis

Incidence	Risk for Childbearing
60 000–120 000 in the UK – approximately 1:600 Most common age 15–35[1]	Variable Risk

EXPLANATION OF CONDITION

Ulcerative colitis (UC) is a chronic autoimmune disease of the bowel, characterised by mucosal inflammation in the colon. UC can be distal disease, confined to the rectum (proctitis), as in 30% of cases[2], or rectum with sigmoid colon (proctosigmoiditis). Alternatively, in 20% of cases the disease can be more extensive, affecting the whole colon as in pancolitis[2]. A severe attack of UC is still a potentially life-threatening illness, due to the risk of haemorrhage caused by widespread mucosal ulceration or toxic megacolon causing perforation. If this happens, emergency colectomy must be performed immediately[2,3].

UC is diagnosed by stool examinations and sigmoidoscopic biopsies, which exclude Crohn's disease or infection.

Of patients with ulcerative colitis:

- 50% will have a relapse each year
- 20–30% will need a colectomy; however this is curative[2]

Symptoms include:

- Visible blood in stool of 90% of people presenting with UC[4]
- Continence problems
- Abdominal pain

UC can present at any age; it is common during reproductive years although aetiology is unknown. It is thought that UC may be caused by environmental and genetic factors[2]. Smoking is known to decrease the risk of UC, although it is not known why[2].

COMPLICATIONS

In addition to the risk of perforation or toxicity, the symptoms and complications all lead to a poor quality of life and body image[5]:

- Weight loss has an adverse effect on body image and self-esteem[6]
- Medical treatments such as corticosteroids or immunosuppressive drugs have their own unpleasant side effects, e.g. weight gain, Cushingoid features, osteoporosis, glaucoma, cataracts and infections[2]
- Ocular, oral, joint or skin changes are noted in some patients[4]
- Children may experience delays in onset of puberty
- Young adults may have trouble in forming intimate relationships
- Dyspareunia and recurrent vaginal candidiasis are more common than in healthy women[7]
- Increased risk of colonic carcinoma, particularly after about 8–10 years of disease
- Frequent laboratory and bowel investigations are necessary, mostly in the second decade of disease[2]

NON-PREGNANCY TREATMENT AND CARE

Treatment is based more on clinical severity of the attack than histology.

Treatment is primarily medical. The most common types of drugs used are aminosalicylates and corticosteroids. The combination of oral and topical aminosalicylates is more effective than monotherapy[4]. Aminosalicylates should be used in treatment of mild disease and steroids should be used for active disease. Long-term use of steroids is undesirable due to the side effects

For those patients with long-term chronic disease, or who are steroid dependent, azathioprine or 6-mercaptopurine (immune suppressants given to transplant recipients), are recommended. Newer agents are reserved for refractory disease (i.e. disease resistant to treatment).

Infliximab is recommended as an option for the treatment of acute exacerbations of severely active ulcerative colitis only in patients in whom ciclosporin is contraindicated or clinically inappropriate[8].

Surgery is considered when a patient with UC does not respond to medical therapy. It is a decision that is made between the patient, the gastroenterologist and the colorectal surgeon. Surgery is also necessary if colonic carcinoma develops. Resection of the colon is then performed to form an ileostomy.

A rectal stump is left in some patients who may be considering the construction of an ileoanal pouch later. This involves removal of the colon and rectum, using the end of the ileum to form a new rectum or reservoir. If pouch surgery is not an option, due to poor sphincter efficiency or anal disease, a total pan-proctocolectomy may be considered, which includes removal of the rectum and closure of the anus[3].

PRE-CONCEPTION ISSUES AND CARE

- Fertility is not adversely affected by UC, with the possible exception of severely active disease[9]. However, voluntary infertility can be high, particularly if patients have had previous gastrointestinal surgery
- Pre-conceptual assessment for clinical activity of disease should be performed in liaison with a gastroenterologist. This should include a full blood count, c-reactive protein, erythrocyte sedimentation rate, liver enzymes and albumin
- Sulfasalazine is a folic acid antagonist that has the potential of causing neural tube defects and other congenital abnormalities. Consequently, pre-conceptual folic acid supplementation is advised and a change to an alternative aminosalicylate preparation, such as mesalazine, that is considered safe in normal doses
- Conception during remission is advisable

Pregnancy Issues

As UC often occurs in young adults, managing the disease in pregnancy is not unusual. The risks of infertility are no different to women who do not suffer from UC[6,9], and 25% of women with UC will conceive following diagnosis[2].

Control during pregnancy is crucial for fetal and maternal health. Women may need to remain on medication to remain in remission, rather than risk an acute flare-up, which could hold more dangers for feto-maternal well being[2]. Flare ups occur most commonly in the first trimester.

Most pregnant women will present with an existing diagnosis of UC, but if new diagnosis is suspected in pregnancy then endoscopy and biopsy are preferable to barium studies.

Risks to pregnancy

- No significant increase in the rate of spontaneous miscarriage when compared with the normal population[9]
- An increased risk of pre-term birth, IUGR and caesarean section with active disease[10]
- If the woman has an ileostomy, there is a significant risk of a hernia or stomal prolapse developing, due to the increased strain on the weak abdominal walls
- Vomiting in pregnancy can also cause herniation of the small bowel

Medical Management and Care

In the event of acute flare-up:

- Intravenous access with fluid and electrolyte replacement to prevent any dehydration or electrolyte imbalance
- FBC, ESR or CRP, serum electrolytes and liver function tests should be measured every 24–48 hours to monitor the severity of flare
- Flexible sigmoidoscopy can be used safely in pregnancy[6]
- Do not manage acute UC any differently than in non-pregnancy
- Azathioprine and corticosteroids to be continued as risks to fetus from disease outweigh risks from the continued therapy. Although azothioprine is known to cross the placenta, the immature fetal liver is unable to convert it into an active metabolite. This is thought to protect against any teratogenic effects[11]
- Emergency colectomy is not encouraged during pregnancy
- An intrapartum care plan to be agreed between the woman and the multidisciplinary team and documented in the notes

Midwifery Management and Care

- Involve the inflammatory bowel disease nurse specialist (if available) as teamwork is fundamental to effective care
- Be aware that severe disease will require hospital admission, mild or moderate disease can be managed as an outpatient
- If hospital admission occurs, monitor the following:
  - stool frequency and condition
  - blood, mucous and consistency
  - four-hourly vital signs[2]
  - levels of abdominal pain and tenderness
- Due to the degree of 'urgency' UC women experience, it is essential that they have easy access to toilet facilities
- These women are prone to malnutrition, and may need referral to a dietician during pregnancy
- Regular weighing is essential

Labour Issues

Mode of delivery should be carefully planned and options discussed with the woman. This discussion will incorporate the multidisciplinary team, so the woman can make an informed decision. Aim for vaginal delivery in most cases, unless severe or chronic disease is present. In these instances, a caesarean section may be offered in order to protect the anal sphincter from damage.

If the woman has already undergone gastrointestinal surgery, e.g. ileoanal pouch formation[2], or has an ileostomy, an elective LSCS may be offered, as an emergency LSCS would be very complex due to the scar tissue from previous surgery. However, most women have been reported to deliver normally without complications to the UC[11]

Medical Management and Care

- Aim for vaginal delivery unless disease is active
- Active disease – consider LSCS to protect the anal sphincter
- Prolonged second stage and difficult instrumental deliveries should be avoided to prevent anal sphincter damage, particularly if future surgery for ileoanal pouch is contemplated
- A senior obstetrician should perform caesarean if there is a history of previous gastrointestinal surgery, as there is a higher risk of bowel damage from previous adhesions

Midwifery Management and Care

- Quiescent disease – normal midwifery management of labour
- Keep woman well hydrated in labour
- Easy access to toilets, or alternative, is essential in labour
- There is no need for the midwife to have any concerns over 'bag' management, if a woman with a stoma is labouring normally; assistance may be needed in emptying the appliance if the woman is unable to mobilise (see Appendix 10.3.1)

Postpartum Issues

- Anaemia may result from rectal bleeding, which is a symptom of active disease
- With haemoglobin already compromised, even the 'normal' bleeding at delivery may be detrimental to the woman's health
- If the disease remains quiescent, there are no significant postpartum issues and a flare up is not common.
- With active disease, the mother may suffer from extreme tiredness; giving birth is a demanding experience, even without a chronic condition causing exhaustion
- Immunosuppressant drugs may be either contraindicated with breast-feeding, or used on a risk–benefit assessment basis, especially azathioprine (see Appendix 11.1.1)

Medical Management and Care

- Treat any anaemia
- If breast-feeding while taking azathioprine or 6-MP it is advisable for the baby to be monitored for clinical signs of immunosuppression and regular complete blood counts should be taken[12,13]
- A 4-hour delay in breast-feeding following oral corticosteroid use is recommended by most manufacturers, particularly if taking more than 20 mg; but this has practical implications. After observation, steroids appear to be safe[6]

Midwifery Management and Care

- Support the mother in her choice of infant feeding, and deflect any guilt she may feel if she is not breast-feeding. However, where appropriate, breast-feeding should be encouraged as a protection for the baby against the autoimmune and heredity aspects of the disease
- Be aware of the extreme tiredness and assist as needed
- Ascertain if the woman has any help at home
- Ensure that the mother and her relatives understand the need for rest

10.4 Crohn's Disease

Incidence	Risk for Childbearing
50–100 per 100 000	Variable Risk
Affects men and women equally	
Most common age 15–25[1]	

EXPLANATION OF CONDITION

Crohn's disease (CD) was identified in 1932 by Dr Burril Crohn. It comprises chronic inflammation, ulceration and scarring anywhere from mouth to rectum, but most commonly the small intestine. It is characterised by patchy inflammation that passes through the wall of the intestine, affecting each layer[2].

Symptoms include[1,2]:

- Colicky abdominal pain
- Urgent diarrhoea, leading to dehydration and nutritional deficiencies
- Severe tiredness
- Weight loss
- Malaise, anorexia and fever

Although the aetiology is unknown at present, it is considered that the condition is in response to environmental triggers, such as infections and drugs. Research shows a familial link with first degree relatives who have inflammatory bowel disease (IBD), but not necessarily the same IBD – some may develop ulcerative colitis (UC), others CD[3,4].

COMPLICATIONS

The symptoms can be embarrassing and cause poor self-esteem, leading to loss of education in the young and difficulties in gaining employment in adults[5]. CD causes greater disability than UC as only 75% of patients are fully capable of work in the year following diagnosis[2].

The main complications comprise:

- Intestinal obstruction caused by adhesions or by visceral distension in the presence of dilation
- Fissures in the anal canal
- Fistulas can develop as the inflammation affects all layers of the bowel
- Abscesses in the pelvis, abdomen or ischiorectal area
- Increased risk of gallstones, renal calculi and chronic pancreatitis
- Arthritis, iritis and painful skin complications often associated with the flare-ups themselves
- Increased risk of bowel carcinoma

NON-PREGNANCY TREATMENT AND CARE

- As there is no known cure, treatment is symptomatic
- Care should always be offered by a gastroenterologist who specialises in IBD
- An individual's own knowledge of their condition should always be respected
- After taking a full history, a general assessment of wellbeing, including BP, pulse, temperature, blood investigations, hydration, weight loss and abdominal examination is needed
- Discourage smoking, as this aggravates the condition[2]
- Colonoscopy is useful in endoscopic and histological assessment of large bowel and distal ileum
- MRI can be performed for assessment of perianal fistulating disease

- Stool culture and microscopy to exclude infective aetiology and rule out concurrent *Clostridium difficile* infection
- ESR and CRP to monitor severity of inflammation

Medical Management

Medical management will depend on the site of disease, activity, course of disease, previous responses to drugs and extra-intestinal manifestations and hence this needs to be individualised:

- Anti-inflammatory drugs containing mesalazine (sulfasalazine) are commonly used as first-line management; steroids are used in tapering doses to treat flares. Other drugs used are:
  - Immunosuppressors such as 6-mercaptopurine (6-MP) or azathioprine
  - Infliximab is an anti-inflammatory drug approved for use in the treatment of moderate to severe disease that is not responding to standard treatment
  - Methotrexate, a cytotoxic drug with anti-inflammatory properties. Only used in severe disease that isn't responding to conventional medicines[2]
- Commonly used antibiotics, which may be indicated in stricture or fistula infection, are:
  - ampicillin
  - cephalosporins
  - tetracycline
  - metronidazole
- NSAIDs should be avoided as they may cause inflammation and bleeding in the small intestine[6]

Surgical Management

Surgery may be required to remove damaged parts of the intestine[1]. However, it is not a cure as with UC, and should only be used in symptomatic disease not responding to medical treatment or for complications such as abscess, perforation, strictures or bleeding in the bowel.

Common types of surgery include:

- **Bowel resection**: removing the affected part of the intestine, usually conservative
- **Strictureplasty**: opening up narrowed sections of bowel
- **Colectomy** and **ileostomy:** the complete removal of the colon and creating a stoma for waste elimination

PRE-CONCEPTION ISSUES AND CARE

- Fertility is generally not affected unless active disease is present[3,7,8]. Active disease can cause inflammation of the Fallopian tubes, ovaries and perianal disease may cause dyspareunia[9]
- Methotrexate is known to affect oogenesis, leading to subfertility. Due to its abortive and teratogenic properties, contraception must be used whilst on methotrexate and for 3 months after stopping it if planning pregnancy[10]
- Due to complications during pregnancy from having active Crohn's disease at conception, planning to conceive when disease is quiescent is associated with a better outcome[3,8,9]
- Crohn's disease causes folate deficiency, as does the use of sulfasalazine, which is a folate antagonist
- Folic acid supplements of 5 mg daily rather than the usual 400 micrograms are needed[3] and supplements should continue throughout the pregnancy

Pregnancy Issues

- One-third of women with inactive disease at conception can expect to relapse during the pregnancy or puerperium; relapse rate similar for non-pregnant patient[3]
- Conception during remission is advised:
  - If conception occurs during active disease, two-thirds of women will continue to have disease activity and two-thirds of these will deteriorate[9,11]
  - Active disease is associated with miscarriage, IUGR and prematurity[3]
- Control of the disease during pregnancy is important, therefore drug therapy should not be discontinued; disease activity is more dangerous than the drugs used
- Any exacerbation of Crohn's disease should be investigated and treated promptly
- Anaemia is common and may be due to iron, folate or vitamin B_{12} deficiency as a result of malabsorption
- Folate deficiency can arise with Crohn's disease, particularly if taking sulfasalazine which interferes with absorption of folate[9]
- Disease requiring surgery is associated with high fetal mortality 18–40%[9] and emergency surgery in pregnancy is associated with a fetal loss of 60%. Any necessary elective surgery should be deferred until after pregnancy[3]

Medical Management and Care

- Proactive maintenance of quiescent disease is preferable to treating exacerbation of Crohn's, as main risks are from *active* disease, not from the medication[9]. Therefore collaborative care by obstetricians and gastroenterologists is required, particularly during the third trimester[9]
- Prompt investigation with serum electrolytes, liver function tests and C-reactive proteins should be performed to assess clinical condition in case of flare of disease
- Corticosteroids can be used orally, intravenously or as rectal enemas, with any flare up of disease; oral and local forms of 5-aminosalicylic acid derivatives and salazopyrin compounds are considered safe in pregnancy; metronidazole is used to treat anal fistulas and perianal disease[9]
- Thiopurines are considered safe and well tolerated during pregnancy[9]
- Methotrexate must be stopped immediately if unplanned pregnancy. Termination of pregnancy should be offered as an option[9]
- Monthly FBC, serum folic acid and vitamin B_{12} levels should be monitored during pregnancy, as there is increased risk of nutritional anaemia due to malabsorption
- Folic acid 5mg daily supplementation to continue throughout pregnancy[9]
- Oral or parental iron therapy or blood transfusion may be required depending on the degree of anaemia
- Sigmoidoscopy can be performed safely during pregnancy but colonoscopy may be deferred until the puerperium; in case of life-threatening complications requiring surgery, the management should be the same as for non-pregnant women[2]

Midwifery Management and Care

- Nutrition is a major component in the treatment of CD as malnutrition is common. Referral to a dietician is advisable
- Involve the IBD nurse specialist who is an expert who can liaise with the mother and the multidisciplinary team

Labour Issues

- Vaginal delivery is not contraindicated unless there is active perianal disease or an ileoanal pouch
- There is evidence that there is a risk of perianal Crohn's disease developing following vaginal birth and episiotomy; if a woman already has perianal CD then delivery by LSCS is more appropriate[9,10]
- Generally the cesarean section rate is increased compared with non-sufferers of CD (15% compared with 10%)[3]

Medical Management and Care

- Mothers with either colostomy or ileostomy can deliver vaginally, although rectal disease or a perianal pouch is an indication for elective caesarean[11]
- Good intrapartum care of the perineum should be encouraged and perineal trauma should be minimised
- A senior obstetrician should perform caesarean section in cases with previous bowel surgery as there is increased risk of injury to bowel, bladder or other viscera due to previous adhesions[12,13]
- If necessary, a colorectal surgeon should be available

Midwifery Management and Care

- An experienced midwife should care for the woman in labour
- Perineal trauma should be minimised

Postpartum issues

- There are no known problems when Crohn's disease is quiescent
- There appears to be a correlation between higher parity, and lower relapse rate and subsequent need for surgical intervention[9]

Medical Management and Care

- Sulfasalazine, oral or topical mesalazine and corticosteroids are considered safe in breast-feeding[11]
- As very small amounts of azathioprine and 6-mercaptopurine metabolites appear in breast milk this should be discussed on an individual basis and babies should be monitored clinically and haematologically for signs of immunosuppression and regular full blood counts should be taken[9,14,15,16]
- Ciclosporin should be avoided when breast-feeding, as there is no safety data available[11]
- Even though infliximab cannot be detected in breast-milk and could be considered safe, the data is limited and the long-term effect on immunological development in the infant is unknown[9]
- Advice should be tailored to the individual woman's circumstances following discussion

Midwifery Management and Care

- Breast-feeding should be encouraged for its benefits (mothers may be concerned if they are currently receiving medication)
- Be alert for signs of anaemia and advise accordingly

10.5 Irritable Bowel Syndrome

Incidence
10–15% of adult population in the UK[1]
86% of those affected are women[2]

Risk for Childbearing
Low Risk

EXPLANATION OF CONDITION

Irritable bowel syndrome (IBS) is a functional disorder of the intestines. IBS appears to be the result of motor disturbances in the intestine that respond to certain stimuli[3]. As there is no clear 'disease' or pathology with IBS, it is diagnosed by excluding other bowel disorders and by ensuring the absence of certain 'red flag' features[1]:

- Rectal bleeding
- Anaemia
- Unexplained weight loss
- Late age of onset or acute onset, particularly if associated with bowel changes
- Family history of bowel cancer or IBD
- Signs of infection
- Abdominal/rectal masses

Blood tests for FBC, ESR, CRP and testing for coeliac disease can be taken to exclude other disease when meeting the IBS criteria[4]. A detailed medical history is taken using the 'Rome III criteria'. This is a symptom-based classification system that assists clinicians in examining the symptoms before coming to a diagnosis[5] (see Appendix 10.5.1).

Symptoms

- Abdominal pain related to defecation
- Altered bowel habits, ranging from diarrhoea to constipation to 'normal'
- Abdominal bloating
- A feeling of incomplete evacuation and mucous in the stools[2]

COMPLICATIONS

- All the symptoms of IBS can erode quality of life, influence relationships with family and friends, and cause absenteeism from work
- Diarrhoea or constipation can aggravate or cause haemorrhoids

NON-PREGNANCY TREATMENT AND CARE

IBS cannot be cured, but patients will have periods of remission between the bouts of disease activity[2]. The most effective way to manage IBS is to remain patient centred.

Maintaining a stool chart that also describes the stools, will aid the doctor in treating the symptoms[2].

Dietary Management

Keeping a dietary history may also reveal problem areas that can be addressed by altering habits. High fibre diets are not always recommended in IBS. If fibre is included in the diet then soluble fibre is preferable to insoluble fibres such as wholemeal flours, and whole grains. Oat based fibre is far more easily digested[6]. Caffeine, alcohol, fat and sorbitol-rich foods (e.g. ice cream, chewing gum, honey and jam) are known to aggravate IBS and should be taken in moderation[2]. Discussion with a dietician can help to identify which foods trigger symptoms. Keeping a food diary can assist with this. IBS can be exacerbated by dietary habits rather than specific foods, e.g. large, rushed or irregular meals[2] are also predictors of symptom intensity; in the absence of stress, improved symptoms can be manifested[7]. Some patients may choose to try probiotics. These may help to alleviate symptoms by enhancing the gut barrier function, inhibiting pathogen binding and modulating the gut inflammatory response[4]. Restrict the intake of caffeinated drinks, alcohol and fizzy drinks, but increase amount of water/non-caffeinated drinks[4].

Psychological Treatment

It has been identified that IBS patients respond positively to the placebo effect of a caring physician. As there are psychological influences on IBS, the most important aspects of treatment are to listen, validate the symptoms, educate the patient and identify reinforcing and coping strategies with each individual[8,9].

Psychosocial factors, such as a history of abuse[10], should be addressed by the physicians caring for these women in a sensitive manner. Some women may require additional psychiatric or psychological intervention. Some of these include relaxation therapy, hypnosis, cognitive behavioural therapy and biofeedback techniques.

Pharmacological Treatment

Psychotropic agents can modify the symptoms of IBS by their action in modulating psychosocial factors, e.g. antidepressant medications (tricyclic antidepressants) in women who have major depression as co-morbidity with IBS. They can also modify the pain threshold in these patients.

The choice of antidepressants will depend on the main presenting complaints and side-effect profiles for the individual patient. Tricyclic antidepressants are likely to be more effective in cases of diarrhoea and abdominal pain, due to its anticholinergic activity. A sedating tricyclic antidepressant may be useful when there are associated sleep problems, whereas selective serotonin re-uptake inhibitors (SSRI) such as fluoxetine may help in cases that have constipation or bloating[11].

Diphenoxylate, an anticholinergic medication, can be used to control pain and diarrhoea. Antidiarrhoeals like loperamide and cholestyramine are used if diarrhoea is a dominant symptom. Lactulose is no longer recommended for constipation in IBS; instead bulk-forming laxatives like ispaghula or sterculia should be used[6].

Antibiotics must be used with caution as some, e.g. erythromycin, can exacerbate IBS[1].

PRE-CONCEPTION ISSUES AND CARE

The individual may find pregnancy easier to cope with if her IBS symptoms are not too severe. Avoiding stress, using individualised coping mechanisms and following dietary advice may all assist in keeping the IBS in abeyance.

Pregnancy Issues

- Normal hormonal changes in pregnancy can alter bowel habits even in the absence of irritable bowel disease
- IBS is not debilitating even though the mother's quality of life is affected

Medical Management and Care

- Diagnosis of IBS during pregnancy is difficult due to the normal physiological changes in the bowel
- Exacerbation of known IBS could also be difficult to diagnose for the same reasons
- Avoid foods that trigger the symptoms
- Antidepressants are sometimes used in the treatment of non-pregnant women for severe pain
- Selective serotonin re-uptake inhibitors (SSRIs) have not been shown to cause any major fetal problems other than irritability in neonates, thought to be due to withdrawal from the drug[3]
- Adequate fluid intake and bulking agents are used to manage constipation
- Loperamide has been used for treatment of diarrhea. In one prospective multicentre study no significant differences were found in the rate of major or minor malformations with matched controls following exposure in the first trimester[12]

Midwifery care

- Give dietary advice as usual, responding to each bowel symptom
  - high fibre diet
  - multiple smaller meals
  - drink plenty of water
  - avoid stimulant drinks, e.g. caffeinated tea and coffee
  - avoid gas-producing food
- Psychological support is paramount, rather than drug therapy in pregnancy

Labour Issues

- There are no significant labour issues with IBS

Medical Management and Care

- There are no specific issues related to IBS although offering early pain relief may help to reduce the stress related to painful labour

Midwifery care

- Supportive care in labour

Postpartum Issues

- No postpartum issues other than to continue with dietary advice and psychological support
- As stress is a major factor in IBS, this could influence symptoms either way, depending on how the individual approaches the experience of having a newborn:
  - some sufferers may be so preoccupied with caring for the new baby that the focus is removed from their own symptoms and consequently they improve
  - other women may find the experience so traumatic, that it has a negative influence on their IBS

Medical Management and Care

- Debriefing individuals who may have had difficult or traumatic birth experiences and dealing with those at risk of postpartum depression may reduce the trigger factors for the worsening of pre-existing IBS

Midwifery care

- Continue with psychological support, demonstrating a caring positive demeanour
- Be ready to acknowledge and validate any symptoms
- Persist with dietary advice

10.6 Haemorrhoids

Incidence
50% of adult UK population at some stage in their life
More frequent in pregnancy[1]

Risk for Childbearing
Low Risk

EXPLANATION OF CONDITION

Within the anal canal lie three fibrovascular cushions of submucosal tissue, which are suspended by connective tissue arising from the internal anal sphincter and the longitudinal muscle of the anal canal. The role of these cushions is to maintain continence. If this connective tissue breaks down, prolapse will occur. Once this has happened the venous pressure will increase and the venous return will be impaired, the cushions then become engorged and dilated[1].

Classification of Haemorrhoids (see Figure 10.6.1)

- First degree – haemorrhoids bleed but do not prolapse
- Second degree – haemorrhoids prolapse on straining but then return spontaneously
- Third degree – haemorrhoids prolapse on straining but then require manual reduction
- Fourth degree – haemorrhoids remain prolapsed and cannot be reduced manually

Rarely, an external haemorrhoid can develop on the outside edge of the anus – this is sometimes called a perianal haematoma.

Predisposing Factors[2]

- Straining to defecate, as with constipation or, by contrast, with chronic diarrhoea
- Pregnancy, due to poor venous return and relaxation of the smooth muscles
- Obesity
- Low-fibre diet
- Weakened pelvic floor[3]

Symptoms[2]

- Rectal bleeding
- Itching round anus
- Pain/discomfort on defecation
- Mucous discharge
- Feeling of incomplete evacuation

COMPLICATIONS

Complications include[4]:

- Strangulation – when the prolapsed haemorrhoid swells considerably so prevents venous return
- Thrombosis – if the blood in the swollen haemorrhoid clots, a thrombosed haemorrhoid forms

Haemorrhoids

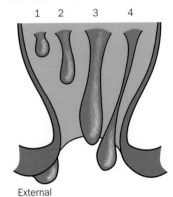

1   2   3   4

External

Figure 10.6.1 Stages of internal and external haemorrhoids. This figure is downloadable from the book companion website at www.wiley.com/go/robson

- Gangrene, if haemorrhoid blood supply is reduced
- Infection, leading to an abscess

NON-PREGNANCY TREATMENT AND CARE

Investigations are needed for correct diagnosis and exclusion of other disorders with rectal bleeding. Haemorrhoids are not always felt by performing a rectal examination; hence proctoscopy or sigmoidoscopy may be undertaken by the doctor. A stool guaiac to detect the presence of blood may be performed. These investigations may need to be performed by a general or colorectal surgeon, as other conditions can present with similar symptoms. Treatment is based on severity of symptoms, and the best treatment is prevention[5].

Conservative Treatment

Mostly treatment is conservative and includes[4]:

- High-fibre diet, including fibre supplements
- Remain well hydrated – at least 2 litres water per day
- Avoid codeine-based analgesics, which are constipating
- Ice packs may be held in place for 15–20 minutes for immediate relief
- Warm baths to relieve itching
- Re-education in toileting habits:
  - do not suppress the need to evacuate
  - do not strain
  - do not spend too long sitting on the toilet

Medical Treatment[1]

- Ointments and creams may ease the symptoms, but are not curative; a plain ointment may ease the itch
- Anaesthetic based creams may relieve the pain
- A steroid-based cream, if there is inflammation, but these are not to be used for a prolonged period of time[6]
- Strong analgesia for an acute attack or complication

Surgical Treatment[1,7]

- Rubber band ligation: a band is placed around the haemorrhoid's base, causing it to become necrotic and fall off
  - usually performed as an outpatient
  - 79% successful with first- to third-degree haemorrhoids[1]
- Sclerotherapy: an injection of phenol into the pedicle causes tissue necrosis and can be used as an alternative to banding in outpatients for first- and second-degree haemorrhoids, but has a high failure rate[6]
- Doppler-guided haemorrhoidal artery ligation: feeding arteries located with a Doppler probe then ligated using absorbable sutures[6]
- Haemorrhoidectomy is recommended for fourth-degree haemorrhoids, or third-degree unresponsive to banding
- Stapled haemorrhoidopexy involves excising a section of anal mucosa, blocking the blood supply so that the haemorrhoids shrink[8]. This has superseded haemorrhoidectomy as there is a more rapid recovery and reduction in post-operative pain

PRE-CONCEPTION ISSUES AND CARE

- Avoid trying to conceive soon after haemorrhoid surgery as extra pressure on the pelvic floor could cause strain on the rectum
- Any conservative treatment would be safe in pregnancy
- Most medical treatments would be safe, with the exception of strong analgesia – this would need further discussion with the pharmacist or GP
- Surgical treatment may be avoided until the postnatal period, in order to assess the extent of the damage

Pregnancy Issues

As it enlarges, the uterus puts pressure on the pelvic veins and the inferior vena cava. This slows the return of blood from the lower half of the body, increasing the pressure on the veins below the level of the uterus and causing them to become more dilated or swollen. This makes the woman more prone to haemorrhoids – possibly her first experience.

- Management will depend on the severity of the condition
- As with non-pregnant treatment, it is necessary to confirm diagnosis and exclude any other more serious disorders, e.g. Crohn's disease and ulcerative colitis

Medical Management and Care

- Antenatal management should be conservative as far as possible with diet modification, local creams and analgesia
- Urgent referral should be arranged for evaluation by surgeons, in women with prolapsed haemorrhoids or any rectal bleeding
- Surgical intervention in pregnancy should be performed only in intractable cases
- Although there are studies published regarding efficacy of rutosides in reducing symptoms in pregnant women with first- and second-degree haemorrhoids, there is insufficient safety data at present; it is advisable to avoid these during pregnancy until further data is available[9]

Midwifery Management and Care

- Conservative treatment may continue, giving the same advice as for a non-pregnant woman – laxatives and high-fibre diet[1,9,10]
- Medical referral if this is the first episode or if the haemorrhoids become more severe
- It is unlikely that any operative measures will be undertaken, as the haemorrhoids may improve after delivery
- Encourage pelvic floor exercises as the pelvic floor will be weakened as a result of pregnancy, exacerbating the severity of the haemorrhoids
- Give advice on measures to avoid constipation

Labour Issues

- Haemorrhoids may prolapse with pushing in the second stage

Medical Management and Care

- In women with symptomatic haemorrhoids, avoid a prolonged second stage

Midwifery Management and Care

- Avoid prolonged active pushing in the second stage
- If the haemorrhoids prolapse, applying a cream may soothe any discomfort

Postpartum Issues

- One-third of women will have exposed thrombosed haemorrhoids following delivery[11]
- Most cases of haemorrhoids in pregnancy will improve by 6 weeks after the birth, but they can be troublesome and painful in the immediate postnatal period
- They must not be dismissed as a *minor disorder*: the woman will be distressed at the discomfort and need advice and support

Medical Management and Care

- Infected episiotomy, constipation and prolonged second stage can exacerbate haemorrhoids and can lead to thrombosis, strangulation or rectal prolapse; prompt treatment with antibiotics and encouraging plenty of hydration and high-fibre diet would help to reduce this risk
- Careful inspection of the perineum and assessment of the haemorrhoids is required to avoid complications and arrange appropriate referral in cases they may need surgical management

Midwifery Management and Care

- The routine postnatal examination by the midwife should include inspection of the perianal area
- Mild creams can be administered, e.g. Anusol
- Warm baths, without added bath products, might ease discomfort
- Ice packs or cold compresses will give some immediate relief; do not use for more than 15–20 minutes
- Avoid post-delivery constipation with advice on diet and fluid intake
- Laxatives may be necessary to ensure a soft stool
- A woman with perineal sutures may be wary of opening her bowels
- Encourage defecation when the urge occurs, as to ignore the urge will increase the impaction of faeces within the bowel making it more difficult to defecate
- Equally, discourage straining to defecate
- Analgesia to be given as needed, but avoid codeine-based analgesics, e.g. co-codamol, due to their constipating effect; NSAIDs (if not contraindicated) will be the best form of analgesia
- Reinforce advice on pelvic floor exercises
- Advise the woman to mention any remaining haemorrhoids to the GP at her 6-week postnatal examination; the GP can then make any necessary referral to a colorectal surgeon
- The GP will also need to know if the woman is able to perform a pelvic floor contraction: if this still has not been seen by this stage, a referral to the obstetric physiotherapist can be made

10.7 Anal Sphincter Disorders

Incidence
2% of adult population[1]
Obstetric anal sphincter injury: up to 11% of vaginal
deliveries[2]
Occult injury: 36% diagnosed following childbirth[3]

Risk for Childbearing
Low Risk

EXPLANATION OF CONDITION

Anal Sphincter Damage

Anal sphincter damage may be muscular or neurological in
origin[4], often leads to faecal incontinence and is most commonly caused by[5]:

- Pelvic floor denervation
- External sphincter weakness
- Degeneration of the smooth muscle of the anal sphincter
  as a result of trauma, as in abuse
- Damage following surgery, e.g. haemorrhoidectomy or
  other sphincter surgery
- Spinal cord injury
- Diabetes, multiple sclerosis
- Structural damage, e.g. obstetric anal sphincter injury

Obstetric Anal Sphincter Injury (OASI)

OASI may be classified as a third- or fourth-degree tear and
includes injury to the perineum involving the anal sphincter
complex (external or internal anal sphincter) and/or to the
rectal mucosa[3].

Risk factors for OASI are[3,6]:

- Instrumental assistance, particularly at first delivery
  (<7% of OASI)
- Prolonged second stage (<4% of OASI)
- Persistent occipito-posterior position (<3% of OASI)
- Episiotomy (<3% of OASI); risk higher if midline[7]
- Previous sphincter damage at first delivery[8]
- High infant weight (over 4 kg) (<2% of OASI)
- Nulliparity (<4% of OASI)
- Rectal compromise due to illness, e.g. ulcerative colitis or
  Crohn's disease
- Race related – Afro-Caribbean women have a lesser inci-
  dence than Caucasian women whereas Asian, Indian and
  Filipino women have an increased risk[2,9]
- High BMI[9]

As many of these risk factors are unpreventable, OASI is
therefore difficult to avoid. The damage can be overt and
identified at delivery. Frequently (36%) damage is covert and
diagnosed during a postpartum endo-anal ultrasound for
investigation of incontinence[10]. Lack of understanding of
perianal anatomy by midwives and doctors is considered a
contributing factor for increase in occult OASI[11].

COMPLICATIONS

The complications of anal sphincter damage are:

- Faecal/flatus incontinence, necessitating use of a pad
- Repeated contact with stools can be an irritant to the
  perianal skin causing pain, itching and sores (ulcers)
- Urgency of defecation
- Lifestyle alterations and social embarrassment

NON-PREGNANCY TREATMENT AND CARE

Due to the embarrassment felt, only one-third of those with
damage are thought to present to their GP with symptoms[10].

A detailed history, anal endosonography and anal manometry will comprise part of the work up to diagnose cause of
the symptoms, and give advice on treatment. Treatment may
involve correction of any predisposing factors.

Medical Treatment

- **Loperamide** will reduce the force of any bowel contractions, also reducing the amount of liquid in the stools that
  may lead to leakage[2]
- **Topical phenylephrine** is being researched to see if
  the resting anal tone is increased; early results are
  encouraging[12]

Surgical Treatment

- **Sphincteroplasty**: overlapping of the anal sphincter
  muscles when caused by OASI[11]. Long-term results not
  always satisfactory[12]
- **Artificial bowel sphincter**: can be created, or the gracillis
  muscle can be repositioned round the anal canal to form
  a new anal sphincter; these two surgical options still have
  considerable morbidity attached to them[11]
- **Colostomy**: may be performed as a last resort

Other Treatments

- **Behavioural techniques** and **biofeedback** teach patients
  how to control their bowel habits and use their pelvic
  floor muscles; physiotherapists are able to teach these
  techniques as an outpatient[13]
- **Sacral nerve stimulation** of the damaged pudendal
  nerve is a successfully established treatment that provides good functional outcome and has minimal
  morbidity[2,14]

PRE-CONCEPTION ISSUES AND CARE

The type of pre-conception counseling will vary depending
on the nature of treatment the patient has been receiving.
This can entail:

- Advice regarding the safety of any medication in pregnancy, especially loperamide and phenylephrine
- The safety of proceeding with any sacral nerve
  stimulation
- The safety of biofeedback in pregnancy, as this involves
  a probe being inserted into the vagina to assist with stimulating the pelvic floor
- Women who have experienced OASI need specific
  counselling regarding future pregnancies and vaginal
  deliveries

Pregnancy Issues

Maternal concerns about vaginal delivery must be addressed early in the antenatal period.

The higher morbidity associated with caesarean section has to be considered, along with the symptoms the woman is experiencing. However, women who have experienced anal incontinence, required a repair for an occult OASI or are found to have significantly abnormal manometry results are at greater risk of further injury from a vaginal delivery, and should be offered a caesarean section[8,15].

Bowel habits often change frequently in pregnancy, due to hormonal changes. Hence, bowel function becomes a priority issue that requires particular attention to avoid the previous symptoms.

Medical Management and Care

* A plan of care must be discussed and clearly documented at booking
* The degree of anal incontinence and previous treatment will influence the decision regarding mode of delivery
* There may be a need for combined care between the colorectal team and the obstetrician

Midwifery Management and Care

* Accurate booking history to identify past obstetric problems including perineal trauma and treatment; it may be necessary to obtain medical records from other areas
* Referral to a consultant unit is crucial in order to plan care and the mode of delivery
* The woman will have many concerns about the impending birth and will need frequent reassurance and support from the midwife
* A focus on dietary needs in pregnancy is important to maintain healthy bowel function
* As iron tablets often disrupt bowel function, advice is needed in relation to foods high in iron, in an attempt to avoid anaemia and the need for iron supplementation
* Folic acid supplementation should be encouraged, as this aids the absorption of any natural iron in the diet

Labour Issues

Unless the caesarean section rate is increased dramatically, OASI will remain difficult to prevent, despite knowing the risk factors involved. Performing caesarean sections purely to protect the perineum, would lead to other risks associated with surgical morbidity. However, for those at greater risk of anal incontinence, elective caesarean section may be recommended[16].

For any overt OASI, experience of the practitioner is an important factor in management of these cases. A junior doctor should not be managing this without supervision.

There is evidence that midwives are poor at recognising third- and fourth-degree tears[8]. There is a need for further education on these issues to improve the recognition of the degree of perineal trauma.

Medical Management and Care

* Clear documentation of the degree of perineal and sphincter trauma from previous deliveries should be highlighted in the notes
* Intrapartum care plan should be documented clearly
* Recommendations for care for repair comprise[2,8]:
    approximation (end to end), or overlapping of the anal sphincter muscles, can be used as a technique. However, the latter reports less faecal urgency/incontinence at 1 year[2]
    polydioxanone sutures have a longer half-life and less chance of causing infection than polypropylene (Vicryl) and are therefore considered preferable
    the operator must be skilled in the repair technique
    broad-spectrum antibiotic cover should be prescribed

Midwifery Management and Care

* There is no evidence that a prophylactic episiotomy is of any benefit as was previously thought, but if necessary a medio-lateral incision must be made[6,17]
* If clinically appropriate, delay pushing until woman feels the urge[2]
* Perineal trauma is not influenced by whether or not the midwife practices perineal protection in the second stage
* It has been found that there is little difference in perineal outcome between the expectant ('hands off') or interventionist ('hands on') technique[18]
* As a third of OASIs are not identified at delivery, it is important to seek more experienced advice if there is any level of uncertainty with regard to the degree of perineal trauma

Postpartum Issues

* Increased awareness of need to question women directly about symptoms of faecal incontinence and dyspareunia following childbirth
* Short-term sequelae of anal sphincter injury include pain, infection, constipation and sexual dysfunction[15]
* Understanding is needed about the embarrassment felt and lifestyle adaptations women have to make. This can lead to anxiety and depression. The fear of incontinence may limit social activity due to the fear of being too far away from a toilet[2]

Medical Management and Care

* One-third of coloproctologists recommend a *defunctioning colostomy* for fourth-degree tears[8] that will allow the bowel to rest
* The woman should be debriefed about the risks of faecal incontinence following anal sphincter injury before discharge from hospital
* A follow-up period of 6–12 months with an expert practitioner
* Anal endosonography is to be recommended following any OASI[19]
* Address any issues regarding anxiety and effects of the injury on continence, body image and sexual function

Midwifery Management and Care

* Midwives need to be aware that a *defunctioning colostomy* is a temporary colostomy while the sphincter heals, and give apt reassurance.
* As the perineum will feel particularly uncomfortable following anal sphincter injury adequate analgesia and assistance with positioning during breast-feeding will be needed
* Dietary advice is essential in order to avoid constipation
* Laxatives to be prescribed, as passage of a hard stool may disrupt the repair

10.8 Obstetric Cholestasis

Incidence
0.7% in multi-ethnic populations in England[1]
1.2–1.5% Indian-Asian or Pakistani-Asian origin[2]

Risk for Childbearing
High Risk

EXPLANATION OF CONDITION

Obstetric cholestasis (OC) can also be known as **intrahepatic cholestasis of pregnancy** (ICP).

The condition was first reported by Aslfield (1883), later by Eppinger (1936), further reported by Thorling (1954) and by the late 1950s clinical features were described by several documented reports[3]. It is thought to be a rare liver disorder that only occurs in pregnancy[4]. Cholestasis is the term used to characterise the disruption and reduction of bile products from the liver and its flow to the intestine[5].

The cause of this condition is unclear[6]. However, current findings suggest a multifactorial phenomenon, with the involvement of genetic environmental and hormonal factors[7]. One theory suggests the liver is unable to cope with high levels of sex steroids during pregnancy[8] therefore causing elevation of liver enzymes and the potential for total hepatic failure.

The condition usually occurs after the 28th week of pregnancy when oestrogen levels are at their highest[9,10] and ceases 1–2 weeks postpartum[11]. During this time the woman can suffer physiologically, psychologically and emotionally from the side-effects of this condition.

Increased risk factors include:

- Environmental factors[12] and seasonal dietary requirements due to climate changes[13]
- Twin pregnancies[14]
- Genetic trait – in some ethnic groups[15] such as descendants of Araucanian Indians[16] in Chile and Quechaun Indians in Bolivia[17]
- Genetic studies have identified gene variants of hepatocanalicular transport proteins and their regulators in some ICP patients[18]
- Subsequent pregnancies are susceptible, manifesting earlier and more severely if jaundice was apparent during the first pregnancy[9]
- Symptoms could recur during menstruation and using the COCP[13]

Signs and symptoms of the condition are:

- Intense pruritus (itching) which mainly affects hands and soles of feet, but can affect face, back, chest and legs and, in rare cases, ears, eyelids and oral cavity
  - itching is more severe at night
  - no visible rash except from excessive itching, which is thought to be from increased levels of bile acids in the blood and liver[11]
- Urinary tract infections
- Pale stools
- Possible jaundice[4]

The diagnosis of OC is confirmed if raised serum bile acids are found and other causes for these results have been excluded. Bile acids are the most sensitive indicator and may precede abnormalities of serum liver function tests[19].

COMPLICATIONS

This condition causes severe liver impairment and may cause liver failure in the woman, but also has effects on the fetus. These may include:

- Increased perinatal morbidity and mortality[20]
- Premature delivery[21]
- Meconium-stained liquor[22]
- Fetal distress and intrauterine death[21]

Therefore, the monitoring of fetal growth and wellbeing throughout the pregnancy is paramount. Such investigations can be carried out by regular ultrasound scans and biophysical profiles. Observation by the woman of her baby's activity and movements on a daily basis is important to illustrate any fetal compromise. Therefore, close monitoring is essential. However; it is not known which variables predict intrauterine death[23].

The associated maternal morbidity can be of significance, with severe pruritus and consequent sleep deprivation[13].

The most serious factor to maternal health is the increased risk of a primary postpartum haemorrhage. This ranges from 2 to 22%[24]. This is caused by altered coagulation due to a deficiency of vitamin K resulting from a lack of intestinal bile[25].

Obstetric cholestasis needs to be considered if a woman complains of a prolonged period of pruritus, which may be apparent after delivery if she had an epidural with opiates. If such symptoms persist for more than 3 months, investigations need to be carried out and the woman should be referred to a hepatologist.

PRE-CONCEPTION ISSUES AND CARE

Unless obstetric cholestasis occurred in a previous pregnancy there is no further management required. If there has been evidence in previous pregnancies the woman should be counselled for the chance of recurrence. There is a greater than 90% chance of recurrence in the UK population[26].

Hepatobiliary ultrasonography should be arranged to investigate cholelithiasis and/or other liver disease[27].

Pregnancy Issues

Pruritus is thought to arise from elevated levels of bile acids and histamine released mainly in the areas of the soles of the feet and the palms of the hands[28].

Women with OC are not generally unwell. The main symptom tends to be the intense pruritus that presents itself mainly at night and without the presence of a rash. Sleep deprivation could occur if pruritus is intense and prevents the woman from sleeping.

Key factors in pregnancy:
- An increased level of bile acids is associated with a higher incidence of premature birth and stillbirth; which has been postulated to be due to the toxic effect on the myocytes[28]
- Risk of stillbirth does not correlate with the onset of pruritus and the association of gestational weeks[29]
- The community midwife is generally the first professional to suspect the possibility of obstetric cholestasis
- There is no single biochemical test to prove the state of the condition or the risks to the fetus[8]
- There is no ideal method for fetal surveillance[30]

Medical Management and Care

Investigations
- Other causes for abnormal LFT and/or bile acids should be excluded
- Blood tests to exclude: CMV, hepatitis A, B, C and Epstein Barr virus infection
- Autoantibody screen to check for primary biliary cirrhosis and chronic active hepatitis should be performed
- Once confirmed – LFTs should be measured weekly[20]

Symptomatic Treatment
- Topical treatment with Diprobase, calamine lotion and aqueous cream with menthol may be used; there is no evidence for or against use in pregnancy but they are considered safe and may provide transient symptomatic relief from pruritus
- Chlorpheniramine may be used for sedation at night but does not relieve pruritus
- Ursodeoxycholic acid may act by displacing bile salts and protect the hepatocyte cell membrane from the toxic effects of bile salts. This is currently the most effective pharmacologic treatment. Although commonly prescribed, there is inadequate evidence to recommend its use to improve pruritus and protect against stillbirth[17]
- Vitamin K, 10 mg orally daily, should be prescribed from diagnosis of OC to delivery to reduce the risk of postpartum haemorrhage and fetal or neonatal bleeding. However, there is no clinical data to suggest this improves fetal outcomes[10]

Midwifery Management and Care
- A detailed history is paramount to highlight any previous history of OC
- Requires management as a high-risk pregnancy with complementary midwifery care, so transfer to a consultant unit may be required
- Measure fetal movements daily[32], with emphasis on pattern of movement for that pregnancy instead of a strict fetal kick count alone
- Regular cardiotocography may be performed although there is no evidence to suggest which pregnancies are most at risk of fetal distress or IUFD[17]
- There is a possibility of a pre-term delivery; an opportunity for the woman to view the neonatal unit would be advisable
- Direct the mother to appropriate support groups and give information leaflets

Labour Issues
- It is recommended that women with OC be delivered at 37–38 weeks' gestation[31] to reduce the risk of perinatal mortality and morbidity
- There are associated risks with pre-term delivery, intrapartum fetal distress and meconium-stained liquor
- Timing and risks need to be considered on an individual basis

Medical Management and Care
- Timing of delivery should be individualised as there is no evidence to support or refute early induction of labour at 37–38 weeks[20]. However, it appears to prevent stillbirth beyond the above gestation[17]
- Continuous electronic fetal monitoring, because of the increased incidence of meconium-stained liquor, abnormal CTG findings and prematurity

Midwifery Management and Care
- Labour should be managed from a midwifery perspective with additional implementation of prescribed treatment and care
- Active third stage management is recommended due to the high risk of postpartum haemorrhage

Postpartum Issues
- Symptoms generally resolve within 1–2 days postnatally
- Persistent abnormalities should be further investigated to determine if there is any underlying liver disease
- There is a high possibility of recurrence in subsequent pregnancies

Medical Management and Care
- Ensure liver function test results return to normal; due to raised levels in normal pregnancy[33] it is advised to defer these tests for ≥10 days[17]
- Women should be advised of the recurrence risk of OC, which can be as high as 90%[29]
- Contraceptive advice to avoid oestrogen-based preparations
- A follow-up should be offered to ensure that LFTs return to normal parameters and counseling should be offered.

Midwifery Management and Care
- Ensure that the mother has full understanding of the implications of OC and the possibility of recurrence, and encourage her to seek pre-conception care prior to a future pregnancy
- Advise the mother of the possibility of OC arising in family members[34]

10.9 Gall Bladder and Pancreatic Disease

Incidence	Risk for Childbearing
Cholelithiasis: about 15% of women ≥35 years of age[1]	Variable Risk

EXPLANATION OF CONDITION

Gall Bladder and Gallstones

The biliary system has a major role to play within the body by storing a liver product called bile. Bile is an alkaline fluid that is secreted by the liver and stored in the gall bladder. Bile pigments and bile salts are excretory products of bile. The bile salts assist in the emulsification of fats in the duodenum so that they may be more easily digested by the pancreatic enzymes.

Disorders within the biliary system generally present in middle age and are more common in women than men. However, the incidence after the age of 50 is equal for men and women[2]. The hormonal milieu of elevated oestrogen and progesterone levels is suggested as the causative factor in the pathophysiology of gallstones[3].

The risk of gallstones is also thought to increase with the number of pregnancies[4]. There are five types of biliary tract disorder:

1. **Cholelithiasis** (gallstones) – two types, cholesterol stones and pigment stones (5–12% of pregnant women)[5,6] *Risk factors associated with gallstones:*

Cholesterol Gallstones	Pigment Gallstones
Female	Rising age
Rising age	Chronic haemolysis
Pregnancy/oral contraception	Alcohol abuse
Obesity	Biliary infection
Stasis of the gall bladder	Total parenteral nutrition
Spinal injury	Stasis of the gall bladder[7]

2. **Acute cholecystitis** – gallstones that can irritate the mucus membrane of the gall bladder or block the opening to the gall bladder causing inflammation
3. **Choledocholithiasis** – gallstones that are present in the common bile duct or hepatic duct
4. **Cholangitis** – obstruction within the bile duct that is associated with a bacterial infection
5. **Carcinoma of the biliary tract** – a rare cause of biliary tract disorder; may also involve the gall bladder

In addition, it is apparent that there is a close correlation between gallstones and pancreatitis. Alcohol abuse and gallstones in non-pregnant women have been allied as the result of pancreatitis[8].

Pancreatic Disease

Pancreatitis is the inflammation of the pancreas which usually results from obstruction of the pancreatic duct. Pancreatitis can be either an acute or chronic problem.

- Acute pancreatitis – an emergency situation that is commonly caused by alcohol abuse, abdominal trauma and gallstones, or it can occasionally be idiopathic
- Chronic pancreatitis – related to acute pancreatitis but usually caused by extreme alcohol abuse

The symptoms may be mild, moderate or severe and include:

- Nausea and vomiting
- Severe upper abdominal pain

COMPLICATIONS

The symptoms may be associated with:

- Shock
- Pyrexia
- Jaundice
- Substantial weight loss

The main complication of any biliary disorder is the obstruction or inflammation of the gall bladder. Gall bladder disease is the second most common indication for non-obstetric surgical intervention in pregnancy[9]. Therefore, by surgically removing the gall bladder the symptoms may be cured. However, the need for cholecystectomy occurs in 1 in 1600 to 1 in 10 000 pregnancies[10].

In the case of acute and chronic pancreatitis, there is inappropriate activation of enzymes in the pancreas, which can result in the destruction of the pancreas, having catastrophic consequences. These include infection, respiratory distress, pseudocyst, abscess or pancreatic fistula formation and extremely brittle diabetes. However, left untreated gallstone pancreatitis has an associated maternal mortality rate as high as 37%[11].

NON-PREGNANCY TREATMENT AND CARE

Often, investigation of biliary disorders may require endoscopic retrograde cholangiopancreatography (ERCP). This may also form part of the treatment. However, the majority of gall bladder cancers are treated palliatively[2].

Acute and chronic pancreatitis is usually treated conservatively, with the exception of pancreatic cancer, which may be treated surgically.

One of the key roles with treatment is the information and support offered by the multidisciplinary team. Good pain relief, antibiotics and fluid resuscitation are key aspects of care.

PRE-CONCEPTION ISSUES AND CARE

It is suggested that, if any gall bladder or pancreatic disease is evident prior to conception, it would be advisable to seek medical opinion so that treatment may be instituted to optimise symptoms prior to pregnancy.

A low cholesterol diet and limited alcohol consumption should be considered prior to conception. Literature suggests that although pregnancy does not predispose to gastrointestinal disorders such as cholecystitis or pancreatitis, pregnancy does increase the risk of cholelithiasis and biliary sludge[12].

Pregnancy Issues

Overall, gall bladder and pancreatic disease impacts on perinatal mortality and morbidity by increasing the incidence of premature delivery[8]. It is therefore vital to have some understanding of the disease process to ensure optimum outcome for mother and fetus.

The symptoms previously mentioned in association with gall bladder disease in a non-pregnant state are mirrored in a pregnancy state. However, acute epigastric pain in pregnancy is a common symptom which can delay diagnosis and management of the condition. Other differential diagnoses include dyspepsia, pre-eclampsia, HELLP syndrome and fatty liver disease.

Although transient, pregnancy does increase the risk of gall bladder disease due to gall bladder stasis and the secretion of bile with increased amounts of cholesterol and decreased amounts of chenodeoxycholic acid[13]. Also, delayed gastric emptying and reduced gastrointestinal motility may contribute to the above.

Gall bladder disease is the second most frequent indication for surgery in pregnancy, after appendicitis[14]. The total bile acid pool increases to an estimated 50% during pregnancy. The percentage of cholic acid increases due to the increased synthesis, whereas the percentages of chenodeoxycholic acid and deoxycholic acid decrease[15].

Medical Management and Care

- A past medical history may reveal previous gall bladder disease or episodes of pancreatitis
- Laboratory diagnosis of gall bladder disease may be suggested by elevated white cell count and elevated liver function tests
- Serial amylase and lipid level tests should be performed to confirm the diagnosis of pancreatitis during pregnancy
- Diagnostic tools such as ultrasound are approximately 95% effective at diagnosing gall bladder problems, avoiding the exposure to radiation with X-rays[17]
- Conservative medical management is primarily used to reduce the risk of spontaneous miscarriage within the first trimester, and pre-term labour within the second and third trimesters. Management includes intravenous hydration, correction of hyperglycaemia, and electrolyte imbalance (mainly hypocalcaemia), analgesia, broad-spectrum antibiotics and a fat-restricted diet
- Women with acute pancreatitis should be managed in an intensive care unit

Surgery
- If possible, surgery should be postponed until after delivery
- Cholecystectomy, laparoscopic cholecystectomy and ERCP have been performed in pregnancy with varying degrees of success[18]. The only adverse effect of surgery has been found to be premature labour contractions[19].
- Surgery after 12 weeks, organogenesis is complete and pregnancy loss rate decreases[20]
- The choice of the procedure will vary depending on operator skills, gestational age and severity of symptoms
- Indications for surgery include: ascending cholangitis, obstruction of the common bile duct or the development of severe pancreatitis and persistent biliary colic
- If laparoscopic surgery is performed during pregnancy, open laparoscopy technique is recommended to avoid injury to the uterus and the large gravid uterus can obstruct safe access to the abdomen and gall bladder fossa[21]

Midwifery Management and Care
- A detailed history is important to ascertain any previous or relevant history that requires further attention
- Advise a low fat, low cholesterol diet and no alcohol
- It is essential to be alert to all the signs and symptoms that are related to gall bladder and pancreatic disease to ensure an urgent referral is made to expedite assessment and treatment
- Prompt identification and hospitalisation of women suffering from acute pancreatitis has been related to a reduction in both maternal and perinatal morbidity and mortality

Labour Issues
- There is a risk of iatrogenic pre-term labour following cholecystectomy and this would need surveillance by the midwives and doctors caring for these women
- It has been recommended that elective non-obstetric surgery be delayed until postpartum[16]

Medical Management and Care
- The decision to interfere surgically is dependent on the individual, taking into account the history of episodes of acute pancreatitis and gestational age
- A study evaluated open and laparoscopic cholesystectomies during pregnancy and did not show significant differences regarding preterm delivery rates, birth weights, or Apgar scores[22]

Midwifery Management and Care
- Supportive care in labour is clearly essential
- If cholecystectomy has been performed anticipate, and if necessary prepare for, a pre-term birth

Postpartum Issues

There are no relevant postpartum issues to take into account for the mother unless cholecystectomy is to be considered.

If the birth was pre-term, then care of the mother with a baby on the neonatal unit should be implemented (see Chapter 1)

Medical Management and Care

Cholecystectomy might be considered postpartum dependent upon symptoms and condition.

Midwifery Management and Care

Supportive care during the postnatal care is required with the assistance of the general practitioner.

10 Gastrointestinal Disorders

PATIENT ORGANISATIONS

Living with Reflux
www.livingwithreflux.org

Irritable Bowel Syndrome Network
Unit 5
53 Mowbray Street
Sheffield S3 8EN
www.ibsnetwork.org.uk

National Association for Colitis and Crohn's Disease
4 Beaumont House
Sutton Road, St Albans
Hertfordshire AL1 5HH
www.nacc.org.uk

Crohn's in Childhood Research Association (CIRCA)
Parkgate House
356 West Barnes Lane
Motspur Park
Surrey KT3 6NB
www.cicra.org

Coeliac UK
Suites A–D, Octagon Court
High Wycombe
Buckinghamshire HP11 2HS
www.coeliac.org.uk

Colostomy Association
15 Station Road
Reading RG1 1LG
www.colostomyassociation.org.uk

Ileostomy and Internal Pouch Support Group
(formally The Ileostomy Association)
Peverill House
1–5 Mill Road
Ballyclare, Co. Antrim
Northern Ireland BT39 9DR
www.the-ia.org.uk

National Advisory Service to Parents of Children with a Stoma (NASPCS)
51 Anderson Drive
Darvel
Ayrshire KA17 0DE
www.naspcs.co.uk

British Liver Trust
Portmann House
44 High Street
Ringwood
Hampshire BH24 1HY
www.britishlivertrust.org.uk

Obstetric Cholestasis Support
www.ocsupport.org.uk

ESSENTIAL READING

Alaedini A and Green PHR 2005 Narrative review: celiac disease: understanding a complex autoimmune disorder. **Annals of Internal Medicine**, 142:289–298

Lancaster Smith M 2004 **Gastrointestinal Problems**. Dartford; Magister Consulting Ltd

Logan R, Harris A, Misiewicz J and Baron J 2002 **ABC of The Upper Gastrointestinal Tract**. Oxford; BMJ books/ Blackwell Publishing Ltd.

McLatchie GR and Leaper DJ 2002 **Oxford Handbook of Clinical Surgery**, 2nd Edn. Oxford; Oxford University Press 293–294

Powerie R, Green M and Camann W 2010 Chapt. 10 Disorders of the gastrointestinal tract in pregnancy in **De Swiet's Medical Disorders in Obstetric Practice**. Oxford; Wiley-Blackwell 256-260

Simon C, Everitt H, Birtwistle J and Stevenson B 2002 **Oxford Handbook of General Practice**. Oxford; Oxford University Press 528–529

Smith ML 2004 **A General Practice Guide to Gastrointestinal Problems**. Dartford; Magister Consulting Ltd

Thompson W and Heaton K 2003 **Fast Facts: Irritable Bowel Syndrome**, 2nd Edn. Oxford; Health Press

References

10.1 Gastro-oesophageal Reflux and Hiatus Hernia

1. Spechler SJ 1992 Epidemiology and natural history of gastro-oesophageal reflux disease. **Digestion**, 51(supplement 1):24–29
2. Welsh A 2005 Hyperemesis, gastrointestinal and liver disorders in pregnancy. **Current Obstetrics and Gynaecology**, 15, 123–131
3. Loffeld RJLF and Van Der Putten ABMM 2002 Newly developing hiatus hernia: a survey in patients undergoing upper gastrointestinal endoscopy. **Journal of Gastroenterology and Hepatology**, 17:542–544
4. NHS Choices 2011 Heartburn and gastrooesophageal reflux http://www.nhs.uk/conditions/gastroesophageal-reflux-disease/Pages/Introduction.aspx [Accessed 17-4-2011]
5. Tytgat GN, Heading RC, Muller–Lissner S, *et al.* 2003 Contemporary understanding and management of reflux and constipation in the general population and pregnancy: a consensus meeting. **Alimentary Pharmacology and Therapeutics**, 18:291–301
6. Coad J and Dunstall M 2002 **Anatomy and Physiology for Midwives**. London; Mosby 243
7. Boon NA, Colledge NR, Walker BR and Hunter JAA 2006 **Davidson's Principles and Practice of Medicine**, 20th Edn. London; Churchill Livingstone/Elsevier 878–881
8. Rubenstein D, Wayne D and Bradley J 2003 **Lecture Notes on Clinical Medicine**, 6th Edn. Oxford; Blackwell Publishing Ltd. 219–220
9. Wilson LJ, Ma W and Hirschowitz BI 1999 Association of obesity with hiatus hernia and esophagitis. **American Journal of Gastroenterology**, 94:2840–2844
10. Sloan S and Kahrilas PJ 1991 Impairment of esophageal emptying with hiatus hernia. **Gastroenterology**, 100:596–605
11. Kumar P and Clarke M 2004 **Clinical Medicine**, 5th Edn. London; Saunders 263–266
12. Smith ML 2004 Chapt.1 Gastro-oesophageal Reflux (GORD) in **A General Practice Guide to Gastrointestinal Problems**. Dartford; Magister Consulting Ltd 8–20
13. Ali R.A.R. and Egan L.J. 2007 Gastroesophageal reflux disease in pregnancy. **Best Practice and Research in Clinical Gastroenterology**, 21:793–806
14. Savarino V, Di Mario F and Scarpignato C 2009 Proton pump inhibitors in GORD. An overview of their pharmacology, efficacy and safety. **Pharmacological Research**, 59:135–153
15. Vakil N 2007 The role of surgery in gastro-oesophageal reflux disease. **Alimentary Pharmacology and Therapeutics**, 25: 1365–1372
16. Reich J, Strom K, Fresco S, Pasquariello J and Barbalinardo J 2010 Routine hiatal hernia repair in laparoscopic gastric banding. **Surgical Technology International**, 20:163–166
17. BNF 2011 **British National Formulary** No.61 www.bnf.org
18. De Swiet M 2002 **Medical Disorders in Obstetric Practice**. Oxford; Blackwell Publishing Ltd. 350–351
19. Briggs GC, Freeman RK and Yaffe SJ 2008 **Drugs in Pregnancy and Lactation** 8th Edn. Lippincott; London
20. Nikfar S, Abdollahi M, Morettti ME, *et al.* 2002 Use of proton pump inhibitors during pregnancy and rates of major malformations. A meta-analysis. **Digestive Diseases Sciences**, 47:1526

10.2 Coeliac Disease

1. Lancaster Smith M 2004 Chapt. 8 Coeliac disease in **Gastrointestinal Problems**. Kent; Magister Consulting
2. Van Heel DA and West J 2006 Recent advances in coeliac disease. **Gut** 55:1037–1046
3. Smith G and Watson R 2005 **Gastrointestinal Nursing**. Oxford; Blackwell Publishing Ltd.
4. Unsworth DJ and Brown DL 1994 Serological screening suggests that adult celiac disease is under diagnosed in the United Kingdom and increases the incidence by up to 12%. **Gut**, 35:61–64
5. Alaedini A and Green PHR 2005 Narrative review: celiac disease: understanding a complex autoimmune disorder. **Annals of Internal Medicine**, 142:289–298
6. Eliakim R and Sherer DM 2001 Celiac disease: fertility and pregnancy. **Gynecologic and Obstetric Investigation**, 51:3–7
7. Saalman R and Fallstrom SP 1996 High incidence of urinary tract infection in patients with coeliac disease. **Arch Dis Child**, 74: 170–171
8. Fanos V, Verlato G, Matti P, Pizzini C and Maffeis C 2002 Increased incidence of urinary tract infections in patiemts with coeliac disease. **Pediatric Nephrology**, 17: 570–571
9. Olen O, Montgomery M, Ekbom A, Bollgren I and Ludvigsson J 2007 Urinary tract infections in pregnant women with coeliac disease. **Scandinavian Journal of Gastroenterology**, 42: 186–193
10. Nash S 2003 Does exclusive breast-feeding reduce the risk of coeliac disease in children? **British Journal of Community Nursing**, 8:127–132
11. Akobeng AK, Ramanan AV, Buchan I and Heller RF 2006 Effect of breast feeding on risk of coeliac disease: a systemic review and meta-analysis of observational studies. **Archives of Diseases of Childhood**, 91:39–43
12. Raisler J, Alexander C and O'Campo P 1999 Breast-feeding and infant illness: a dose-response relationship? **American Journal of Public Health**, 89:25–30

10.3 Ulcerative Colitis

1. NACC 2004 **Ulcerative Colitis** http://www.nacc.org.uk/ontent/ibd/ucBG.asp
2. Carter MJ, Lob AJ and Travis SPL 2004 Guidelines for the management of inflammatory bowel disease in adults. **Gut**, 53:1–16
3. Kornbluth A and Sachar D 2004 Ulcerative colitis practice guidelines in adults (update): American College of Gastroenterology, Practice Parameters Committee. **American Journal of Gastroenterology**, 99:1371–1385
4. Stange, EF, Travis SPL, Vermeire, S *et al.* 2008 European evidence-based consensus on the diagnosis and management of ulcerative colitis: definitions and diagnosis. **Journal of Crohn's and Colitis**, 2:1–23
5. Reddy S and Wolf J 2001 Management issues in women with inflammatory bowel disease. **Journal of the American Osteopathic Association**, 101s17–s22
6. Alstead EM 2002 Inflammatory bowel disease in pregnancy. **Postgraduate Medical Journal**, 78:23–26
7. Moody G, Probert G, Srivasta E, *et al.* 1992 Sexual dysfunction in women with Crohn's disease, a hidden problem. **Digestion**, 52:179–183
8. NICE 2089 Infliximab for acute exacerbations of ulcerative colitis. **NICE technology appraisal guidance 163**. London; National Institute for Health and Clinical Excellence. www.nice.org.uk
9. Hudson M, Flett G, Sinclair TS *et al.* 1997 Fertility and pregnancy in inflammatory bowel disease. **International Journal of Gynaecology and Obstetrics**, 58:229–237
10. Kornfeld D, Cnattingius S, Ekbom A 1997 Pregnancy outcomes in women with inflammatory bowel disease – a population-based cohort study. **American Journal of Obstetrics and Gynaecology**, 177:942–946
11. Williamson C and Girliing J 2011 Chapt. 47 Hepatic and gastrointestinal disease in **High Risk Pregnancy, Management Options**, 4th Edition. Elsevier Saunders

193

12. Khare M, Lott J, Currie A and Howarth E 2003 Is it safe to continue azathioprine in a breast-feeding mother? **Journal of Obstetrics and Gynaecology**, 23(supplement 1):S53

13. Sau A, Clarke S, Bass J, Kaiser A, Marinaki A and Nelson-Piercy C. 2007 Azathioprine and breast-feeding – is it safe? **British Journal of Obstetrics and Gynaecology**, 114:498–501

10.4 Crohn's Disease

1. NACC 2004 **Crohn's Disease**. http://www.nacc.org.uk/content/ibd/ucBG.asp

2. Carter MJ, Lobo AJ and Travis SPL 2004 Guidelines for the management of inflammatory bowel disease in adults. **Gut**, 53:1–16

3. Alstead EM 2002 Inflammatory bowel disease in pregnancy. **Postgraduate Medical Journal**, 78:23–26

4. Bruno M 2004 Irritable bowel syndrome and inflammatory bowel disease in pregnancy. **Journal of Perinatal and Neonatal Nursing**, 18:341–350

5. Irvine J, Feagan B, Rochon J, et al. 1994 Quality of life: a valid and reliable measure of therapeutic efficacy in the treatment of inflammatory bowel disease. **Gastroenterology**, 106:287–296

6. Feagins LA and Cryer BL 2010 Do non-steroidal anti-inflammatory drugs cause exacerbations of inflammatory bowel disease? **Digestive Diseases and Sciences**, 55:226–232

7. Hudson M, Flett G, Sinclair TS, et al. 1997 Fertility and pregnancy in inflammatory bowel disease. **International Journal of Gynaecology and Obstetrics**, 58:229–237

8. Alstead E and Nelson-Piercy C 2003 Inflammatory bowel disease in pregnancy. **Gut**, 52:159–161

9. Van Assche G, Dignass A, Panes J et al. (European Crohn's and Colitis Organisation [ECCO]) 2010 The second European evidence-based Consensus on the diagnosis and management of Crohn's disease: Special situations. **Journal of Crohn's and Colitis**, 4, 63–101

10. ABPI Medicines Compendium 2009b Summary of product characteristics for Methotrexate 10 mg tablets. **Electronic Medicines Compendium**. Datapharm Communications Ltd

11. Caprilli R, Gassull A, Escher J C, et al. 2006 European evidence based consensus on the diagnosis and management of Crohn's disease: special situations. **Gut**, 55:36–58

12. Brandt L, Estabrook S and Reinus J 1995 Results of a survey to evaluate whether vaginal delivery and episiotomy lead to perineal involvement in women with Crohn's disease. **American Journal of Gastroenterology**, 90:1918–1922

13. Ilnyckyj A, Blanchard J, Rawsthorne P and Bernstein C 1999 Perianal Crohn's disease and pregnancy: role of the mode of delivery. **American Journal of Gastroenterology**, 94:3274–3278

14. Khare M, Lott J, Currie A and Howarth E 2003 Is it safe to continue azathioprine in a breast-feeding mother? **Journal of Obstetrics and Gynaecology**, 23(supplement 1):S53

15. Sau A, Clarke S, Bass J, Kaiser A, Marinaki A and Nelson-Piercy C. 2007 Azathioprine and breast-feeding – is it safe? **British Journal of Obstetrics and Gynaecology**, 114:498–501

16. Singh M , Qualie J, Currie A, Howarth ES, and Khare MM. 2011 Is breast-feeding safe with azathioprine? **Obstetric Medicine**, 4:104–107

10.5 Irritable Bowel Syndrome

1. Agrawal A and Whorwell P 2006 Irritable bowel syndrome: diagnosis and management. **British Medical Journal**, 332(7536):280–283

2. Thompson W and Heaton K 2003 **Fast Facts: Irritable Bowel Syndrome**, 2nd Edn. Oxford; Health Press Ltd

3. Bruno M 2004 Irritable bowel syndrome and inflammatory bowel disease in pregnancy. **Journal of Perinatal and Neonatal Nursing**, 18:341–350

4. NICE 2010 **CG61 Irritable Bowel Syndrome: NICE guideline**. London; National Institute for Health and Clinical Excellence. www.nice.org.uk

5. Drossman DA 2006 The Functional Gastrointestinal Disorders and the Rome III Process. **Gastroenterology**, 130:1377–1390

6. http://www.cks.nhs.uk/irritable_bowel_syndrome

7. Bennett E, Tennant C, Piesse C, Badcock C and Kellow J 1998 Level of chronic life stress predicts clinical outcome in irritable bowel syndrome. **Gut**, 43:256–261

8. Grundfast M and Komar M 2001 Irritable bowel syndrome. **Journal of American Osteopathic Association**, 101 April supplement: S1–S5

9. Drossman DA 2005 Brain imaging and its implications for studying centrally targeted treatments in irritable bowel syndrome: a primer for gastroenterologists. **Gut**, 54: 569–573

10. Ringel Y, Drossman DA, Leserman J, et al. IBS diagnosis and a history of abuse have synergistic effect on the perigenual cingulate activation in response to rectal distension. **Gastroenterology** 2003;124:A531

11. Gaynes BN and Drossman DA 1999 The role of psychosocial factors in irritable bowel syndrome. **Baillière's Clinical Gastroenterology**, 13:437–452

12. Emarson A, Mastroiacovo P, Arnon J, et al. 2000 Prospective, controlled multicentre study of loperamide in pregnancy. **Canadian Journal of Gastroenterology**, 14:185–187

10.6 Haemorrhoids

1. Nisar P and Schofield J 2003 Managing haemorrhoids. **British Medical Journal**, 327(7419):847–851

2. Simon C, Everitt H, Birtwistle J and Stevenson B 2002 **Oxford Handbook of General Practice**. Oxford; Oxford University Press 528–529

3. Bruck C, Lubowski D and King D 1988 Do patients with haemorrhoids have pelvic floor denervation? **International Journal of Colorectal Disease**, 3:10–14

4. Prodigy Guidance – Haemorrhoids. UK Department of Health. **Prodigy**. www.prodigy.nhs.uk [Accessed 12-06-06]

5. Brisinda G 2000 How to treat haemorrhoids. **British Medical Journal**, 321(7261):582–583

6. Acheson A, Scholefield J 2008 Management of Haemorrhoids. **British Medical Journal** 336: 380–383

7. McLatchie GR and Leaper DJ 2002 **Oxford Handbook of Clinical Surgery**, 2nd Edn. Oxford; Oxford University Press 293–294

8. NICE 2003 **Circular stapled haemorrhoidectomy. National Institute for Health and Clinical Excellence**. www.nice.org.uk [Accessed 12–06–06]

9. Quijano C and Abalso E 2005 Conservative management of symptomatic and/or complicated haemorrhoids in pregnancy and the puerperium. **The Cochrane Database for Systematic Reviews**, July 20, No. 3:CD04077

10. Alonso-Coello P, Guyatt G, Heel-Andsell D, et al. 2005 Laxatives for the treatment of haemorrhoids. **The Cochrane Database for Systematic Reviews**. Issue 4, Art. No:CD004649. DOI:10.1002/14651858.CD004649.pub2

11. Abramowitz L, Sobhani I, Benifla J, et al. 2002 Anal fissure and thrombosed external haemorrhoids before and after delivery. **Diseases of the Colon and Rectum**, 45:650–655

10.7 Anal Sphincter Disorders

1. Perry S, Shaw C, McGrother C, et al. and the Leicestershire MRC Incontinence Study Team 2002 Prevalence of faecal incontinence in adults aged 40 years or more living in the community. **Gut**, 50: 480–484

2. Dudding T, Vaizey C and Kamm M 2008 Obstetric anal sphincter injury: incidence, risk factors and management. **Annals of Surgery**, 247:224–237

3. RCOG 2007 **Greentop Guidelines No. 29: Management of Third and Fourth Degree Perineal Tears Following Vaginal Delivery**. London; Royal College of Obstetricians and Gynaecologists

4. Cook TA and Mortensen N 1998 Management of faecal incontinence following obstetric injury. **British Journal of Surgery**, 85:293–299

5. Vaizey C, Kamm M and Bartrum C 1997 Primary degeneration of the internal anal sphincter as a cause of passive faecal incontinence. **Lancet**, 349:612–615

6. O'Herlihy C 2003 Obstetric perineal injury: risk factors and strategies for prevention. **Seminars in Perinatology**, 27:13–19

7. Eogan M, Daly L, O'Connell P and O'Herlihy C 2006 Does the angle of the episiotomy affect the incidence of anal sphincter injury? **British Journal of Obstetrics and Gynaecology**, 113:190

8. Faltin D, Sangali M, Roche B, Floris L, Boulvain M and Weil A 2001 Does a second delivery increase the risk of anal incontinence? **British Journal of Obstetrics and Gynaecology**, 108:684

9. Burgio K, Borello-France D, Richter H *et al.* 2007 Risk factors for fecal and urinary incontinence after childbirth: The Childbirth and Pelvic Symptoms Study. **The American Journal of Gastroenterology**, 102:1998–2004. Epub 2007 Jun 15

10. Andrews V, Sultan AH, Thakor R, *et al.* 2006 Occult anal sphincter injuries – myth or reality? **British Journal of Obstetrics and Gynaecology**, 113: 195–200

11. Sultan A, Kamm M and Hudson C 1995 Obstetric perineal trauma: an audit of training. **Journal of Obstetrics and Gynaecology**, 15:19–23

12. Cheetham M, Kamm M and Phillips R 2001 Topical phenylephrine increases anal canal resting pressure in patients with faecal incontinence. **Gut**, 48:356–359

13. Norton C and Kamm M 2001 Anal sphincter biofeedback and pelvic floor exercises for faecal incontinence in adults – a systematic review. **Alimentary Pharmacology and Therapeutics**, 15: 1147–1154

14. Kenefick N, Vaizey C, Cohen R, Nicholls R and Kamm M 2002 Medium-term results of permanent sacral nerve stimulation for faecal incontinence. **British Journal of Surgery**, 89:896–901

15. Fitzpatrick M and O'Herlihy, C 2005 Short-term and long-term effects of obstetric anal sphincter injury. **Current Opinion in Obstetrics and Gynaecology**, 17:605–610

16. Faradi A, Willis S, Schelzig P, Siggelkow W, Schumpelick V and Rath W 2002 Anal sphincter injury during vaginal delivery – an argument for caesarean section on request? **Journal of Perinatal Medicine**, 30:379–387

17. Power D, Fitzpatrick M and O'Herlihy C 2006 Obstetric anal sphincter injury: how to avoid, how to repair: a literature review. **Journal of Family Practitioners**, 55:193–200

18. De Souza Caroci da Costa A and Gonzalez Riesco M 2006 A comparison of 'hands off' versus 'hands on' techniques for decreasing perineal laceration during birth. **Journal of Midwifery and Women's Health**, 51:106–111

19. De Parades V, Etienney I, Thabut D, *et al.* 2004 Anal sphincter injury after forceps delivery: myth or reality? A prospective ultrasound study of 93 females. **Diseases of the Colon and Rectum**, 47:24–34

10.8 Obstetric Cholestasis

1. Kenyon AP, Girling J, Nelson-Piercy C, Williamson C, Seed PT and Poston L 2002 Pruritus in pregnancy and the identification of obstetric cholestasis risk: a prospective prevalence study of 6531 women. **Journal of Obstetrics and Gynaecology**, 22(supplement 1):S15

2. Abedin P, Weaver JB, Eggintin E 1999 Intrahepatic cholestasis of pregnancy: prevalence and ethnic distribution. **Ethnic Health**, 4:35–37

3. Raine-Fenning N and Kilby N 1997 Obstetric cholestasis. **Fetal Maternal Medicine**, 9:1–17

4. Turner A 2000 Obstetric cholestasis: symptoms, causes and treatments. **British Journal of Midwifery**, 8:530

5. British Liver Trust 2004 **Obstetric Cholestasis: A Liver Disease in Pregnancy**. Ringwood; British Liver Trust

6. Milkiewicz P, Elias E and Williamson C 2002 Obstetric cholestasis. **British Medical Journal**, 324(7330):123–124

7. Geenes V and Williamson C 2009 Intraheptic cholestasis of pregnancy. **World Journal of Gastroenterology** 15:2049–2066

8. Fagan EA 1994 Intrahepatic cholestasis of pregnancy: timely intervention reduces perinatal mortality. **British Medical Journal**, 309(6964):1243–1244

9. Chambers J 1996 Obstetric cholestasis – a cause of unexplained stillbirth? **Changing Childbirth Update**, 5:4

10. Williamson C and Girling J 2011 Chapt. 47 Hepatic and gastrointestinal disease in James DK, Steer PJ, Weiner CP and Gonik B (Eds) **High Risk Pregnancy Management Options**, 4th Edn Elsevier Saunders; Nottingham

11. Redfearn J 1994 Obstetric cholestasis. **Midwifery Matters**, 62:14

12. Waine C 1995 Beware of itching during late pregnancy. **Practitioner**, 239:97–99

13. Coombes J 2000 Cholestasis in pregnancy: a challenging disorder. **British Journal of Midwifery**, 8:565–570

14. Lamment F, Marschall HU, Glantz A and Matern S 2000 Intrahepatic cholestasis of pregnancy: molecular pathogenesis, diagnosis and management. **Journal of Hepatology**, 33: 1012–1021

15. Reyes H, Gonzalez M and Ribalta J 1978 Prevalence of ICP in Chile. **Annals of Internal Medicine**, 88:487–493

16. Reyes H 1992 The spectrum of liver and gastrointestinal disease seen in cholestasis of pregnancy. **Gastroenterology Clinics of North America**, 21:905–921

17. RCOG 2006 **Guideline No. 43 Obstetric Cholestasis**. London; Royal College of Obstetricians and Gynaecologists 1–10

18. Pusl T and Beuers U 2007 Intrahepatic Cholestasis of pregnancy. **Orphanet Journal of Rare Disorders**, 2:26

19. Lee RH, Kwok KM, Ingles S, *et al.* 2008 Pregnancy outcomes during an era of aggressive management for intrahepatic cholestasis of pregnancy. **American Journal of Perinatology**, 25: 341–345

20. Saleh MM and Abdo KR 2006 Consenus on the management of obstetric cholestasis? National UK Survey. **Royal College of Obstetrics and Gynaecology**, 114: 99–103

21. Heinonen S and Kirkinen P 1999 Pregnancy outcome with intraheptic cholestasis. **Obstetetrics and Gynecology**, 94:189–193

22. Brites D 2002 Intrahepatic cholestasis of pregnancy: changes in maternal fetal bile acid balance and improvement by ursodeoxycholic acid. **Annals of Hepatology**, 1: 20–28

23. Savander M, Ropponen A, Avela K, *et al.* 2003 Genetic evidence of heterogeneity in intrahepatic cholestasis of pregnancy. **Gut**, 52: 1025–1029

24. Kenyon AP, Nelson-Piery C, Girling J, Williamson C, Tribe RM and Shennan AH 2002 Obstetric cholestasis outcome with active management: a series of 70 cases. **British Journal of Obstetrics and Gynaecology**, 109: 282-288

25. European Association for the study of the Liver 2009 EASL Clinical Practice Guidelines management of cholestatic liver diseases. **Journal of Hepatology**, 51: 237–267

26. Roncaglia N, Arreghini A and Locatelli A 2002 Obstetric cholestasis: outcome with active management. **European Journal of Obstetrics and Gynaecology and Reproductive Biology**, 100:167–170

27. Williamson C, Hems LM and Goulis DG 2004 Clinical outcome in a series of cases of obstetric cholestasis – identified via a patient support group. **British Journal of Obstetrics and Gynaecology**, 111:676–681

28. Chin GY 2003 Dermatoses of pregnancy. **Journal of Paediatrics, Obstetrics and Gynaecology**, 29:22–27

29. Welsh A 2005 Hyperemesis, gastrointestinal and liver disorders in pregnancy. **Current Obstetrics and Gynaecology**, 15:123–131

30. Kondrackierie J, Kupcinskas L 2008 Intrahepatic cholestasis of pregnancy – current achievements and unsolved problems. **World Journal of Gastroenterology**, 14:5781-5788

31. Fagan EA 2002 Disorders of the liver, biliary system and pancreas in Swiet MD (Ed.) **Medical Disorders in Obstetric Practice**, 4th Edn. Oxford; Blackwell Publishing Ltd. 282–345

32. Rioseco AJ, Ivankovic MB and Manzur A 1994 Intrahepatic cholestasis of pregnancy: a retrospective case–control study of perinatal outcome. **American Journal of Obstetrics and Gynecology**, 170:890–895

33. David AL, Kotecha M and Girling JC 2000 Factors influencing postnatal liver function tests. **British Journal of Obstetrics and Gynaecology**, 107:1421–1426

34. British Liver Trust 2004 **Obstetric Cholestasis**. Ringwood; British Liver Trust

10.9 Gall Bladder and Pancreatic Disease

1. Landon MB 2004 Diseases of the liver, biliary system and pancreas in Creasy RK and Resnik R (Eds) **Maternal-Fetal Medicine, Principles and Practice**, 5th Edn. Pennsylvania; Saunders Elsevier 1127–1145

2. Summerfield JA 2000 Diseases of the gallbladder and biliary tree in Leadingham JGG and Worrell DA (Eds) **Concise Oxford Textbook of Medicine**. Oxford; Oxford University Press 609–613

3. Noridelle B, Gilo MD, Amin D and Landy H 2009 Appendicitis and cholecystitis in pregnancy. **Clinical Obstetrics and Gynecology**, 52:586–596

4. Tsimoyiannis EC, Antonion NC, Tsabonlas C, *et al.* 1994 Cholelithiasis during pregnancy and lactation. **Prospective Study, European Journal of Surgery**, 160:627–31

5. Valdivieso V, Covarrubias C, Siegel F, *et al.* 1993 Pregnancy and choleithiasis: pathogenesis and natural course of gallstones diagnosed in early puerperium. **Hepatology**, 17:1–4

6. Basso L, McCollum PT, Darling MR, *et al.* 1992 A descriptive study of pregnant women with gallstones. Relation to dietary and social habits, education, physical activity, height & weight. **European Journal of Epidemiology**, 8:629–633

7. Smith G and Watson R 2005 **Gastrointestinal Nursing**. Oxford; Blackwell Publishing Ltd.

8. Ramin KD, Ramin SM, Richey SD and Cunningham FG 1995 Acute pancreatitis in pregnancy. **American Journal of Obstetrics and Gynaecology**, 173:187–191

9. Sharp HT 1994 Gastrointestinal surgical conditions during pregnancy. **Clinical Obstetrics and Gynaecology**, 37: 306–315

10. Elerding SC 1993 Laparoscopic cholecystectomy in pregnancy. **American Journal of Surgery**, 165: 625–627

11. Mendez-Sarchez Nahum, Chavez Tapia N and Uribe M 2006 Pregnancy and gallbladder disease. **Annals of Hepatology**, 5: 227–230

12. Maringhini A, Ciambra M, Baccelliere P, *et al.* 1993 Biliary sludge and gallstones in pregnancy: incidence, risk factors and natural history. **Annals of Internal Medicine**, 119:116

13. Blum A, Tatour I, Monir M *et al.* 2005 Gallstones in pregnancy and their complications : postpartum acute pancreatitis and acute peritonitis. **European Journal of Internal Medicine**, 16:473–6

14. Yates MR and Baron TH 1999 Biliary tract disease in pregnancy. **Clinical Liver Disease**, 3:131–146

15. Kern F Jr, Everson GT, DeMark B *et al.* 1982 Biliary lipids, bile acids and gall bladder function in the human female: effects of contraceptive steroids. **Journal of Laboratory and Clinical Medicine**, 99:798–805

16. Chohan L and Kilpatrick C 2009 Laparoscopy in pregnancy. A literature review. **Clinical Obstetrics and Gynecology**, 52:557–569

17. Chang T and Lepanto L 1992 Ultrasonography in the emergency setting. **Emergency Medicine Clinics of North America**, 10:1–25

18. Angelini DJ 2002 Gallbladder and pancreatic disease during pregnancy. **Journal of Perinatal and Neonatal Nursing**, 15:1–12

19. Lu EJ, Curet MJ, El-Sayed YY, *et al.* 2004 Medical versus surgical management of biliary tract disease in pregnancy. **American Journal of Surgery**, 188:755–759

20. O'Rourke N and Kodali BS 2006 Laparoscopic surgery during pregnancy. **Current Opinion in Anesthesiology**, 19:254–259

21. Sungler P, Heinerman PM, Steiner H, *et al.* 2000 Laparoscopic cholecystectomy and interventional endoscopy for gallstone complications during pregnancy. **Surgical Endoscopy**, 14:267–71

22. Affleck DG, Handrahan DL, Egger MJ, *et al.* 1999 The laparoscopic management of appendicitis and cholelithiasis during pregnancy. **American Journal of Surgery**, 178:523–529

Appendix References

Appendix 10.5.1 Management Algorithm of Irritable Bowel Syndrome

1. NICE 2010 **CG61 Irritable Bowel Syndrome: NICE guideline**. London; National Institute for Health and Clinical Excellence. www.nice.org.uk

2. Drossman DA 2006 The Functional Gastrointestinal Disorders and the Rome III Process. **Gastroenterology**, 130:1377–1390

Appendix 10.3.1 Care of a Stoma

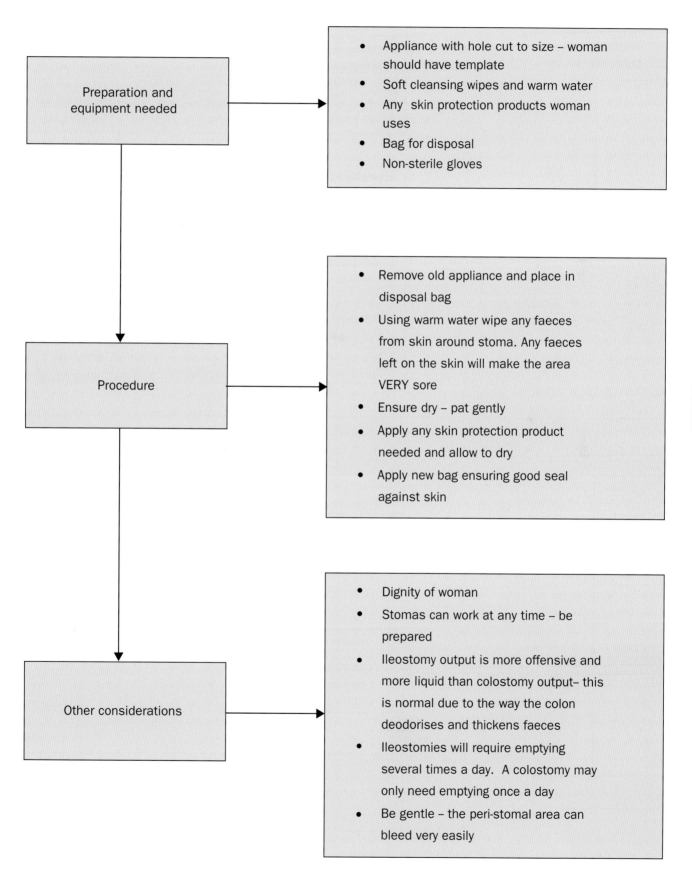

Preparation and equipment needed

- Appliance with hole cut to size – woman should have template
- Soft cleansing wipes and warm water
- Any skin protection products woman uses
- Bag for disposal
- Non-sterile gloves

Procedure

- Remove old appliance and place in disposal bag
- Using warm water wipe any faeces from skin around stoma. Any faeces left on the skin will make the area VERY sore
- Ensure dry – pat gently
- Apply any skin protection product needed and allow to dry
- Apply new bag ensuring good seal against skin

Other considerations

- Dignity of woman
- Stomas can work at any time – be prepared
- Ileostomy output is more offensive and more liquid than colostomy output– this is normal due to the way the colon deodorises and thickens faeces
- Ileostomies will require emptying several times a day. A colostomy may only need emptying once a day
- Be gentle – the peri-stomal area can bleed very easily

197

S. E. Robson and J. Waugh

Appendix 10.5.1 Management Algorithm of Irritable Bowel Syndrome

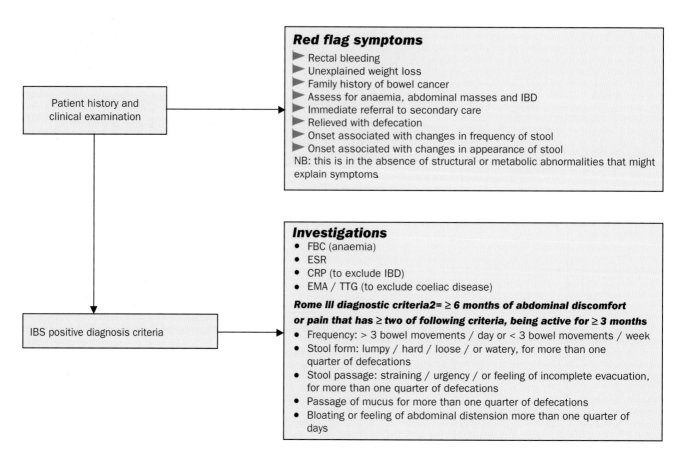

Patient history and clinical examination

Red flag symptoms
▶ Rectal bleeding
▶ Unexplained weight loss
▶ Family history of bowel cancer
▶ Assess for anaemia, abdominal masses and IBD
▶ Immediate referral to secondary care
▶ Relieved with defecation
▶ Onset associated with changes in frequency of stool
▶ Onset associated with changes in appearance of stool
NB: this is in the absence of structural or metabolic abnormalities that might explain symptoms

IBS positive diagnosis criteria

Investigations
- FBC (anaemia)
- ESR
- CRP (to exclude IBD)
- EMA / TTG (to exclude coeliac disease)

Rome III diagnostic criteria2= ≥ 6 months of abdominal discomfort or pain that has ≥ two of following criteria, being active for ≥ 3 months
- Frequency: > 3 bowel movements / day or < 3 bowel movements / week
- Stool form: lumpy / hard / loose / or watery, for more than one quarter of defecations
- Stool passage: straining / urgency / or feeling of incomplete evacuation, for more than one quarter of defecations
- Passage of mucus for more than one quarter of defecations
- Bloating or feeling of abdominal distension more than one quarter of days

198

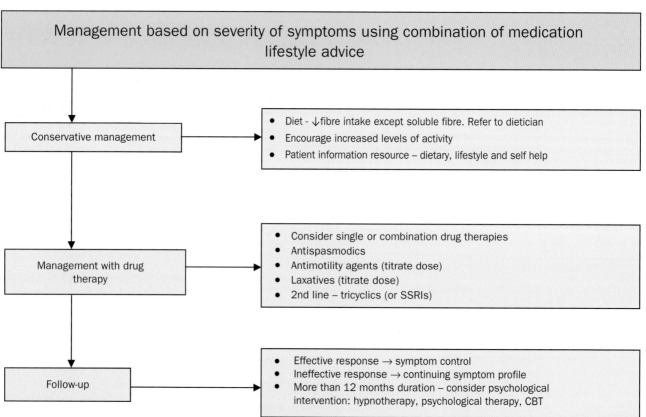

Management based on severity of symptoms using combination of medication lifestyle advice

Conservative management
- Diet - ↓fibre intake except soluble fibre. Refer to dietician
- Encourage increased levels of activity
- Patient information resource – dietary, lifestyle and self help

Management with drug therapy
- Consider single or combination drug therapies
- Antispasmodics
- Antimotility agents (titrate dose)
- Laxatives (titrate dose)
- 2nd line – tricyclics (or SSRIs)

Follow-up
- Effective response → symptom control
- Ineffective response → continuing symptom profile
- More than 12 months duration – consider psychological intervention: hypnotherapy, psychological therapy, CBT

Adapted from several sources, mainly: [1]NICE Clinical Guideline No 61 and [2]Drossman 2006. This figure is downloadable from the book companion website at www.wiley.com/go/robson

AUTOIMMUNE DISORDERS

S. Elizabeth Robson[1]
and Julie Goddard[2]

[1]De Montfort University, Leicester, UK
[2]Calderdale Royal Hospital, Halifax, UK

11.1 Rheumatoid Arthritis
11.2 Raynaud's Phenomenon
11.3 Systemic Lupus Erythematosus
11.4 Antiphospholipid (Hughes) Syndrome

11.1 Rheumatoid Arthritis

Incidence
Women 36:100 000; Men 14:100 000 UK[1]

Risk for Childbearing
Variable Risk

Population Prevalence
Women 1.16%; Men 0.44% UK[1] (similar in USA and Northern Europe)[2]

EXPLANATION OF CONDITION

Rheumatoid arthritis (RA) arises when IgM autoantibodies (**rheumatoid factor**) activate the complement system to inflame the synovial membrane of joints, tendons, bursae and often the pericardium of the heart. Inflammation is accompanied by an influx of inflammatory cytokines, including tumor necrosis factor (TNF) alpha[3], which induce synovial membrane to thicken (**hyperplasia**) and be thrown into folds (**pannus**) with a subsequent increase of synovial fluid, causing painful swelling and restricted movement. Cells of the synovial membrane (synoviocytes) invade the joint cartilage where they secrete enzymes initiating destructive changes in bone and cartilage[3,4].

Finger and toe joints are usually affected first with subsequent involvement of larger synovial joints. Onset can be chronic, over several weeks, with early morning stiffness, swelling of joints and progressive joint pain. Alternatively onset can be acute, with fever and generalised illness. On occasion a **palindromic** pattern might present with pain and inflammation appearing to 'flit' from one joint to another, which can be misdiagnosed as more trivial aches and pains. There are usually periods of remission and relapses[5]. Tiredness results with a temptation to snack on carbohydrate foods and avoid exertion, with the inherent risk of obesity[6].

RA is three times more common in women and the incidence increases with age. It can occur in children as juvenile idiopathic arthritis (JIA) or juvenile rheumatoid arthritis (JRH).

There is a genetic predisposition in around 50% of cases[7,8], and infection is implicated in 10-20% cases[7–9] Risk factors include winter, smoking, obesity, blood transfusion and pet ownership[7]. The oral contraceptive pill may offer protection or delay the onset[10]. Whilst it is rare for RA to present in pregnancy[11] onset is associated with the puerperium, particularly in women who breast-feed after their first delivery[9].

Diagnosis is made by clinical examination and laboratory results showing raised erythrocyte sedimentation rate (ESR) or inflammatory markers, and a positive rheumatoid factor in some cases[6]. Prognostic criteria are under review[12] but currently, with modern management, 20% have mild disease, 75% moderate disease with relapses and remissions and 5% have severe destructive disease[5].

COMPLICATIONS

- Reduced movement of affected joints
- Wasting of small muscles of the hand
- Osteoporosis and fractures[5]
- Swelling of soft tissue around the joints
- Ruptured tendons or joints (Baker's cysts)
- Spinal cord compression
- Neuropathy
- Infection (secondary to steroids)
- Secondary anaemia
- Sjögren's syndrome (dry eyes)
- Secondary Raynaud's phenomenon (see Section 11.2)
- Scleroderma (see Section 11.2)
- Lungs develop pleural effusion and nodules
- Heart develops asymptomatic pericarditis
- Reduced life expectancy from cardiac complications[5]

When JIA was followed up in adulthood[13], 83% of those affected were sexually active, but affected by:

- Relationship instability and sexual problems
- Detrimental effect on body image
- Short stature (associated with caesarean section)
- Reduced hip mobility (associated with caesarean section)

NON-PREGNANCY TREATMENT AND CARE

Modern management advocates disease-modifying anti-rheumatic drugs (DMARDs) used at disease onset[14] to control disease activity and reduce cardiovascular mortality[15] with monitoring for side effects[5]. TNF inhibitors can be started after a 6-month trial on two DMARDs if the condition worsens[5]. Examples of drugs include:

- **NSAIDs** to control symptoms
  - aspirin
  - indometacin (Indomod)
  - ibuprofen (Brufen, Nurofen)
  - naproxen (Naprosyn)
  - phenylacetic acid (Diclofenac)
  - ketoprofen (Ketocid)
- **Steroids** to reduce inflammation
  - prednisolone (Deltacortril)
- **DMARDs** to modify disease
  - azathioprine (Imuran)
  - ciclosporine (Neoral)
  - gold (Myocrisin, Ridaura)
  - hydroxychloroquine (Plaquenil)
  - leflunomide (Arava)
  - methotrexate (Maxtrex)
  - penicillamine (Distamine)
  - sulfasalazine (Salazopyrin)
- **TNF inhibitors** to suppress the immune response
  - etanercept (Enbrel)
  - infliximab (Remicade)
- **Contraception** is essential as fertility is normal and some of the above drugs are contraindicated in pregnancy[16]
- **Diet**: specific diets are not supported by evidence and fasting followed by a vegetarian diet risks malnutrition[17]
- **Physiotherapy**
  - assessment, with the provision of aids to enhance mobility
  - exercises and/or hydrotherapy to maintain joint function and muscle power
  - splints to support joints during disease flare

PRE-CONCEPTION ISSUES AND CARE

Re-refer to the rheumatologist for a risk benefit analysis to maintain or alter drug therapy, ideally in consultation with a consultant in maternal medicine. Azathioprine, hydroxychloroquine and sulfasalazine might be continued. Other DMARDs can be replaced by steroids[18]. Paracetamol for pain relief[3].

Avoid methotrexate[18]. Leflunomide should be stopped, with effective contraceptive cover, for 2 years prior to conception or until plasma levels fall below 0.02 mg/l[18] (see Appendix 11.1.1).

Folic acid 0.4 mg is important, as folate deficiency results from long-term DMARD usage[19].

Assess weight; if necessary implement obesity reduction measures. Encourage a vitamin- and iron-rich diet (see Appendix 1.2). Promote smoking cessation, and regular exercise.

Pregnancy Issues

- Women on aggressive RA therapy have improved health and sexual function, therefore risk unplanned pregnancy
- TNF inhibitors have drug-related teratogenic risk to the fetus[20] (see Appendix 11.1.1)
- Third trimester use of NSAIDs is associated with fetal and obstetric complications (see Appendix 11.1.1)
- Mothers may use a favoured diet or complementary therapy to 'control' their condition, which might not be sanctioned for use in pregnancy
- Remission of symptoms is experienced in 70% of cases in pregnancy[21]
- Some may have positive experience of hydrotherapy for RA treatment and may be attracted to the idea of 'waterbirth'
- Existing complications, such as anaemia and infection, can be exacerbated by pregnancy
- Affected joints risk becoming unstable due to joint laxity and altered weight distribution[22]
- Risk of subluxation of cervical vertebrae C1–2[21]; which is often under-recognised
- Psycho-social dilemmas may arise as the woman and her family raise fears of parenthood affected by potential disability
- There is conflicting information about increased miscarriage risk; this aside there appears to be no significant risk of preterm birth, pre-eclampsia or IUGR[3]

Medical Management and Care

- Obstetrician and rheumatologist share care; appointments at 2–4 week intervals[18]
- DMARDs are reviewed. Avoid D-penicillamine and methotrexate[18]. Azathioprine, hydroxychloroquine and sulfasalazine may be continued. Other DMARDs can be replaced with steroids
- NSAIDs are best avoided[18], especially in third trimester (see Appendix 11.1.1) and paracetamol is preferred for pain relief[23]
- Steroids, e.g. prednisolone, are prescribed for worsening disease[18]
- Counselling and screening for fetal congenital abnormalities may be required for women who conceive whilst on TNF inhibitors or other contraindicated drugs
- Refer to anaesthetist if there is severe RA, limited abduction of hips or if subluxation (partial dislocation) of cervical vertebrae are suspected

Midwifery Management and Care

- Detailed booking history to identify past and present drug therapy, and use of complementary therapies
- Book for consultant unit care and hospital confinement
- Assess expectations and discuss options on a medical model of care
- Support medical treatment, whilst giving positive yet realistic reassurance
- Advice on the altered state of health in pregnancy with RA
- Confer with multiprofessional team, such as OT for specific aids and advice
- Assess nutritional status; advise a well-balanced, iron- and folate-rich diet; discourage unorthodox nutritional practices which could potentially be harmful[24]
- Regular FBC investigations to detect anaemia at an early stage to implement treatment with iron, B_{12} and folate tablets[25]
- Assess prospective ability to care for herself and the baby[25]
- Consider home antenatal or parentcraft visits for serious disability[25]
- If the mother requests water immersion during labour or birth, discuss with the obstetrician; a risk analysis must be carried out especially if there is restriction of mobility or muscle weakness; a hoist must be available in labour

Labour Issues

- Mobility restriction with a theoretical risk of DVT for immobile mothers
- Problems with abduction of hips, especially a problem for lithotomy position. In extreme cases caesarean section is indicated
- At risk of subluxation of cervical vertebrae if this was not assessed previously[23]
- Theoretical risk of difficult iv cannulation, especially if there is scleroderma (see Raynaud's phenomenon, Section 11.2) in which case, there can also be problems with intubation should a general anaesthetic be required

Medical Management and Care

- Consider use of additional steroid cover in labour
- If scleroderma co-exists, refer to anaesthetist early in labour
- Avoid lithotomy position whenever possible

Midwifery Management and Care

- Passive leg exercises to prevent DVT[25]
- Left lateral position should be considered for delivery[25]
- Mother's partner to support her limbs[25]
- If lithotomy position is used, lift legs together and slowly with time for abduction
- If the waterpool is used a risk assessment specific to the medical condition should be carried out, and a hoist must be available
- Labour should otherwise be managed on a normal basis by the midwife[25]

Postpartum Issues

- RA disease will flare postpartum in 70% cases[21], which can be accompanied by depression
- Neonate has theoretical risk of premature closure of ductus arteriosus if the mother was taking NSAIDs
- Breast-feeding may delay the return to the pre-pregnancy drug regimen
- If the mother has disability or muscle weakness her maternal coping skills with handling and feeding the baby may be impeded
- Mothers with disability and reduced mobility are at risk of VTE postpartum (see Section 15.2)

Medical Management and Care

- Confer with the rheumatologist who is likely to reduce the steroid dosage slowly and return to pre-pregnancy drug regimen, unless breast-feeding
- Keep breast-feeding mothers on steroids
- Neonatal examination to be conducted by a paediatrician if mother has received NSAIDs or other drugs with a potentially adverse effect on the neonate
- VTE risk assessment if mobility is affected (see Table 15.2.1)

Midwifery Management and Care[25]

- Encourage mobility and assist with handling baby whilst in hospital
- Assess ability to care for self and baby on activities of daily living
- If necessary ask the physiotherapist to visit on the postnatal ward
- Advise mother about the potential exacerbation of RA, and to contact her rheumatologist at first symptoms
- Arrange drugs to take home and a rheumatology outpatient appointment
- Promote breast-feeding in a realistic manner
- Contraceptive advice
- Be alert for signs of depression

11.2 Raynaud's Phenomenon

Incidence
2–5% adults worldwide, especially cold climates[1,2]
14–21% UK patients attending General Practice[3,4]
Primary phenomenon has a female excess[5,6]

Risk for Childbearing
Low Risk for Primary Raynaud's phenomenon
High Risk for Secondary Raynaud's phenomenon

EXPLANATION OF CONDITION

Maurice Raynaud first described a cold-induced transient, painful cessation of blood flow to the fingers and toes with triphasic colour changes in 1862[6]. The peripheral blood circulation becomes congested following arteriolar spasm under sympathetic nervous control on exposure to a cold temperature or stress[7]. Attacks usually subside after a few minutes. The middle fingers are most commonly affected, but not the thumb[8], and sometimes toes, ears, and the tip of the nose. Colour changes comprise[6,7]:

- **White** – becomes painful due to ischaemia
- **Blue** – becomes numb due to cyanosis
- **Red** – becomes painful when reperfusion of blood occurs

The condition is probably under-recognised, as only 2% of sufferers consult a doctor[4] and many try natural remedies before conventional treatment[9]. Of unknown aetiology[10], there are varying associations with cigarette and alcohol consumption[11,12] and a strong correlation with anxiety traits[13]. There are two types: primary and secondary.

Primary Raynaud's Phenomenon (PRP) (90% of cases[2])

- Young women mainly affected, onset commonly at puberty[1,2]
- Can affect children, even in early childhood[14], with a female predominance[15,16]
- Familial[17,18] in 26% of cases[19]
- Migraine headache (see Section 8.1) in 15–27% of cases[20,21]
- Condition may go into remission[10,22]
- If nailform and autoantibody tests are normal (90% of PRP) the condition is benign[1]; reassurance and advice can be given[2,23] and the condition managed by the GP usually without drug treatment[2, 9]
- If nailform and autoantibody tests are abnormal (10% of PRP) there is risk of a defined connective tissue disease developing within 10 years[2,10], especially if there was a higher age of onset[24], hence consultant referral is indicated

Secondary Raynaud's Phenomenon (SRP) (10% of Cases[2])

Usually presents later in life as it arises from occupational hazards or another medical condition and drug therapy. Common associations:

- Hand vibration injury (repetitive strain)[4]
- Carpal tunnel syndrome[20]
- Beta-blocker use[1,20]
- Systemic lupus erythematosus (SLE) in 10–45% of cases[5]
- Sjögren's syndrome (dry eyes and mouth) in 33% of cases[5]
- Rheumatoid arthritis in 10–20% of cases[5] (see Section 11.1)
- Scleroderma (*systemic sclerosis, scleroma*) >90% of cases[5]
  - literally 'hard skin' which becomes thick and taut with a waxy appearance due to swelling of collagen fibres and constriction of the peripheral capillary blood vessels
  - Renal, respiratory and gastrointestinal tracts progressively affected[25]
  - 5-year survival rate in 37–74% of cases[26]
  - Uncommon in nulliparous women, very rare in pregnancy, and 87% had their last pregnancy ≤5 years before the onset of scleroderma[25]
- Other connective tissue diseases

COMPLICATIONS

Only a small number of those with primary Raynaud's will go on to develop connective tissue disease, usually 10 years from the onset of Raynauds[27]. Those with SRP, and the chronically sick and disabled, risk complications which include:

- Chilblains and mouth ulcers
- Skin rashes
- Livedo reticularis (red/blue skin mottling)[7]
- Cyanosis and ulceration of tips of fingers and toes which, with SRP, can lead to gangrene in extreme cases[7]

NB: Midwives are most likely to care for mothers with primary Raynaud's phenomenon and minimal complications.

NON-PREGNANCY TREATMENT AND CARE

As Raynaud's can precede connective tissue disease, especially scleroderma[10,22], investigations are required:

- Blood tests for FBC, ESR, and autoantibody screen
- Nailform capillary test using an ophthalmoscope[9]

NB: If these are abnormal, underlying connective tissue disease is implied, so keep under review or refer to a specialist centre[9]

Advice

- Avoid extremes of temperature[28]
- Wear warm clothing[28]
- Cease smoking and minimise caffeine intake[28]
- Undertake regular exercise[28]
- Mention this condition when seeking contraceptive advice – the combined contraceptive pill may be contraindicated
- Relaxation techniques if stress is a contributing factor[23]

Drug Therapy (more likely with (SRP)

- Many patients try natural remedies before prescribed drugs[9]
- Vasodilator nifedipine (Adalat, Tenif)[9,23]
- Calcium channel blockers[23]
- Other treatment is dependent on the underlying condition.

NB: Put an alert note on case notes, as she should not take beta-adrenoceptor antagonists or vasoconstrictor drugs

PRE-CONCEPTION ISSUES AND CARE

Primary Raynaud's

- Combined oral contraceptive pill might be contraindicated
- Risk–benefit assessment for cessation of drugs periconception
- Promote smoking cessation
- Advise that PRP is unlikely to affect a forthcoming pregnancy

Secondary Raynaud's (as Above, Plus)

- Management and implications for childbearing depends upon the co-existing condition
- Scleroderma has functional problems with coitus[28] and its potential mortality may raise significant dilemmas about termination or continuation of a pregnancy
- If Sjögren's syndrome symptoms are apparent investigate for anti-Ro/-La antibodies, which cross the placenta with a 10% risk of neonatal lupus syndrome (see Section 11.3)

Pregnancy Issues

Symptoms are likely to improve due to:
- Increased blood volume
- Reduced arteriolar spasm from a relaxing effect of progesterone on the blood vessel walls[29,30]
- rise in maternal core temperature as the fetus enlarges, which increases blood flow to the periphery and encourages vasodilatation to assist with heat loss[30]

Women may already be taking natural remedies such as evening primrose or fish oils[9]; a randomised controlled trial (RCT) with *Ginkgo biloba* showed a reduction in frequency of attacks in primary Raynaud's but no indication of its safety in pregnancy[31].

PRP
- No known adverse effect on pregnancy. One study demonstrated an increased incidence of pre-term birth with no adverse fetal outcomes[32]

SRP
- Pregnancy problems and outcome is dependent upon the co-existing condition.

Scleroderma Associated With[29]
- Maternal pulmonary hypertension
- Maternal renal disease
- Miscarriage
- IUGR

Medical Management and Care
- **PRP**: usual antenatal care
- **SRP**: antenatal care at a combined or specialist clinic; liaison with physician as indicated
- Risk–benefit assessment for the first trimester use of nifedipine and other drugs[29]
- **Sjögren's syndrome**: test for anti-Ro and anti-La antibodies
- **Scleroderma**: management depends upon the progression and severity of the condition; such complex variables are outside the scope of this book

Midwifery Management and Care[36]

PRP
Mother can have low-risk care and the phenomenon is not a contraindication for home birth. The midwife should:
- Reinforce the general advice of the pre-pregnant state
- Advise on avoidance of complementary therapies due to lack of evidence on safety in pregnancy
- Encourage smoking cessation
- Advocate minimal caffeine products
- Advise on avoidance of extremes of temperature
- Encourage regular, well-balanced meals and hot drinks
- Promote breast-feeding, and explain about Raynaud's 'attack' on the nipple
- Be alert for pre-term labour, and advise mother on the signs
- Use astute observational skills to identify the potential for other co-existing conditions, then refer to an appropriate doctor

SRP
Antenatal care is shared with physicians, as per the co-existing conditions. The midwife needs to:
- Give advice and care as for PRP above
- Reinforce any medical advice and treatment given
- Seek information on recent treatments
- Advise on potential side effects of drugs
- Observe to identify deterioration of the co-existing condition

Labour Issues

Raynaud's
- Ergometrine and syntometrine are vasoconstrictive, hence their routine use should be avoided[30]

Scleroderma – Risks Of:
- Pre-term labour[29]
- Difficulties with iv cannulation[29]
- Problems with intubation[29]

Medical Management and Care
- **PRP**: labour can be managed normally by the midwife
- **SRP**: as per the co-existing condition
- **Scleroderma**: anaesthetist needs to assess mother in advance

Midwifery Management and Care[36]
- Labour can be managed from a normal perspective by the midwife
- Implement any prescribed treatment and care for a co-existing condition
- Oxytocin for active third stage management; ergometrine reserved for emergency use with haemorrhage

Postpartum Issues
- Maternal blood volume returns to its pre-pregnancy state after 3 days[30] and the protective effect for Raynaud's attacks will subside acutely
- Raynaud's attack on the nipple has been reported in pregnancy[33] and breast-feeding[34] being misdiagnosed as thrush and contributing to breast-feeding failure[35]
- Raynaud's is a familial condition[27] associated with anxiety[13]. Whilst childhood Raynaud's usually presents at 5–16 years[16], it has been reported in toddlers[15]; hence an anxious mother could worry that her baby might develop the condition
- Additional support is required if the neonate is admitted to a neonatal unit

Medical Management and Care
- Evaluate necessity for pre-pregnancy drugs once breast-feeding has ceased
- If Sjögren's symptoms are present, be alert for neonatal lupus, which usually presents in the baby as a florid facial rash with an 'owl eyes' appearance and carries a risk of congenital heart block[37]
- If the above neonatal features present, initiate maternal investigations[26,37]

Midwifery Management and Care[36]
- Avoid the use of ice cubes or a cold compress around the nipple
- Examine nipples if pain is reported, and do not dismiss as 'thrush'
- The mother should be advised:
  - that her old symptoms are likely to return
  - that the baby should be dressed sensibly in warm baby clothing for outdoors, including hat and mittens, as would any other baby
  - to avoid a reactionary tendency to over-wrap and over-heat the baby giving a theoretical increased risk of sudden infant death syndrome (SIDS)

11.3 Systemic Lupus Erythematosus

Incidence
26 in 100000 of UK population[1] with 90% female dominance[2]
Afro-Caribbean, Asian and Chinese have greater susceptibility[2]

Risk for Childbearing
High Risk

EXPLANATION OF CONDITION

With lupus erythematosus, the body produces autoantibodies against its own connective tissue. Shortened to *lupus*, there are several variations of which the two most common are:

1. **Discoid lupus erythematosus** (DLE): only skin is affected, with red scaly patches well-defined on the face and neck. Alopecia (hair loss) results, leading to scarring on the scalp. Both are made worse by sunlight[3]; treatment is by avoiding intense sunlight and sunbeds[3] and the application of topical corticosteroids or hydroxychloroquinine[4]

2. **Systemic lupus erythematosus** (SLE): the most common variation affecting the entire body including serous membrane, kidneys, joints, and skin[2]. Presenting symptoms[2] often include:
   i   Classic 'butterfly rash' (malar rash) on cheeks
   ii Weight loss
   iii Fatigue and headaches
   iv Fever with flu-like symptoms
   v   Arthralgia (joint pain without swelling)

Lupus has periods of remission, and when active is termed 'lupus flare' which is often triggered by infection, exposure to sunlight or oestrogen increase – as may occur when prescribed the oral contraceptive pill. It can be difficult to differentiate between a flare and infection[2].

Diagnosis is based using clinical criteria[5] and investigations. Skin biopsy is used to detect SLE autoantibodies reacting with its complementary antigen[6]. Patients usually test positive for antinuclear antibody (ANA) and often DNA antibodies (70–80%). A raised ESR is common, and a positive rheumatoid factor is found in 25%. A false positive test for syphilis is found in 33%[7] and some have antiphospholipid antibodies[8], which can result in a co-existing antiphospholipid syndrome[2] with thrombo-embolic sequelae[8].

There is no cure for SLE and treatment aims to control symptoms and prevent progression. With modern treatment the survival rate has increased to 15 years in 80% of cases[9]. Death usually results from generalised disease, infection or cardiovascular disease.

COMPLICATIONS

Some of the following manifestations may be experienced[2,8]:

- Acute and chronic infection
- Nausea, vomiting and diarrhoea
- Alopecia (hair loss)
- Photosensitivity
- Arthritis and sometimes early morning stiffness
- SRP (see Section 11.2)
- Sjögren's syndrome (dry eyes/mouth) (see Section 11.2)
- Ulceration of mouth, nose and vagina
- Fatigue and myalgia (muscle pain)
- Jaccoud's arthropathy (deformed joints due to lax ligaments)
- Renal disease (lupus nephritis) in 40–75% of cases
- Pleurisy (often asymptomatic)
- Ischaemic heart disease
- Pulmonary hypertension
- Pericarditis (often asymptomatic)

- Anaemia – as a result of chronic infections[6]
- Leucopenia (reduced leucocyte count)
- Thrombocytopenia
- Neuro-psychiatric states, e.g. cerebrovascular accident[2], migraine, epilepsy[10] and depressive or manic symptoms[11] and dementia[10]

NON-PREGNANCY TREATMENT AND CARE

Advice for the Woman

- Avoid sunlight and use sun block
- Avoid infection situations
- Avoid unplanned pregnancy and seek pre-conception care
- Avoid stress and get adequate rest (may need to adapt job)
- Use analgesics as required
- Protect against cold if Raynaud's phenomenon occurs
- Eat a well-balanced diet
- Have a positive self-image (e.g. camouflage make-up)

Monitor

- Urinalysis for blood and protein (indicates renal disease)
- Regular blood pressure measurement
- Screening for diabetes
- Assessing osteoporosis risk (from prolonged steroid use)
- Investigations for antiphospholipid (Hughes) syndrome
- Blood tests for FBC, ESR, WBC, U&E, creatinine, C3 and C4 complement and anti-DNA titre[5,8]
- LFT if taking azathioprine

Medical Treatment

- Corticosteroids for disease flare, e.g. prednisolone[7]
- NSAIDs for pain, fever and arthritis[7]
- DMARDs to arrest disease progression
  ○ methotrexate
  ○ cyclophosphamide[2]
  ○ azathioprine
  ○ mycophenolate
- Antimalarial drugs (e.g. hydroxychloroquine) for skin disease, fatigue and arthralgia[7,8]

PRE-CONCEPTION ISSUES AND CARE

- Pre-conception counselling is essential to allow accurate assessment of the woman's disease, permitting discussion of the potential complications of pregnancy – including pre-eclampsia, intra-uterine growth restriction and premature birth
- Refer to obstetrician and rheumatologist with specialist expertise in SLE/pregnancy to facilitate the above and review current medication and adjust as required
- Advise conception during a period of disease remission as this decreases the risk of pregnancy complications. SLE does not appear to affect fertility[12] so contraceptive advice is important
- Women with active lupus nephritis at conception have a higher risk of decreasing renal function during pregnancy which may occasionally be permanent[13]

Pregnancy Issues

- The risk of pregnancy complications depends on the level of disease activity and the presence of lupus nephritis, hypertension, anti-Ro/La antibodies and antiphospholipid antibodies
- Pregnancy complications are generally reduced if the lupus is mild or stable, particularly at conception[13,14]
- Fetal loss has reduced from 50% to 20% with modern management, but there is still an increased risk[13,15] of:
  - IUGR
  - pre-term birth (iatrogenic or spontaneous)
  - IUFD
  - miscarriage
  - risk of congenital abnormalities – linked with some drug treatment (see Appendix 11.1.1)
- The risk of a lupus flare during pregnancy is 15–60%. It is unclear whether pregnancy increases the risk of a flare as studies show conflicting results[13]
- Lupus nephritis increases the risk of pre-eclampsia to 25–35%[16] and increases the chance of pre-term birth to around 30%[17]
- There is an increased risk of hypertensive disease of pregnancy[16]
- Differentiating between lupus flare and pre-eclampsia can be challenging
- Lupus flare is associated with premature delivery[15,18,19]
- Risk of fetal loss is increased with hypertensive disease and a raised antiphospholipid antibody titre. The presence of lupus anticoagulant has the greatest association with recurrent fetal loss[13]

Medical Management and Care

- Women should be under the combined care of a high risk obstetrician and rheumatologist/physician with expertise in the management of SLE
- Ascertain baseline levels for FBC, U&E, LFT, platelets, anti-DNA antibodies and complement early in pregnancy. Repeat as clinically indicated
- Assess proteinuria baseline level by 24-hour urine collection to allow detection of increased levels later in pregnancy suggesting pre-eclampsia or renal flare
- Check anti-Ro/La antibody status if not known – women with these antibodies have a 2–5% chance[8,22] of their first baby developing in-utero congenital heart block (CHB), rising to 16% with subsequent pregnancies[13,23]; fetal monitoring with echocardiography is advocated[9] and corticosteroid use is debated[22,23]
- Review medications – some DMARDs may be replaced by other drugs, such as NSAIDs or steroids, if this was not done pre-conception; continue hydroxychloroquine as stopping may increase risk of a flare
- Commence aspirin post-conception for women with lupus nephritis to reduce the risk of pre-eclampsia. Consider additional low molecular weight heparin for women with antiphospholipid antibodies and a poor obstetric history (see Section 11.4)
- Treat disease flare promptly with steroids[13,24]
- Serial ultrasound scans to detect congenital abnormalities (particularly if conceived on potential teratogenic drug), assess uterine artery Doppler (risk of pre-eclampsia) and monitor for development of IUGR
- Anticipate elective delivery at the earliest sign of disease flare, significant pre-eclampsia or renal deterioration, preparing for a pre-term infant

Midwifery Management and Care

As a high-risk pregnancy, book for multidisciplinary antenatal care at a combined clinic[21] and delivery at a hospital with a neonatal unit. The midwife should also:
- At booking history, record manifestations of the condition and medication
- Warn of possible false positive result for syphilis if Wassermann test is used
- Explain the risk of miscarriage or pre-term delivery, and the necessity to contact delivery suite for any signs of labour
- Address the mother's concerns, accepting that she has insight into her condition and may be the first to recognise her altered health state
- Conduct astute observations at each antenatal visit, especially urinalysis and blood pressure
- Refer to medical team if proteinuria is detected, as this may indicate renal flare
- Promote a well-balanced, iron-rich diet to prevent anaemia
- Encourage gentle exercise to reduce risk of DVT

Labour Issues

- Mothers with SLE remains 'high-risk' in labour, but most should be able to deliver vaginally[12] in the absence of obstetric complications or lupus flare

Medical Management and Care

- TED stockings are required for operative delivery
- Consider the need for additional steroids to cover delivery

Midwifery Management and Care

- Continuous EFM throughout labour
- Midwife can manage and conduct normal, term vaginal birth

Postpartum Issues

- Increased risk of lupus flare[21]
- The mother may need prompt return to her pre-pregnancy drug regimen, and these drugs might pass into breast milk (Appendix 11.1.1)
- Lactation might be suppressed by corticosteroids and disease activity[20]
- Prolactin released may lead to exacerbation of the condition[12]
- Breast-feeding contributes to maternal fatigue
- A neuropsychiatric state could be wrongly identified as postnatal depression
- Neonates born to anti-Ro or anti-La positive mothers risk neonatal lupus in 5% of cases[8], presenting with a discoid, facial 'owl eyes' rash at 2–3 weeks of age and resolves spontaneously within 6 months
- 2% risk of neonatal congenital heart block, possibly diagnosed antenatally[21]

Medical Management and Care

- Bottle-feeding mothers are returned to pre-pregnancy drug regimen
- Steroids are increased for 'postpartum flare' and breast-feeding
- The oestrogen-based contraceptive pill should be avoided
- Neonatal examination prior to discharge by paediatrician not midwife
- Post-delivery ECG for babies born to Ro and La positive mothers

Midwifery Management and Care[24]

- Postnatal observations and visits should be continued for 10 postnatal days, and for longer if the mother is unwell being alert for lupus flare[21]
- Seek paediatric/pharmaceutical advice on drugs and breast-feeding
- Thorough neonatal examinations, reporting any neonatal facial rashes promptly
- Be alert for the baby experiencing any cardiopulmonary problems
- Reinforce medical advice and treatment
- Should psychiatric symptoms present, do not dismiss as the 'baby blues' and refer promptly to medical staff
- Encourage breast-feeding realistically, giving support if she has to cease
- Alert the mother to the risk of neonatal lupus, and advise her to avoid excess sunlight exposure for the baby

11.4 Antiphospholipid (Hughes) Syndrome

Incidence	Risk for Childbearing
>1% healthy adults have antibodies without disease[1] 40% of patients with SLE have antiphospholipid syndrome antibodies[2] 15% women with recurrent miscarriage have antibodies[3]	High Risk

EXPLANATION OF CONDITION

Antiphospholipid syndrome (APS) is alternatively known as **Hughes syndrome**, after Graham Hughes who first described the condition in 1984 in patients with SLE[4]. There is no racial predominance and the prevalence increases with age[1]. The condition is an acquired thrombophilia (clotting disorder) associated with previous thrombosis, or obstetric complications including placental insufficiency, recurrent miscarriage, late fetal loss, pre-eclampsia, and pre-term delivery[5].

Phospholipids are fat molecules within cell membranes, and are found in the lining of blood vessels. With APS, autoantibodies called antiphospholipid antibodies (APA) are produced which bind to the phospholipid of cell membranes causing inflammation and damage. When blood vessels are affected the damage is termed vasculopathy, and clots can form in the narrowed, damaged vessels.

APA indicates the presence of one or both of two autoantibodies: lupus anticoagulant (LA) and anticardiolipin antibodies (aCL)[6]. Cardiolipin is a component of the Wasserman reaction which tests for syphilis[7], hence there may be a false positive result for syphilis in geographical areas still using this test.

These autoantibodies (LA or aCL) bind to endothelial cells, platelets and monocytes, and initiate an increase of thromboxane A2 and tissue factor. This leads to activation of the complement cascade and provoke thrombosis in any organ/vessel of the body, including the placenta[8]. In simple terms a patient with APS has 'sticky blood' being prone to thrombotic disorders and their complications.

Revised Sapporo Classification Criteria For APS[9]

Clinical Criteria
Vascular Thrombosis

- One or more clinical episodes of arterial, venous or capillary thrombosis in any tissue/organ

Pregnancy Morbidity

- One or more unexplained deaths of a morphologically normal fetus after 10 weeks gestation
- One or more pre-term births before 34 weeks gestation due to pre-eclampsia or placental insufficiency
- Three of more unexplained consecutive miscarriages prior to 10 weeks gestation

Laboratory Criteria

- LA present on at least two occasions at least 12 weeks apart
- aCL, IgG or IgM in medium/high titre present on at least two occasions at least 12 weeks apart
- Anti-β2 glycoprotein-I, IgG or IgM, present on at least two occasions at least 12 weeks apart

NB: There must be at least one clinical **and** one laboratory criterion to make a diagnosis of APS.

Other Clinical Manifestations of APS

- **Cardiac disease:** valve dysfunction (usually mitral valve), endocarditis, coronary artery disease, pulmonary hypertension[10]
- **Renal disease:** nephropathy, renal artery stenosis, hypertension
- **Haematological:** thrombocytopenia, haemolytic anaemia
- **Neurological:** migraine, epilepsy, chorea. Some cases of APS may have been misdiagnosed as multiple sclerosis[11]
- **Psychiatric:** depression, cognitive impairment, vascular dementia[11]
- **Dermatological:** leg ulcers, distal gangrene, livedo reticularis (present in 25% of APS patients)[12]

This thrombotic disease can manifest in several forms detailed below.

Primary Antiphospholipid Syndrome (PAPS)

This syndrome occurs in isolation[13] and manifests as one of:

- Arterial or venous thrombo-embolic disease
- Three or more consecutive miscarriages prior to 10 weeks gestation
- Unexplained loss of a normal fetus >10 weeks gestation
- Premature birth prior to 34 weeks gestation due to pre-eclampsia or placental insufficiency
- In the presence of the laboratory findings detailed above

Secondary Antiphospholipid Syndrome (SAPS)

This condition is associated with infection or autoimmune disease, especially SLE[8,13] and thrombocytopenia[14]. It manifests as above.

Catastrophic Antiphospholipid Syndrome (CAPS)

This is rare, but develops rapidly, with small vessel thrombosis causing multi-organ failure, deep vein thombosis (DVT), pulmonary embolism and stroke, resulting in a high mortality rate[15]. In 50% of cases patients had PAPS and 45% SLE[15]. Six per cent of cases present in pregnancy or the puerperium[16].

There are other clinical manifestations of APS, including livedo reticularis (see Figure 11.4.1), migraine (Chapter 8.1), valvular heart disease (Chapter 4.4) and haemolytic anaemia (Chapter 14).

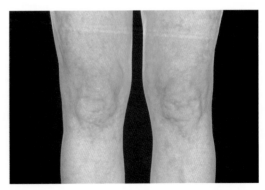

Figure 11.4.1 Livedo reticularis is characterised by persistent patchy reddish-blue mottling of the legs that is exacerbated by cold (Adebajo, 2009). This figure is downloadable from the book companion website at www.wiley.com/go/robson

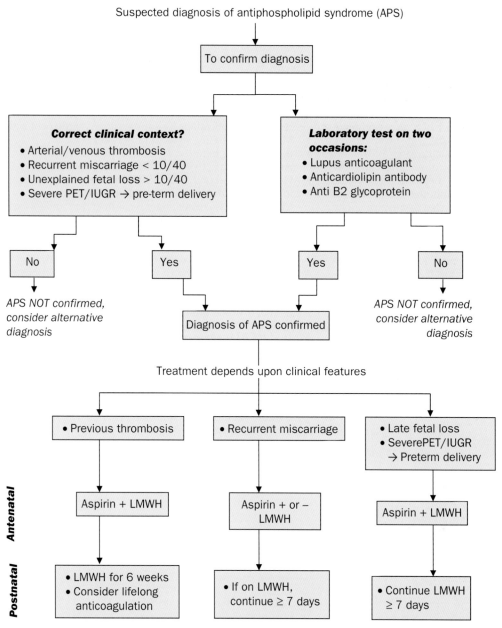

Figure 11.4.2 Antiphospholipid syndrome and pregnancy. PET, pre-eclampsia toxaemia. IUGR, intrauterine growth retardation. LMWH, low molecular weight heparin. This figure is downloadable from the book companion website at www.wiley.com/go/robson

NON-PREGNANCY TREATMENT AND CARE

Medical Treatment

Treatment of anti-phospholipid syndrome outside pregnancy aims to prevent thrombosis and its subsequent complications. The type of treatment depends on whether the patient requires primary or secondary thromboprophylaxis and may include the following:

- Daily aspirin
- Low molecular weight heparin *sc* injection
- Warfarin tablets

Patients with previous thrombosis might require life-long anti-coagulation[1].

PRE-CONCEPTION ISSUES AND CARE

- Women with a previous history of the following conditions should be offered screening for antiphospholipid antibodies prior to pregnancy: SLE, thrombosis, recurrent early miscarriages, severe intra-uterine growth restriction, early onset pre-eclampsia, intra-uterine death or premature delivery associated with IUGR. Figure 11.4.2

gives a management algorithm for suspected APS diagnosis

- Women known to have APS should ideally be referred to a multidisciplinary team with expertise in the condition for pre-conception counselling. This allows assessment and discussion of the risks of pregnancy, and planning of pregnancy care.
- Women with APS should be informed of their individual risk of the following pregnancy complications:
  - thrombosis
  - stroke
  - pre-eclampsia
  - IUGR
  - placental abruption
  - miscarriage
  - pre-term delivery and consequent neonatal morbidity[6]
- Confirm antibody levels[6]
- Assess for anaemia, thrombocytopenia, SLE and underlying renal disease[6]
- Advise aspirin (75 mg) pre- and post-conception
- Commence low molecular weight heparin, if required, with a positive pregnancy test
- Discontinue warfarin and commence low molecular weight heparin, as warfarin is teratogenic in the first trimester of pregnancy[6]

Pregnancy Issues
- Untreated APS increases the risk of adverse obstetric outcomes
- Women with thrombotic APS have higher rates of pregnancy complications than those with obstetric APS[5]
- The rate of fetal loss is directly related to the antibody titre[6]
- Untreated the chance of a successful pregnancy is around 20%, with treatment the chance of a live birth increases to 70–80%[6]
- Treatment with low dose aspirin and low molecular weight heparin (LMWH) is recommended[16] although some recent studies have suggested that aspirin alone is as effective at improving successful pregnancy outcome for some groups of women[17,18]
- Those treated are still susceptible to pre-eclampsia and IUGR[19], and thrombocytopenia may worsen[6]
- Although rare, catastrophic APS can be triggered by infection, anticoagulation withdrawal, surgery, neoplasia and lupus 'flares' in pregnancy or the puerperium[16]
- Warfarin is avoided in the first trimester as it is teratogenic, and second/third trimester use should be justified on clinical grounds[6]

Additional Complications[6,7,20,21]:
- IUGR
- Placental abruption
- Thrombosis in any organ or tissue
- Pre-eclampsia
- HELLP syndrome
- Local bruising from injection sites
- Treatment side effects – e.g. rare osteoporosis risk with LMWH

Medical Management and Care
- Regular review in high risk obstetric clinic, including input from obstetrician, physician, haematologist and anaesthetist
- See Figure 11.4.2 for the management algorithm
- Early dating scan[6], and regular/serial scans to detect IUGR
- Uterine artery waveforms[6] at 20 and 24 weeks – if normal consider cessation of heparin (if no previous history of thrombosis)
- Aspirin and/or LMWH to improve pregnancy outcome (heparin reduces complications by suppressing complement action[25])
- Monitor closely for signs of pre-eclampsia
- Blood tests as required – FBC and platelet count
- Anti-factor Xa activity may be monitored to adjust LMWH dose
- Heparin, or second/third trimester warfarin, to prevent thrombosis in women with previous thrombotic complications
- Corticosteroids are no longer recommended[6] unless a co-existing condition such as ITP or SLE necessitates their use
- Immunoglobulin, as IVIG, might be tried in specialist centres[6] for women with previously poor outcomes on aspirin and LMWH
- Prompt identification and treatment of infection
- Counselling about the prognosis of pregnancy, potential for further medical complications and chance of pre-term delivery
- Discuss and initiate an intrapartum care plan with the mother and members of the multi-disciplinary team

Midwifery Management and Care
- An accurate booking history should be taken, and the mother booked for care at a consultant unit with specialist maternal medicine clinics
- Midwives need to understand the condition to collaborate with doctors in explanations, care planning, or to support potentially grieving parents
- Educate mothers to self-administer heparin injections correctly and encourage them to persevere with therapy
- Encourage regular clinic attendance, with close surveillance of blood pressure and urinalysis to detect pre-eclampsia promptly[6]
- Get the mother fitted for TED stockings in readiness for labour
- Mother to have midwifery contact within a high-risk clinic situation

Labour Issues
- There is a risk of intrapartum fetal asphyxia, particularly if pre-eclampsia or IUGR present[22]
- Women who are admitted in spontaneous labour, or for a planned delivery, will have been advised to omit their LMWH injection at the onset of contractions to avoid the problem of having an anticoagulant effect at the time of delivery and facilitate the use of epidural anaesthesia
- Aspirin in pregnancy does not affect intrapartum use of regional anaesthesia[6]

Medical Management and Care
- Omit heparin to allow for regional analgesia
- Advise continuous CTG monitoring

Midwifery Management and Care
- Ensure that the woman is seen by an anaesthetist early in labour
- Ensure adequate hydration and IVI may be necessary
- TED stockings throughout labour
- Encourage mobility and leg care
- Continuous fetal heart monitoring
- Active management of third stage
- Competent, prompt suturing of perineal tears or episiotomy

Postpartum Issues
- The effect of maternal APS on the neonate is debated and APS itself is rare in neonates[23] hence some centres recommend paediatric follow-up until transplacentally-acquired antibodies are undetectable[24]
- The postpartum period is a risk time for thrombosis for normal mothers, and the risk is increased with APS
- The baby might be admitted to a neonatal care unit if small for gestational age or pre-term

Medical Management and Care
- Those previously on long-term warfarin need this recommenced and LWMH stopped once the international normalised ratio is >2.0[26]
- Mothers with previous thrombosis need heparin or warfarin for 6 weeks[26]
- Mothers without previous thrombosis need heparin for at least 7 days[27]
- Avoid COCP because of thrombo-embolic risk[28]

Midwifery Management and Care
- Liaise with multidisciplinary team because not all mothers are for early discharge
- Be alert for thrombosis or catastrophic APS, and encourage early mobilisation
- Advise that it is safe to breast-feed on warfarin or heparin therapy having first conferred with the paediatrician and or pharmacist
- Additional support is needed for the mother and partner if the baby is on NNU
- Ensure relevant maternal and neonatal follow-up appointments have been made prior to discharge, and that above anti-coagulants have been obtained to take out

11 Autoimmune Disorders

PATIENT ORGANISATIONS

American College of Rheumatology
1800 Century Place, Suite 250
Atlanta, GA 30345, USA
www.rheumatology.org

ARC–Arthritis Research Campaign
www.arc.org.uk

Australian Rheumatology Association
145 Macquarie Street
Sydney NSW 2000
www.rheumatology.org.au

Arthritis Care
18 Stephenson Way
London NW1 2HD
http://www.arthritiscare.org.uk

Arthritis Foundation
PO Box 7669
Atlanta, GA 30357-0669, USA
www.arthritis.org

Hughes Syndrome Foundation
Louise Coote Lupus Unit
Gassiot House
St Thomas's Hospital
London SE1 7EH
www.hughes-syndrome.org

Lupus UK
St James House
Eastern Road
Romford
Essex RM1 3NH
www.lupusuk.com

NRAS – National Rheumatoid Arthritis Society
11 College Avenue
Maidenhead
Berkshire SL6 6AR
www.rheumatoid.org.uk

Raynaud's and Scleroderma Association Trust
112 Crewe Road
Alsagar
Cheshire ST7 2JA
www.raynauds.org.uk

St Thomas's Lupus Trust
St Thomas's Hospital
London SE1 7EH
www.lupus.org.uk

ESSENTIAL READING

Adebajo A 2010 **ABC of Rheumatology**, 4th Edn. Oxford; BMJ Books/Wiley-Blackwell

Barwich A 2004 **Lupus - A Guide for Nurses and other Health Professionals**. Romford: Lupus UK

Greer I, Nelson-Piercy C and Walters B 2007 **Maternal Medicine: Medical Problems in Pregnancy**. London; Elsevier

Hakim A, Clunie G and Haq I (2006) **Oxford Handbook of Rheumatology**, 2nd Edn. Oxford; Oxford University Press

Hughes G 2001 **Hughes Syndrome – A patient's guide**. London; Springer

Isaacs J and Moreland L 2011 **Fast facts: Rheumatoid Arthritis**. 2nd Edn. Oxford; Health Press

Isenberg D and Morrow J 1995 **Friendly Fire: Explaining Autoimmune Disease**. Oxford; Oxford University Press

Khare M and Nelson-Piercy C 2003 Acquired thrombophilias and pregnancy. **Best Practice and Research in Obstetrics and Gynaecology**, 17:491–507

Lupus UK 2012 **Lupus: A Guide to Pregnancy**. Romford: Lupus UK. Also 16 other factsheets direct from Lupus UK. www.medical.lupusuk.org.uk

Moots R and Jones N 2004 **Your Questions Answered: Rheumatoid Arthritis**. London; Churchill Livingstone

Norton Y 2009 **Lupus: Diagnosis and Treament**. Romford; Lupus UK. Direct from Lupus UK. www.medical.lupusuk.org.uk

Ostensen M and 28 authors 2006 Anti-inflammatory and immunosuppressive drugs and reproduction. **Arthritis Research & Therapy**, 8:209–228

http://arthritis-research.com/content/8/3/209

http://www.bnf.org

http://www.prodigy.nhs.uk

http://www.raynauds.demon.co.uk

References

11.1 Rheumatoid Arthritis

1. Symmons DP 2005 Looking back – aetiology, occurrence and mortality. **Rheumatology (Oxford)**, 44(Suppl.4):iv 14–17
2. Tobon GJ, Youinou P and Saraux A 2009 The environment, geo-epidemiology, and autoimmune disease: Rheumatoid Arthritis. **Autoimmunity Reviews**, doi.10.1016/j.autrev.2009.11.019
3. Clowse M, Petri M and James A 2010 Rheumatologic disorders in pregnancy, in **De Swiet's Medical Disorders in Obstetric Practice** 5th Edn. Oxford; Wiley-Blackwell 209–221
4. Isaacs JD and Moreland LW 2009 **Fast Facts – Rheumatoid Arthritis**. Oxford; Health Press Ltd 23–36
5. Hakim A, Clunie G and Haq I 2006 **Oxford Handbook of Rheumatology**, 2nd Edn. Oxford; Oxford University Press 256
6. Kinder AJ 2006 **Consultant rheumatologist at University Hospitals of Leicester – Personal communication on 16 May**
7. Silman A and Oliver J 2010 Epidemiology of rheumatic diseases in Adebajo A (Ed.) **ABC of Rheumatology**, 4th Edn. Oxford: BMJ Books/Wiley-Blackwell 167–170
8. Colebatch AN and Edwards CJ 2010 The influence of early life factors on the risk of developing rheumatoid arthritis. **Clinical and Experimental Immunology**, 163;11–16
9. Soderlin M, Bergsten U and Svennsson B 2011 Patient reported events preceding the onset of rheumatoid arthritis: possible clues to aetiology. **Musculoskeletal Care**, 9:25–31
10. Silman AJ and Pearson JE 2002 Epidemiology and genetics of rheumatoid arthritis. **Arthritis Research and Therapy**, 4(Suppl.3):265–272
11. Wallenius M, Skomsvoll J, Salvesen K, *et al.* 2010 Postpartum onset of rheumatoid arthritis and other chronic arthritides: results from a patient register linked to medical birth registry. **Annals of Rheumatic Disease**, 69:332–336
12. Scott DL 2002 The diagnosis and prognosis of early arthritis: rationale for new prognostic criteria. **Arthritis and Rheumatism** 46:286–290
13. Packham JC and Hall MA 2002 Long-term follow-up of 246 juvenile idiopathic arthritis: social function, relationships and sexual activity. **Rheumatology (Oxford)**, 41:1440–1443
14. Nell VP, Machold KP, Eberl G, Stamm TA, Uffmann M and Smolen JS 2004 Benefit of very early referral and very early therapy with disease-modifying anti-rheumatic drugs in patients with early rheumatoid arthritis. **Rheumatology**, 43:906–914
15. Wise EM and Issacs JD 2005 Management of rheumatoid arthritis in primary care – an educational need. **Rheumatology**, 44: 1337–1338
16. Clowse M 2010 Managing contraception and pregnancy in the rheumatologic diseases. **Best Practice and Research Clinical Rheumatology**, 24:373–385
17. Ernst E 2004 Musculoskeletal conditions and complementary/alternative medicine. **Best Practice and Research: Clinical Rheumatology**, 18:539–556
18. Denny J, Troy FP and Branch W 2011 Autoimmune Diseases in **High Risk Pregnancy Management Options**, 4th Edn. London; Elsevier 783–786
19. Silman A 2006 **Pregnancy and Arthritis: An information booklet**. Arthritis and Rheumatism Campaign www.arc.org.uk/about_arth/booklets/6060/6060.htm [Accessed 26-2-06]
20. Kinder AJ, Edwards J, Samanta A and Nichol F 2004 Pregnancy in a rheumatoid arthritis patient on infliximab and methotrexate. **Rheumatology (Oxford)**, 43:1195–1196
21. Borchers A, Naguwa S, Keen C and Gershwin ME 2010 The implications of autoimmunity and pregnancy. **Journal of Autoimmunity**, 34:287–299
22. Barron WM and Lindheimer MD 2000 **Medical Disorders During Pregnancy**, 3rd Edn. London; Mosby-Harcourt 375–376
23. Yee C-S, Gordon C and Khamashta M 2007 Immunological diseases in Greer A, Nelson-Piercy and Walters B (Eds) **Maternal Medicine: Medical Problems in Pregnancy**. London; Elsevier
24. Shepherd AA 2006 Nutrition and rheumatoid arthritis. **Complete Nutrition**, 6:16–18
25. Robson SE and Hodgett S 2008 Autoimmune disorders in Robson SE and Waugh J (Eds) **Medical Disorders in Pregnancy: A Manual For Midwives**. Oxford; Blackwell Publishing Ltd. 138–139

11.2 Raynaud's Phenomenon

1. Suter LG, Murabito JM, Felson DT and Fraenkel L 2005 The incidence and natural history of Raynaud's phenomenon in the community. **Arthritis and Rheumatism**, 52, 1259–1263
2. Denton CP and Black C 2010 Chapt. 19 Raynaud's phenomenon and scleroderma in Adebajo A (Ed.) **ABC of Rheumatology**, 4th Edn. Oxford; BMJ Books/Wiley-Blackwell 123–128
3. Silman A, Holligan S, Brennan P and Maddison P 1990 Prevalence of Raynaud's Phenomenon in general practice. **BMJ**, 301:590–592
4. Palmer K, Griffin M, Syddall H, Pannett B, Cooper C and Coggon D 2000 Prevalence of Raynaud's phenomenon in Great Britain and its relation to hand transmitted vibration: a national postal survey. **Occupational and Environmental Medicine**, 57:448–452
5. Block JA and Sequeira W 2001 Raynaud's phenomenon. **Lancet**, 357(9273):2042–2048
6. Herrick A 2005 Pathogenesis of Raynaud's Phenomenon. **Rheumatology**, 44:587–596
7. Cooke J and Marshall J 2005 Mechanisms of Raynaud's disease. **Vascular Medicine**, 10:293–307
8. Chikura B, Moore T, Manning J, Vail A and Herrick A 2008 Sparing of the thumb in Raynaud's phenomenon. **Rheumatology**, 47;219–221
9. Black C 2008 **Raynaud's and Scleroderma: An update for the GP**. Alsagar, Raynaud's and Scleroderma Association. www.raynauds.org.uk
10. Hirschl M, Hirschl K, Lenz M *et al.* 2006 Transition from primary Raynaud's phenomenon to secondary Raynaud's phenomenon identified by diagnosis of an associated disease: results of 10 years of prospective surveillance. **Arthritis and Rheumatism**, 54:1974–1981
11. Palesch YY, Valter I, Carpentier PH and Maricq HR 1999 Association between cigarette and alcohol consumption and Raynaud's phenomenon. **Journal of Clinical Epidemiology**, 52:321–328
12. Suter LG, Murabito JM, Felson DT and Fraenkel L 2007 Smoking, alcohol consumption, and Raynaud's phenomenon in middle age. **American Journal of Medicine**, 120:264–271
13. Brown K, Middaugh S, Haythornthwaite J and Bielroy L 2001 The effect of stress, anxiety and outdoor temperature on the frequency and severity of Raynaud's attacks: the Raynaud's Treatment Study. **Journal of Behavioural Medicine**, 24:137–153
14. Herrick A and Jayson M 1991 Primary Raynaud's Phenomenon in early childhood. **British Journal of Rheumatology**, 30: 223–225
15. Nigrovic PA, Fuhlbrigge RC and Sundel RP 2003 Raynaud's phenomenon in children: a retrospective review of 123 patients. **Pediatrics**, 111, 715–721
16. Kone-Paut I, Olivar E, Elbhar C, Garnier JM and Berbis P 2002 Raynaud's disease in children: a study of 23 cases. **Archives de Pediatrie**, 9:365–370
17. Planchon B, Pistorius MA, Beurrier P and De Faucal P 1994 Primary Raynaud's Phenomenon: age of onset and pathogenesis in a prospective study of 424 patients. **Angiography**, 45:677–686
18. Wigley F 2002 Raynaud's Phenomenon. **New England Journal of Medicine**, 347:1001–1008

19. Freedman R and Mayes M 1996 Familial aggregation of primary Raynaud's Disease. **Arthritis and Rheumatism**, 39:118–1191

20. Brand F, Larson M, Kannel W and McGuirk J 1997 The occurence of Raynaud's phenomenon in a general population: the Framlingham study. **Vascular Medicine**, 2:296–301

21. O'Keeffe S, Tsapatsaris N and Beetham W 1992 Increased prevalence of migraine and chest pain in patients with primary Raynaud Disease. **Annals of Internal Medicine**, 116:985–989

22. Carpentier PH, Satger B, Poensin D and Maricq HR 2006 Incidence and natural history of Raynaud phenomenon: a long-term follow-up (14 years) of a random sample from the general population. **Journal of Vascular Surgery**, 44:1023–1028

23. Garcia-Carrasco M, Jimenez-Hernandez M, Escarcega RO *et al.* 2008 Treatment of Raynaud's phenomenon. **Autoimmunity Reviews**, 8:62–68

24. Ziegler S, Brunner M, Eigenbauer E and Minar E 2003 Long-term outcome of primary Raynaud's phenomenon and its conversion to connective tissue disease: a 12-year retrospective patient analysis. **Scandinavian Journal of Rheumatology**, 32:343–347

25. Artlett CM, Rasheed M, Russo-Stieglitz KE, Sawaya HHB and Jimenez SA 2002 Influence of prior pregnancies on disease course and cause of death in systemic sclerosis. **Annals of the Rheumatic Diseases**, 61:346–350

26. Hakim A, Clunie G and Haq I 2006 **Oxford Handbook of Rheumatology**. Oxford; Oxford University Press

27. Spencer-Green G 1998 Outcomes of primary Raynaud Phenomenon. **Archives of Internal Medicine**, 158:595–600

28. Raynaud's and Scleroderma Association 2011 http://www.raynauds.org.uk/raynauds/coping-with-raynauds [Accessed 27-2-2011]

29. Nelson-Piercy C 2002 **Handbook of Obstetric Medicine**. London; Martin Dunitz 151–153

30. Coad J 2001 **Anatomy and Physiology for Midwives**. London; Mosby 233

31. Muir AH, Robb R, McLaren M *et al.* 2002 The use of Ginkgo biloba in Raynaud's disease: a double-blind placebo-controlled trial. **Vascular Medicine**, 7:265–267

32. Kahl LE, Blair C, Ramsey-Goldman R and Steen VD 1990 Pregnancy outcomes in women with primary Raynaud's phenomenon. **Arthritis and Rheumatism**, 33:1249–1255

33. Hardwick JCR, McMurtrie F and Melrose EB 2002 Raynaud's syndrome of the nipple in pregnancy. **European Journal of Obstetrics and Reproductive Biology**, 102:217–218

34. Lawlor-Smith L and Lawlor-Smith C 1997 Vasospasm of the nipple – a manifestation of Raynaud's phenomenon: case reports. **British Medical Journal**, 314:644

35. Anderson JE, Held N and Wright K 2004 Raynaud's phenomenon of the nipple: a treatable cause of painful breast-feeding. **Pediatrics**, 113:360–364

36. Robson SE and Hodgett S 2008 Raynaud's Phenomenon in Robson SE and Waugh J (Eds) **Medical Disorders in Pregnancy: A Manual For Midwives**. Oxford; Blackwell Publishing Ltd. 140–141

37. BSSA 2003 **Sjogren's Syndrome – A Concise Guide to Diagnosis and Management for Health Care Professionals**. British Sjogren's Association

11.3 Systemic Lupus Erythematosus

1. O'Neill S and Cervera R 2010 Systemic lupus erythematosus. Best practice and research. **Clinical Rheumatology**, 24:841–855

2. Gordon C and Ramsey-Goldman R 2010 Chapt. 18 Systemic lupus erythematosus and lupus-like syndromes in Adebajo A (Ed.) **ABC of Rheumatology**, 4th Edn. Oxford; BMJ Books/ Wiley-Blackwell 114–122

3. Lupus UK 2011 **Factsheet: Lupus – The skin and Hair**. Romford; Lupus UK

4. Jessop S, Whitelaw D and Jordaan F 2000 Drugs for discoid lupus erythematosus. **The Cochrane Database of Systematic Reviews**. Issue 2. Art.No.:CD002954.DOI:10.1002/14651858

5. Hughes GRV 2011 **The Diagnosis to Lupus**. Romford; Lupus UK

6. Higgins C 2007 **Understanding Laboratory Investigations**. 2nd Edn. Oxford; Blackwell Publishing Ltd.

7. Kumar P and Clarke M 2004 **Clinical Medicine**, 5th Edn. London; Saunders 557–560

8. Hakim A, Clunie G and Haq I 2006 **Oxford Handbook of Rheumatology**. Oxford; Oxford University Press 322–340

9. Rahman A and Isenberg DA 2008 Systemic lupus erythematosus. **New England Journal of Medicine**, 358:929–939

10. Sofat N, Malik O and Higgens CS 2006 Neurological involvement in patients with rheumatic disease. **Quarterly Journal of Medicine**, 99:69–79

11. Puandare KN, Wagle AC and Parker SR 1999 Psychiatric morbidity in patients with systemic lupus erythematosus. **Quarterly Journal of Medicine**, 92:283–286

12. Ostensen M 2004 New insights into sexual functioning and fertility in rheumatic diseases. **Best Practice and Research: Clinical Rheumatology**, 18:219–232

13. Denny J, Troy FP and Branch W 2011 Autoimmune diseases in **High Risk Pregnancy Management Options** 4th Edn. London; Elsevier 783–786

14. Lupus UK 2011 **Factsheet: Lupus and Pregnancy**. Romford: Lupus UK

15. Burrow GN, Duffy GN and Copel JA 2004 **Medical Complications During Pregnancy**, 6th Edn. Philadelphia; Elsevier Saunders 432–438

16. Stratta P, Canavese C and Quaglia M 2006 Pregnancy in patients with kidney disease. **Journal of Nephrology**, 19:135–142

17. Imbasciati E, Tincani A, Gregorini G, *et al.* 2009 Pregnancy in women with pre-existing lupus nephritis: predictors of fetal and maternal outcome. **Nephrology Dialysis Transplantation**, 24:519–525

18. Clowse M, Petri M and James A 2010 Rheumatologic disorders in pregnancy, in **De Swiet's Medical Disorders in Obstetric Practice** 5th Edn. Oxford; Wiley-Blackwell 209–221

19. Ruiz–Irastoraz G, Khamashta MA, Castinellio G and Hughes GRV 2001 Systemic lupus erythematosus. **Lancet**, 357(9261): 1027–1032

20. Barron WM and Lindheimer MD 2000 **Medical Disorders During Pregnancy**, 3rd Edn. London; Mosby 360–374

21. Yee C, Gordon C, Khamashata M, Foster R and D'Cruz D 2007 Chapt. 10 Connective tissue diseases in Greer I, Nelson-Piercy C and Walters B (Eds) **Maternal Medicne: Medical Problems in Pregnancy**. London; Elsevier 191–205

22. Shonohara K, Miyagawa S, Fujita T, *et al.* 1999 Neonatal lupus erythematosus: results of maternal corticosteroid therapy. **Obstetrics and Gynaecology**, 93:952–957

23. Costedoat-Chalumeau N, Amoura Z, Thi Hong DL, *et al.* 2003 Questions about dexamethasone use for prevention of anti-SSA related congenital heart block. **Annals of Rheumatic Diseases**, 62:1010–1012

24. Robson SE and Hodgett S 2008 Autoimmune disorders in Robson SE and Waugh J (Eds) **Medical Disorders in Pregnancy: A Manual For Midwives**. Oxford; Blackwell Publishing Ltd. 142–143

11.4 Antiphospholipid (Hughes) Syndrome

1. Petrie M 2000 Epidemiology of the Antiphospholipid Antibody Syndrome. **Journal of Autoimmunity**, 15:145–151

2. Mok CC, Tang SSK, To CH, *et al.* 2005 Incidence and risk factors of thromboembolism in systemic lupus erythematosus: a comparison of three ethnic groups. **Arthritis and Rheumatism**, 52:2774–2782

3. RCOG 2003 **Guideline No.17: The Investigation and Treatment of Couples with Recurrent Miscarriage**. London; Royal College of Obstetricians and Gynaecologists. 4.5.2

4. Hughes 1984 Autoantibodies in lupus and its variants: experience in 1000 patients. **British Medical Journal**, 289(6441): 339–342

5. Bramham K, Hunt BJ, Germain S, *et al.* 2010 Pregnancy outcome in different clinical phenotypes of antiphospholipis syndrome. **Lupus**, 19:58–64

6. Khare M and Nelson-Piercy C 2003 Acquired thrombophilias and pregnancy. **Best Practice and Research in Obstetrics and Gynaecology**, 17:491–507

7. Branch DW and Khamashata MA 2003 Antiphospholipid syndrome: obstetric diagnosis, management and controversies. **Obstetrics and Gynaecology**, 101:1333–1344

8. Ruiz-Irastorza G, Crowther M, Branch W and Khamashata M 2010 Antiphospholipid syndrome. **Lancet**, 376:1498–1509

9. Miyakis S, Lockshin MD, Atsumi T, *et al.* 2006 International consensus statement on an update of the classification criteria for definite antiphospholipid syndrome (APS). **Journal of Thrombosis and Haemostasis**, 4:295–306

10. McMillan E, Martin WL, Waugh J, *et al.* 2002 Management of pregnancy in women with pulmonary hypertension secondary to SLE and anti-phospholipid syndrome. **Lupus** 11:392–398

11. Sanna G, Bertolaccini ML and Khamashta MA 2006 Unusual clinical manifestations of the antiphospholipid syndrome. **Current Rheumatology Reviews**, 2:387–394

12. Frances C, Niang S, Laffitte E, *et al.* 2005 Dermatologic manifestations of the antiphospholipid syndrome: two hundred consecutive cases. **Arthritis and Rheumatism**, 52:1785–1793

13. Nimmo MC and Carter CJ 2003 The antiphospholipid syndrome: a riddle wrapped in a mystery inside an enigma. **Clinical and Applied Immunology Reviews**, 4:125–140

14. Bidot CJ, Wenche J, Lawrence L, *et al.* 2004 Antiphospholipid antibodies in immune thrombocytopenic purpura tend to emerge in exacerbation and decline in remission. **British Journal of Haematology**, 128:366–371

15. Asherson RA 2006 New subsets of the antiphospholipid syndrome in 2006: Pre-APS (probable APS) microangiopathic anti phospholipid syndrome (MAPS). **Rheumatologia**, 20:119–129

16. Tenedios F, Erkan D and Lockshin MD 2006 Cardiac manifestations in the antiphospholipid syndrome. **Rheumatic Disease Clinics of North America**, 32:491–507

17. Laskin CA, Spitzer KA, Clark CA *et al.* 2009 Low molecular weight heparin and aspirin for recurrent pregnancy loss: results from the randomised controlled HepASA trial. **Journal of Rheumatology**, 36:279–287

18. Farquharson RG, Quenby S, Greaves M 2002 Antiphospholipid syndrome in pregnancy: a randomised controlled trial of treatment. **Obstetrics and Gynaecology**, 100:408–413

19. Carbillon L, Sauvet M, Fain O and Aurousseau 2005 Letter. **Journal of Reproductive Immunology**, 65:89–90

20. Tincani A, Branch W, Piette JC, *et al.* 2003 Treatment of pregnant patients with antiphospholipid syndrome. **Lupus**, 12:524–529

21. Miesbach W, Glizinger A, Gokpinar B, Claus D and Scharrer I 2006 Prevalence of antiphospholipid antibodies in patients with neurological symptoms. **Clinical Neurology and Neurosurgery**, 108:135–142

22. Shehata HA and Nelson-Piercy C 2001 Connective tissue diseases in pregnancy. **Current Obstetrics and Gynaecology**, 11:329–335

23. Cimez R and Descloux E 2006 Pediatric antiphospholipid syndrome. **Rheumatic Disease Clinics of North America**, 32:553–573

24. Motta M, Tincani A, Locjacono A, *et al.* 2004 Neonatal outcome in patients with rheumatic disease. **Lupus**, 13:718–723

25. Girardi G, Redecha P and Salmon JE 2004 Heparin prevents anti phospholipid syndrome antibody-induced fetal loss by inhibiting complement activation. **Nature Medicine**, 10:1222–1226

26. Nelson-Piercy C 2002 **Handbook of Obstetric Medicine**. London; Martin Dunitz 146–151

27. RCOG 2009 **Green Top Guideline No.37a Thrombosis and Embolism during Pregnancy and the Puerperium, Reducing the Risk**. London; Royal College of Obstetricians and Gynaecologists

28. Lakasing L and Khamashta M 2001 Contraceptive practices in women with systemic lupus erythematosus and/or antiphospholipid syndrome: what advice should we be giving? **British Journal of Family Planning**, 27:7–12

Figure Reference

Adebajo A 2009 **ABC of Rheumatology**, 4th Edn. Oxford; BMJ Books/Wiley-Blackwell

Appendix References

1. Ostensen M, Khamashta M, Lockshin M, *et al.* 2006 Anti-inflammatory and immunosuppressive drugs and reproduction. **Arthritis Research and Therapy**, 8:209–228 http://arthritis–research.com/content/8/3/209

2. Briggs GG, Freeman RK and Yaffe SJ 2011 **Drugs in Pregnancy and Lactation**, 8th Edn. Philadelphia; Lippincott

3. BNF 2010 **British National Formulary**. Issue 60 http://www.bnf.org/bnf/ [Accessed 20-12-2010]

4. Weiner CP and Buhimschi C 2009 **Drugs for Pregnant and Lactating Women**,2nd edn. London; Churchill Livingstone

5. MIMS 2010 **Monthly Index of Medical Specialities (October)**. London; Haymarket Medical Publications

6. Khare M, Lott J and Howarth E 2003 Is it safe to continue azathioprine in breast feeding mothers? **Journal of Obstetrics and Gynaecology**, 23(Suppl. 1).S53

7. Sau A, Clarke S, Bass J, *et al.* 2007 Azathioprine and breastfeeding – is it safe? **British Journal of Obstetrics and Gynaecology**, 114:498–501

8. Prodigy 2006 www.prodigy.nhs.uk/pk.uk/raynauds_phenomenon/extended_information/management_issues [Accessed 16-05-2006]

9. NTIS 2006 **Exposure to Nifedipine during Pregnancy**. National Teratology Information Service, Regional Drug and Therapeutics Centre

Appendix 11.1.1 Drugs for Autoimmune Disease – An Overview for Midwives

This table gives midwives an **overview** of autoimmune drug use at different pregnancy stages. These drugs are prescribed, by a doctor, in pregnancy, if the expected benefit to the mother outweighs any effect upon the fetus.

Type of Drug	Name	RISK		Notes
		Pregnancy	Breast-feeding	
NSAIDs Non-steroidal anti-inflammatory drugs to control symptoms	Aspirin – low dose	Safe[1]	Safe[1]	Aspirin does not cross the placenta, and single use is considered safe in breastfeeding[1–5]
	Aspirin – standard	C	Potential toxicity Use with caution[2]	
	Ibruprofen (Brufen, Nurofen)	B	Compatible[2]	Regular use with children is associated with Reye's syndrome[3,6]
	Naproxen (Naprosyn)	B	Probably compatible[2]	*Regular* NSAID use in third trimester is associated with fetal:
	Indometacin (Indomod)	B	Probably compatible[2]	• ductus arteriosus constriction[1]
	Phenylacetic acid (Diclofenac)	B	Probably compatible[2]	• impaired renal function[1] Breast-feeding *prior* to a maternal dose
	Ketocid (Ketoprofen)	B	Probably compatible[2]	minimises infant exposure[1]
DMARDs Disease-modifying anti-rheumatic drugs to modify disease	Azathioprine (Imuran)	D	Potential toxicity[2] Human/animal data suggest risk[2]	Transplant patients continue use[3] Pregnancy dosage ≤2 mg/kg/day[1] Evidence is emerging for breast-feeding use based on a risk–benefit analysis[6,7]
	Ciclosporin (Neoral)	C	Potential toxicity[2] Limited risk data[2]	Use in pregnancy to be supervised by specialist clinic Present in breast milk[1,3]
	Gold (Myocrisin, Ridaura)	C	Probably compatible[2]	Prolonged elimination time in breast milk[2]
	Hydroxychloroquine (Plaquenil)	C	Compatible[2]	Use in pregnancy to be supervised by specialist clinic[3]
	Leflunomide (Arava)	X	Potential toxicity[2] Contraindicated[2]	Pregnancy should not be attempted until plasma level ≤0.02 mg[3–5]
	Methotrexate (Maxtrex)	X	Toxicity reported[2] Contraindicated[2]	Avoid pregnancy for ≥3 months after ceasing treatment[3] Folate supplements required throughout pregnancy[1]
	Penicillamine (Distamine)	D	Potential toxicity[2] Limited risk data[2]	Fetal anomalies found in rodents[4] Continue use in second and third trimesters with Wilson's disease[2,4]
	Sulfasalazine (Salazopyrin)	B	Limited data[2] Use with caution[2]	Theoretical risk of neonatal haemolysis, so folate supplements are required[1,3–5]
TNF Tumour necrosis factor to inhibit immune response	Etanercept (Enbrel)	B	Limited data[2] Probably compatible[2]	Limited data so most advise avoidance or caution with use in pregnancy
	Infliximab (Remicade)	C	Limited data[2] Contraindicated[2]	Avoid pregnancy for ≥6 months after ceasing treatment[1,3–5] Manufacturer advises against use in breast-feeding[2]
Steroids to reduce inflammation	Prednisolone (Deltacortril)	C	Compatible[2]	Neonate unaffected if maternal dose ≤40 mg daily Benefit usually outweighs risk[1]
Vasodilators	Nifedipine (Adalat)	C	Limited data[2] Probably compatible[2]	Modified release version is preferred in pregnancy[8] Antenatal exposure is *not* grounds for invasive prenatal screening[9]

A, little or no risk (human studies)[2]; **B**, little risk (animal studies)[2]; **C**, some adverse effects (animal studies); used if benefit outweighs risk[2]; **D**, positive evidence of risk (human studies); used with serious conditions[2]; **X**, risk outweighs possible benefits, contraindicated in pregnancy[2]

Midwives: Mothers should be advised to continue with existing medication until a doctor with experience of prescribing such medications in pregnancy has been consulted, because sudden cessation of any medication without careful thought for substitution can be associated with a poor pregnancy outcome. This especially applies to mothers with renal transplants and systemic lupus erythematosus.

Doctors: This simple table cannot address factors for prescribing, and a more authoritative source **must** be used, e.g.:
- Weiner CP and Buhimschi C 2009 **Drugs for Pregnant and Lactating Women**, 2nd Edn. London; Churchill Livingstone
- Ostensen M, Khamashta M, Lockshin M *et al.* 2006 Anti-inflammatory and immunosuppressive drugs and reproduction. **Arthritis Research and Therapy**, 8:209–28. http://arthritis–research.com/content/8/3/209

INFECTIOUS CONDITIONS

Karen Watkins[1], Veronica Johnson-Roffey[2], Juliet Houghton[3] and S. Elizabeth Robson[4]

[1]The Royal Cornwall Hospital, Truro, UK
[2]Three Shires Hospital, Northampton, UK
[3]CHIVA/South Africa Support and Mentoring Initiative, Durban, South Africa
[4]De Montfort University, Leicester, UK

Medical Disorders in Pregnancy: A Manual for Midwives, Second Edition. Edited by S. Elizabeth Robson and Jason Waugh.
© 2013 John Wiley & Sons, Ltd. Published 2013 by John Wiley & Sons, Ltd.

S. E. Robson and J. Waugh

12.1 Viral Hepatitis

Incidence	Risk for Childbearing
Viral hepatitis C – estimated at 250–500 million worldwide Viral hepatitis B – over 350 million worldwide are carriers[1,2]	Variable Risk: *in utero* and peripartum transmission are both possible for hepatitis B and C

EXPLANATION OF CONDITION

Viral hepatitis describes a group of blood-borne viruses denoted as A, B, C, D or E, which can cause hepatocellular necrosis and inflammation (see Appendix 12.1.1). The infections can be either acute or chronic in nature. The most important of these to health workers are hepatitis B (HBV) and hepatitis C (HCV).

These viruses are found in blood, but can also be found in other bodily fluids (including semen and saliva). They are most commonly transmitted through unprotected sexual intercourse, by sharing injecting equipment or from a mother to her infant *in utero* or during delivery – known as vertical transmission. Breast-feeding poses a low risk if nipples are not cracked or bleeding[3].

Both viruses can lead to serious illness, including cirrhosis of the liver and even death, but this is more commonly seen with hepatitis B. Both infections may also resolve spontaneously and have no adverse effects[4,5].

Treatments for hepatitis B include interferon or lamivudine[6], but prevention of infection remains the primary aim and can usually be achieved through immunisation[7,8]. Prevention of infection with hepatitis B for the majority of newborns can be effectively instituted through immunisation commenced at birth[9]. There is no immunisation against hepatitis C, but new treatments are proving to be successful in eradicating the virus.

COMPLICATIONS

The key complication associated with hepatitis B is **chronic hepatitis**, the key features of which include:

- Chronic liver disease including:
  - spider naevi
  - finger clubbing
  - jaundice
  - hepatosplenomegaly and ascites
  - skin bruising[4]
- Liver cirrhosis
- Liver failure
- Hepatocellular carcinoma

Fulminant hepatitis is rare in hepatitis C infection[4,5], but occurs more commonly with co-infection with hepatitis A[10]. Vertical transmission (*in utero* or peripartum) is a complication for acutely infectious hepatitis B carriers, as, in this situation, over 90% of infants born to HBV infectious mothers will become chronic carriers unless immunised[8,11]. They then risk developing cirrhosis and hepatocellular carcinoma.

The risk of vertical transmission of hepatitis C infection is currently around 5–6%, and is related to the amount of hepatitis C virus the mother has in her bloodstream during pregnancy and delivery[12,13].

NON-PREGNANCY TREATMENT AND CARE

- All women with HCV or HBV require ongoing medical care to monitor for any progressing liver disease
- Women should be advised to stop or reduce alcohol consumption, and to avoid taking over-the-counter or herbal medicines without first seeking medical advice
- Women identified as HBV infected should be offered assessment and immunisation for previous and current sexual partners and close family contacts
- Barrier methods of contraception should be advocated until immunisation of the sexual partner is complete
- Detailed explanation of the condition should be given, with emphasis on routes of transmission
- Carriers should be advised not to donate blood or organs

There are now effective treatments for chronic hepatitis C, primarily the use of pegylated interferon in combination with ribavirin. This treatment is successful in clearing infection in up to 55% of patients[11].

Hepatitis B and acute hepatitis C are both notifiable diseases in the UK. Notification forms are completed by a doctor.

PRE-CONCEPTION ISSUES AND CARE

Any woman found to have either HBV or HCV should be advised to seek specialist opinion prior to conception, to ensure that she is in optimum health for pregnancy.

When a woman is known to have HBV prior to conception, it is important to identify whether she is chronically infected or acutely infectious. Those women in whom hepatitis B e-antigen (HBeAg) is detected are most infectious[6]. Those with antibody to HBeAg (anti-HBe) are generally of low infectivity.

Mothers should be counselled of the importance of immunisation of their newborn and, if they are HbeAg positive, the need for hepatitis B immunoglobulin (HBIG). It has been established that the administration of immunisation and HBIG in high risk infants reduces the vertical transmission risk by 90%[14,15]. There is no vaccine to prevent HCV infection.

- Women known to have HCV prior to conception should have their general health and lifestyle assessed (including liver function), and immunisation against hepatitis A and B should be offered
- Screening of sexual partners and existing children should be initiated
- Increasing migration to the UK from high prevalence countries is increasing the rates of hepatitis infections seen here
- Vaccination for hepatitis A and B are often required for travel to high prevalence countries and should be administered prior to pregnancy
- Vaccination differentials are outlined in Appendix 12.1.1

Pregnancy Issues
- All pregnant women are routinely screened for hepatitis B and this might be how it is first diagnosed
- Women deemed to be at higher risk for hepatitis C (i.e. partners of carriers, those from high prevalence areas, intravenous drug users and sex workers) should be tested for this and results clearly documented in maternity notes/hand-held records
- Women with a positive result should be counselled about the risk to sexual partners, other family members and their baby; written in formation should also be provided
- Consent for immunisation against hepatitis B (and the need for HBIG where appropriate) should be negotiated and agreed prior to delivery
- Vaccine (+/− HBIG) should be ordered in advance and stored in the labour ward fridge

Medical Management and Care

Hepatitis B
- Establish high- or low-infectivity of the client
- Counsel for risks to partner, children and infant
- Obtain consent for hepatitis B immunisation (+/− HBIG)
- Document delivery and immunisation plan in maternal notes

Hepatitis C
- Counsel for risks to partner, children and infant
- Explain screening for partner, children and infant
- Document delivery plan in maternal notes

Midwifery Management and Care

Hepatitis B
- Counsel for risks to partner, children and infant
- Ensure the mother is informed of risks and benefits of immunisation (+/− HBIG)
- Advise of safety of breast-feeding (including abstinence if nipples are cracked or bleeding)

Hepatitis C
- Counsel for risk to partner, children and infant
- Stress importance of follow-up care for all
- Advise of safety of breast-feeding (including abstinence if nipples are cracked or bleeding)

Labour Issues
- Labour and delivery should be planned and instigated with adherence to 'Control of Infection' guidelines provided by the hospital
- Invasive procedures, such as use of fetal scalp electrodes or fetal blood sampling, pose a significant risk of vertical transmission to the fetus
- Consideration of patient confidentiality should be paramount at all times to prevent inappropriate disclosure of diagnosis or undue anxiety during labour and delivery

Medical Management and Care

Hepatitis B and C
- Avoid fetal blood sampling due to the risk of vertical transmission
- No clear benefit of caesarean section
- Apart from the infection issues the labour can otherwise be managed normally by the midwife

Midwifery Management and Care

Hepatitis B and C
- The woman and her birth partner should be reassured about planned interventions and the rationale for these and kept informed and reassured throughout labour
- Avoid fetal scalp electrode use due to the risk of vertical transmission
- Ensure that 'Control of Infection' guidelines are adhered to

Postpartum Issues
- No evidence that HCV or HBV are transmitted via breast milk, so breast-feeding should still be promoted
- Transmission of infection occurs via blood, so breast-feeding mothers with cracked or bleeding nipples present a significant transmission risk to the neonate
- Infants born to HBV-infected mothers should be immunised with the accelerated immunisation schedule (at birth, 1 month, 2 months and 12 months of age)
- If the mother is hepatitis B e-antigen (HBeAg) positive, hepatitis B immunoglobulin (HBIG) should also be given to the infant
- Bathing the infant immediately after birth will further decrease the transmission risk

Medical Management and Care
- Ensure referrals to appropriate services are in place to provide follow-up for the mother and her infant
- Communicate with relevant health professionals with consent

Midwifery Management and Care
- Bathe the infant shortly after delivery
- Provide support for successful initiation of breast-feeding (if wished)
- Examine the breast-feeding mother's nipples daily to detect cracking
- If cracked or bleeding nipples occur, mothers should temporarily abstain until healing has occurred

Hepatitis B
- Ensure that first vaccine (+/− HBIG) is administered to the infant before transfer to the postnatal ward or discharge home

12.2 Human Immunodeficiency Virus

Incidence	Risk for Childbearing
86 500 known cases in the UK[1], of which 1645 are children (to end of March 2010)[2]	Low Risk – with interventions/no breast-feeding Variable Risk – without interventions plus breast-feeding

EXPLANATION OF CONDITION

Human immunodeficiency virus (HIV) is a retrovirus that is transmitted sexually (through unprotected sexual intercourse), parenterally (via shared injecting equipment or blood transfusion/organ receipt) or from a mother to her infant through vertical transmission (during pregnancy, delivery or breast-feeding). HIV infects the CD4 T-lymphocytes (an essential component of the immune system) rendering them ineffective at fighting infections, and leads to a gradual deterioration in immune function. This leaves the body susceptible to any form of infection, including those commonly present in the body that are usually contained by the immune system (known as opportunistic infections)[3].

The advent of anti-retroviral therapy (ART) has enabled the replication of HIV to be suppressed to such a level that the CD4 count can recover. HIV is therefore now viewed as a chronic infection that is manageable with medications.

In the UK, prevalence of HIV in pregnant women has increased every year since 2006. In untreated women, the risk of transmission is related to maternal health, obstetric factors and infant prematurity. The only obstetric factors that consistently show a risk of transmission are mode of delivery, duration of membrane rupture and delivery before 32 weeks gestation[4,5].

The rate of mother-to-child transmission in the UK is now in the region of 1.2%. This was not significantly affected by maternal ART or zidovudine monotherapy, or mode of delivery[4-6].

COMPLICATIONS

HIV may take many years to damage the immune system, but if untreated it will ultimately lead to the development of AIDS (acquired immune deficiency syndrome), a collection of diseases (including opportunistic infections) that ultimately may result in the premature death of the woman[2]. Early identification of women with HIV allows for the preservation of the immune system and the introduction of antiretroviral therapy before she becomes unwell[3].

HIV positive women have a small increased risk of adverse effects during pregnancy, including:

- Miscarriage
- Stillbirth
- Fetal abnormality
- Perinatal mortality
- Neonatal death
- IUGR
- Low birth weight
- Premature delivery[4,6]

NON-PREGNANCY TREATMENT AND CARE

HIV is now viewed as a chronic disease, and many women do not require drug therapy for many years after contracting HIV. Regular monitoring by their specialist team will ensure that their immune function is monitored, and treatment initiated when their clinical or immunological condition dictates. Standard treatment for non-pregnant women is three antiretroviral medicines (known as combination therapy) and is usually started once the CD4 count falls below 0.35×10^9/ml or the patient displays signs of advancing clinical disease[7].

Sexually active women are also advised to seek routine sexual health screening, to reduce the risk of onward transmission of HIV and other sexually transmitted infections. Annual screening for cervical cancer is also recommended, as HIV-positive women are four or five times more likely to develop cervical cancer[8].

Psychological and emotional support remain a key aspect of routine HIV care. The importance disclosure to their sexual partner[4] and adhering to their ART prescription are encouraged. Comprehensive on-going education about their illness, treatment options and family planning choices should also be provided.

PRE-CONCEPTION ISSUES AND CARE

The three key aspects to consider are:

1. Minimising the risk of HIV transmission between discordant couples
2. Management of any fertility issues
3. Health and medication needs[4]

Couples wishing to conceive should be advised against unprotected sexual intercourse (regardless of the man's HIV status). They should be provided with quills, syringes and sterile containers, with advice on self-insemination techniques during the fertile period of the menstrual cycle.

There is limited data on genital infections among HIV positive women[9] but sexually-transmitted infection rates in sub-Saharan Africa (where the majority of UK HIV infections originate) are known to be high[10,11]. Women are therefore advised to seek regular check-ups at a genito-urinary medicine clinic[12], as *Chlamydia trachomatis*, *Neisseria gonorrhoeae*, *Ureaplasma urealyticum*, and bacterial vaginosis are all associated with chorioamnionitis, which may lead to premature rupture of membranes, premature delivery and an increased risk of vertical transmission of HIV[13,14].

Where infections are diagnosed, sexual partners should be screened and treated as required.

Other infectious viral and bacterial diseases are outlined in Appendices 12.2.1 and 12.2.2.

Pregnancy Issues

- All HIV positive women should be routinely screened for sexually transmitted infection at presentation and in the third trimester[2]
  - cervical cytology should routinely be performed
  - *Treponema* serology should also be repeated in the third trimester
- A full assessment of the psycho-social issues should be undertaken to ensure adequate and appropriate support
- Disclosure of HIV to partners is advised, but is often challenging and complex and should therefore be viewed as a process rather than an event; never assume that anyone other than the woman knows her HIV status
- Sensitive handling of exclusive formula feeding must be provided
- Disclosure of HIV infection to other health care professionals is on a 'need to know' basis, and rationale for disclosure should be provided and consent sought (where appropriate)
- Support of adherence to antiretroviral medication is crucial if medications are to be taken correctly

Medical Management and Care

- Sexually transmitted infection screen at presentation and in the third trimester
- Cervical cytology should also be performed
- *Treponema* serology should be repeated in the third trimester
- Genotypic resistance testing is recommended before starting zidovudine and prior to delivery to identify viral mutations
- Referral to paediatric team and other services as required
- Initiate and continue dialogue around disclosure of HIV diagnosis to partner and/or health care professionals

Midwifery Management and Care

- Be aware that HIV screening at the booking interview may be the first time that HIV has been raised as an issue, and how some women discover they are HIV positive, hence diplomacy and informed consent are important.
- Promote attendance for other sexually transmitted infection screenings
- Provide sensitive advice around risk of HIV transmission through breast-feeding, and advise exclusive formula feeding to all HIV positive mothers
- Refer to available services for assistance with the purchasing of infant formula (where available)
- Ensure documentation is maintained around all aspects of pregnancy care, including who their HIV diagnosis has been disclosed to
- Provide support and monitoring of antiretroviral medication and promote adherence

Labour Issues

- All women should have a plan for their expected mode of delivery; invasive fetal monitoring should be avoided due to the risk of transferring maternal HIV infection to the baby
- Prophylactic intravenous antibiotics should be considered to reduce the incidence of chorio-amnionitis or post-caesarean infection
- Sensitivity around inadvertent disclosure of diagnosis is crucial (through notes, prescriptions, etc.) and local control of infection guidelines must be followed correctly

Medical Management and Care

- Elective vaginal delivery is an option for women with an HIV viral load <50 cps/ml
- Elective caesarean section should be planned for 38 weeks
- Avoid invasive procedures (including fetal scalp monitoring and artificial rupture of membranes)
- Consider intrapartum antibiotics

Midwifery Management and Care

- Home confinement not advised
- Avoid invasive procedures (see above)
- Follow local control of infection guidelines
- Administration of intravenous zidovudine as indicated
- Bathe the baby immediately after delivery
- Maintain discretion around HIV diagnosis

Postpartum Issues

- Postnatal depression is a risk for HIV positive women due to compounding pressures associated with HIV, housing or financial difficulties, immigration uncertainties or social isolation. Early referral to appropriate psychology or mental health services is advised
- Many women discover their HIV infection during antenatal screening, and pregnancy becomes a stressful and medically invasive process. Supporting women to remain in health care during and following their delivery is therefore crucial for their long-term wellbeing.

Medical Management and Care

- Short-term antiretroviral therapy should be discontinued after delivery when viral load <50 copies/ml
- Consider the half-life of each drug prior to discontinuation to avoid inadvertent monotherapy
- ART commenced prior to pregnancy should continue postnatally
- Liaise with health professionals to ensure maternal and neonatal HIV follow-up is arranged

Midwifery Management and Care

- Ensure neonatal antiretroviral therapy prescription is completed and administered within 6 hours of delivery
- EDTA blood from both mother and baby (*not* cord blood) on first or second postpartum days
- Ensure postnatal HIV appointments have been arranged

12.3 Malaria

Incidence	Risk for Childbearing
Estimated 225 million cases worldwide 78 100 deaths annually, mostly children <5 years and pregnant women[1]	Variable Risk – uncomplicated malaria High Risk – severe malaria

EXPLANATION OF CONDITION

Malaria is a protozoal infection that is potentially fatal. Transmission occurs mainly in tropical and sub-tropical countries, especially in Africa. More than 1000 cases of malaria are imported into the UK annually[2,3].

Malaria is caused by four protozoal species: *Plasmodium falciparum, P. malariae, P. ovale* and *P. vivax. P. falciparum* is present in most of the endemic areas and is associated with most deaths; the remaining three being more localised[1,4]. Those people residing in, or travelling to, a malaria area risk infection. Partial immunity develops with repeated attacks but is lost with lack of exposure, especially after emigration. Sickle cell trait offers some protection, with those affected by *P. falciparum* more likely to survive acute illness if they have sickle cell trait[5,6].

Malaria parasites present in the infected *Anopheles* mosquito saliva are transmitted from person to person by its bite. Transmission can also occur by infected blood transfusions, organ transplant, sharing contaminated needles and, rarely, from mother to baby during delivery[5,7]. Parasites within a victim's blood are carried to liver cells where they invade, grow and multiply. Eventually parasites are released back into the circulation to infect and destroy red blood cells[4] (Figure 12.3.1).

Incubation period varies and symptoms can occur in the first week of exposure; *P. falciparum* has the shortest incubation period. Suspect malaria in anyone who has travelled to a malaria area in the previous year and exhibits symptoms. *P. ovale, P. malariae* and *P. vivax* produce dormant stages, thus may be symptomatic over a year after exposure[3,4].

Symptoms of uncomplicated malaria comprise:

- Sweats
- Periodic fevers
- Headache
- Malaise
- Aching muscles
- Joint pain
- Rigors
- Vomiting
- Enlarged spleen
- Mild jaundice[4]

Symptoms may be misdiagnosed for conditions such as meningitis. Correct diagnosis is made by microscopy to demonstrate *Plasmodium* parasites in peripheral blood samples[8,9].

COMPLICATIONS

P. falciparum infection in immunosuppressed, young and pregnant patients leads to severe (complicated) malaria, often presenting within days of the initial symptoms. Complications occur singly or in combinations[3], as:

- Coma (cerebral malaria)
- Severe anaemia and jaundice
- Pulmonary oedema and respiratory distress
- Renal failure
- Hypoglycaemia and convulsions
- Disseminated intravascular coagulation
- Hyperpyrexia
- Hyperparasitaemia
- Malarial haemoglobinuria

NON-PREGNANCY TREATMENT AND CARE

Due to antimalarial drug resistance, specialist expert medical advice should be sought before treatment, e.g. from the *HPA Malaria Reference Laboratory – 020 7636 3924*.

Treatment in the UK usually commences after diagnosis is confirmed by blood test. However, if severe malaria is strongly suspected treatment might have to commence before laboratory diagnosis. Treatment is with the appropriate antimalarial drug, and choice of drug treatment is dependent on the woman's clinical status, the infecting *Plasmodium* species and its drug susceptibility[3,10,15]. In the UK, hospitalisation is usually advised until the strain of malaria is identified. Patients with *P. falciparum* malaria will usually require longer hospitalisation due to potential manifestation of severe complications.

Currently the drugs used in the UK for the treatment and prophylaxis of malaria include:

- Malarone (atovaquone plus proguanil)
- Doxycycline
- Chloroquine
- Proguanil
- Quinine
- Artesunate
- Mefloquine

These drugs are used individually or in combination[10,16].

Good patient care includes monitoring vital signs, intake/output, blood glucose and general conditions of the patient to observe for the signs of severe malaria, which will need specialist treatment. Ensure adequate patient follow-up after discharge.

NB: *Delay in diagnosis and treatment could be fatal.*

PRE-CONCEPTION ISSUES AND CARE

Anyone travelling to a malaria endemic area should pay particular attention to preventative measures: awareness of risk, avoiding mosquito bites, taking appropriate prophylaxis and seeking immediate medical attention if symptoms develop within and up to a year after travel[11].

Prophylaxis is dependent on the areas to be visited, so encourage compliance with treatment. At-risk groups include anyone originating from an endemic area, recent immigrants and long-term travellers such as those in the forces[11,12].

Pregnant women are at greater risk of developing severe malaria with adverse effects of drugs on the fetus, so advise women to avoid conceiving for up to 12 weeks after completing prophylaxis. Those wishing to conceive sooner should consider whether travel to a malaria area is necessary[11].

Advise avoidance of insect bites by:

- Using insect repellents
- Sleeping under a pyrethroid-impregnated mosquito net
- Using knockdown insecticide sprays in room at night
- Wearing long sleeves, trousers and socks[11]

Pregnancy Issues

In pregnancy, immunity is reduced, rendering the mother susceptible either to infection or to a relapse. This is especially so during a first pregnancy, but also the second trimester of all pregnancies. *P. falciparum* in particular can have a significant impact on maternal, fetal and neonatal health and is a medical emergency.

Even if no clinical symptoms are shown women can still develop placental parasitaemia, and relapses of *P. vivax* and *P. ovale* can also occur in pregnancy[11,12,14].

Adverse effects of malaria on pregnancy are:
- *Maternal effects* – complications as mentioned above
  - anaemia makes woman more susceptible to other infections
  - women with co-existing HIV are more likely to suffer maternal and fetal complications and malaria infections in placenta may increase fetal transmission of HIV[13]
- *Fetal effects*
  - miscarriage
  - stillbirth
  - low birth weight
  - prematurity
  - fetal acidosis
  - congenital malaria
  - neonatal death[13,14,17]
- Management in pregnancy involves treating the malaria, monitoring for and managing any complications, surveillance of fetal wellbeing and management of labour[17]

Medical Management and Care

Prevention of Malaria in Pregnancy
Advise not to travel to malaria area while pregnant but if necessary stress correct prophylaxis and give preventative advice. Some antimalarials contraindicated in pregnancy, therefore seek expert advice, e.g. from *HPA Malaria Reference Laboratory – 020 7636 3924* for the UK[6,10,17].

Management of Malaria in Pregnancy
- Confirm infection by demonstrating malaria parasites in peripheral blood on thick and thin films
- If symptomatic, admit immediately for prompt specialist management, treatment and monitoring of complications, such as anaemia, renal failure, hypoglycaemia and DIC[13,17]
- Fluid replacement should be carefully monitored because of the risk of pulmonary oedema
- 50% glucose may need to be given for hypoglycaemia and blood transfusion if anaemia causes cardiovascular compromise
- Treat pyrexia promptly as may cause pre-term labour
- Severe malaria is a medical emergency and should be managed in a HDU/ITU with multidisciplinary input
- Fetal surveillance
  - monitor for pre-term labour and give steroids for lung maturation if needed
  - monitor fetal wellbeing by CTG and ultrasound
- Induction of labour may be necessary if fetal and maternal health concerns

Midwifery Management and Care
- Booking history should always include travel and prophylaxis history
- Advise against travel to malaria areas unless strictly necessary
- Advise to seek immediate medical help if symptoms develop abroad or on return, as infection is possible even if prophylaxis was taken
- Be aware that some symptoms of malaria resemble pre-eclampsia
- Seek medical advice immediately for concerns about mother or baby

Labour Issues
- Monitoring for fetal distress in labour is important due to adverse maternal condition
- There is increased risk of PPH[17] and infection
- Pulmonary oedema, if not already present, can occur immediately after delivery if the woman is severely anaemic[17]

Medical Management and Care
- Manage according to medical condition
- Obstetric intervention may become necessary if fetal distress detected
- Fetal heart rate abnormalities may improve on correction of maternal pyrexia or hypoglycaemia, otherwise delivery may be required

Midwifery Management and Care
- Manage according to medical condition at time of labour
- Active management of third stage with regard to increased risk of PPH
- Careful observations of vital signs and temperature in mother
- Attention to strict infection control precautions
- Cord blood should be taken post-delivery and sent to the laboratory for a *blood smear* to diagnose or exclude congenital malaria

Postpartum Issues
- Risk of secondary postpartum haemorrhage (PPH)[17]
- Theoretical, but rare, risk of congenital malaria in the baby[18]
- Possible complications associated with low-birth-weight infant
- Some antimalarial drugs are contraindicated in breast-feeding[10,11,15,19]

Medical Management and Care
- Be alert for signs of pulmonary oedema such as acute breathlessness, which could develop immediately after birth and should be treated
- Prompt medical intervention if PPH occurs
- Observe for anaemia and instigate prompt treatment if necessary

Midwifery Management and Care
- Manage according to medical condition
- Mother and baby are not for early discharge home
- Continue observation of mother's vital signs
- Observe for PPH
- Observations of neonate for signs of fever, respiratory distress or jaundice, which could be suggestive of congenital malaria[18,20]
- Care of possible low-birth-weight baby
- Confer with paediatrician and pharmacist about safety of maternal drugs whilst breast-feeding
- Paediatrician, not midwife, for the neonatal 'discharge' examination

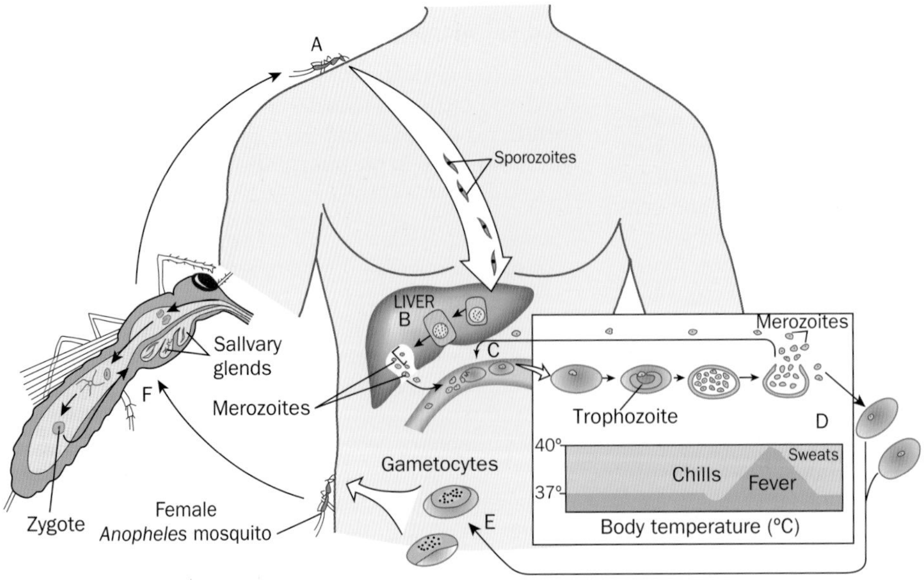

Figure 12.3.1 The lifecycle of the malaria parasite *Plasmodium* (Black, 2008). A, Female Anopheles mosquito bites a person and transmits sporozoites (from its salivary glands) which travel in the blood to the liver. B, In the liver the sporozites multiply and become merozoites which are shed into the blood when the liver cells rupture. C, The merozoites enter the erythrocytes (red blood cells) and become trophozoites which feed and form more merozoites. D, The red blood cells rupture releasing the merozoites which affect other blood cells; and the patient experiences chills, high fever and sweating. E, Merozoites infect other erythrocytes and after several such asexual cycles the sexual phase begins and gametocytes are produced. F, An uninfected Anopheles mosquito bites the malaria-infected person and ingests gametocytes which give rise to infective sporozoites in the salivary glands. This mosquito bites another person, and the cycle recommences. This figure is downloadable from the book companion website at www.wiley.com/go/robson

12.4 Chickenpox

Incidence	Risk for Childbearing
Complicates three in 1000 pregnancies[1]	High Risk

EXPLANATION OF CONDITION

Chickenpox, also known as **varicella**, is a common childhood illness caused by infection with *Varicella zoster* virus. This is a DNA virus from the herpes family. The mode of transmission is mainly via respiratory droplets or by direct contact and is therefore highly contagious. Reactivation of the virus, which has remained latent in the dorsal root or cranial nerve ganglion, causes shingles. This often occurs many years after the initial infection. Chickenpox may be acquired by contact with shingles but this is less common.

Clinical features of chickenpox include a mild febrile illness, associated with malaise and the development of a characteristic vesicular rash. The rash is pruritic, the vesicles appear in waves and typically vesicles, pustules and crusted lesions appear together. The illness usually lasts 7–10 days. There is increased morbidity and mortality in pregnancy compared with being non-pregnant, especially as the pregnancy advances[2].

Shingles is characterised by an eruption of painful vesicles covering an area of skin corresponding to one or two sensory nerves, particularly the thoracic nerves, but may affect the cranial nerves, e.g. ophthalmic. If the dorsal root ganglion is affected then the rash may extend from the middle of the back to the chest wall.

The incubation period is 10–12 days. However, the infective period extends from 48 hours prior to the appearance of the rash until all the vesicles have crusted over.

Immunity is solid and long-lasting and as the infection is so commonly acquired in childhood over 90% of the antenatal population is immune to the virus[3]. Of those with uncertainty regarding their immune status, 80% will have IgG antibodies on serum testing and will therefore be immune[4].

COMPLICATIONS

Chickenpox is generally a mild, self-limiting illness in childhood. However, it can be a much more serious condition in adults, with pneumonia being relatively common and encephalitis and hepatitis being other possible complications. Up to 10% of pregnant women with chickenpox develop pneumonia and it is associated with a higher mortality and morbidity than in the non-pregnant patient. The severity of the pneumonia increases as the pregnancy progresses[2] and many of these women will require hospital admission.

Fetal risks include the risk of **fetal varicella syndrome** (FVS) if the infection is acquired within the first 20 weeks of pregnancy, and **varicella infection of the newborn** (VIN) if the infection is acquired within the last 4 weeks of the pregnancy[5]. Chickenpox has not been associated with an increased risk of miscarriage[6].

The risk of FVS is approximately 1% (<0.5% if the infection is acquired in the first trimester) and is associated with:

- Skin loss or scarring
- Eye defects, including cataracts
- Hypoplasia of the limbs
- Neurological abnormalities[6,7]

Some features of FVS can be detected prenatally by ultrasound examination of the fetus and these include:

- Shortening of the long bones
- Hydrocephalus
- Microcephalus
- IUGR[8]

There have been very occasional reports of FVS occurring at 20–28 weeks gestation[9]. However, the risk is likely to be extremely small. At 20–36 weeks of gestation the risk is the possibility of the infant developing shingles, which may present subsequently in the first few years of his/her life.

VIN can occur when maternal infection is acquired within four weeks of delivery or immediately after. Approximately half of the babies born will be infected, with a quarter of them developing chickenpox. If, however, the delivery is within one week of the rash developing, or just prior to the onset of the rash, then passively-acquired antibodies in the baby are low and severe chickenpox infection, which may be fatal, can occur in the baby[10].

There does not appear to be any risk to the fetus of shingles in pregnancy[7].

NON-PREGNANCY TREATMENT AND CARE

As chickenpox in childhood is a mild, self-limiting illness all that is generally required is control of the pyrexia and pruritus, e.g. with paracetamol and antihistamines if necessary. Care needs to be taken to avoid secondary infection of the lesions; advice on hygiene should be given and antibiotics if secondary infection does occur. As adults tend to have a more severe illness, oral aciclovir may be given within 24 hours of developing the rash[11]. If complications develop then hospital admission may be required.

PRE-CONCEPTION ISSUES AND CARE

A vaccine exists for chickenpox and is available for women in the UK who are planning a pregnancy and are found to be seronegative for VZV IgG. This is not, however, at present, a national screening recommendation in the UK[12]. The vaccine is contraindicated in pregnancy and pregnancy should be avoided for 3 months after vaccination.

Women who have not had chickenpox should be advised to avoid contact with chickenpox in the peri-conception period, and to report any possible contact to their midwife or doctor.

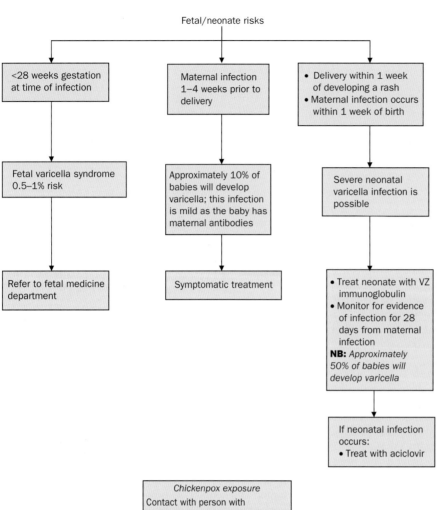

Figure 12.4.1 Chickenpox risk to fetus and neonate. This figure is downloadable from the book companion website at www.wiley.com/go/robson

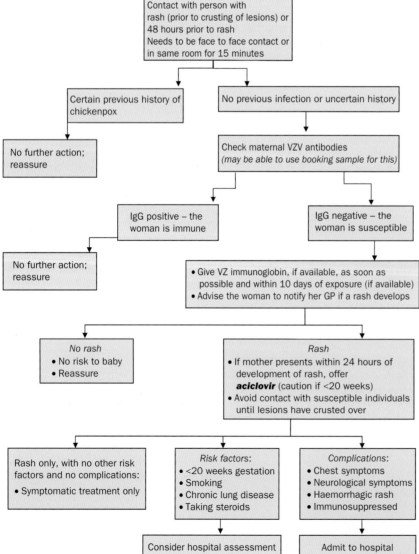

Figure 12.4.2 Management of chickenpox during pregnancy. This figure is downloadable from the book companion website at www.wiley.com/go/robson

Pregnancy Issues

Varicella zoster immunoglobulin (VZIg) should be used to prevent chickenpox in susceptible women who have had significant exposure. It should be given within 10 days of exposure for maximal effect[12]. It has no place in treatment once chickenpox has developed.

Oral aciclovir decreases the duration and severity of symptoms in women who develop chickenpox in pregnancy. To be effective it needs to be given within 24 hours of the rash developing. It may also decrease the risk of serious complications[12]. Due to the theoretical risk of teratogenicity, it should be used with caution prior to 20 weeks[12].

Women with chickenpox in pregnancy should be alerted to the possible complications that may occur and should report any respiratory or neurological symptoms or any bleeding immediately so that hospital admission may be considered. Hospital admission may also be required if the mother is in the latter stages of pregnancy, if she smokes or is taking steroids or is immunosuppressed[13].

Neonatology involvement is very important and the mother should be given the opportunity to discuss possible neonatal complications and plans for investigation and treatment of the neonate, post delivery. Figure 12.4.1 outlines the risks to the fetus and neonate.

Medical Management and Care

- If a mother presents with chickenpox within the first 20 weeks she should be counselled regarding the risks of FVS (0.5–1%); although amniocentesis can identify VZ DNA, it should not routinely be advised due to the low risk of FVS. A detailed ultrasound examination should be arranged at least 5 weeks after infection to try to detect features of FVS
- If complications arise the mother should be managed in hospital by a multi disciplinary team involving obstetrician, virologist and neonatologist[12]

Midwifery Management and Care (see Figure 12.4.2 for management algorithm)

If a Women Reports Contact with Chickenpox:
- Ask if previous infection – if so, reassure
- If not, check if significant exposure – was the diagnosis definite; did exposure occur when uncrusted lesions were present or 48 hours prior to development of the rash; was there face to face contact with infected person?
- If yes – arrange for booking blood samples to be tested for *Varicella zoster* virus IgG or send serum for testing
- If IgG negative – arrange for VZIg to be given as soon as possible (within 10 days)
- Inform the woman to notify her doctor or midwife if she develops a rash, irrespective of whether she had VZIg or not

If a Woman Presents with Chickenpox in Pregnancy:
- Arrange for her to be given oral aciclovir if >20 weeks gestation and if she has presented within 24 hours of the onset of the rash
- Consider whether factors indicating hospital admission are present, and discuss with obstetrician if in doubt
- Inform the woman to report any new symptoms immediately, e.g. chest symptoms, bleeding
- If the woman is less than 20 weeks pregnant, refer to obstetrician for counselling regarding the risks of FVS
- Counsel her to avoid contact with anyone at risk of developing severe chickenpox, e.g. other pregnant women, including attending antenatal classes
- Advise on use of topical soothing agents and possible use of antihistamines
- Ensure women who remain at home are reviewed regularly

Labour Issues

- Delivery should be avoided during the acute illness
- There is a risk of serious maternal complications including DIC
- For the neonate, there is the risk of severe varicella of the newborn, with significant morbidity and possible mortality[10]

Medical Management and Care

- Supportive treatment should be given if labour occurs in the viraemic period
- Intravenous aciclovir is recommended in this situation[12]

Midwifery Management and Care

- The woman should be closely observed for the development of the complications of chickenpox, in particular DIC
- Ascertain if the paediatrician is to review the baby post delivery

Postpartum Issues

The highest risk to the neonate is when delivery occurs within 5 days of maternal infection or if the mother develops chickenpox within 2 days of delivery. In this situation the baby should be given VZIg and monitored. If chickenpox does develop then the baby should be treated with aciclovir[12].

- Any baby born to a seronegative mother who has significant exposure to chickenpox in the first 7 days of its life should be given VZIg[12]
- Premature babies (less than 28 weeks gestation) are at risk of chickenpox because of inadequate transfer of maternal antibodies at this gestation; if exposure has occurred VZIg should be given[12]

Medical Management and Care

- If maternal infection occurred in the first 20 weeks of pregnancy then neonatal blood should be sent for *Varicella zoster* virus IgM antibody testing[12] and the baby should have a neonatal ophthalmic examination soon after birth
- If delivery occurred during the acute maternal illness the neonatologists should be involved to treat and observe the baby appropriately
- If severe maternal complications arise then the woman may require transfer to the intensive care unit for further monitoring and supportive treatment

Midwifery Management and Care

- The woman should continue to be monitored for complications
- If infective, woman and baby should be isolated from other mothers and babies on the ward but not from each other[14]
- Breast-feeding is not contraindicated and should be encouraged[14]

12.5 Toxoplasmosis

Incidence	Risk for Childbearing
Worldwide: estimated 1 billion exposed to parasite[1]	High Risk – acute infection
UK: approximately 400 cases diagnosed annually[1]	Variable Risk – chronic infection

EXPLANATION OF CONDITION

Toxoplasmosis is a common parasitic infection, caused by the protozoan parasite *Toxoplasma gondii*, which was discovered in 1908[1-3]. It is found in a wide variety of animals, but the reservoir is the cat and other felines in whose gut the parasite completes its sexual stage by producing oocysts (egg cysts). Cats acquire the infection by eating infected birds or rodents. For up to 2 weeks following primary infection they pass the oocysts, which remain viable in the soil for up to 18 months, in their faeces. If other animals and humans eat these oocysts they hatch and the parasite moves from the gut to invade tissues and cause toxoplasmosis.

Toxoplasmosis potentially poses a significant health risk to the fetus during pregnancy and to people with impaired immunity, i.e. HIV disease. It can cause congenital mental retardation, chorioretinitis and encephalitis[1,2,4-6].

Humans acquire the infection by:

- Ingestion of undercooked meat (mainly mutton or pork)
- Ingesting unwashed, uncooked vegetables and fruits
- Hand to mouth contact with faeces of infected cats
  - cleaning out litter tray
  - gardening
- Blood transfusion or organ transplant
- Drinking unpasteurised milk[2,4-6]

Person to person transmission does not occur except vertically from pregnant woman to the fetus or, rarely, by organ transplant or blood transfusion.

The incubation period is 10–25 days[2,6]. After the initial acute infection the parasite becomes inactive and remains dormant, giving lifelong protection, but can be reactivated if the immune system becomes impaired. Generally, reactivation in a seropositive woman carries very little or no risk of transmission to the fetus[4].

The majority of healthy sufferers have little or no symptoms or a mild flu-like illness, sometimes mistaken for glandular fever. These symptoms include:

- Headache
- Sore throat
- Fever
- Fatigue
- Swollen glands
- Night sweats
- Muscle aches

Diagnosis is confirmed by history of clinical symptoms and examination of blood or other body fluid to detect IgG and IgM antibodies. Raised levels of IgG antibodies indicate past infection and raised IgM indicate current infection. Other means of diagnosis, such as demonstration of cysts in the placenta or lymph tissue, have also been used[1,2,4,6].

COMPLICATIONS

First and Second Trimester Acquired Infection

- Miscarriage
- Congenital hydrocephalus
- Mental retardation

- Deafness and blindness
- Growth problems

Third Trimester Acquired Infection

- Retinochoroiditis developing later[4,7]
- Stillbirth[4,7]

In about 40% of new infections in pregnancy the fetus is infected, with most cases occurring in the third trimester, in which case the baby can appear 'normal' at birth. The earlier in pregnancy that the infection occurs the more severe the disease in the neonate.

NON-PREGNANCY TREATMENT AND CARE

Most cases are asymptomatic and patients will make a full recovery requiring no treatment. However, some people, e.g. those who are immunocompromised, may develop severe symptoms and in these cases specialist treatment advice should be sought from an infectious disease or microbiology department.

For those requiring treatment this is usually with a combination of pyrimethamine and sulfadiazine or clindamycin. Pyrimethamine is a folate antagonist, so weekly blood counts should be taken and folinic acid supplement given[8].

Advise patients to get plenty of rest, take medication as prescribed and report any unusual side effects of medication.

If maternal diagnosis is confirmed during early pregnancy, spiramycin may be given to the mother to try and reduce the risk of transmission to the fetus[4,7]. If there is concern that the baby may already be infected, and the woman is more than 15 weeks pregnant, then she may be offered amniocentesis, or cordocentesis at 20–22 weeks, both preceded by thorough counselling as to the implications.

If the fetus is affected, a termination of pregnancy may be offered or alternatively continue pregnancy with treatment using pyrimethamine and sulfadiazine and folinic acid supplement. Unfortunately this may have side effects. Drug treatment will reduce the severity of infection in the fetus but will not reverse any harm which may already have occurred[4,6].

PRE-CONCEPTION ISSUES AND CARE

Emphasis should be on prevention. In addition to the usual advice on maintaining a healthy lifestyle, healthy diet, folic acid supplement and avoiding infections, women should be educated about toxoplasmosis and methods of minimising the risk of contracting this infection before, during and after pregnancy by[1-7]:

- Avoid eating under-cooked meats
- Wash fruits and vegetables thoroughly
- Wash hands and utensils after preparing raw meat
- Feed cat with dry or canned food instead of raw meat
- Wash hands after handling cat, if it is necessary to handle cat litter tray wear gloves and wash hands afterwards
- Disinfect cat litter box with boiling water for 5 minutes
- Avoid handling stray or ill cats
- Wear gloves when gardening and wash hands afterwards

Women with an active infection should be advised to avoid becoming pregnant until treatment is completed.

Pregnancy Issues

Management of pregnancy is aimed at preventing vertical transmission.

During pregnancy spiramycin is used to treat toxoplasmosis. It will reduce the risk of transmission of infection. It is not effective if the baby is already infected. However, if tests reveal fetal infection and the pregnancy is to continue then pyrimethamine and sulfadiazine may be suggested[8].

Pyrimethamine can cause suppression of bone marrow, is a folate antagonist and terratogenic in animals. Sulfadiazine can cause macular papular rash and should be discontinued immediately should this occur[6,8].

An ultrasound scan may also highlight any obvious physical abnormalities, such as hydrops or microcephaly in the fetus. Termination of pregnancy is an option for some women, when an infected fetus with severe abnormalities has been confirmed[7].

France and Austria conduct routine antenatal toxoplasmosis screening, but not the UK, where cost effectiveness is not proven[9] because prevalence is low.

Medical Management and Care
- Consider toxoplasmosis if a pregnant woman develops a glandular-fever-like illness; test for IgG and IgM antibodies
- Obtain specialist microbiological or infectious diseases advice on treatment
- Consider congenital toxoplasmosis if mother has positive serology
- Discuss screening of fetus using amniocentesis or cordocentesis and implications with mother, including consideration of termination of pregnancy
- Fetal ultrasound may be used to demonstrate any abnormality such as IUGR, fetal hydrops, microcephaly, intracranial calcification or hepatosplenomegaly[7]
- Ultrasound examination should be performed at least monthly to monitor for any signs of fetal infection

Midwifery Management and Care
- Advise how to avoid toxoplasmosis exposure during pregnancy
- Advise woman to seek medical advice if they experience fever or flu-like symptoms or if concerned that she could have acquired infection
- If the toxoplasmosis infection is chronic, with no other fetal or maternal concerns, manage as a low-risk pregnancy
- If infection is acute, treat as high-risk pregnancy that will require intense fetal monitoring and treatment of mother to prevent vertical transmission to the fetus
- Women with acute infection, and hence an 'at risk' fetus, may decide to terminate the pregnancy and will require counselling and support[10]
- Some women will decide to continue pregnancy and have prophylactic antibiotics to try and prevent fetal infection; reinforce any advice and instructions regarding treatment
- If amniocentesis or cordocentesis or other investigation is to be carried out, reassure and support mother and ensure she understands procedures[10]
- If the fetus is not infected, and there are no other maternal or fetal complications, home confinement is not contraindicated

Labour Issues

Delivery should follow normal practice unless there are any gross fetal abnormalities, such as hydrocephalus, or any maternal concerns which will necessitate medical intervention.

Medical Management and Care
- Normal midwifery care, unless any concerns arise requiring medical intervention for birth

Midwifery Management and Care
- Manage from normal perspective unless medical concerns arise
- Be aware that the parents may express anxiety, and want answers about the baby's prognosis immediately after birth; hence the baby may need to be seen by a paediatrician sooner rather than later

Postpartum Issues

Breast-feeding has not been demonstrated to be a means of toxoplasmosis transmission in humans[4]. However, if the baby is not infected, but the mother is receiving treatment, check compatibility of drugs with breast-feeding.

Babies born to women with confirmed toxoplasmosis in pregnancy will be monitored closely by paediatricians, with repeated investigations in first year of life. If still seropositive at one year of age, with abnormal clinical findings, then congenital toxoplasmosis is confirmed and therapy should continue[11].

Medical Management and Care
- Treatment of the neonate usually continues for the first year of life
- Consider congenital toxoplasmosis if mother had positive serology
- Refer to paediatricians for follow-up
- The neonate will need clinical, serological, neurological and ophthalmic assessment to rule out or confirm congenital infection[4]

Midwifery Management and Care
- Support prompt commencement of breast-feeding
- Reinforce any advice on medication given for mother and baby
- Care of baby according to condition
- If congenital toxoplasmosis confirmed, or suspected, initiate communication with health visitor or specialist nurse and the community team, because long-term follow-up will be necessary

12.6 Listeriosis

Incidence	Risk for Childbearing
Varies worldwide, but within European Union 0.31 cases per million population reported annually[1]	High Risk

EXPLANATION OF CONDITION

In 2009 in England and Wales, 213 cases of listeriosis infections were reported to the Health Protection Agency, of which 34 were pregnancy related[2]. In Scotland, 17 cases in pregnancy were reported[3].

This is an uncommon but potentially serious infection in humans. It is caused primarily by eating food contaminated with the bacterium *Listeria monocytogenes,* a Gram-positive bacillus that has also been identified in natural environments, such as soil, water, intestinal tract of animals and sewage. Humans may be asymptomatic carriers in their intestinal flora. Human listeriosis was recognised in the late 1920s and demonstrated to be a food-borne infection in 1981. Food stored in a refrigerator can still be a hazard, as *L. monocytogenes,* can grow at low temperatures[4-7].

L. monocytogenes is found in a variety of raw foods, such as uncooked meats, raw fish, poultry and vegetables and in some processed foods that become contaminated after processing, i.e. cook–chill meats, salads, soft cheeses and pâté. Unpasteurised milk and food made from it has also been implicated[6,7]. Most cases are sporadic; however, some outbreaks have been associated with contaminated food[8].

Transmission from person to person is rare *except* for vertical transmission from mother to fetus transplacentally or during delivery. Papular lesions may occur on hands and arms from contact with infectious material, i.e. sick or dead animals. A few cases due to hospital cross-infection and nosocomial infection in nurseries have been reported[6,7,9,10].

L. monocytogenes infections are most harmful to pregnant women, newborns, the elderly and those with weakened immune systems due to HIV infection or cancer[6,11]. The incubation period varies widely, but is reported to be on average 21 days in adults, intrauterine infections 30 days and in neonates just a few days[6,7]. Infection can be asymptomatic, but if symptoms manifest in healthy adults these are usually mild and include fever, muscle ache, nausea or diarrhoea.

Isolating *L. monocytogenes* in cerebrospinal fluid or blood culture confirms the diagnosis. The bacterium may also be identified in meconium, amniotic fluid and placenta samples.

COMPLICATIONS

In the immunocompromised, elderly, or pregnant listeriosis can be more serious and can cause meningitis or septicaemia thus giving rise to symptoms such as fever, headache, neck stiffness, loss of balance or confusion[6,12].

While infection in the mother might be asymptomatic or mild, in the fetus and neonate it is usually serious. Transplacental infections during the very early stage of pregnancy might lead to spontaneous abortion and fetal infection later in pregnancy may lead to premature birth, stillbirth or death in the first few days of life[6,13-16]. Neonatal listeriosis has two stages of clinical onset presentation.

Early Onset

- Birth is usually premature and the disease is due to intra-uterine infection
- Symptoms occur within hours to first 5 days of birth and fatality is high

- Symptoms include:
  - meconium staining
  - respiratory distress
  - fever
  - rash
  - lethargy
  - vomiting
  - poor feeding
  - jaundice

Late Onset

- Most likely due to infection around birth
- Usually a term infant, well at birth, develops symptoms after 5–7 days presenting as meningitis or septicaemia
- Neurodevelopment delay and hydrocephalus have also been reported in those with meningitis[4,13,14,16]

NON-PREGNANCY TREATMENT AND CARE

Currently first-line treatment is with ampicillin, sometimes combined with gentamicin. Several other antibiotics are also available as second-line treatment[17].

Advise the woman to complete the course of antibiotics, get plenty of rest, good fluid intake and a healthy diet. Advise on good hygiene measures to prevent spread.

In the UK this is a notifiable disease if identified as food-borne 'food poisoning', which should be reported to the Health Protection Agency by the clinician.

PRE-CONCEPTION ISSUES AND CARE

All women preparing for pregnancy should be advised to maintain a healthy lifestyle, eat a well-balanced diet and avoid known infection risks. Additional advice should be given on avoidance of contracting listeriosis, and to report any symptoms of infection to the doctor immediately in order to aid investigation and early treatment. Women with a known infection should always make sure that the infection is treated successfully if possible before becoming pregnant.

Measures to reduce risk of listeriosis are:

- Completely cook raw meat and poultry before eating
- Wash all fruits and raw vegetables
- Keep uncooked meats separate from cooked foods, ready to eat foods and vegetables
- Avoid unpasteurised milk or foods made from it
- Wash hands, utensils and chopping boards after dealing with uncooked foods
- Eat ready-prepared and perishable foods as soon as possible while still in date
- If re-heating food make sure it is piping hot all through as cooking destroys this bacteria[4,6,12]
- Avoid eating *soft* cheeses such as brie, camembert, blue-veined and Mexican-style cheeses, meat spreads and pâté
- Avoid delicatessen-counter food unless thoroughly heated

Whilst they are not a main source of infection, it is still wise to avoid contact with sheep during lambing and aborted animal fetuses and silage on farms[4,6,12].

Pregnancy Issues
- Emphasis should be on prevention and early detection of listeriosis
- Prompt identification and treatment of listeriosis during pregnancy can lead to a successful pregnancy outcome[16]
- Maternal infection during pregnancy can lead to complications as discussed previously
- Diagnosis is made by culturing the organism from blood, placenta or liquor
- Maternal symptoms may be mild, can be overlooked and therefore go untreated, thus leaving fetus at risk of contracting infection *in utero or at birth*
- A child born to a woman diagnosed with *L. monocytogenes* infection during pregnancy could be at risk of developing early or late neonatal listeriosis (see earlier) so confinement in hospital consultant unit should be discussed with the mother to be

Medical Management and Care
- Be aware that any febrile illness in pregnancy, amnionitis or pre-term labour, particularly with meconium staining of liquor could be due to *L. monocytogenes* infection
- If diagnosed, the mother requires hospital admission for immediate intravenous antibiotic treatment and observation

Midwifery Management and Care
- There is no routine screening for listeriosis in the UK
- Women should be advised to seek medical advice immediately if they develop any flu-like symptoms during pregnancy
- Advise on which foods to avoid during pregnancy, good food and kitchen hygiene measures (as discussed under pre-conception care)
- If maternal listeriosis is suspected or diagnosed, there should be regular monitoring of maternal and fetal wellbeing throughout pregnancy to detect early any abnormalities such as signs of pre-term labour

Labour Issues
- There is an increased risk of premature birth or stillborn baby in mothers with listeriosis
- Characteristics of listeriosis infections in the neonate can be similar to those caused by group B Streptococci
- Sometimes in neonatal *L. monocytogenes* infection there may be micro-abscesses seen on the fetal surface of the placenta as well as on the skin of the neonate[14,16]

Medical Management and Care
- Medical management as necessary if pre-term labour
- If mother and fetus well, and pregnancy is full-term, midwife can manage labour; if maternal or fetal complications present or develop then manage accordingly

Midwifery Management and Care
- Summon medical aid immediately if any concern such as fetal compromise arises
- After delivery examine placenta and note any signs of chorioamnionitis (e.g. a yellow or green tint of membranes and chorion), or signs of micro-abscesses, all of which may indicate early onset infection in the neonate of a woman who has been treated for listeriosis
- Send samples for culture if abnormality present
- Observe newborn for signs of infection, respiratory distress or any other complications

Postpartum Issues
- Early and late onset listeriosis may become evident
- Signs of early onset occur within hours to 5 days of birth, and late onset from 5–7 days after birth (symptoms as described earlier)
- There have been reports of nosocomial infections of *L. monocytogenes* infections in nurseries[9,10]
- Breast-feeding is rarely contraindicated[18]
- Signs and symptoms of early and late onset listeriosis in the baby include those of meningitis or septicaemia:
  - fever
  - rash
  - irritability
  - lethargy
  - poor feeding
  - bulging fontanelle

Medical Management and Care
- Test baby for *L. monocytogenes* if mother was affected during, or immediately prior to, this pregnancy
- Commence antibiotic treatment if necessary

Midwifery Management and Care
- Observe for signs of early- and late-onset neonatal listeriosis, i.e. signs of respiratory distress soon after birth
- Advise parents what signs to look for
- Strict adherence to infection control precautions to prevent nosocomial infections in nursery
- If pre-term delivery, attention to the specialist care of such infants
- If mother intends to breast-feed, help to establish lactation promptly
- Support and keep parents/family informed
- Good communication between hospital and community staff on transfer home
- Continue observation for signs and symptoms of late-onset listeriosis, extending the period of home visits by the midwife if indicated

12.7 Herpes Simplex Virus

Incidence
Genital herpes in women has increased twenty-fold over the last 30 years[1]
Neonatal herpes – 1.7 per 100 000 UK live births[2]

Risk for Childbearing
High Risk

EXPLANATION OF CONDITION

Herpes simplex virus (HSV) can manifest itself in a variety of different ways and can be due to primary infection, when the virus is first encountered, or reactivation of the latent virus.

The clinical manifestations of a primary infection include:

- **Gingivo-stomatitis**: vesicles appear on the inside of the mouth
- **Herpetic whitlow**: seen as a lesion on the fingers
- **Conjunctivitis** or **keratitis** (inflammation of the cornea)
- **Genital herpes**: as vesicular eruption on the genital area
- **Neonatal herpes**: as generalised infection (see below)

The virus then remains dormant in either the trigeminal or sacral ganglion until reactivated, causing recurrent infection. This manifests itself in the form of cold sores (**orolabial herpes**), keratitis or recurrent genital herpes. Neonatal herpes is caused by transmission to the neonate at or around delivery and is associated with a high morbidity and mortality[3].

Orolabial herpes is usually caused by HSV type 1. Genital herpes (GH) can be caused by HSV 1 or HSV 2[4]. Symptoms of GH include blistering and painful ulceration of the external genitalia, which may involve the cervix and rectum, and systemic symptoms, e.g. myalgia, inguinal lymphadenopathy[4]. Symptoms are commoner in primary infection and often more extensive. Prior infection with HSV 1 modifies the clinical manifestation of HSV 2[4]. The patient may be asymptomatic or may only present with systemic symptoms. Reactivation can be provoked by stress, menstruation, and other viral infections.

The virus is spread by close person contact, kissing or sexual contact, and there is a peak in the incidence during adolescence due to kissing. Asymptomatic viral shedding occurs with genital HSV 1 and 2 but more so with HSV 2[4]. It occurs most commonly in the first year after infection and can cause transmission of the virus[4].

COMPLICATIONS

Urinary Retention

- Catheterisation may be needed if conservative measures (analgesics/topic anaesthetics) fail
- Suprapubic catheterisation is preferred to transurethral[4]

Herpes Hepatitis

- Most cases caused by primary HSV 2 infection
- Clinical features are:
  - fever
  - abdominal pain
  - abnormal liver transaminases
  - high mortality rate
- Treatment comprises iv antiviral therapy and hospitalisation[5]

Encephalitis/Meningitis

- This is a rare but serious complication
- Clinical features are:
  - fever
  - headache
  - confusion
- Treatment with iv antiviral therapy required

Neonatal Herpes

- Can be caused by HSV 1 or HSV 2 and is characterised by severe generalised infection in the neonate[6]
- Affected babies can present with:
  - jaundice
  - hepatosplenomegaly
  - thrombocytopenia
  - vesicular lesions on the skin
- Risk is greatest with primary GH during late pregnancy as the baby will not have acquired protective antibodies from the mother[3]

NON-PREGNANCY TREATMENT AND CARE

Primary herpetic gingivo-stomatitis is treated by soft diet, encouraging adequate fluid intake and analgesia, including the use of local analgesic mouthwashes. Chlorhexidine mouthwash will help to prevent secondary infection[7]. If the lesions are severe, an antiviral, such as aciclovir, may be used orally[7]. Aciclovir cream can be used for cold sores (recurrent orolabial herpes infection) and should be commenced at the first sign of an attack, ideally before vesicles appear[7].

For GH it is important that the diagnosis is made as this will have implications for women if an episode were to occur in a future pregnancy. Ideally it would be valuable to determine whether the infection was due to HSV 1 or 2 as it would then be possible to determine whether a future attack in pregnancy was a primary infection with that type or a recurrence[4]. The virus can be isolated and typed by swabs taken from the base of an ulcer, ensuring that the swab is sent rapidly to the laboratory. The diagnosis can also be made by serological testing but viral detection remains the method of choice[4].

Primary or secondary GH is usually treated by an oral antiviral drug, e.g. aciclovir, and should be started within 5 days of the onset of the episode[7]. These have been shown to decrease the severity and duration of the episode and are more effective than topical antiviral agents. General hygiene advice needs to be given also and includes the use of saline baths[4]. Analgesia, with or without topical anaesthetic agents, is often required[4] and the patient advised to seek advice if they are unable to pass urine. Hospitalisation may be required for complications.

If the patient experiences regular attacks of recurrent GH, suppressive antiviral therapy may be required, e.g. with aciclovir. This should initially be used for up to a year and then the recurrence frequency should be reassessed[4]. Patients should abstain from sexual contact during an attack.

PRE-CONCEPTION ISSUES AND CARE

- If women are known to have a history of genital herpes then reassurance should be given that the risk of transmission to the neonate with recurrent episodes is very small
- Women in whom there is no history of GH, but whose partner has a positive history, are advised to abstain from sexual intercourse at times when he has a recurrence[6]. This will not completely prevent transmission to the woman, as asymptomatic viral shedding at times when there is no evidence of an attack can lead to transmission[8]. Use of condoms has been proposed but not formally assessed[4].
- Identifying women who are susceptible to acquiring primary GH in pregnancy by serological testing has not been found to be cost effective in the UK[9].

Pregnancy Issues

- Aims:
  - give symptomatic relief of infection
  - monitor for and treat any complications
  - prevent neonatal herpes in the newborn
- Check for other sexually transmitted diseases in cases of primary herpes
- Aciclovir has not been shown to be teratogenic; however, it is not licensed in pregnancy and it should be used with caution in the first 20 weeks[6]
- Oral or iv aciclovir should be used in standard doses in line with the clinical condition[4]
- Women who have had their first episode of genital herpes in the first or second trimester or who have recurrent genital herpes, can take oral aciclovir for the last 4 weeks of pregnancy to try and prevent a recurrence at term[10]
- Determination of whether any episode is a primary infection or a recurrence is extremely important and has implications for the mode of delivery (see below)
- Recurrences of genital herpes in pregnancy are likely to be brief and uncomplicated

Medical Management and Care

Primary Genital Herpes in Pregnancy

- Swabs should be sent to confirm diagnosis and referral to a genitourinary physician made[4]
- Blood should also be sent if the lesions present within 6 weeks of delivery as the presence of antibodies of the same type as the HSV isolated from genital swabs would confirm this episode to be a recurrence rather than a primary infection
- A full screen for other sexually transmitted diseases should be undertaken
- The woman should be given counselling, support and written information[4]
- A 5-day course of oral aciclovir should be considered if symptoms are severe and iv aciclovir used if there is disseminated infection[6] (aciclovir is rarely indicated for treatment of recurrent episodes of genital herpes during pregnancy)
- The woman should be warned of the possible complications and to report any deterioration in her condition
- Discuss the need for LSCS if infection has occurred within 6 weeks of delivery

Midwifery Management and Care

- A history of HSV infection should be obtained at booking and the woman warned to report any symptoms of genital herpes if they arise, in which case she should be referred for confirmation, treatment and counselling
- General hygiene advice and advice regarding pain relief should be given if an episode occurs
- Be aware of confidentiality issues including possibility of withholding details on patient-held records

Labour Issues

The mode of delivery depends upon whether the episode is primary or a recurrence and how near to delivery the primary infection was.

When the first episode of genital herpes occurs at the time of delivery and if the baby is delivered vaginally in the presence of active lesions, the risk of neonatal herpes is around 40%[6]. In view of this LSCS is recommended if primary genital herpes occurs at or up to 6 weeks prior to delivery.

If a woman has a recurrence around the time of delivery, the risk to the baby of neonatal herpes is small[11,12], and vaginal delivery is now considered safe[6].

For women with a history of recurrent genital herpes, who would opt for caesarean delivery if HSV lesions were detected at the onset of labour, daily suppressive aciclovir given from 36 weeks of gestation until delivery may be given to reduce the likelihood of HSV lesions at term.

Medical Management and Care

- Discuss the benefits of caesarean section if primary genital herpes occurs at, or within, 6 weeks of delivery. This is not the case if the infection occurs in the first or second trimesters[4,6]
- If a woman has primary herpes during labour, or within the previous 6 weeks, and opts for a vaginal delivery, then invasive procedures such as fetal blood sampling, the use of fetal scalp electrodes and instrumental deliveries avoided[6]
- Intravenous aciclovir should be considered in labour and for the neonate[6]
- Women who have a recurrence of genital herpes in pregnancy should be reassured that vaginal delivery is safe and that in the absence of active lesions there is no indication for a LSCS
- If a woman has active lesions of recurrent genital herpes at the onset of labour then the mode of delivery should be discussed with her, but she should be informed that the risks to the baby are small and should be set against the risks of LSCS[6]

Midwifery Management and Care

- Examination of all women during vaginal assessment for any possible sign of genital herpes should be made at the beginning of labour[4] and the medical staff alerted if any concerns

Postpartum issues

- The neonatologists should be informed of any women who delivered within 6 weeks of primary genital herpes infection, irrespective of mode of delivery – and the baby observed and treated appropriately[6]
- Care of the perineum is important in the presence of active lesions
- There is a risk of postnatal transmission of HSV to the baby due to contact with HSV infection such as orolabial herpes or herpetic whitlow[6]
- If symptoms 'flare' in the puerperium there may be dysuria or an inability to micturate

Medical Management and Care

- The baby should be assessed and the need for aciclovir in the baby determined

Midwifery Management and Care

- Advice on perineal hygiene should be given
- Ensure adequate bladder care, and ascertain ease and frequency of micturition
- Mothers, family members and healthcare worker with active HSV infection, including 'cold sores', should avoid contact with newborn babies[6]

12.8 Streptococcal Sepsis

Incidence	Risk for Childbearing
52 UK cases of Streptococcus A puerperal sepsis in 2003[1]	High Risk
13 UK maternal deaths 2006–2008 from group A streptoccal sepsis[2]	

EXPLANATION OF CONDITION

Rebecca Lancefield in 1933[3] classified the Streptococcus bacteria into sub-groups denoted by letter. This classification system is still used internationally. Of most significance in childbearing are Lancefield Groups A and B.

Group A – *Streptococcus pyogenes* (GAS): 5–30% of the UK population are asymptomatic carriers[4] and GAS causes impetigo, scarlet fever, rheumatic fever, and tonsillitis[5,6]. It is the most common cause of sore throats in childhood[2]. This community acquired infection is more common in winter and spring[1,7] and can cause severe, sudden illness in the otherwise fit and healthy[1].

Historically, GAS caused epidemic puerperal sepsis prior to the advent of hand-washing techniques and antisepsis[8,5]. Whilst puerperal sepsis declined in high income countries[7] it persisted elsewhere[6]. A virulent strain has recently developed[9] contributing to the re-emergence of invasive GAS and associated diseases, including maternal sepsis, in high income countries.

Group B – *Streptococcus agalactiae* (GBS): 10–30% of women carry GBS in their vaginal flora[10] and a debate persists about routine screening in pregnancy[11]. A vaccine is currently being tested[10]. Maternal infection is rarely life threatening, often presenting as urinary tract or wound infections[12]. However, GBS is the leading cause of neonatal sepsis and meningitis[10].

Neonatal GBS is acquired by 'vertical transmission' in labour and the affected baby presents within days of birth with lethargy, pyrexia and respiratory distress[10].

There is moderate evidence that antibiotic prophylaxis is beneficial for women at high risk of neonatal GBS infection[13]. If GBS is found in the urine on midstream specimen then this should be treated and the woman offered antibiotic prophylaxis in labour[11]. There is no need to treat asymptomatic vaginal carriage. However, prophylactic antibiotics should be offered in labour[11]. Other risk factors for early neonatal infection include prematurity, prelabour rupture of membranes >18 hours, pyrexia >38°C in labour and previous affected baby. Intrapartum prophylactic antibiotics should be considered if one or more risk factors are present[11].

As GBS rarely causes significant maternal infection, the rest of this section will discuss the diagnosis and management of maternal sepsis with GAS.

COMPLICATIONS

Genital Tract Sepsis

Historically, severe sepsis was mainly a postpartum event (puerperal sepsis). However, it is now widely recognised that genital tract infection can be acquired during pregnancy, labour, the puerperium or after surgery[2]. The main causative organism is GAS[2].

Sepsis in early pregnancy is associated with septic miscarriage, termination of pregnancy, premature rupture of membranes and chorioamnionitis[2].

Infection in the third trimester may present with a short history of flu-like symptoms, tachycardia and an abnormal CTG. This may lead to emergency caesarean section with an increased risk of an atonic uterus, major haemorrhage, cardiac arrest or adult respiratory distress syndrome (ARDS), fetal infection and asphyxia, maternal and/or perinatal

death[2]. Recognition of the severity of the infection and prompt treatment prior to caesarean section may prevent this.

GAS sepsis is associated with prolonged rupture of membranes, emergency CS, and retained products of conception[14]. It has a high case fatality rate (7.7% of maternal sepsis), often requiring ICU admission[8].

Early symptoms and signs of sepsis are[10,14]:

- Vomiting
- Diarrhoea
- Abdominal pain
- Lymphangitis (reddened streaks due to inflamed lymphatic vessels beneath the skin)[10]
- Tachycardia
- Increased respiratory rate
- Pyrexia

Necrotising Fasciitis **(Haemolytic Gangrene)**[7]

The infection starts in a layer of fascia and spreads rapidly destroying tissue.

Toxic Shock Syndrome

If unrecognised and untreated the infection can progress to **septicaemia.** Initially a systemic inflammatory response syndrome (SIRS) occurs, leading to a fall in blood pressure (hypotension), tachycardia, collapse of blood vessels and reduced perfusion of the peripheries (**septic shock**).

Cyanosis, organ dysfunction, and increased thrombotic risk follow. Multiple organ failure results leading to death. Septicaemia alone has 50–70% mortality[10].

Puerperal Sepsis

Defined by WHO[15] as: infection of the genital tract occurring at any time between the rupture of membranes or labour, and the 42nd day postpartum in which two or more of the following are present:

- Pelvic pain
- Oral temperature ≥38.5°C on any occasion
- Abnormal vaginal discharge, e.g. presence of pus
- Abnormal smell/foul odour of discharge
- Delay in the rate of reduction of the size of the uterus (<2 cm/day during the first 8 days)

NON-PREGNANCY TREATMENT AND CARE

- Blood culture to determine organism
- Specific antibiotic therapy
- Elevation and stabilisation of blood pressure
- Intense observation

PRE-CONCEPTION ISSUES AND CARE

Woman who have previously had septicaemia and/or genital tract sepsis are at increased risk of infection in pregnancy. The risk of infection depend upon issues such as general state of health, immunosuppression, drug misuse, social living factors, and pre-existing medical conditions, e.g. sickle cell disease. Ideally optimum heath should be attained before contraception is ceased.

Pregnancy Issues

- UK CMACE report showed 13 out of 26 maternal deaths due to genital tract sepsis were caused by GAS[2]. A similar picture is emerging in Japan, Australia and the Netherlands[1,8,16]
- Acquisition of GAS occurs mainly in winter or spring[1,7] and is associated with respiratory tract infections
- Affected UK and Japanese women either had, or worked with, children[2,7], suggesting children as a source of infection
- Risk factors include pre-existing medical disorders, especially sickle cell disease and ethnicity (particularly Black African)[2]
- The uterine myometrium is extremely sensitive to bacterial infection in late pregnancy and a generalised streptococcal illness could result in a myometritis which irritates the myometrium causing intense contractions similar to abruptio placentae and risking preterm labour[7]
- Fluid overload may lead to fatal pulmonary or cerebral oedema[2]

Common Symptoms of Genital Tract Sepsis:
- Fever, flu-like illness
- Diarrhoea and vomiting
- Abdominal pain
- Abnormal CTG/absent fetal heart beat
- Rash/red streaks in the skin/mottling
- Vaginal discharge
- Wound inflammation and pain

Be aware that symptoms can mimic a placental abruption

Medical Management and Care

Appropriate antibiotic prophylaxis for women with sickle cell disease[2], for women requiring ERPoC, or for women with pre-term premature rupture of the membranes (PPROM). Prompt treatment with antibiotics if miscarriage associated with sepsis[16]

If symptoms present, initial investigations[2]:
- Full blood picture
- C-reactive protein
- U&E
- Liver function tests
- Coagulation screen
- Arterial blood gases and lactate
- Blood cultures (preferably two), taken prior to antibiotic administration
- High and low vaginal swabs
- MSU
- Throat swab

Immediate aggressive treatment with iv broad spectrum antibiotics within first hour (golden hour) of recognising sepsis[18] with a full loading dose. Adjust drugs and dosages as results become available. This regimen should be reviewed daily[2].

Involve critical care team /anesthetists early.

Midwifery Management and Care

- Antenatal education to raise awareness of signs and seriousness of infection
- Personal and perineal hygiene
- General house cleaning especially toilet handles and seat
- Avoiding unnecessary contact with potentially ill children

If a mother reports symptoms of feeling unwell, especially sore throat:
- Observations of temperature, pulse, respiration, blood pressure, and urinalysis
- Refer to a doctor early if signs of sepsis
- Assist with taking and recording of above investigations
- Frequent observations recorded on a MEOWS chart
- Strict hourly recording of fluid balance
- Care of IVI and drug administration
- Basic nursing care
- Keep relatives informed of current condition of woman
- Report any worsening of condition to medical staff

Labour Issues

Streptococcal sepsis is due to GAS (GBS rarely causes severe maternal sepsis[12])

Risk of GAS infection increases after prolonged rupture of membranes, emergency caesarean section and retained products[14]

If there is a persistent septic focus surgery may be required and may include:
- Caesarean section
- ERPoC
- Laparotomy
- Hysterectomy[2]

Following delivery or surgery transfer to intensive care is likely

Medical Management and Care

- Appropriate antibiotic prophylaxis for caesarean section[16], repair of 3rd and 4th degree tears[16], manual removal of placental and pre-term labour[2,16]
- If symptoms present in labour, investigations and treatment as above
- If surgery is required stabilise condition first if possible, cross-match adequate blood and avoid multiple doses of carboprost
- If a laparotomy is felt to be necessary, involve a GI surgeon and consider a mid-line incision

Midwifery Management and Care

- Effective hygiene throughout labour to prevent acquisition of infection
- Regular observations and accurate recording throughout labour
- Prepare for possible surgery
- Adhere to local high risk protocols and give care as above

Postnatal Issues

Contamination of the perineum or a wound, is more likely if the mother or her family have throat infections and a hand to perineum transmission results.

Although the infection might have been acquired during the intrapartum period, the illness may present postnatally once the mother has been discharged home.

Symptoms are as above plus poor involution of the uterus, pain in the supra-pubic area, and heavy or offensive smelling lochia.

If illness is suspected the midwife should not delegate observations or care to an unqualified assistant.

Puerperal sepsis is not longer a notifiable disease in the UK,[17] but it may be in other countries.

Medical Management and Care

If infection presents postnatally investigations as above, with the addition of:
- Perineal and rectal swabs
- Culture breast milk

Management and treatment as above. Neonatologist to assess baby if concerns.

Midwifery Management and Care

Prevention:
All the advice of the antenatal period but emphasise washing hands BEFORE and after using the toilet in hospital and at home.

Detection:
- Thorough systematic postnatal examination of all mothers
- Be alert for the sudden presentation of symptoms and illness
- Vigilant observations as above, with accurate recording

Action:
- Medical aid must be sought as a matter of priority and the midwife should not leave the mother. Save key items such as sanitary pads
- Make arrangements for care of the baby, while accompanying a mother in an ambulance
- Realistic reassurance of mother and her family

12 Infectious Disease

PATIENT ORGANISATIONS

Children's Liver Disease Trust
36 Great Charles Street
Birmingham B3 3JY
www.childliverdisease.org

British Liver Trust
Ransomes Europark
Ipswich IP3 9GQ
www.britishlivertrust.org.uk

Hepatitis Foundation International
504 Blick Drive
Silver Spring
MD 20904, USA
www.HepatitisFoundation.org

Hepatitis C Trust
27 Crosby Row
London SE1 3YD
www.hepcuk.info

NHS Hepatitis C
www.hepc.nhs.uk

Human Immunodeficiency Virus
Children's HIV Association (CHIVA)
www.bhiva.org/chiva

Children with AIDS Charity (CWAC)
Lion House
3 Plough Yard
London EC2A 3LP
info@cwac.org

Terence Higgins Trust (THT)
52–54 Grays Inn Road
London WC1X 8JU
www.tht.org.uk

Tommy's Pregnancy Information Service
(Toxoplasmosis Support Network)
http://www.tommys.org/Page.aspx?pid=193

International Herpes Alliance
www.herpesalliance.org

Group B Strep Support
PO Box 203
Haywards Heath
West Sussex RH16 1GF
www.gbss.org.uk

Surviving Sepsis Campaign
http://www.survivingsepsis.org/About_the_Campaign/
Pages/default.aspx

ESSENTIAL READING

British HIV Association (BHIVA) for latest HIV in pregnancy guidelines. http://www.bhiva.org/ClinicalGuidelines.aspx

Clinical Effectiveness Group 2001 **National Guideline on the Management of Genital Herpes.** Association of Genitourinary Medicine and the Medical Society for the Study of Venereal Diseases

Department of Health 2004 **Hepatitis C: Essential Information for Professionals and Guidance on Testing**. London: DoH. www.dh.gov.uk/publications

Doroshenko A, Sherrard J and Pollard A 2006 Syphilis in pregnancy care and the neonatal period. **International Journal of STD and AIDS**, 17:221–226 (reprinted in **MIDIRS**, 16:491–496).

Gilling-Smith C and Almeida P 2003 HIV, Hepatitis B and Hepatitis C and Infertility: Reducing Risk. Educational Bulletin by the Practice and Policy Committee of the BFS. **Human Fertility**, 6:106–122.

Health Protection Agency **Pregnancy and Tuberculosis.** www.hpa.org.uk/infections/topics_az/tb/menu.htm

Kennedy J 2003 **HIV in Pregnancy and Childbirth**, 2nd Edn. Hale; Books for Midwives Press/Elsevier

Royal College of Obstetricians and Gynaecologists Clinical Guidelines, No. 13: Chickenpox in Pregnancy; No. 30: Management of genital herpes in pregnancy; No. 36: Prevention of early onset neonatal group B streptococcal disease www.rcog.org.uk

The Cat Group Policy Statement No.6. **Cats and Toxoplasmosis** The Cat Group, High Street, Tisbury, Wiltshire SP3 6LD. http://www.thecatgroup.org.uk/

World Health Organisation 2010 Guidelines for the Treatment of Malaria 2nd Edn. Geneva: WHO. http://www.who.int/malaria/publications/atoz/9789241547925/en/index.html

http://www.cdc.gov/malaria/

http://www.hpa.org.uk/Topics/InfectiousDiseases/InfectionsAZ/Malaria/Guidelines/

http://www.hpa.org.uk/Topics/InfectiousDiseases/InfectionsAZ/Toxoplasmosis/GeneralInformation/toxop010InformationforHealthProfessional/

http://www.rcog.org.uk/womens-health/clinical-guidance/infection-and-pregnancy-study-group-statement

References

12.1 Viral Hepatitis

1. Worman HJ. **The Liver Disorders and Hepatitis Sourcebook**. Maidenhead; McGraw-Hill Education
2. Hoofnagle JH 1990 Chronic hepatitis B. **New England Journal Medicine**, 323:337–339
3. Hill JB, Sheffield JS, Kim MJ, *et al.* 2002 Risk of hepatitis B transmission in breast–fed infants of chronic hepatitis B carriers. **Obstetrics and Gynaecology**, 99:1049–1052
4. Hoofnagle JH 1997 Hepatitis C: the clinical spectrum of disease. **Hepatology**, 26(Suppl. 1):15S–20S
5. Seeff LB 1997 Natural history of hepatitis C. **Hepatology**, 26(Suppl. 1):21S–28S
6. **Hepatitis Prevention and Treatment (Milestones in Drug Therapy)**. Joseph M Colacino, Beverly A Heinz (Eds). 2004. Birkhauser Verlag Press, Basel-Boston-Berlin
7. Department of Health 2002 **Getting Ahead of the Curve: A Strategy for Combating Infectious Diseases**. London; DH
8. Salisbury TM and Begg N (Eds) 1996 *Hepatitis B* in **Immunisation Against Infectious Disease**. London; HMSO 95–108
9. Kane M 1995 Global programme for the control of hepatitis B infection. **Vaccine**, 13(Suppl. 1):S47–49
10. Vento S, Garfano T, Renzeni Ce, *et al* 1998 Fulminant hepatitis associated with hepatitis A virus superinfection in patients with hepatitis C. **New England Journal of Medicine**, 338: 286-290
11. Brook MG, Lever AM, Griffiths P, *et al.* 1989 Antenatal screening for hepatitis B is medically and economically effective in the prevention of vertical transmission: three years experience in a London hospital. **Quarterly Journal of Medicine**, 264:313–317
12. Department of Health 2004 **Hepatitis C: Essential Information for Professionals and Guidance on Testing**. London; DH
13. Giacchino R, Tasso L, Timitilli A, *et al.* 1998 Vertical transmission of hepatitis C virus infection: usefulness of viraemia detection in HIV-seronegative hepatitis C virus-seropositive mothers. **Journal of Pediatrics**, 132:167–169
14. Seow HF 1999 Hepatitis B and C in pregnancy. **Current Obstetrics and Gynecology**, 9:216–223
15. Andre FE, Zuckerman AJ 1994 Review: protective efficacy of hepatitis B vaccines in neonates. **Journal of Medical Virology**, 44: 144–151

12.2 Human Immunodeficiency Virus

1. Health Protection Report HIV in the United Kingdom: 2010 Report. Volume 4 Number 47 Published on: 26 November 2010
2. Collaborative HIV Paediatric Study (CHIPS). Summary data to the end of March 2009. Available at: www.chipscohort.ac.uk/summary_data.asp (Accessed 1-1-2011)
3. Patman R, Sankar KN, Elawad B, Handy P and Price DA (Eds) 2010 **Oxford Handbook of Genitourinary Medicine, HIV and AIDS (Oxford Handbooks Series)**. Oxford; Oxford University Press
4. De Ruiter A, *et al.* 2008 British HIV Association and Children's HIV Association guidelines on the management of HIV infection in pregnant women 2008. **HIV Medicine**, 9:452–502
5. Brocklehurst P and French R 1998The association between maternal HIV infection and perinatal outcome: a systematic review of the literature and meta-analysis. **British Journal of Obstetrics and Gynaecology**, 105: 836–848
6. European Collaborative Study 2000 Swiss mother and Child HIV Cohort Study. Combination antiretroviral therapy and duration of pregnancy. **AIDS**, 14: 2913–2930
7. Gazzard BG *et al.* 2008 British HIV Association guidelines for the treatment of HIV-1-infected adults with antiretroviral therapy. **HIV Medicine**, 9:563–608

8. Wright TC Jr, Ellerbrock TV, Chiasson MA, Van Devanter N, Sun XW 1994 Cervical intraepithelial neoplasia in women infected with human immunodeficiency virus: prevalence, risk factors, and validity of Papanicolaou smears. New York Cervical Disease Study. **Obstetrics and Gynecology**, 84:591–597
9. Madge S, Phillips AN, Griffioen A, *et al.* 1998 Demographic, clinical and social factors associated with an immunodeficiency virus infection and other sexually transmitted diseases in a cohort of women from the United Kingdom and Ireland. MRC Collaborative Study of women with HIV. **International Journal of Epidemiology**, 27:1068–1071
10. Corbett EL, Steketee RW, Ter Kuile FO, *et al.* 2002 HIV-1/AIDS and the control of other infectious diseases in Africa. *Lancet* 359:2177–2187
11. Leroy V, De Clerq A, Ladner J, *et al.* 1995 Should screening of genital infections be part of antenatal care in areas of high HIV prevalence? A prospective cohort study from Kigali, Rwanda, 1992–1993. The Pregnancy and HIV (EGE) Group. **Genitourinary Medicine**, 71:207–211
12. Hillier SL, Martius J, Krohn M *et al.* 1988 A case-control study of chorioamniotic infection and histologic chorioamnionitis in prematurity. **New England Journal of Medicine**, 319:972–978
13. Goldenberg RL, Hauth JC and Andrews WW 2000 Intrauterine infection and preterm delivery. **New England Journal of Medicine**, 342: 1500–1507
14. Hillier SL, Nugent RP, Eschenbach DA *et al.* 1995 Association between bacterial vaginosis and preterm delivery of a low-birthweight infant. **New England Journal of Medicine**, 333: 1737–1742

12.3 Malaria

1. WHO 2010 The World Malaria Report 2010. http://www.who.int/malaria/world_malaria_report_2010/en/index.html [Accessed 23-12-2010]
2. http://www.hpa.org.uk/Topics/InfectiousDiseases/Infections AZ/Malaria/EpidemiologicalData/malaEpi10CasesandDeaths/ [Accessed 22-12-10]
3. The NHS Clinical Knowledge Summaries (formerly PRODIGY) http://www.cks.nhs.uk/clinical_topics/by_clinical_specialty/infections_and_infestations [Accessed 22-12-10]
4. http://www.cdc.gov/malaria/about/facts.html [Accessed 22-12-10]
5. Wyler DJ 1992 **Plasmodium and Babesia** in Gorbach SL, Bartlett JG and Blacklow NR (Eds) Infectious Diseases. Philadelphia: WB Saunders 1967–1975
6. Wellcome Trust 2005 Sickle Cell Trait Offers Malaria Immunity to Children. http://malaria.wellcome.ac.uk/doc_WTD023878.html [Accessed 22-12-10]
7. http://www.cdc.gov/malaria/about/faqs.html [Accessed 22-12-10]
8. Stephen L and Hoffman DM 1992 Diagnosis, treatment, and prevention of malaria. **Medical Clinics of North America**, 76:1327–1355
9. Franco A and Ernest JM 2011 Parasitic infections in James DK, Steer JS, Weiner CP and Gonik B (Eds) **High Risk Pregnancy Management Options**, 4th Edn. London: WB Saunders 548–551
10. BNF 60, 2010 **British National Formulary**. London: British Medical Association and Royal Pharmaceutical Society of Great Britain
11. Chiodini P, Hill D, Lalloo D, *et al.* 2007 on behalf of Health Protection Agency Advisory Committee on Malaria Prevention for UK Travellers. Guidelines for malaria prevention in travellers from the United Kingdom. http://www.hpa.org.uk/Publications/

InfectiousDiseases/TravelHealth/0701Malariaprevention
fortravellersfromtheUK/ [Accessed 23-12-10]

12. WHO 2006 **The Africa Malaria Report**. Geneva; World Health Organization

13. Brabin BJ, Warsame M, Uddenfeldt-Wort U, Dellicour S, Hill J and Gies S 2008 Monitoring and evaluation of malaria in pregnancy-developing a rational basis for control. **Malaria Journal**, 7(suppl.1):s6

14. Whitty CJ, Edmonds S and Mutabingwa TK 2005 Malaria in pregnancy. **British Journal of Obstetrics and Gynaecology**, 112:1189–1195

15. http://www.cdc.gov/malaria/pdf/clinicalguidance.pdf [Accessed 23-12-10]

16. Lalloo DG, Shingadia D, Pasvol G, *et al.* 2007 HPA Advisory Committee on Malaria prevention in UK Travellers. UK malaria treatment guidelines. **Journal of Infection**, 54:111–121

17. WHO 2010 **Guidelines for the treatment of malaria**, 2nd Edn. Geneva; World Health Organization. Available: http://www. who.int/malaria/publications/atoz/9789241547925/en/index. html [Accessed 22-12-10]

18. Hashemzadeh A and Heydarian F 2005 Congenital malaria in a neonate. **Archives of Iranian Medicine**, 8:226–228

19. http://www.hpa.org.uk/web/HPAwebFile/HPAweb_C/ 1194947318515 [Accessed 23-12-10]

20. http://malariasite.com/malaria/pregnancy.htm [Accessed 23-12-10]

12.4 Chickenpox

1. Miller E, Marshall R and Vurdien JE 1993 Epidemiology, outcome and control of *Varicella zoster* virus infection. **Reviews in Medical Microbiology**, 4:222–230

2. Smego RA and Asperilla MO 1991 Use of acyclovir for varicella pneumonia during pregnancy. **Obstetrics and Gynaecology**, 78:1112–1116

3. O'Riordan M, O'Gorman C, Morgan C, *et al.* 2000 Sera prevalence of *Varicella zoster* virus in pregnant women in Dublin. **Irish Journal of Medical Science**, 169:288

4. McGregor JA, Mark S, Crawford GP and Levin MJ 1987 *Varicella zoster* antibody testing in the care of pregnant women exposed to varicella. **American Journal of Obstetrics and Gynecology**, 157:281–284

5. Paryani SG and Arvin AM 1986 Intrauterine infection with *Varicella zoster* virus after maternal varicella. **New England Journal of Medicine**, 314:1542–1546

6. Pastuszak Al, Levy M, Schick RN, *et al.* 1994 Outcome after maternal varicella infection in the first 20 weeks of pregnancy. **New England Journal of Medicine**, 330:901–905

7. Enders G, Miller E, Cradock-Watson J, Bolley I and Ridehalgh MK 1994 Consequences of varicella and *Herpes zoster* in pregnancy: prospective study of 1739 cases. **Lancet**, 343:1548–1551

8. Pretorrius DH, Hayward I, Jones KL and Stamm E 1992 Sonographic evaluation of pregnancies with maternal varicella infection. **Journal of Ultrasound Medicine**, 11:459–463

9. Anon 2005 Chickenpox, pregnancy and the newborn: a follow-up. **Drugs and Therapeutics Bulletin**, 43:94–95

10. Miller E, Cradock-Watson JE and Ridehalgh MK 1989 Outcome in newborn babies given anti-*Varicella zoster* immunoglobulin after perinatal maternal infection with *Varicella zoster* virus. **Lancet**, 2:371–373

11. BNF 49 2005 **British National Formulary**. London; British Medical Association and Royal Pharmaceutical Society of Great Britain

12. RCOG 2001 **Clinical Guideline No.13, Chickenpox in Pregnancy**. London; Royal College of Obstetricians and Gynaecologists

13. Nathwani D, Maclean A, Conway S and Carrington D 1998 Varicella infections in pregnancy and the newborn. **Journal of Infection**, 36(Suppl.1):59–71

14. Anon 2005 Chickenpox, pregnancy and the newborn. **Drugs and Therapeutics Bulletin**, 43:69–72

12.5 Toxoplasmosis

1. http://www.hpa.org.uk/Topics/InfectiousDiseases/Infections AZ/Toxoplasmosis/GeneralInformation/toxop010Informationfor HealthProfessional/ [Accessed 04-01-2011]

2. Hawker J, Begg N, Blair I, Reintjes R and Weinberg J 2005 **Communicable Disease Control Handbook**, 2nd Edn. Oxford; Blackwell Publishing Ltd. 215–217

3. http://www.nhs.uk/chq/pages/1107.aspx?CategoryID=54&SubCategoryID=137 [Accessed 06-01-2011]

4. Remington J, McLeod R, Wilson C and Desmonts G 2010 Toxoplasmosis in Remington J, Jerome Klein J, Wilson C, Victor Nizet V, Maldonado Y (Eds) **Infectious Diseases of the Fetus and Newborn Infant**, 7th Edn. Amsterdam: Elsevier 918–1028

5. Shetty N, Tang JW and Andrews J 2009 **Infectious Disease: Pathogenesis, Prevention and Case Studies**. Oxford; Wiley-Blackwell 349–352

6. Kravetz JD, Federman DG 2005 Toxoplasmosis in pregnancy. **The American Journal of Medicine**, 118:212–216

7. Franco A and Ernest JM 2011 **Parasitic infection** in James DK, Steer JS, Weiner CP and Gonik B (Eds) **High Risk Pregnancy Management Options**, 4th Edn. London: WB Saunders 555–558

8. BNF 60, 2010 **British National Formulary**. London: British Medical Association and Royal Pharmaceutical Society of Great Britain

9. Miron D, Raz R and Luder A 2002 Congenital toxoplasmosis in Israel: to screen or not to screen. **Israel Medical Association Journal**, 4, 119–122

10. Personal View 1991 Controversy breeds ignorance. **British Medical Journal**, 302:973

11. Naessens A, Jenum PA, Pollak A, *et al.* 1999 Diagnosis of congenital toxoplasmosis in the neonatal period: a Multicenter evaluation. **The Journal of Pediatrics**, 135:714–719

12.6 Listeriosis

1. European Centre for Disease Prevention And Control 2010 Annual epidemiological report on communicable disease in Europe. http://www.ecdc.europa.eu/en/publications/Publications/1011_ SUR_Annual_Epidemiological_Report_on_Communicable_ Diseases_in_Europe.pdf [Accessed 02-01-2011]

2. http://www.hpa.org.uk/Topics/InfectiousDiseases/Infections AZ/Listeria/EpidemiologicalData/listeCaseReports19832009/ [Accessed 02-01-2011]

3. http://www.hps.scot.nhs.uk/ewr/subjectsummary.aspx?subjectid =99 [Accessed 02-01-2011]

4. Braden CR 2003 Listeriosis. **Paediatric Infectious Disease Journal**, 22:745–746

5. http://www.hpa.org.uk/listeriafactsheet [Accessed 01-01-2011]

6. Hawker J, Begg N, Blair I, Reintjes R and Weinberg J 2005 **Communicable Disease Control Handbook**, 2nd Edn. Oxford; Blackwell Publishing Ltd. 148–150

7. Shetty N, Tang JW, Andrews J 2009 **Infectious Disease: Pathogenesis, Prevention and Case Studies**. Oxford; Wiley-Blackwell 338–340

8. Lundén J, Tolvanen R and Korkeala H 2004 Human listeriosis linked to dairy products in Europe. **Journal of Dairy Science**, 87:E6–E12

9. Nelson KE, Warren D, Tomasi AM, Raju TN and Vidyasagar D 1985 Transmission of neonatal listeriosis in a delivery room. **American Journal of Diseases of Children**, 139:903–5

10. Hanssler L, Rosenthal E and Fitza B 1990 Listeriosis in newborn infants. **Klinical Padiatric**, 202:379–382

11. http://www.merckmanuals.com/professional/sec18/ch261/ ch261l.html [Accessed 02-01-2011]

12. http://www.cdc.gov/nczved/divisions/dfbmd/diseases/ listeriosis/ [Accessed 02-01-2011]

13. Sweet RL and Gibbs RS 2002 **Infectious Diseases of the Female Genital Tract**. Philadelphia; Lippincott Williams & Wilkins 474–477

14. Silver HM 1998 Listeriosis during pregnancy. **Obstetrical and Gynecological Survey**, 53:737–740

15. Nolla-Salas J, Bosch J, Gasser I, *et al.* 1999 Perinatal listeriosis: a population-based multicenter study in Barcelona, Spain (1990–1996). **Obstetrical and Gynecological Survey**, 54:358–360

16. Mylonakis E, Paliou M, Hohmann EL, Calderwood S and Wing EJ 2002 Listeriosis during pregnancy: a case series and review of 222 cases. **Medicine**, 81:260–269

17. Temple ME and Nahata MC 2000 Treatment of listeriosis. **The Annals of Pharmacotherapy**, 34:656–661
18. American Academy of Pediatrics 2005 Breast-feeding and the use of human milk. **Pediatrics**, 115:496–506

12.7 Herpes Simplex Virus

1. HPA 2004 Epidemiological data – genital herpes. **Health Protection Agency** www.hpa.org.uk [Accessed: 22-04-2006]
2. Tookey P and Peckham CS 1996 Neonatal *Herpes simplex* virus infection in the British Isles. **Paediatric Perinatal Epidemiology**, 10:432–442
3. Brown ZA, Selke S, Zeh J, *et al.* 1997 The acquisition of *Herpes simplex* virus during pregnancy. **New England Journal of Medicine**, 337:509–515
4. Clinical Effectiveness Group 2001 National guideline on the management of genital herpes. Clinical Effectiveness Group – **Association for Genitourinary Medicine and the Medical Society for the Study of Venereal Diseases**
5. Nelson-Piercy C 2002 **Handbook of Obstetric Medicine**, 2nd Edn. London; Taylor and Francis
6. RCOG 2002 **Guideline No. 30 Management of Genital Herpes in Pregnancy**. Royal College of Obstetrics and Gynaecology
7. BNF 49 2005 **British National Formulary**. London; British Medical Association and Royal Pharmaceutical Society of Great Britain
8. Mertz GJ, Benedetti J, Ashley R, Selke SA and Corey L 1992 Risk factors for the sexual transmission of genital herpes. **Annals of Internal Medicine**, 116:197–202
9. Qutub M, Klapper P, Vallely P and Cleator G 2001 Genital herpes in pregnancy: is screening cost-effective? **International Journal of Sexually Transmitted Disease and AIDS**, 12:14–16
10. Sheffield JS, Hollier LM, Hill JB, Stuart GS and Wendel GD 2003 Acyclovir prophylaxis to prevent *Herpes simplex* virus recurrence at delivery: a systematic review. **Obstetrics and Gynaecology**, 102:1396–1403
11. Prober CG, Sullender WM, Yasukawa LL, Au DS, Yeager AS and Arvin AM 1987 Low risk of *Herpes simplex* virus infections in neonates exposed to the virus at the time of vaginal delivery to mothers with recurrent genital *Herpes simplex* virus infections. **New England Journal of Medicine**, 316: 240–244
12. Brown ZA, Benedetti J, *et al.* 1991 Neonatal herpes simplex virus infection in relation to asymptomatic maternal infection at the time of labor. **New England Journal of Medicine**, 324:1247–1252

12.8 Streptococcal Sepsis

1. Lamagni T *et al.* 2008 Epidemiology of severe *Streptococcus pyogenes* disease in Europe **Journal of Clinical Microbiology**, 46: 2359–2367. http://www.ncbi.nlm.nih.gov/pmc/articles/PMC2446932/ [Accessed 26-5-2011]
2. Harper A 2011 **Chapt. 7 Sepsis** in Lewis G (Ed.) **Saving Mothers Lives: Reviewing maternal deaths to make motherhood safer 2006–2008** 85–96
3. Lancefield RC 1933 A serological differentiation of human and other groups of hemolytic streptococci. **Journal of Experimental Medicine**, 57:571–595 http://www.jem.org/cgi/content/abstract/57/4/571.
4. Health Protection Agency 2004 Interim UK guidelines for management of close community contacts of invasive group A streptococcal disease. **Communicable Disease and Public Health**, 7:354–361
5. Sosa M 2009 Streptoccal A infection remerging and virulent. **Journal of Perinatal Nursing**, 23:141–147
6. VanDillen J *et al.* 2010 Maternal sepsis: epidemiology, etiology and outcome. **Current Opinion in Infectious Diseases**, 2:249–254
7. Udagawa H, Oshio Y and Shimizu Y 1999 Serious streptoccal infection around delivery. **Obstetrics and Gynaecology**, 94: 153–157
8. Kramer H, Schutte J, Zwart J, Schuitemaker N, Steegers E and Van Roosmalen J 2009 Maternal mortality and severe morbidity from sepsis in the Netherlands. **Acta Obstetrica et Gynecologica**, 88: 647–653

9. Lynskey N, Lawrenson R and Sriskandan S 2011 New understanding in Streptoccus pyogenes. **Current Opinion in Infectious Diseases**, 24:196–202
10. Black J 2008 **Microbiology Principles and Explorations**, 7th Edn. Hoboken; John Wiley & Sons, Inc. 719–720
11. RCOG 2003 **Guideline No. 36: Prevention of Early Onset Neonatal Group B Streptococcal Disease**. http://www.rcog.org.uk/womens-health/clinical-guidance/prevention-early-onset-neonatal-group-b-streptococcal-disease-green [Accessed 28-5-2011]
12. Walker T and Estrada B 2001 Antibiotic prophylaxis for neonatal group B streptoccal disease. http://www.medscape.com/viewarticle/410190 [Accessed 28-5-2011]
13. Gilbert R 2003 Prenatal screening for group B streptoccal infection: gaps in the evidence. **International Journal of Epidemiology**, 33: 2–8
14. Greer I, Nelson-Piercy C and Walters B 2007 **Maternal Medicine: Medical Problems in Pregnancy**. London; Elsevier 318
15. Dolea C and Stein C 2003 Global burden of maternal sepsis in the year 2000 – Evidence and Information for Policy (EIP), **World Health Organization**, Geneva, July 2003. http://www.who.int/healthinfo/statistics/bod_maternalsepsis.pdf [Accessed 22-5-2011]
16. NSW Health 2010 Safety Notice 017/10 Group A Streptococcal Maternal Sepsis. New South Wales Department of Health. http://www.health.nsw.gov.au/resources/quality/sabs/pdf/sn_017_10.pdf [Accessed 28-5-2011]
17. Steer PJ 2011 Is infection making a comeback in maternity care? **British Journal of Obstetrics and Gynaeology**, 118:i–ii http://onlinelibrary.wiley.com/doi/10.1111/j.1471-0528.2010.02826.x/full
18. Dellinger R, Levy M, Carlet J et al 2008 Surviving Sepsis Campaign. **Critical Care Medicine**; 36 296–327

Figure Reference

Black JG 2008 **Microbiology: Principles and Explorations**, 7th Edn. International Student Version. Oxford; Wiley-Blackwell

Appendices References

Appendix 12.1.1 The ABC of Hepatitis
1. Hepatitis Foundation International 2007 ABC of Hepatitis. www.hepatitisfoundation.org [Accessed 02-07-2007]

Appendices 12.2.1 and 12.2.2
1. Koch WC, Harger JH, Barnstein B, *et al.* 1998 Serological and virologic evidence for frequent intrauterine transmission of human parvovirus B19 with a primary maternal infection during pregnancy. **Journal of Pediatric Infectious Disease**, 17:489–494
2. Miller E, Fairley CK, Cohen BJ, *et al.* 1998 Immediate and long term outcome of human parvovirus B19 infection in pregnancy. **British Journal of Obstetrics and Gynaecology**, 105:174–178
3. Clinical Effectiveness Group 2002 UK National Guidelines on the Management of Early Syphilis. www.bashh.org/guidelines
4. Health Protection Agency 2006 Pregnancy and Tuberculosis www.hpa.org.uk/infections/topics_az/tb/menu.htm

Appendix 12.1.1 The ABC of Hepatitis[1]

	Hepatitis A (HAV)	Hepatitis B (HBV)	Hepatitis C (HCV)	Hepatitis D (HDV)	Hepatitis E (HEV)
What is it?	HAV is a virus that causes inflammation of the liver. It does not lead to chronic disease.	HBV is a virus that causes inflammation of the liver. It can cause liver cell damage, leading to cirrhosis and cancer.	HCV is a virus that causes inflammation of the liver. It can cause liver cell damage, leading to cirrhosis and cancer.	HDV is a virus that causes inflammation of the liver. It only infects those persons with HBV.	HEV is a virus that causes inflammation of the liver. It is rare in the U.S. Rarely it can cause chronic disease
Incubation Period	2 to 7 weeks. Average 4 weeks.	6 to 23 weeks. Average 17 weeks.	2 to 25 weeks. Average 7 to 9 wks.	2 to 8 weeks.	2 to 9 weeks. Average 40 days.
How is it Spread?	Transmitted by fecal/oral (anal/oral sex) route, close person to person contact or ingestion of contaminated food and water. Hand to mouth after contact with feces, such as changing diapers.	Contact with infected blood, seminal fluid, vaginal secretions, contaminated needles, including tattoo and body-piercing tools. Infected mother to newborn. Human bite. Sexual contact.	Contact with infected blood, contaminated iv needles, razors, and tattoo and body-piercing tools, Infected mother to newborn. Not easily spread through sex.	Contact with infected blood, contaminated needles. Sexual contact with HDV infected person.	Transmitted through fecal/oral route. Outbreaks associated with contaminated water supply in other countries.
Symptoms	Children may have none. Adults usually have light stools, dark urine, fatigue, fever, nausea, vomiting, abdominal pain, and jaundice.	May have none. Some persons have mild flu like symptoms, dark urine, light stools, jaundice, fatigue and fever.	Same as HBV	Same as HBV	Same as HAV
Treatment of Chronic Disease	Not applicable	Peginterferon, entecavir, and tenofovir are first-line treatment options.	Peginterferon with ribavirin and serine protease adjuncts.	Peginterferon with varying success.	Ribavirin for chronic hepatitis E but needs confirmation
Vaccine	Two doses of vaccine to anyone over 1 year of age.	Three doses may be given to persons of any age.	None for HCV. Should receive Hepatitis A and B vaccines	HBV vaccine prevents HDV infection.	None commercially available
Who is at Risk?	Household or sexual contact with an infected person or living in an area with HAV outbreak. Travelers to developing countries, persons engaging in anal/oral sex and injection drug users.	Infants born to infected mother, having sex with an infected person or multiple partners, injection drug users, emergency responders, healthcare workers, persons engaging in anal/oral sex, and hemodialysis patients.	Blood transfusion recipients before 1992, healthcare workers, injection drug users, hemodialysis patients, infants born to infected mother, multiple sex partners.	Injection drug users, persons engaging in anal/oral sex and those having sex with an HDV infected patient.	Travelers to developing countries, especially pregnant women.
Prevention	Vaccination or Immune Globulin within 2 weeks of exposure. Washing hands with soap and water after going to the toilet. Use household bleach (10 parts water to 1 part bleach) to clean surfaces contaminated with feces, such as changing tables. Safer sex.	Vaccination provides protection for 20 plus years. Clean up blood with household bleach and wear protective gloves. Do not share razors, toothbrushes, or needles. Safer sex. Hepatitis B immune globulin for vaccine non-responders after exposure.	Clean up spilled blood with household bleach. Wear gloves when touching blood. Do not share razors, toothbrushes, or needles with anyone. Safer sex.	Hepatitis B vaccine to prevent HBV/HDV infection. Safer sex.	Avoid drinking or using potentially contaminated water.

Grid 11 |

HEPATITIS FOUNDATION INTERNATIONAL
504 Blick Drive, Silver Spring, MD 20904, USA
Tel: 1-800-891-0707 Fax: 301-622-4702
Website: www.hepatitisfoundation.org
Reproduced with kind permission

Appendix 12.2.1 Other Infectious Viral Diseases

General Details	Symptoms and Signs	Fetal Risks	Trimester of Risk	Management
Rubella RNA togavirus known as German measles Most UK women are vaccinated, hence protected from infection IP – up to 21 days (typically 7–10 days) Infective from 7 days before rash to 7 days after rash	May be symptomless May present with: · Macular rash (spreads from ears and face) · Mild febrile illness · Pharyngitis · Lymphadenopathy · Arthralgia	Congenital defects: · Ocular defects (e.g. cataracts) · Sensorineural hearing impairment · Cardiac abnormalities (e.g. patent ductus arteriosus) · Hepatosplenomegaly · Jaundice · Thrombocytopenic purpura · Low birth weight · Mental retardation	First trimester mainly: nearly all pregnancies are affected if acquired in the first 10 weeks 13–16 weeks: less risk, mainly sensorineural deafness	Ensure women are immune pre-pregnancy If not immune, immunise after delivery If infected in first 16 weeks refer for multi-disciplinary counselling to plan for further management Termination of pregnancy should be discussed
Human parvovirus B19 DNA virus causes *Erythema infectiosum*, also known as *fifth disease or slapped cheek syndrome* IP – 4–20 days Infective mainly before symptoms arise Infection gives life-long immunity; 50–60% adults immune Outbreaks occur and can last for several months	Often symptomless In children: · Febrile illness · Maculopapular rash (causing flushing of cheeks) Adult women are particularly likely to complain of arthralgia or arthritis which may last a couple of weeks and predominantly affects the peripheral joints	Fetal infection is usually benign and self-limiting Asymptomatic infection occurs in approximately 50% following maternal infection[1] · Miscarriage, risk increased by approx 10%[2] · Fetal anaemia · Hydrops fetalis, approximately 3% risk[2] · Fetal death There is no risk of congenital abnormality[2]	Risk to fetus is in the first 20 weeks only The interval between infection and development of hydrops fetalis is 2–7 weeks, with an average of 5 weeks[2]	Serological testing to confirm diagnosis Monitoring of fetus post maternal infection is by ultrasound assessment at 1–2 weekly intervals for up to 12 weeks If evidence of hydrops fetalis: fetal blood sampling and intrauterine blood transfusion when appropriate
Cytomegalovirus (CMV) DNA virus; member of the herpes family Reactivation and reinfection are common The virus can be transmitted: · Transplacentally intrapartum (by exposure to virus in cervix) · Postnatally (in breast milk) · Cross-infection (especially from other babies in nurseries)	Often symptomless May take the form of a glandular-fever-like illness with: · Fever · Hepatitis · Lymphocytosis (but no pharyngitis) It may cause hepatitis or other abnormal liver function It causes a more severe and widespread disease in immunosuppressed patients	Most commonly asymptomatic infection with no long-term sequelae Associations include: · Mental retardation · Microcephaly · Hepatosplenomegaly · Jaundice · Thrombocytopenic purpura · Low birth weight · Chorioretinitis	All trimesters Most infected fetuses not affected About 5–10% of infected newborns are symptomatic at birth	Diagnosis can be made from viral culture from urine, nasopharynx or blood, or by serological tests Discuss invasive testing to establish fetal infection Consider termination of pregnancy if early gestation and fetal infection confirmed Ultrasound surveillance of the infected or at *risk* fetus; arrange paediatric follow-up of infected neonates
Measles RNA virus; paramyxovirus IP – 10–14 days Immunity life long Well-established vaccination programme **NB**: Vaccine contraindicated in pregnancy	Usually a self-limiting illness in children with: · Fever · Rash · Cough More severe illness in adults with possible complications of: · Pneumonia · Hepatitis · Encephalitis	Not associated with congenital abnormalities Newborn delivered to a woman with active disease may develop severe neonatal measles Maternal pyrexia may precipitate premature delivery	Throughout pregnancy	Treat pyrexia aggressively, e.g. with paracetamol and cold sponging, and be alert for signs of pre-term labour

IP, incubation period

Appendix 12.2.2 Other Infectious Bacterial Diseases

General Details	Symptoms and Signs	Fetal Risks	Management
Syphilis Caused by the spirochaete Treponema *pallidum* Incubation period 10–90 days Classified as congenital or acquired	Characterised by stage: Primary syphilis · Primary anogenital chancre (ulcer) · Lymphadenopathy Secondary syphilis · Widespread maculopapular rash · Lymphadenopathy · Mucocutaneous lesions · Condylomata lata (wart-like genital lesions) Late syphilis · Gummatous lesions which may affect respiratory tract, skin, bones, joints · Possible cardiac and CNS (*neurosyphilis*) complications	70–100% of fetuses will be infected if the woman has untreated primary syphilis in pregnancy; one third of these fetuses will die *in utero*. Congenital syphilis *Early features* include skin lesions, e.g. rash, raised moist mucocutaneous lesions, 'snuffles', periostitis, hepatosplenomegaly, lymphadenopathy, osteochondritis. *Late features* include interstitial keratitis, deafness and characteristic facial features, e.g. Hutchinson's incisor, mulberry molars, frontal bossing, short maxilla, saddlenose deformity and protuberance of the mandible.	All pregnant women should be screened for syphilis at the initial antenatal visit. Those that screen positive should be managed by genitourinary physicians, obstetricians and midwives and treatment needs to be commenced promptly. First line treatment: im procaine penicillin G for 10 days[3] (erythromycin or azithromycin if penicillin allergy – treatment of baby needed if either of these are used). All babies of women treated for syphilis, either in pregnancy or in the past, should have paediatric follow-up for evidence of congenital syphilis, and serology performed[3].
Tuberculosis Caused by Mycobacterium *tuberculosis* and, rarely, Mycobacterium *bovis* Transmission is by respiratory droplets. However, M. bovis is acquired by ingestion of contaminated milk Seen as acid-alcohol fast bacilli in a Ziehl-Neelsen stain	Infection often subclinical. Approximately 5% of newly-infected people develop clinically-active disease. This is more likely if immunosuppressed or at the extremes of life. HIV is a significant risk factor for TB and complicates management. Active TB normally manifests as pulmonary TB. The symptoms and signs include malaise, night-sweats, productive cough and haemoptysis. However, it may be asymptomatic. Miliary TB occurs when the bacilli invade blood vessels and disseminate to multiple organs. This is rare but more common if immunosuppressed.	There is no increase in congenital malformations or fetal damage when rifampicin, isoniazid, ethambutol and pyrazinamide are used. Streptomycin, however, has been shown to cause fetal sensorineural deafness when used at any stage in pregnancy and must therefore be avoided. Congenital TB is rare. However, it is more common if the woman has miliary TB and is associated with increased neonatal mortality. Delays in diagnosis can result in an increase in prematurity, low birth weight and perinatal mortality[4]. If the woman is diagnosed and treated early the outcome is good[4].	Clinical infection is diagnosed by detecting acid-fast bacilli in sputum or evidence on chest X-ray. Any woman with symptoms suggestive of TB should be screened or if there has been prolonged close contact with newly-diagnosed infectious TB. Aim to diagnose and treat women prior to pregnancy. If detected in pregnancy treatment should be started without delay and coordinated by the local TB specialist and is likely to require 6 months of treatment[4]. It is rarely necessary to separate the neonate at delivery. If the infant has been exposed to infectious TB then it will require treatment. The neonatologist and TB specialist should be involved.

METABOLIC DISORDERS

Rowena Doughty[1] and Jason Waugh[2]

[1]De Montfort University, Leicester, UK
[2]Royal Victoria Infirmary, Newcastle upon Tyne, UK

13.1 Obesity
13.2 Phenylketonuria
13.3 Hyperemesis Gravidarum
13.4 Acute Fatty Liver of Pregnancy

Medical Disorders in Pregnancy: A Manual for Midwives, Second Edition. Edited by S. Elizabeth Robson and Jason Waugh.
© 2013 John Wiley & Sons, Ltd. Published 2013 by John Wiley & Sons, Ltd.

13.1 Obesity

Incidence
Obesity is an increasing phenomenon worldwide
In pregnancy the incidence is around 16–19% in the UK[1]

Risk for Childbearing
High Risk – throughout the childbearing period, especially if
co-morbidities are present or complications occur

EXPLANATION OF CONDITION

Obesity is considered to be one of the most significant health concerns affecting current society, where an individual's risk of serious morbidity and/or mortality is directly related to their increasing weight through the development of disease pathways attributable to obesity, although these pathways are unclear as individuals of normal weight also develop these conditions. The trend in the rate of obesity is upward, with an estimated 50% of women of childbearing age being classed as obese by 2050[2]. Obesity was a factor in 35% of maternal deaths[3] and has a significant influence on pregnancy outcomes[4].

- Defined as the excessive accumulation of fat within the fat cells as a result of discrepancy between energy intake and energy expenditure, obesity is a complex interplay between biology, hormonal, and emotional and psychosocial issues
- It is diagnosed using the body mass index (BMI) classification as recommended by NICE, which is the weight in kilograms divided by the square of the height in metres (see Appendix 13.1.1)
- Obesity is defined as a BMI ≥30, with underweight as <18.5, normal weight 18.5–24.9 and overweight 25–29.9. Obesity can be further subdivided into Class 1 (BMI 30.0–34.9), Class 2 (BMI 35.0–39.9) and Class 3 or morbid obesity (BMI ≥40)
- Of similar significance is the distribution of body fat, especially an increased waist-to-hip ratio; thought to be more valuable than weight alone and suggestive of disordered glucose tolerance

Obesity is also associated with:

- Gender – more common in women than men
- Postcode – there are more cases in the north of the country than in the south of the UK
- Lifestyle – increasing sedentary occupations, reliance on the car, fast food, etc.
- Mental wellbeing – depression may be linked with obesity
- Social class – rates of obesity increase as the social class lowers
- Ethnicity – increased obesity seen in certain ethnic groups, e.g. Afro-Caribbean
- Genetics – some obesity has an inherited component, although this accounts for only a small proportion of cases

COMPLICATIONS

There is a continuous relationship between obesity and morbidity and mortality and it is a common risk factor in many conditions, especially:

- Metabolic (e.g. type 2 diabetes)
- Circulatory (e.g. cardiovascular disease)
- Degenerative (e.g. osteoarthritis)

These conditions are usually associated with advancing age, although with increases in childhood obesity the age of presentation of many of these conditions is lowering.

Many of these diseases have a negative effect on life expectancy and there are increased morbidity rates for individuals

with obesity. The amplified health and social welfare costs for society in managing obesity-related conditions is also a concern, especially due to shifting population demographics. Individuals with obesity also suffer from discrimination and stigma directly attributed to their size, which may lead to lower self-esteem and self-confidence; many individuals with obesity report an overall poorer quality of life[5-7].

For women, obesity increases the risk of gynaecological complications, e.g. endometrial cancer, infertility and menorrhagia through menstrual disturbances and ovulation disorders. In the presence of sub-fertility, to increase the chances of spontaneous conception through regular menses or to increase the sensitivity of ovulation-induction techniques, women with obesity are recommended to achieve a moderate weight loss of at least 5%[8].

Therefore, weight loss to achieve a normal BMI has short- and long-term health benefits.

NON-PREGNANCY TREATMENT AND CARE

The management aim is to attain a steady weight loss until the BMI is within the normal range. Slow weight loss is more sustainable in both the short- and long-term. This is achieved through education about what constitutes a healthy diet and eating patterns and lowered overall energy intakes. Moderate exercise in combination with a well-balanced, energy-restricted diet has been shown to increase weight-loss success rates by:

- Increasing overall muscle mass (which consumes more energy than fat)
- Producing a sense of wellbeing
- Depressing the appetite
- Increasing the overall metabolic rate

Studies have also shown that behavioural and cognitive therapy combined with the above can augment success rates[9]. Group therapy, e.g. Weight Watchers, may also improve success rates.

Some obese individuals resort to surgery. There are two main types of surgical techniques: restrictive, e.g. gastric banding, and malabsorptive, e.g. stomach stapling. Bariatric surgery increases the risk of malnutrition, anaemia and vitamin deficiencies which may negatively affect pregnancy[10]. There has also been renewed interest in diet pills, e.g. orlistat (a lipase inhibitor) and sibutramine (a centrally-acting appetite suppressant), although these must be prescribed and supervised closely by the medical team and are contraindicated in pregnancy[11].

PRE-CONCEPTION ISSUES AND CARE

Because of the strong association with maternal mortality/morbidity and the problems outlined in this chapter, pre-conception support and advice should be available for all women with a BMI ≥30 in order that they achieve a normal BMI prior to pregnancy[4]. Bariatric surgery to achieve weight loss does improve a woman's fertility if obese[12]. Encourage all women with obesity to take 5 mg of folic acid supplementation pre-conceptually and during the first trimester[4].

Pregnancy Issues

Obesity is a significant risk factor during pregnancy and increases the risk of many disorders that have a direct influence on pregnancy outcome:

- Early miscarriage
- Gestational diabetes and pregnancy hypertension/pre-eclampsia[13–16]
- Venous thrombo-embolism[2]
- Anaesthetic problems, e.g. tracheal intubation or epidural/spinal insertion[2]

Especially if maternal complications develop, the fetus/neonate is also at risk of:

- Neural tube defects[16]
- Late stillbirth[3] and neonatal death[17]
- Fetal macrosomia[18]
- Fetal trauma[2]
- Neonatal unit admissions

Obesity creates issues pertaining to the value and reliability of certain aspects of care during the antenatal period:

- Difficulties in performing amniocentesis[19]
- Difficulties in achieving venous access
- Difficulties in performing an abdominal palpation[20]
- Difficulties in obtaining ultrasound data for fetal anomalies[21] and growth

Assess risk throughout pregnancy and re-assess if circumstances change. Prompt referral to the appropriate specialist is important: escalate any concerns if complications occur.

Medical Management and Care

- It is important to identify those women who have co-morbidities directly attributed to their obesity, in particular GDM (offer a Gamma-GT [GTT][4]) and hypertension
- The presence of related conditions will directly influence their care needs; a multidisciplinary team approach to management during pregnancy is advised[2]
- Women with a BMI ≥40 should have an antenatal anaesthetic referral screen[4]
- Encourage all women with obesity to take 10 mg of a vitamin D supplement throughout pregnancy and while breast-feeding[4]

Midwifery Management and Care

- All women have their BMI calculated as part of a full risk assessment performed at booking and women found to have a BMI ≥30 should be referred to a consultant to discuss intrapartum risks and management strategies[4]
- Women with a BMI ≥35 should be booked in a consultant-led environment[4]
- All women should receive advice about healthy eating in pregnancy[4,26]; seek out and access any locally provided support groups focusing on obese women in pregnancy, which include specialist midwives and dieticians
- There are no evidence-based UK guidelines on recommended weight gain ranges during pregnancy and dieting in pregnancy should be avoided[27]
- Moderate exercise should be encouraged, unless the woman is experiencing other signs or symptoms, i.e. dyspnoea[28]
- Individualised advice, especially options for fetal anomaly screening, is important, taking into account the effects of weight on biochemical results
- Careful observation of the maternal and fetal status is important during pregnancy to detect complications; community monitoring for pre-eclampsia at least every 3 weeks between 24 and 32 weeks for women with a BMI ≥35 is recommended[4]
- Ascertain mobility; assess risks of potential intrapartum moving and handling/environmental concerns in preparation for birth[4]
- Continuity of care and support to foster self-esteem and self-confidence

Labour Issues

Obesity is a significant risk factor during the intrapartum period:

- Increased rates of prolonged labour[22]
- Risks associated with macrosomia, e.g. shoulder dystocia[2,13]
- Increased rates of operative birth[2] especially for primigravida[23]
- Difficulties in undertaking instrumental and operative procedures[13]
- Difficulty siting an epidural or spinal for labour or caesarean section

Medical Management and Care

- Encourage birth in a consultant-led environment[4]
- Avoid induction of labour where possible and aim for a vaginal birth[4]
- Strongly consider thrombo-embolic prophylaxis[21] and secure venous access on admission if BMI >40[4]
- Consider the differences in labour progression in obese women before resorting to augmentation[22]

Midwifery Management and Care[29]

- Effective midwifery support in labour is important; women with a BMI ≥40 should receive continuous midwifery care in labour[4]
- Encourage changes in maternal position throughout labour
- Avoid dehydration in labour (risk of venous thrombo-embolism)
- Observe progress – use the partogram carefully throughout labour
- Fetal scalp electrode for difficulty with abdominal auscultation of the fetal heart

Postpartum Issues

Obesity has a direct influence on short and long-term health and wellbeing, especially:

- Venous thrombo-embolism; obesity in the presence of two other persisting risk factors should prompt the need for thrombo-prophylaxis for 3–5 days[2,24]
- Longer post-operative recovery and increased rates of post-operative complications, e.g. infections of wound and urinary tract[4]
- Women who are obese during pregnancy tend to retain fat centrally on their abdomen postnatally, which may result in increased morbidity and mortality in later life[25]
- Lower rates of breast-feeding
- Contraceptive choices will be influenced by the presence of complications

Medical Management and Care

- Multidisciplinary approach to the management of associated conditions
- Encourage women to lose excess weight to achieve a healthy BMI prior to any subsequent pregnancy[4]

Midwifery Management and Care

- May need increased post-operative analgesia[30]
- Early mobilisation[4]; continue thrombo-embolic prophylaxis until fully mobile[4]
- Encourage and support breast-feeding to help mobilise fat stores: tailor breast-feeding advice to meet individual needs; suggest underarm positioning at the breast
- Review postpartum weight at the 6–8 week check and consider referral to the MDT for support and advice regarding weight reduction and moderate exercise[27]
- Consider referral for cognitive and behavioural therapy and consider providing extended midwifery postnatal care[31]
- The combined contraceptive pill may not be as effective in obese women
- Repeat GTT at 6 weeks postnatal if GDM diagnosed during pregnancy[4,26]

13.2 Phenylketonuria

Incidence	Risk for Childbearing
1 in 10 000 live births worldwide, but is more common in Northern European countries and Caucasian races[1]	High Risk – for pre-conceptual, antenatal and neonatal care Low Risk – for labour

EXPLANATION OF CONDITION

Phenylketonuria (PKU) is an autosomal recessively inherited inborn error of amino acid metabolism, caused by mutations in the gene for phenylalanine hydroxylase, found on chromosome 12. Phenylketonuria, as a disease, was first recognised in the 1930s, but maternal PKU syndrome as a complication was not documented until the 1950s[2].

There are two main types of phenylketonuria:

1. **Type 1 or Classical phenylketonuria** – the more serious form of the disease, discussed below
2. **Type 2 or Hyperphenylalaninaemia** – a less severe form, with lower serum phenylalanine levels and fewer complications

Phenylalanine hydroxylase is an enzyme produced by the liver that converts the amino acid phenylalanine, which is found in dietary protein, to another amino acid called tyrosine. Amino acids are important building blocks for proteins, which are vital for growth and wellbeing. In individuals with PKU, phenylalanine and its by-products accumulate in the body and will result in neurological symptoms and irreversible damage to nerve cells within the developing brain and nervous system.

As this is a recessively inherited disorder[3]:

- A woman with PKU whose partner does not carry the affected gene for PKU will produce unaffected children
  - the couple will always pass on the affected gene to their infants, who will be carriers
  - carriers do not exhibit signs of PKU – a child would need to inherit both affected genes to inherit and express symptoms of PKU
- A woman with PKU whose partner also carries an affected gene for PKU will have a one in two chance of having an affected child
- If a woman's partner also has PKU, all children conceived will have PKU
- Individuals who are both carriers of the PKU gene will have a one in four chance of conceiving a child with PKU

COMPLICATIONS

Complications will occur in affected individuals unless screening to detect the condition and management to control the condition is instigated. The earlier treatment begins the less affected the child will be; some limited evidence suggests that the diet should be modified within the first month of life for best results[4].

A neonate will appear normal at birth, as the mother will have processed phenylalanine through her bodily systems during pregnancy. Symptoms in untreated affected infants will begin to appear from 3–4 months of age onwards. These include:

- Abnormal movements
- Developmental delay
- Decreased muscle tone
- Difficulty walking
- Microcephaly
- Learning disabilities
- Seizures
- Psychosis
- Reduction in IQ
- Skin conditions, e.g. eczema
- Pale skin

Attention deficit hyperactivity disorder (ADHD) is also associated with biological insults such as PKU; this is thought to be dose-related and associated with high levels both before birth and in the neonatal period[5].

NON-PREGNANCY TREATMENT AND CARE

All mothers of newborn infants are offered screening for the condition in their baby within the first week of life[1].

Treatment of affected infants consists of a low phenylalanine diet and a supplement of synthetic amino acids (protein substitutes) and vitamins, minerals and trace elements, with food exchanges. This modified diet should continue throughout childhood and some studies suggest this should continue into adulthood[6]. Foods that are naturally high in phenylalanine include meat, dairy produce and nuts, while foods that are low in phenylalanine are generally fruit and vegetables and are considered to be phenylalanine-free foods[7]. A traffic-light approach to foods is taken.

The diet is restrictive and studies have shown that it is difficult to adhere to[8]; social support has been shown to improve compliance so support by the midwife in pregnancy, as part of the multidisciplinary team, is crucially important.

Gene therapy, as an alternative to dietary management, is in the experimental stage and may be available in the future[9].

PRE-CONCEPTION ISSUES AND CARE

To prevent maternal PKU syndrome women with PKU are advised to return to the restricted diet when planning to conceive or as soon as possible when pregnant.

This has been shown in many studies to prevent or lessen the effects on the neonate[10–12]. It can take 1–2 weeks to reduce phenylalanine levels to a therapeutic range of 60–200 mmol/l on commencing the diet.

As many pregnancies are unplanned the advice to remain on the restrictive diet during adulthood[6] is important for women of child-bearing age as the aim is to achieve low blood phenylalanine levels early, ideally pre-conception.

Pregnancy Issues

Women with PKU who have not continued on their low phenylalanine diet need to resume the diet ideally pre-conceptually or as early as possible antenatally[10–12]. This lessens the risk of maternal PKU syndrome, which can affect the fetus and increase the risk of:

- Congenital heart disease[13]
- Microcephaly
- Cranio-facial abnormalities
- IUGR

The frequency and severity of abnormality rises with increasing phenylalanine levels[11].

- It is important to maintain blood phenylalanine levels at <200 μmol/l[3,8]
- Untreated levels of phenylalanine of 1200 μmol/l have been reported
- Women who are given increased support tend to attain earlier metabolic control[8]

The woman is allowed around three to six exchanges daily in the first 20 weeks, but this may be increased in the latter half of pregnancy, under dietetic advice. It is also essential that the woman with PKU eats significant calories to maintain metabolic control and avoids catabolism, where the body will breakdown protein and release phenylalanine[14].

Medical Management and Care

- Pre-conception care is essential to optimise maternal levels before conception
- In women with PKU who conceive on normal diets, early recourse to the restrictive diet has been shown to reduce fetal effects
- Referral to a wider multidisciplinary team as necessary, e.g. physician, dietician, geneticist, clinical nurse specialist
- Early booking facilitates first and second trimester screening for associated congenital abnormalities and appropriate counselling
- Serial ultrasound assessment to screen for IUGR

Monitoring of PKU status is advised

- Twice-weekly phenylalanine self-blood-testing by the woman
- Regular venous blood testing, i.e. Hb, FBC, copper, zinc, selenium, calcium, albumin, phosphates, ferritin, vitamin B_{12} and tyrosine
- Monthly 24-hour phenylalanine profile

Midwifery Management and Care

- Support by a known midwife may help dietary compliance rates and attendance at clinics, which will improve pregnancy outcomes[16]
- Shared care is necessary during the antenatal period
- Place of birth is dependent on presence of fetal complications, e.g. IUGR when birthing in a consultant-led environment with neonatal unit facilities would be advised
- If no complications develop by term then giving birth in a midwifery-led environment may be possible
- Full information on risks and management, both through discussion and in written format should be provided
- If antenatal in-patient care is needed, attendance to diet is vitally important, so seek advice from a dietician on admission

Labour Issues

There are no special requirements for women with PKU during labour. Place of birth and care in labour will depend on the presence of complications, e.g. IUGR.

Babies of women with PKU are not screened immediately after birth, as levels of phenylalanine are higher immediately after birth and would result in false positive screening results[3].

Medical Management and Care

- No significant implications for delivery
- Babies will require neonatal assessment at delivery

Midwifery Management and Care

- Decisions about the place of birth are dependent upon the presence or absence of complications
- Complications should be managed in accordance with local unit guidelines
- Provide good-quality, midwifery-led care for low-risk women

Postpartum Issues

The routine screening of all neonates for PKU by the Newborn Blood Spot Screening Test began in 1969. The neonatal screening test that is offered to all babies between 5 and 8 days will detect almost 100% of cases of PKU. As this is a screening test, any babies who screen positive will need diagnostic follow-up. Screening for all neonates has been shown to be cost-effective[15].

Breast-feeding of babies with PKU is not prohibited, but supplements of phenylalanine-free formula feeds are required to lessen the risk of neurological damage.

A low phenylalanine diet should be commenced within the first month of life to lessen the effects of the condition[4].

Medical Management and Care

- Re-affirm the need for pre-conception care ahead of any further pregnancies

Midwifery Management and Care

- Ensure all women are informed about the Newborn Blood Spot Screening Test – this subject should be discussed antenatally as well as pre-test, giving women and their partners adequate time to ask questions
- Women whose infants have PKU can still breast-feed and should be supported
- A small study suggests that alternate feeds of a phenylalanine-free formula feed, rather than at every feed, would allow for breast-feeding[17]
- If a woman with PKU chooses to revert to a 'normal' diet postnatally, this circumstance should not preclude her breast-feeding[3]
- Women with PKU should be reminded, in the late postnatal period, about the value of pre-conceptual care for a prospective pregnancy

13.3 Hyperemesis Gravidarum

Incidence	**Risk for Childbearing**
Occurs in up to 2% of all pregnancies[1]	Moderate to high risk antenatally, especially if poorly managed or untreated.

EXPLANATION OF CONDITION

Nausea and vomiting of pregnancy (NVP) is a common symptom experienced by women[2], especially during early pregnancy. Nausea occurs in up to 70% of women from around 4–6 weeks gestation: 45% experience nausea and vomiting, while the other 25% experience nausea alone, with 85% of cases experiencing more than two episodes a day and 55% experiencing more than three episodes a day. Symptoms usually resolve by the end of the first trimester, although around 10–20% of these women experience symptoms throughout pregnancy.

Eating tends to reduce symptoms in 50% of cases, but 30% find the experience so debilitating that they need to take time off work. One in 150 women with NVP will develop hyperemesis gravidarum (HG), a more serious condition, and require admission to hospital.

There are several reasons as to why the majority of pregnant women experience NVP. The effect of the rise in human chorionic gonadotrophin (hCG) during the first trimester has been implicated as a cause, although the link has not been clearly established. Raised oestrogen levels are often associated with nausea and vomiting and the rise in progesterone relaxes smooth muscle within the gastrointestinal tract, which delays gastric emptying and sphincter contractibility. It has also been suggested that NVP is an evolutionary development designed to protect the embryo from the absorption of potential harmful substances, e.g. toxins and teratogens during early pregnancy. NVP also stimulates early placental growth; there is subsequently less maternal food assimilation, a lower rate of maternal tissue growth and a resultant shift of nutrients towards placental functioning. The latter suggests that NVP is a symptom that is associated with positive pregnancy outcomes and women should be reassured[3].

Interestingly, an absence of NVP symptoms is associated with an increase in rates of spontaneous abortion[4], especially in older mothers, and the risk increases as symptom duration decreases. So women should be reassured that NVP is a positive symptom and not an experience to be concerned about.

COMPLICATIONS

However, hyperemesis gravidarum (HG) is an extreme form of NVP and occurs in between 0.5 and 2% of all pregnant women[1]. It is the major reason for admission to hospital during early pregnancy and is defined as the occurrence of three or more episodes of vomiting per day, with significant maternal weight loss, i.e. >5% of pre-pregnancy weight and ketonuria[5]. Diagnosis is usually made on the woman's history and clinical examination.

The cause of HG is unclear, but it appears to be multifactorial; a complex interplay between physical and psychological factors[6–8]. Differential diagnoses, which need to be investigated and excluded, include urinary tract infections, e.g. pyelonephritis, gastro-oesophageal reflux disease (GORD), pancreatitis, Addison's disease, helicobacter[9] and CNS pathologies.

If inadequately treated HG can lead to serious maternal and fetal morbidity. There are two types: type 1 which is nausea and vomiting without metabolic changes and type 2, which is nausea and vomiting with metabolic changes – the latter is more serious and if untreated can be life-threatening.

The presence of certain factors increase the incidence of HG, e.g. primigravida, extremes of BMI[10], the presence of eating disorders pre-pregnancy, multiple gestation and is associated with a history of psychiatric conditions, e.g. PTSD and depression[7]. It is also associated with hydatidiform mole, so it is important to exclude this during initial investigations. HG also seen as a consequence of bariatric surgery[11]. Maternal smoking appears to protect against the occurrence of HG[10].

Signs and symptoms include weight loss through the breakdown of stored body fat and muscle mass, resulting in muscle wasting, tachycardia, low BP and postural hypotension and sometimes ptyalism. Blood tests – U&Es, TFTs and LFTs – will show marked changes in biochemical and hormonal markers. Raised serum leptin levels may be a significant marker in HG[12]. Electrolyte changes are the result of dehydration and starvation. The women's urine will be concentrated and ketones will be present on dipstick testing. She will also have inelastic skin, a coated tongue and sunken eyes.

If untreated, or inadequately managed, significant morbidity and mortality can occur due to:

- Hyponatraemia
- Alkalosis
- Thrombo-embolism
- Wernicke's encephalopathy[13] – a vitamin B_1 deficiency – women will exhibit confusion and ataxia – this has a 10–15% mortality rate
- Maternal distress and anxiety[6,14]

The effect on the fetus was initially thought to increase miscarriage and stillbirth rates, but current evidence suggests an absence of fetal adverse outcomes, so long as weight gain in later pregnancy is adequate[15,16].

NON-PREGNANCY TREATMENT AND CARE

This condition is specific to pregnancy.

PRE-CONCEPTION ISSUES AND CARE

The literature suggests a link between HG with extremes of BMI[10] and psychiatric co-morbidities[7], both of which may benefit from pre-conception counseling in order to maximise a woman's physical health and emotional wellbeing before pregnancy. This may reduce the incidence of HG. If HG occurred in a previous pregnancy a robust relationship between a woman and her GP is important[17].

Pregnancy Issues

It is important that the condition is recognised promptly and if severe, the woman is referred to a consultant-led environment.

Research has identified a stigma associated with HG[13], where women have experienced unhelpful attitudes from healthcare practitioners. It appears that women with HG need more acknowledgement of their symptoms by staff and more support is needed to manage the altered family, social and occupational impacts of both NVP and HG[8,18].

Pharmaceutical treatments include:

- Antihistamines – these are considered to be safe in pregnancy and effective, but can cause drowsiness
- Metaclopramide - although there is limited information on their safety it is considered to be effective[19], but may cause drowsiness and restlessness

All medications should be prescribed and monitored through medical supervision during pregnancy. However, many women worry about the possible teratogenic effects of medication taken during early pregnancy and this may increase anxiety and emotional distress.

Alternative therapies for NVP have been reviewed[1]:

- Acupressure – limited effectiveness – pressure on the P6 point found at three fingers breadth above the wrist
- Acupuncture – not effective – limited evidence
- Ginger – 1000 mg a day - may help, but the evidence is limited and not consistent; may cause heartburn and clotting problems by inhibiting platelet aggregation
- Vitamin B_6 – limited evidence
- Massage – considered to be a robust addition to the traditional management of HG[20]

Medical Management and Care

- If severe admit to a maternity ward
- Manage mild or moderate cases in the community environment
- Blood tests – U&Es, TFTs and LFTs[21]
- Exclude other pathology, e.g. gastroenteritis
- Treat with iv rehydration and anti-emetics initially; as the condition resolves change to oral hydration and rectal or oral anti-emetics
- Correct any electrolyte imbalances
- Consider vitamin supplementation, e.g. thiamine
- Assess the risk of venous thrombo-embolism and consider prophylaxis
- Assess fetal wellbeing – ultrasound to exclude a molar pregnancy and to detect a multiple pregnancy for instance
- Consider the use of oral steroid therapy for intractable cases and multiple admissions (prednisolone 5–30 mg/day in divided doses)

Midwifery Management and Care

- Take a full and comprehensive medical, psychiatric and obstetric history on admission
- Assess maternal wellbeing – assess vital signs, test urine, assess weight loss, etc. and assess the psychosocial impact of the condition
- Provide psychological support to reduce stress and anxiety

As the Pregnancy Progresses:

- Assess fetal wellbeing as the pregnancy continues – monitor fetal growth and wellbeing, especially if NVP persists throughout the pregnancy
- Prompt referral for ultrasound for fetal growth if concerned
- Assess incidence of NVP at every antenatal appointment and consider these cases as a legitimate reason to weigh the woman during pregnancy
- Provide emotional support and consider a referral for psychosomatic counselling
- Give individualised nutritional advice, e.g. smaller and more frequent meals, importance of an adequate fluid intake, meals based around carbohydrates rather than fats
- Refer to a dietician for specialised input to ensure the woman's nutritional needs are met
- Consider individual lifestyle adaptations to accommodate the family, social and occupational impact of HG

Labour Issues

- This is usually an early pregnancy experience – see above

Medical Management and Care

- Obstetric management depends on the presence of morbidity and complications, e.g. IUGR

Midwifery Management and Care

- Unless there have been complications arising from HG, continuity of care in a low risk environment would reduce stress and anxiety
- Ensure adequate hydration during labour, especially if NVP is still present

Postpartum Issues

- The hormones associated with the pregnancy will subside during the early postpartum period and the NVP should also subside
- Symptoms may recur in a subsequent pregnancy, although it is more common in the first pregnancy

Medical Management and Care

- The symptoms of NVP should subside following the birth
- If symptoms persist further investigations may be required to exclude other pathology

Midwifery Management and Care

- If the woman wishes to breast-feed, consider any medications that she may be taking and seek advice from the pharmacist
- Consider psychology referral for longer term emotional support

S. E. Robson and J. Waugh

13.4 Acute Fatty Liver of Pregnancy

Incidence	Risk for Childbearing
Rare complication affecting 1 in 700 to 1 in 1300 pregnancies[1]	High risk, especially third trimester with high maternal/fetal mortality

EXPLANATION OF CONDITION

Acute fatty liver of pregnancy (AFLP) is a rare, but very serious, condition. Its aetiology is unclear, but it has links with pre-eclampsia and there is some evidence that suggests that it may be part of the same illness. Another suggestion is the effect of female hormones, i.e. oestrogen on the liver mitochondria[2]. However, current thinking suggests that there may be a link with an abnormality in the mitochondrial fatty acid oxidation in the fetus (long-chain 3-hydroxyacyl-CoA dehydrogenase – LCHAD), especially if the mother is heterozygous[2,6]. The un-metabolised chains enter the maternal circulation and accumulate in the maternal liver, causing microvesicular infiltration resulting in hepatic failure[2-6]. Women having their first child, with multiple pregnancies and with raised BMIs are also at increased risk[1,7,8].

Symptoms usually present themselves typically after 30 weeks gestation[7-9] and common signs and symptoms include:

- Nausea and vomiting
- Fever
- Pruritus
- Right upper quadrant abdominal pain
- Headache
- Tiredness
- Confusion
- Jaundice
- Flu-like symptoms
- Lack of appetite
- Ascites
- Mild hypertension and proteinuria
- Liver failure and hepatic encephalopathy
- Symptoms of diabetes insipidus, e.g. polyuria and polydipsia
- Hypoglycaemia
- Hyperuricaemia

Diagnosis hinges on the clinical picture and the presence of abnormal LFTs, in particular a gross increase in conjugated hyperbilirubinaemia and a marked increase in the transaminases – ALT and AST, but with normal platelet counts, which would exclude a diagnosis of HELLP syndrome[10-12]. Occasionally, ultrasound or MRI scans of the liver are used and may show fatty infiltration of the liver, which may aid the diagnosis. Liver biopsy is not usually indicated though, due to the risks associated with the coagulopathy.

COMPLICATIONS

The clinical picture can deteriorate rapidly and prompt management is needed to secure optimal maternal and fetal outcomes. Maternal and fetal mortality and morbidity rates have decreased over the last few decades[13].

Complications can include:

- Renal and hepatic failure
- Adult respiratory distress syndrome (RDS)
- Pancreatitis
- Hypoglycaemia
- Infection and sepsis
- Haemorrhage – gastro-intestinal, i.e. ulceration, Mallory–Weiss syndrome
- Coagulopathy
- Stillbirth
- PPH

NON-PREGNANCY TREATMENT AND CARE

This condition is specific to pregnancy.

PRE-CONCEPTION ISSUES AND CARE

It is unlikely to recur in a subsequent pregnancy[10]. However, it might be useful to test for the genetic abnormality of fatty acid oxidation (LCHAD), as recurrence is more likely in these women[11].

Diagnosis of LCHAD in a fetus in a subsequent pregnancy can be achieved through the enzyme immune assay of amniocytes and analysing DNA obtained through CVS.

Pregnancy Issues

- Prompt recognition and management of the condition is important to reduce maternal and fetal morbidity and mortality[1]
- AFLP has a prodromal phase of 1–21 days[9], after which jaundice and hepatic failure occurs

Medical Management and Care

- AFLP needs prompt diagnosis
- Alternative diagnoses such as HELLP needs to be excluded through biochemical analysis
- Involve a specialist hepatologist at an early stage

Midwifery Management and Care

- Admit to a consultant-led unit with NNU facilities
- Any woman who presents in the third trimester with flu-like symptoms should be investigated
- Taking a full history is important to aid diagnosis
- Observe for signs of DIC and hypoglycaemia which are common complications

Labour Issues

- Fetal compromise is common in AFLP, but the pathology is unclear[9,10]. Studies suggest that it is because of placental hypoperfusion due to maternal hypotension, low-grade coagulopathy and hypoglycaemia
- Multidisciplinary team input provides the optimal clinical environment

Medical Management and Care

- As above
- Once the diagnosis has been made delivery of the fetus is expedited
- Operative birth versus induction of labour – which is better is unclear and depends on the maternal and fetal condition

Midwifery Management and Care

- If the labour is induced then close observation of the maternal and fetal condition is important
- Meconium-stained liquor and fetal distress is common
- Careful fluid balance is important to prevent pulmonary and cerebral oedema
- Avoid episiotomy

Postpartum Issues

- AFLP is a reversible form of hepatic disease and in most women who develop the condition, if supportive measures are promptly instigated, hepatic function is restored in the majority of cases[1]
- Careful observation of the neonate, who is at increased risk of hypoketotic hypoglycaemia, fatty liver, cardiac problems and neuropathy, is recommended[11]. These babies are also more susceptible to SIDS

Medical Management and Care

- Postnatal care is best carried out in a critical care unit (CCU)
- Supportive care involves correction of coagulopathy, treatment of hypoglycaemia, broad spectrum antibiotics and anti-fungal medication, renal support
- Observation and biochemistry analysis is needed to detect encephalopathy, pancreatitis and renal/hepatic failure is required
- After 48 hours the condition should improve

Midwifery Management and Care

- Postnatal wound infection is common, so evidence-based wound care and observation is important
- Closely observe the lochia as PPH is a common complication
- The majority of women also require a blood transfusion as part of postnatal care
- Provide support and communication between NNU and CCU and the parents
- Inform the parents of the genetic risk of recurrence
- Oral contraceptives are best avoided as a form of contraception

13 Metabolic Disorders

PATIENT ORGANISATIONS

National Obesity Observatory (NOO)
www.noo.org.uk/

Weight Wise
www.bdaweightwise.com

The Obesity Awareness and Solutions Trust (TOAST)
The Latton Bush Centre
Southern Way
Harlow
Essex CM18 7BL
www.toast-uk.org.uk

The National Society for Phenylketonuria
(Charity Number: 373670)
www.nspku.org

PKU.com
www.pku.com

Children's PKU Network
www.pkunetwork.org

PKU Teens – It's all in the genes!
www.pkuteens.co.uk

USEFUL WEBSITES

Association for the Study of Obesity
www.aso.org.uk/portal.aspx

National Obesity Forum
www.nationalobesityforum.org.uk/

UK Newborn Screening Programme Centre
www.newbornscreening-bloodspot.org.uk

ESSENTIAL READING

CMACE 2010 **Maternal Obesity in the UK: Findings from a National Project**. London; CMACE

CMACE/RCOG 2010 **CMACE/RCOG Joint Guideline Management of Women with Obesity in Pregnancy** http://www.rcog.org.uk/files/rcog-corp/CMACERCOGJoint GuidelineManagementWomenObesityPregnancya.pdf

Department of Health 2006 Care Pathways for the Management of Overweight and Obesity. Adult Care Pathway (Primary Care)
www.dh.gov.uk/asserRoot/04/13/44/12/04134412.pdf

Lewis G (Ed) 2007 **Saving Mothers' Lives: Reviewing Maternal Deaths to Make Motherhood Safer. 7th Report of the Confidential Enquiries into Maternal and Child Health**. London; CEMACH 25–29

Modder J and Fitzsimmons K 2010 **Management of Women with Obesity in Pregnancy**. CMACE/RCOG Joint Guidance

NICE 2003 **Antenatal Care Clinical Guideline No. 6**. London; National Institute for Health and Clinical Excellence. www.nice.org.uk

NICE 2006. **Guidance on the Prevention, Identification, Assessment and Management of Overweight and Obesity in Adults and Children**. London; National Institute for Health and Clinical Excellence. www.nice.org.uk

NICE 2010 **Weight Management Before, During and After Pregnancy**. London; National Institute for Health and Clinical Excellence. www.nice.org.uk

RCOG 2001 Thromboembolic Disease in Pregnancy and the Puerperium: Acute Management – Green Top Guideline. www.rcog.org

RCOG 2004 **Thromboprophylaxis During Pregnancy, Labour and After Vaginal Delivery** – Guideline No. 37. www.rcog.org

RCOG 2006 **Exercise in Pregnancy Statement** No. 4. www.rcog.org

13.1 Obesity

1. Kanagalingam MG, Forouhi NG, Greer IA, *et al.* 2005 Changes in booking body mass index over a decade: retrospective analysis from a Glasgow maternity hospital. **British Journal of Obstetrics and Gynaecology**, 112:1431–1433

2. Foresight 2007 **Tackling Obesities: Future Choices** www.bis.gov.uk/assets/bispartners/foresight/docs/obesity/17.pdf p34

3. Lewis G (Ed.) 2007 **Saving Mothers' Lives: Reviewing Maternal Deaths to Make Motherhood Safer. 7th Report of the Confidential Enquiries into Maternal and Child Health**. London; CEMACH 25–29

4. Modder J and Fitzsimmons K 2010 **Management of Women with Obesity in Pregnancy**. CMACE/RCOG Joint Guidance

5. Ogden J and Clementi C 2010 The experience of being obese and the many consequences of stigma. **Journal of Obesity** doi:10.1155/2010/429098

6. Puhl R and Brownell K 2003 Psychosocial origins of obesity stigma: toward changing a powerful and pervasive bias. **The International Association for the Study of Obesity**, 4:213–227

7. Puhl R and Brownell K 2006 Confronting and coping with weight stigma: an investigation of overweight and obese adults. **Obesity**, 14:1802–1814

8. Mulders A, Laven J, Eijkemans M, *et al.* 2003 Patients predictors for outcome of gonadotrophin ovulation induction in women with normogonadotrophic anovulatory infertility: a mega-analysis. **Human Reproduction Update**, 9:429–449

9. Shaw K, O'Rouke P and Kenardy C 2005 Psychological interventions for overweight or obesity. **The Cochrane Database of Systematic Reviews**, Issue 1

10. Harris A and Barger MK 2010 Specialised care for women pregnant after bariatric surgery. **Journal of Midwifery and Women's Health**, 55:529–539

11. NICE 2006 **Clinical Guideline – Obesity – Guidance on the Prevention, Identification, Assessment and Management of Overweight and Obesity in Adults and Children**. London; National Institute for Health and Clinical Excellence. www.nice.org.uk/guidance/CG43/guidance/pdf/English/download.dspx

12. Merhi ZO, Jindal S, Pollack E and Lieman H 2011 Pregnancy following bariatric surgery. **Expert Review of Obstetrics and Gynecology**, 6:57–67

13. Andreasen K, Anderson M and Schantz A 2004 Obesity in pregnancy. **Acta Obstetrica et Gynecologica Scandinavica**, 83:1022–1029

14. Duckitt K and Harrington D 2005 Risk factors for pre-eclampsia at antenatal booking: systematic review of controlled studies. **British Medical Journal**, 330(7491):565

15. Erez-Weiss I, Erez O, Shoham-Vaedi I, *et al.* 2005 The association between maternal obesity, glucose intolerance and hypertensive disorders of pregnancy in non-diabetic pregnant women. **Hypertensive Pregnancy**, 25:125–136

16. Shaw G, Todoroff K, Schaffer D, *et al.* 2000 Maternal height and pre-pregnancy body mass index as risk factors for selected congenital anomalies. **Paediatric and Perinatal Epidemiology**, 14:234–239

17. Kristensen J, Vestergaard M, Wisborg K, *et al.* 2005 Pre pregnancy weight and the risk of stillbirth and neonatal death. **British Journal of Obstetrics and Gynaecology**, 112:403–408

18. Yogev Y, Langar O, Xenakis E, *et al.* 2005 The association between glucose challenge test, obesity and pregnancy outcome in 6390 non-diabetic women. **The Journal of Maternal-Fetal and Neonatal Medicine**, 17:29–34

19. Irvine L and Shaw R 2006 The impact of obesity on obstetric outcomes. **Current Obstetrics and Gynaecology**, 16:242–246

20. Farrell T, Holmes R and Stone P 2002 The effect of body mass index on three methods of fetal weight estimation. **British Journal of Obstetrics and Gynaecology**, 109:651–657

21. Martinez–Frias ML, Frias JP, Bermejo E, *et al.* 2005 Pre-gestational body mass index predicts an increased risk of congenital malformations in infants of mothers with gestational diabetes. **Diabetes Medicine**, 22:775–781

22. Vahratian A, Zhang J, Troendle J, *et al.* 2004 Maternal pre pregnancy overweight and obesity and the pattern of labour progression in term nulliparous women. **American College of Obstetricians and Gynecologists**, 104:943–951

23. Dempsey J, Ashiny Z, Qui C, *et al.* 2005 Maternal pre-pregnancy overweight status and obesity as risk factors for caesarean delivery. **The Journal of Maternal-Fetal and Neonatal Medicine**, 17:179–185

24. RCOG 2004 **Clinical Guideline No. 37 Thromboprophylaxis During Pregnancy, Labour and After Vaginal Delivery**. London; Royal College of Obstetricians and Gynaecologists

25. Soltani H and Fraser R 2002 Pregnancy as a cause of obesity – myth or reality? **RCM Midwives Journal**, 5:193–195

26. CMACE 2010 **Maternal Obesity in the UK: Findings from a National Project**. London; CMACE

27. NICE 2010 **Weight Management Before, During and After Pregnancy**. London; National Institute for Health and Clinical Excellence. www.nice.org.uk

28. RCOG 2006 **Statement No. 4 Exercise in Pregnancy**. London; Royal College of Obstetricians and Gynaecologists

29. Gates S, Brocklehurst P and Davis L 2002 Prophylaxis for venous thromboembolic disease in pregnancy and the early postnatal period. **The Cochrane Database of Systematic Reviews 2006**, Issue 1

30. Fraser RB 2006 Obesity complicating pregnancy. **Current Obstetrics and Gynaecology**, 16:295–298

31. Walker L, Sterling B and Timmerman G 2004 Retention of pregnancy related weight in the early postpartum period: implications for women's health services. **Journal of Obstetric, Gynecologic and Neonatal Nursing**, 34:418–427

13.2 Phenylketonuria

1. UK Newborn Screening Programme 2005 Why are newborn babies screened for phenylketonuria? www.newbornscreening-bloodspot.org.uk

2. Levy H 2003 Historical background for the maternal PKU syndrome. **Paediatrics**, 112:1516–1517

3. National Society for Phenylketonuria (UK) 2005 Pregnancy in women with phenylketonuria (PKU). www.nspku.org

4. Politt R, Green A and McCabe A, *et al.* 1997 Neonatal screening for inborn errors of metabolism: cost, yield and outcome. **Health Technology Assessment**, 1:1–203

5. Antshel K and Waisbren S 2003 Developmental timing of exposure to elevated levels of phenylalanine is associated with ADHD symptom expression. **Journal of Abnormal Child Psychology**, 31:565–574

6. Poustie VJ and Rutherford P 1999 Dietary interventions for phenylketonuria. **The Cochrane Database of Systematic Reviews**, Issue 3 2006

7. Weetch E and McDonald A 2006 The determination of phenylalanine content of foods suitable for phenylketonuria. **Journal of Human Nutrition and Dietetics**, 19:229

8. Rohr F, Munier A, Sullivan D, Bailey I, *et al.* 2004 The resource mothers study of maternal phenylketonuria: preliminary findings. **Journal of Inherited Metabolic Disorders**, 27:145–155

9. Duig Z, Georgieu P and Thony B 2006 Administration-route and gender-independent long-term therapeutic correction of PKU in

a mouse model by recombinant adeno-associated virus 8 pseudotyped vector-mediated gene transfer. **Gene Therapy**, 13:587–593

10. Lee P, Ridout D, Walker J, *et al.* 2005 Maternal PKU: a report from the UK Registry 1978–1997. **Archives of Disease in Childhood**, 90:143–146

11. Matalon K, Acosta P and Azen C 2003 Role of nutrition in pregnancy with PKU and birth defects. **Pediatrics**, 112:1534–1536

12. Waisbren S and Azen C 2003 Cognitive and behavioural development in maternal PKU offspring. **Pediatrics**, 112:1544–1547

13. Levy H, Guldberg P, Guttlerr F, *et al.* 2001 Congenital heart disease in maternal PKU: report from the maternal phenylketonuria collaborative study. **Pediatric Research**, 49:636–642

14. Acosta P, Matalon K, Castiglioni L, *et al.* 2001 Intake of major nutrients by women in the maternal PKU (MPKU): study and effects on plasma phenylalanine concentrations. **American Journal of Clinical Nutrition**, 73:792–796

15. Geelhoed E, Lewis B, Hounsome D, *et al.* 2005 Economic evaluation of neonatal screening for PKU and congenital hypothyroidism. **Journal of Paediatrics and Child Health**, 41:575–579

16. MacDonald A and Asplin D 2006 Phenylketonuria: practical dietary management. **Journal of Family Health Care**, 16:83–85

17. Van Rijn M, Bekhof J and Dijkstra T 2003 A different approach to breast-feeding for the infant with PKU. **European Journal of Paediatrics**, 162:323–326

13.3 Hyperemesis Gravidarum

1. Matthews A, Dowswell T, Haas D, *et al.* 2010 Interventions for Nausea and Vomiting in Early Pregnancy. **The Cochrane Library** 2010 Issue 9

2. Cuckson C and Germain S 2011 Hyperemesis, gastro-intestinal and liver disorders in pregnancy. **Obstetrics, Gynaecology and Reproductive Medicine**, 21:80–85

3. Coad J and Dunstall M 2005 **Anatomy and Physiology for Midwives**. 2nd Edn. Edinburgh; Churchill Livingstone

4. Chan R, Olshan A, Savitz A, *et al.* 2010 Severity and duration of nausea and vomiting symptoms in pregnancy and spontaneous abortion. **Human Reproduction**, 25:2907–2912

5. Jueckstock J, Kaestner R and Mylonas I 2010 Managing hyperemesis gravidarum: a multimodal challenge. **BMC Medicine**, 8:46

6. Tan P, Vani S, Lim B, *et al.* 2010 Anxiety and depression in hyperemesis gravidarum: prevalence, risk factors and correlation with clinical severity. **European Journal of Obstrtrics and Gynaecology and Reproductive Biology**, 149:153–158

7. Seng J, Schrot J, De Ven C, *et al.* 2007 Service use data analysis of pre-pregnancy psychiatric and somatic diagnoses in women with hyperemesis gravidarum. **Journal of Psychosomatic Obstetrics and Gynaecology**, 28:209–217

8. Harris A and Barger MK 2010 Specialised care for women pregnant after bariatric surgery. **Journal of Midwifery and Women's Health**, 55:529–539

9. Mansour G and Nashaat E 2009 Helicobacter pylori and hyperemesis gravidarum. **International Federation of Gynaecology and Obstetrics** doi:10.106/j.ifgo.2009.03.006

10. Aka N, Atalay S, Sayharman S, *et al.* 2006 Leptin and leptin receptor levels in pregnant women with hyperemesis gravidarum. **Australian and New Zealand Journal of Obstetrics and Gynaecology**, 46: 274–277

11. Michel M, Alanio E, Bois E, *et al.* 2009 Wenicke encephalopathy complicating hyperemesis gravidarum: a case report. **European Journal of Obstetrics and Gynaecology and Reproductive Biology** doi: 10.1016/j.ejogrb.2009.10.017

12. Power Z, Thomson A and Waterman H 2010 Understanding the stigma of hyperemesis gravidarum: qualitative findings from an action research study. **Birth**, 37:237–244

13. Loiuk C, Hernandez-Diaz S and Werler M 2006 Nausea and vomiting in pregnancy: maternal characteristics and risk factors. **Paediatric and Perinatal Epidemiology**, 20:270–278

14. Tan P, Jacob R, Quek K and Omar S 2007 Pregnancy outcome in hyperemesis gravidarum and the effect of laboratory clinical indicators of hyperemesis severity. **Journal of Obstetric and Gynaecology Research**, 33:457–464

15. Swallow B, Lindow S, Mason E and Hay D 2004 Psychological health in early pregnancy: relationship with nausea and vomiting. **Journal of Obstetrics and Gynaecology**, 24:28–32

16. Vikanes A, Grjibovski A, Vangen S, *et al.* 2010 Maternal body composition, smoking and hyperemesis gravidarum. **Annals Epidemiology**, 20:592–598

17. Munch S and Schmitz M 2007 The Hyperemesis Beliefs Scale (HBS): a new instrument for assessing beliefs about severe nausea and vomiting in pregnancy. **Journal of Psychosomatic Obstetrics and Gynaecology**, 28:219–229

18. Locock L, Alexander J and Rozmovits L 2008 Women's responses to nausea and vomiting in pregnancy. **Midwifery**, 24:143–152

19. Matok I, Gorodischer R, Koren G, *et al.* 2009 The safety of metaclopramide use in the first trimester of pregnancy. **New England Journal of Medicine**, 360:2528–2535

20. Agren A and Berg M 2006 Tactile massage and severe nausea and vomiting during pregnancy – women's experiences. **Scandinavian Journal of Caring Sciences**, 20:169–176

21. Ballard S 2011 Blood tests for investigating maternal wellbeing 4: when nausea and vomiting in pregnancy becomes pathological: hyperemesis gravidarum. **The Practising Midwife**, 14:37–41

13.4 Acute Fatty Liver of Pregnancy

1. UKOSS, Knight M, Nelson-Piercy C, *et al.* 2008 A prospective national study of acute fatty liver of pregnancy in the UK. Gut Online, 10.1136/gut.2008.148676

2. Treem WR, Rinaldo P, Hale DE, *et al.* 1994 Acute fatty liver of pregnancy and long chain 3-hydroxyacyl-coenzyme A dehydrogenase deficiency. **Hepatology**, 19:339–345

3. Tyni T, Rapola J, Paetau A, Palotie A and Pihko H 1996 Pathology of long chain 3-hydroxyacyl-CoA dehydrogenase deficiency with the g1528c mutation. **Neuromuscular Disorder**, 6:327–337

4. Kompare M, Rizzo W 2008 Mitochondrial fatty acid oxidation disorders. **Seminars in Pediatric Neurology**, 15:140–149

5. Bellig LL 2004 Maternal acute fatty liver of pregnancy and the associated risk for long-chain 3 hydroxy acyl-coenzyme a dehydrogenase deficiency in infants. **Advances in Neonatal Care**, 4:26–32

6. Tyni T, Pihko H 1999 Long-chain 3-hydroxyacyl-CoA dehydrogenase deficiencies. **Acta Paediatrica**, 88:237–245.

7. Ch'ng CL, Morgan M, Hainsworth I, *et al.* 2002 Prospective study of liver dysfunction in pregnancy in Southwest Wales. **Gut**, 51:876–580.

8. Hin Hin Ko and Yoshida E 2006 Acute fatty liver in pregnancy. **Canadian Journal of Gastroenterology**, 20:25–30

9. Williams J, Mozurkewich E, Chilimigras J, *et al.* 2008 Critical care in obstetrics: pregnancy-specific conditions. **Best Practice and Research Clinical Obstetrics and Gynaecology**, 22:825–846

10. Ranjan V and Smith N 1997 Acute fatty liver of pregnancy. **Journal of Obstetrics and Gynaecology**, 17:285–286

11. Sinha P, Kyle P and Gubbala P 2010 Acute fatty liver of pregnancy. **Internet Journal of Gynaecology and Obstetrics**, 13:1–4

12. Pateman K and O'Brien P 2008 Acute fatty liver of pregnancy. **British Journal of Midwifery**, 16:242–243

13. CMACE 2011 **Saving Mother's Lives: Reviewing Maternal Deaths to Make Motherhood Safer: 2006–2008**. London: CMACE

Appendix References

1. Department of Health 2006 **Care Pathways for the Management of Overweight and Obesity**. www.dh.gov.uk

2. World Health Organization 2000 Obesity: preventing and managing the global epidemic: report of a WHO consultation. **World Health Organization Technical Report Series**, 894:i–253

Appendix 13.1.1 Body Mass Index

WORLD HEALTH ORGANIZATION – BODY MASS INDEX[1]

The Body Mass Index (BMI) is an index of weight-for-height. It is assessed by calculating the woman's weight in kilograms divided by the square of her height in metres (kg/m^2)

Body Mass Index Range	Classification	Risk of Associated Comorbidities[1]
<18.5	Underweight	Low risk, but at increased risk of other medical problems
18.5–24.9	Normal weight	Average
25.0–29.9	Overweight	Mildly increased
30.0–34.9	Class I - Obese	High
35.0–39.9	Class II - Obese	High
40.0	Class III - Extreme Obesity	Very high

Maternal Obesity is defined by the World Health Organization[2] as a BMI of $\geq 30\,kg/m^2$ at the first antenatal consultation

HAEMATOLOGICAL DISORDERS

14

Abena Addo[1], Christina Oppenheimer[2] and S. Elizabeth Robson[1]

[1]De Montfort University, Leicester, UK
[2]University Hospitals of Leicester NHS Trust, Leicester, UK

Medical Disorders in Pregnancy: A Manual for Midwives, Second Edition. Edited by S. Elizabeth Robson and Jason Waugh.
© 2013 John Wiley & Sons, Ltd. Published 2013 by John Wiley & Sons, Ltd.

14.1 Iron Deficiency Anaemia

Incidence	Risk for Childbearing
5–10% pregnant women from industrialised countries[1]	Variable Risk

EXPLANATION OF CONDITION

Iron deficiency is the commonest cause of anaemia amongst women of child-bearing age and in particular pregnant women (51%) worldwide[2].

Symptoms vary from mild tiredness to potentially hazardous palpitations, breathlessness or symptoms of high output cardiac failure. In humans, mineral iron is present in all cells and carries oxygen to the tissues from the lungs in the form of haemoglobin (Hb), facilitates oxygen use in muscles as myoglobin, and also in cytochromes within cells for enzyme reactions in tissues.

Women have approximately 2.3 g total body iron of which most (80%) is found in the red blood cell mass as haemoglobin (Hb). Total body iron is determined by intake, loss and storage of this mineral. Any iron not in use is stored as the soluble protein complex ferritin, present primarily in the liver, bone marrow, spleen and skeletal muscle. Normal absorption mechanisms in the gastrointestinal system of the body are required to maintain the balance between functional iron (Hb) and stored iron levels. The body is able to absorb 1–2 mg iron daily from the diet, with the aid of absorption enhancers in the diet and a satisfactory rate of red blood cell production. The main factor controlling iron absorption is the amount of iron stored in the body and the type of iron in one's diet[3].

Anaemia results in a reduction in the oxygen-carrying capacity of the blood. Iron deficiency anaemia is defined by a low serum ferritin concentration of <30 micrograms/l and haemoglobin <11.0, 10.5 and 10.5 g/dl in the first, second and third trimesters respectively[2,4,5]. Red blood cells are microcytic (small) and hypochromic (pale) on microscopic examination (see Figures 14.1.1 and 14.1.2). Iron deficiency anaemia arises from an increase in iron requirements or inadequate iron absorption.

Iron requirements are increased to deal with:

- Growth
- Menstruation
- Blood loss/donation
- Pregnancy
- Haemolytic disorders
- Drugs that cause haemolysis (e.g. antiretrovirals)
- Genitourinary tract infections
- Hookworm infestation

Anaemia caused by inadequate iron absorption occurs from:

- Diet low in haem iron
- Malabsorption
- Gastric surgery
- Malaria infection resulting in poor use of dietary iron

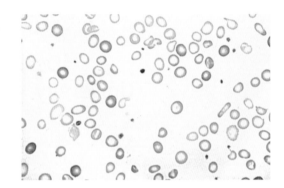

Figure 14.1.2 The peripheral blood film in severe iron deficiency anaemia. The cells are microlytic (small) and hypochromic (pale) with occasional target cells (Hoffbrand, 2011). This figure is downloadable from the book companion website at www.wiley.com/go/robson

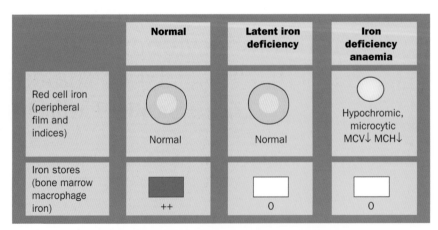

	Normal	Latent iron deficiency	Iron deficiency anaemia
Red cell iron (peripheral film and indices)	Normal	Normal	Hypochromic, microcytic MCV↓ MCH↓
Iron stores (bone marrow macrophage iron)	++	0	0

Figure 14.1.1 The development of iron deficiency anaemia. Reticuloendothelial (macrophage) stores are lost completely before anaemia develops (Hoffbrand, 2011). MCH, mean corpuscular haemoglobin. MCV, mean corpuscular volume. This figure is downloadable from the book companion website at www.wiley.com/go/robson

The amount of functional iron in the body and the concentration of the iron-containing protein Hb in circulating red blood cells are measured by two simple blood tests, Hb and haematocrit and ferritin concentration.

Haemoglobin Concentration and Haematocrit

Haemoglobin and haematocrit (HCT) are both late indicators of anaemia. Haematocrit indicates the proportion of whole blood occupied by the red blood cells, and falls only after the Hb concentration has also fallen. Mean cell volume (MCV) is also important as it falls in iron deficiency, but needs further testing to distinguish it from other causes of microcytosis (see Section 14.6 Thalassaemia).

Serum Ferritin Concentration

Serum ferritin concentration is an early indicator of the status of iron stores and the most specific indicator of depleted iron stores routinely available. A serum ferritin concentration of ≤30 micrograms/l confirms iron deficiency among women who test positive for anaemia on the basis of Hb concentration or haematocrit[6]. Serum ferritin can be raised in infection and may need repeating for a definitive diagnosis of iron deficiency. Caution is advised in interpretation of normal levels in pregnancy since a low normal level (30–50 micrograms/l) may still indicate iron deficiency. Use of other tests should be confirmed with local laboratories.

COMPLICATIONS

Iron deficiency can interfere with vital body functions leading to morbidity and mortality including:

- Palpitations
- Tiredness
- Irritability
- Depression
- Breathlessness
- Poor memory
- Muscle aches
- Poor appetite
- Cardiac failure
- Increased vulnerability if small amounts of blood are lost

NON-PREGNANCY TREATMENT AND CARE

Encourage iron-rich foods in the diet and treat with iron supplementation 60–120 mg/day for 4 weeks[7]. If no response to treatment, investigate using other tests: reticulocyte count and serum ferritin concentration. Conditions such as sickle cell trait or thalassaemia minor in women of African, Mediterranean or Southeast Asian ancestry cause mild anaemia unresponsive to iron therapy. The normal Hb level for this group can be as low as 10 g/dl. However, the lowest normal Hb in healthy non-pregnant women is defined as 12.0 g/dl[2]. Iron absorption can be increased in a vegetarian diet by careful planning of meals to include other sources of iron and enhancers of iron absorption[8].

PRE-CONCEPTION ISSUES AND CARE

A non-pregnant woman of reproductive age has an average iron requirement of 1.3 mg/day. This increases when pregnant by an extra requirement of 3.0 mg/day mainly for increases in maternal red cell mass, placental and fetal growth, blood loss at delivery, physiological intestinal blood loss and menstruating loss over the child-bearing years. A further iron requirement of 6–8 mg/day occurs after 32 weeks' gestation.

Provide culture-specific dietary advice with information on iron body stores and avoidance of absorption inhibitors, e.g. tea, bread and chapatti. A reliable system for investigation of anaemia and monitoring of response to treatment is paramount[2].

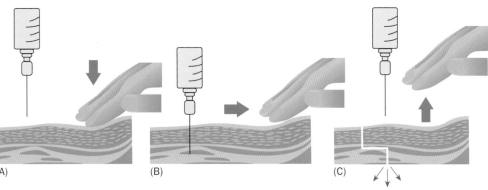

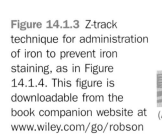

Figure 14.1.3 Z-track technique for administration of iron to prevent iron staining, as in Figure 14.1.4. This figure is downloadable from the book companion website at www.wiley.com/go/robson

(A)　　　　　(B)　　　　　(C)

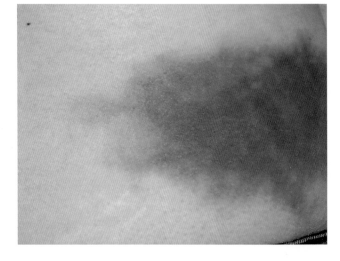

Figure 14.1.4 Iron-stained skin of a pregnant woman (© C. Oppenheimer). This figure is downloadable from the book companion website at www.wiley.com/go/robson

Pregnancy Issues

- Prevention of anaemia by early recognition of iron deficiency in those at risk is paramount
- Anaemia in the third trimester increases the risk of poor recovery from blood loss at birth, as well as tachycardia, shortness of breath and maternal exhaustion
- Parenteral iron, intravenous or intramuscular using the z-track technique (Figure 14.1.3), is used in cases of non-compliance or malabsorption, but contraindicated in cases of allergy
- Be aware of potential skin staining when administering iron, if the z-track technique is not used (see Figure 14.1.4)
- A rise in reticulocyte counts and Hb of 0.8 g/dl/week occurs 5–10 days after starting oral iron treatment[9]; the increase in Hb is similar for parenteral iron[10]
- Randomised controlled trials have been inconclusive on the effect of universal iron supplementation in pregnancy versus adverse maternal and fetal outcomes[11]
- Ensuring normal Hb and adequate iron stores is part of promoting higher likelihood of normality

Medical Management and Care

- Assess cause of anaemia by adequate dietary and medical history and appropriate testing. See algorithm for management (Figure 14.1.5)
- Prescribe ferrous sulfate 200 mg 2–3 times daily, or a proprietary combined iron and folate tablet with a higher elemental iron content until Hb normalises and thereafter to replenish stores. Advise to take iron preparations on 'an empty stomach' with orange or apple juice
- If required, im or iv dose is calculated according to iron deficit and body weight
- Administer iron dextran or sucrose iv in 0.9% sodium chloride infusion as total or divided doses
- Consider blood transfusion only if severe anaemia in a situation with a high risk of blood loss (blood products and transfusion are outlined in Appendix 14.1.1)

Midwifery Management and Care

- Severe/chronically anaemic women to be booked at consultant unit
- Encourage consumption of iron-rich foods with orange juice to enhance iron absorption, and provide information on nutrition in pregnancy[12]
- Be aware that inhibitors of iron absorption include polyphenols (in certain vegetables), tannins (in tea), phytates (in bran) and calcium (in dairy products)
- Screen all women at booking visit and at 28 weeks' gestation[13] and ensure the result is acted upon
- Women with known anaemia need testing at each antenatal visit
- Ensure anaphylactic emergency treatment is available during parenteral iron administration
- Treat selectively with iron[1,7] and folate preparations[14] and if needed reduce gastrointestinal complaints[15]

Labour Issues

Risk of:
- Maternal exhaustion
- Exacerbation of anaemia by excessive blood loss:
    - multiple birth
    - prolonged labour
    - instrumental delivery
    - caesarean section
    - grand multiparity
- Shortness of breath
- Tachycardia

Medical Management and Care

- Group and save serum on admission to labour
- Assess risk factors for excessive blood loss

Midwifery Management and Care

- Care in consultant-led unit
- Active third stage of labour – syntometrine and IVI of oxytocin
- Await FBC results before advocating eating and drinking in labour
- Vigilant monitoring of labour progress
- Prompt referral to obstetrician if slow progress develops
- Avoid directed pushing where possible
- All perineal trauma to be sutured

Postpartum Issues

Maternal Considerations
- Mother is at risk of:
    - postpartum haemorrhage
    - infection
    - poor wound healing
    - postnatal depression
    - lethargy
    - breast-feeding difficulties
- Mother requires return of Hb to normal level before planning further pregnancies

Neonatal Considerations
- Fetus obtains iron from placental transfer regardless of maternal iron stores, hence is unlikely to be anaemic
- Potential for IUGR or pre-term neonate with associated problems[16,17]

Medical Management and Care

- Reassure mother that the baby is unlikely to be anaemic
- Continue the maintenance dose of oral iron for up to 3 months postpartum to replenish stores
- See algorithm for management (Figure 14.1.5)

Midwifery Management and Care

- Be alert for signs of postpartum haemorrhage, infection and side effects of iron supplementation
- Postnatal assessment – FBC to identify any extra requirements
- Promote breast-feeding realistically with options to rest, e.g. express breast milk so that baby can be fed by other family members
- Consider social circumstances and use support such as *Home Start*, family and friends for basic housework
- Reassure mother that baby unlikely to be anaemic.
- Advise an iron-rich diet to improve iron stores (see Patient Organisation page for link to diet sheets)
- Be alert for signs of postnatal depression and continue postnatal visiting if indicated
- Contraceptive advice to ensure adequate spacing of pregnancies

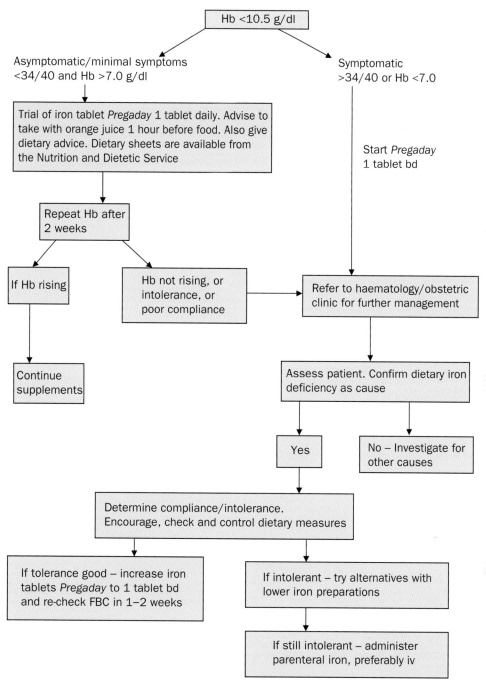

Figure 14.1.5 Protocol* for community management of anaemia in pregnancy. * Clinical protocol used for University Hospitals of Leicester, adapted and used with permission. This figure is downloadable from the book companion website at www.wiley.com/go/robson

14.2 Megaloblastic Anaemia

Incidence	**Risk for Childbearing**
Complicates a third of pregnancies worldwide UK incidence is 0.2–5%[1]	Variable Risk

EXPLANATION OF CONDITION

Megaloblastic anaemia is an acquired condition characterised by **macrocytosis** – the MCV of the red blood cells (erythrocytes) is above the normal range of 80–95 femtolitres (fl). It is called **megaloblastic** because the developing red blood cells in the bone marrow are larger than normal and have immature nuclei. A full blood count may reveal an increased number of immature red blood cells (megaloblasts) in the blood, reduced platelets and haemoglobin levels unresponsive to treatment with iron supplements, as well as the raised MCV.

Megaloblastic anaemia is usually caused by deficiency of folic acid or vitamin B_{12} (cyanocobalamin), but more rarely may be drug-induced or associated with myelodysplastic syndrome. It is also possible to see a non-megaloblastic macrocytic picture in liver disease, hypothyroidism and alcoholism.

In pregnancy a relative macrocytosis is common and normal.

Folate deficiency is associated with nutritional and socio-economic status[2] and may cause complications in pregnancy. Megaloblastic anaemia develops insidiously following:

- Poor dietary folate intake
- Excessive alcohol consumption[3,4]
- Increased cell turnover due to:
  - pregnancy (demands of mother and fetus)
  - chronic haemolytic anaemia (e.g. sickle cell anaemia, hereditary spherocytosis)
  - chronic inflammatory conditions
- Renal loss
  - chronic renal failure
  - dialysis
- Malabsorption disorders, e.g. gluten-induced enteropathy (coeliac disease)
- Drug-induced
  - some anticonvulsants
  - sulfasalazine
  - methotrexate

Mainly stored in the liver, cellular folates help to build DNA and protein in all tissues. This includes those required for growth of the fetus, placenta, maternal red cell mass and uterine development in pregnancy. Folate is found in beans, rice and green vegetables and some food stuffs have folic acid supplemented.

Vitamin B_{12} deficiency is caused by veganism or poor quality diet, pernicious anaemia, gastrectomy or ileal resection (as occurs with Crohn's disease).

COMPLICATIONS

The consequences of true megaloblastic anaemia include:

- Pallor and jaundice
- Increasingly severe anaemia
- Heart failure
- Pancytopenia (low white cell and platelet counts)

Other complications of vitamin B_{12} deficiency include:

- Neuropathy involving peripheral nerves and spinal cord
- Psychiatric disturbances
- Visual disturbance
- Fetal neural tube defects

Both deficiencies can cause epithelial disturbance, e.g. the smooth painful tongue (glossitis), and, if low serum homocysteine levels are present (part of this metabolic pathway), arterial obstruction and venous thrombosis.

NON-PREGNANCY TREATMENT AND CARE

Advise a diet rich in vitamin B_{12} and folate, such as cheese, cereals, leafy green vegetables, fortified cereals, fruit and egg yolks. The recommended daily intake of folate is 3 micrograms/kg of body weight for non-pregnant and non-lactating women.

A daily intake of 5 mg folic acid is recommended for women with hereditary haemolytic disorders, epileptics on anticonvulsants and women of reproductive age with a family history of neural tube defects who are planning a pregnancy[4-6].

PRE-CONCEPTION ISSUES AND CARE

Estimated dietary requirements of folates in pregnancy are 100–600 micrograms/day with an average daily intake of 237 micrograms/day[7,8].

An association exists between periconceptual folic acid deficiency and neural tube defect, cleft lip and cleft palate in the fetus[5], hence the recommended folic acid supplementation of 400 micrograms/day for the first 3 months preconceptually and throughout the first trimester[4,9].

A daily oral supplementation of 5 mg folic acid is recommended for those with a previously affected fetus and family history of neural tube defects and to epileptics[4,10].

Other factors such as genetic factors, pre-conceptual diabetes and first trimester hyperglycaemia and drugs such as sodium valproate used for epilepsy also contribute to the development of megaloblastic anaemia. Also relevant are the increased demands of pregnancy, multiple pregnancy, grand multiparity or frequent pregnancies[3] which may exacerbate other factors or in extreme cases precipitate megaloblastic anaemia.

Pregnancy Issues

It is important to remember that both macrocytosis (raised MCV) and low B_{12} levels (normal range in pregnancy down to 150 micrograms/l) are most likely to be normal in pregnancy.

With megaloblastic anaemia the drop in haemoglobin and platelet levels is exaggerated. However, serum ferritin can remain normal[2]. Leucopenia[1], which is worsened when there is infection, is present.

Folate deficiency is associated with:
- Cervical dysplasia
- Loss of appetite and maternal weight loss
- Glossitis
- Increased risk of neural tube defects
- Increased risk of fetal cleft palate
- IUGR

Vomiting in pregnancy makes the increased demands of pregnancy worse, especially in the presence of multiple pregnancy, where there is more folate transfer from mother to fetus[10] leading to further depletion of folate stores.

Average daily folate requirements rise in pregnancy from 50 micrograms/day to 400 micrograms/day which can be met through a normal diet. However, note that folates are vulnerable to heat, being easily destroyed during cooking.

Any additional needs such as multiple pregnancy or taking antiepileptic drugs further cause this to be exceeded and supplements are needed.

Medical Management and Care
- Full blood count; assess serum and red cell folate levels[9]
- Mild/moderate anaemia – synthetic oral folic acid 5–10 mg/day
- Folic acid oral or im supplement may be prescribed
- Vigilant screening for congenital abnormalities – ultrasound scan
- Further investigations for associated conditions if megaloblastic anaemia presents for the first time in pregnancy[4], but ensure this is true megaloblastic anaemia; obstetrician may need to liaise with physician/haematologist
- Infection screening may be indicated
- IUGR – consider serial ultrasound scanning
- NICE recommend routine supplementation of oral folic acid 400 micrograms/day prior to pregnancy and in the first trimester[9]

Midwifery Management and Care
- Midwife to take thorough booking history to identify any current treatment and co-existing conditions that may influence megaloblastic anaemia, e.g. haemoglobinopathies, dietary restriction
- All such mothers should be booked at a consultant unit
- Weigh at each antenatal appointment if there is any suggestion of weight loss or loss of appetite
- Conduct a nutritional assessment referring to a dietician if indicated
- Promote a folate-rich diet and taking of prescribed supplements
- Encourage attendance at antenatal parent education with an emphasis on food preparation
- Assess for signs of infection and refer for treatment promptly
- Severe anaemia is treated with folic acid 5–10 mg/day im oral iron (and blood transfusion as a last resort)
- Counselling about the increased risks of congenital anomalies is advised if confirmed folate deficiency in the first trimester
- Be alert for IUGR and refer as appropriate
- Be alert for APH and advise mother to seek prompt help if symptoms present, including giving of emergency telephone numbers
- Prepare mother for the possibility of blood transfusion in labour

Labour Issues
- Increased risk of prematurity and low birth weight in severe cases
- Theoretical risk of postpartum haemorrhage in extreme B_{12}/folate deficiency; however, this is rare.
- Maternal tiredness is more likely at the onset of labour

Medical Management and Care
- If symptomatic anaemia presents, repeat full blood count with cross-matched blood available if needed
- No specific recommendations in labour and birth if blood count is stable

Midwifery Management and Care
- Encourage mobilisation and maintain hydration to combat tiredness
- Actively manage third-stage labour to reduce blood loss at birth, especially if symptoms of anaemia persist
- Alert neonatal team if premature birth is imminent

Postpartum Issues
- Human milk has a folate content of 5 micrograms/dl, therefore red cell folate levels are further depleted in lactating women
- Women with folate deficiency diagnosed prenatally should continue supplementation for several weeks postpartum
- Adequate inter-pregnancy interval is advised to encourage woman to fully recover and maintain good folate reserves

Medical Management and Care
- Indices of folate metabolism return to pre-pregnant values within 6 weeks of delivery
- Haematological follow-up may be needed

Midwifery Management and Care
- Continue to promote a diet rich in folates
- Full blood count to determine haemoglobin status, red cell folate concentrations, reticulocyte count and blood film recommended if symptomatic anaemia occurs
- Provide contraceptive advice and consider further discussion with women suffering from epilepsy and malabsorption disorders
- Continuation of folate supplementation advised for those with hereditary haemolytic disorders and epilepsy

14.3 Disseminated Intravascular Coagulation

Incidence	Risk for Childbearing
Rare, less than 1:1000 pregnancies[1]	High Risk

EXPLANATION OF CONDITION

Disseminated intravascular coagulation (DIC), also known as consumptive coagulopathy, is an acquired disorder of haemostasis, which often heralds the onset of multi-organ failure[2].

Underlying causes[3]:

- **Infection** – especially *Escherichia coli, Neisseria meningitidis, Streptococcus pneumoniae* and malaria
- **Cancer** – especially lungs, pancreas[3], gynaecological[4]
- **Trauma, burns, surgery** and **snake bite**[5]
- **Pregnancy** – especially:
  - placental abruption
  - major haemorrhage
  - pre-eclampsia
  - retained dead fetus or placenta
  - amniotic fluid embolism[3]

Endothelial damage arising from one of the above results in thromboplastins being released from the damaged cells[6], *triggering* the extrinsic pathway to initiate a coagulation cascade[3]. With DIC, the tissue damage is so severe that blood clotting occurs at the original site *and* throughout the vascular tree, hence the term *disseminated* intravascular coagulation. This process consumes large quantities of fibrinogen, thrombocytes (platelets) and clotting factors V and VIII[3]. The microthrombi produced occlude some small blood vessels, resulting in ischaemic damage (dead tissue) to body organs[6]. The damaged tissue releases more thromboplastins and a vicious cycle develops[6].

Eventually all the clotting factors and platelets are consumed and bleeding results[5]. The patient is in the ironic situation of having both widespread blood clotting *and* a clotting deficiency. Bleeding occurs, petechiae develop in the skin and, if untreated, **major haemorrhage** can result[7,8].

DIC can be subclinical, only detected on laboratory investigations, or may present with massive haemorrhage[7,9]. Bleeding is observed at vascular access points, GI tract, nose, genitourinary tract, intravenous cannulation sites and wounds[8]. Investigations[2] reveal:

- Increase in prothrombin time
- Increase in partial thromboplastin time
- Increase in fibrin degradation products
- Decrease in platelets
- Decrease in fibrinogen

COMPLICATIONS

- **Damaged kidneys** – renal failure and anuria[6]
- **Damaged liver** – liver failure and jaundice[6]
- **Damaged lungs** – dyspnoea and cyanosis[6]
- **Brain damage** – convulsions or coma[6]
- **Retinal damage** – damaged sight or blindness[6]
- **Pituitary damage** – Sheehan's syndrome[6]
- **Major haemorrhage** – hypovolaemia then death

NON-PREGNANCY TREATMENT AND CARE

- DIC is essentially a clinical diagnosis; laboratory tests confirm the diagnosis and guide replacement of blood component[7]
- Coagulation screen comprising:
  - whole blood film
  - FBC, especially platelet count[8]
  - fibrinogen degradation products/D-dimers[5,8,9]
  - prothrombin time (normal 10–14 seconds)[8]
  - thrombin time (normal 1–15 seconds)[8]
  - partial thromboplastin time (normal 35–45 seconds)
  - fibrinogen levels (normal 2.5–4 g/l)[8]
- Insert indwelling urinary catheter, ideally with a measuring chamber, and monitor urinary output
- Strict monitoring and recording of fluid balance
- Repeat the coagulation screen as clinically indicated
- Central venous pressure (CVP) monitoring[10]
- IVI fresh frozen plasma[2], which contains all the clotting factors[11]
- IVI platelets[6]
- IVI packed cells (blood)[6,11]
- Identify and treat the underlying cause if possible[2]
- Institute high dependency care, transfer if necessary
- Respiratory support if indicated[12]
- Intravenous antibiotics for suspected septicaemia[2]
- Correct exacerbating factors, especially:
  - dehydration
  - acidosis
  - renal failure
  - hypoxia[2]
- Analgesia[12]
- Anticoagulation with heparin rarely used and requires supervision by a haematologist[5,9]
- Concentrates of blood factors (antithrombins and/or protein C) are effective in the non-pregnant state
- Recombinant activated protein C is used for sepsis in non-pregnant patients[9]
- Steroids may be used for precipitating factors

PRE-CONCEPTION ISSUES AND CARE

If a woman had DIC in a previous pregnancy, the recurrence risk will be that of the precipitating cause. Follow-up and de-briefing of any woman who had acute DIC is essential.

Women with chronic DIC may be at high risk of pregnancy complications and need to be assessed and advised by a haematologist before cessation of contraception.

Pregnancy Issues

The activated coagulation system in pregnancy reduces the threshold for DIC[13], putting the mother at risk.

Associated with DIC in Pregnancy:
- Miscarriage, particularly septic
- Septic, illegal termination[4,14]
- Hydatidiform mole[10]
- Placenta accreta and PPH[10]
- Retained dead fetus[7,10]
- Acute fatty liver of pregnancy[10]
- Placental abruption – most common cause
- Placenta praevia[4,10]
- Pre-eclampsia[4,10]
- HELLP syndrome[4]
- Amniotic fluid embolism[7,10]
- Mismatched blood transfusion[7,10]
- Breast/ovarian/uterine cancer[4]

Possible Clinical Presentations:
- One of the above trigger factors
- Haemorrhage
- Ecchymoses (discoloured skin patches)
- Haematuria
- Shock
- Thrombotic complications in the brain, kidneys or lungs
- Acute pulmonary hypertension if the trigger was amniotic fluid embolism[13]

Maternal Mortality Associated with DIC:
- Placental abruption = 1%[10]
- Infection/shock = 50–80%[10]

Accurate record keeping is of paramount importance.

Medical Management and Care

General
- All women with an associated condition (see opposite) should have a full blood count and coagulation screen[13]
- Before attributing a platelet count of $\leq100 \times 10^9/1$ to gestational thrombocytopenia, other causes of a reduced platelet count should be excluded[13], especially DIC

If DIC Presents Acutely with Haemorrhage
- Multidisciplinary team approach, so call haematologist and anaesthetist
- Precipitating factor must be identified and treated immediately[13]
- Investigations – as for non-pregnancy (previous page)
- Blood samples for group and cross-match are especially important as operative delivery may be imminent
- Treatment – as for non-pregnancy (previous page)
- If haemorrhage commences, implement the institution's **major obstetric haemorrhage protocol**

Midwifery Management and Care
- Be aware that DIC can present chronically or acutely, the latter leading to major obstetric haemorrhage (a life-threatening event) and that the midwife might be the first to recognise the problem

If DIC Presents Acutely with Haemorrhage:
- Remain with the mother, giving reassurance and oxygen, whilst preparing for an acute emergency
- **Send for medical aid**
- Initiate observations of vital signs, including measurement of blood loss and retaining blood-soaked items for inspection later
- Summon an assistant to prepare an IVI with blood giving set, and venepuncture equipment for the above blood samples
- Summon an assistant to attend the baby if the mother has delivered
- Insert indwelling urinary catheter and monitor fluid balance strictly
- Once medical aid arrives the midwife's role is to assist the medical team and to care for the mother and baby
- If there is a fetus or placental tissue *in utero*, the mother is likely to be transferred to obstetric theatre, otherwise, the mother should be transferred to high-dependency care area, which may well be delivery suite

Labour Issues

Labour and delivery needs to be planned and attended by senior obstetric and anaesthetic staff. If vaginal delivery can be achieved within a reasonable time frame this should be attempted. This will depend upon feto-maternal wellbeing.

Epidural and spinal anaesthesia are generally contraindicated. Hence, general anaesthetic is likely for operative delivery.

Medical Management and Care
- Caesarean section may be required[13]
- Evacuation of the uterus if there are retained feto-placental products
- Close liaison with haematologist and blood bank

Midwifery Management and Care
- Prepare for, and assist with, an emergency delivery
- Keep mother nil by mouth in case of general anaesthetic
- If a vaginal delivery – active management of the third stage and all perineal trauma must be sutured promptly
- Vigilant examination of the placenta and ascertain if it, or cord blood samples, need to be sent to the laboratory
- Accurate estimation of blood loss, observe for clotting and possibly retain for inspection by the medical team

Postpartum Issues
- The coagulation imbalance usually resolves 24–48 hours post-delivery, and the low platelet count (thrombocytopenia) within a week[11]
- The baby may have been admitted to NNU

Medical Management and Care
- Obstetric postnatal review – debrief; advice for future pregnancies

Midwifery Management and Care
- Careful post-operative care paying particular attention to wound and cannulation sites for signs of bleeding
- Post-operative observations might be continued longer than usual
- Assist the mother to visit her baby on NNU

14.4 Von Willebrand's Disease and Other Bleeding Disorders

Incidence	Risk for Childbearing
1% of the UK population have low von Willebrand Factor[1] 7–20% of women with menorrhagia have von Willebrand's Disease[2]	VWD Type 1 and 2 – Variable Risk VWD Type 3 – High Risk

EXPLANATION OF CONDITION

A familial haematological disorder, characterised by bleeding, was described in 1926 by von Willebrand in Finland[3], hence the term **von Willebrand's disease** (VWD). This is a condition in which there is either a defect, or deficiency, of the von Willebrand factor (VWF), a carrier protein for clotting factor VIII[4]. There are three[5] basic types:

1. **Type 1** – 75% of cases[4]; partial quantitative deficiency of normal VWF[1,5]
2. **Type 2** – 20% of cases[4]; qualitative deficiencies of VWF of which there are four variations[1]
3. **Type 3 (Severe)** – 5% of cases[4]; almost complete deficiency of VWF and reduced factor VIII[1,5]

VWD is the most common inherited bleeding disorder in pregnancy[6], and is inherited as an autosomal dominant condition. Hence, children of either gender may inherit the clotting deficiency[7]. However, women are more likely to present with symptomatic VWD due to menstruation and childbearing[4]. There are no ethnic differences[8].

Non-pregnant patients usually present as young adults with excess bleeding, in the form of:

- Epistaxis (nosebleeds)[1,5]
- Menorrhagia (heavy and prolonged periods)[1,2,5,9]
- Bleeding after dental extraction or surgery[1,5]
- Bruising[1,5]

Screening tests[8] entail:

- FBC – usually normal but a mild thrombocytopenia may occur in Type 2 patients[8]
- Serum ferritin
- Clotting screen – prothrombin time is normal, but the activated partial thromboplastin time may be prolonged
- Bleeding time – usually prolonged, but may be normal in mild forms of VWD[8]
- Platelet aggregation test – measures platelet efficiency[8]
- Von Willebrand factor antigen, factor VIII, Ristocetin cofactor (RiCof)

Other Bleeding Disorders

- **Factor XI deficiency** – similar problems to VWD Type 3
- **Haemophilia A and B** – female carriers can have low levels, and an associated bleeding risk
  - Bleeding history and non-pregnant levels of factor VIII or IX should be identified

COMPLICATIONS

- Haemorrhage (severity varies from VWD Type 1 to 3)
- Joint bleeding and pain (in VWD Type 3)
- Anaemia and fatigue
- Pregnancy problems

NON-PREGNANCY TREATMENT AND CARE

Common Treatments

- Combined oral contraceptive pill (COCP) – to increase levels of factor VIII and von Willebrand factor, reduce menstrual blood volume, and prevent pregnancy[8]
- Iron supplementation – if clinical condition necessitates
- Vaccination against hepatitis A and B[5]
- Tranexamic acid (to inhibit bleeding) – slows the breakdown of blood clots; tablet form, or syrup for children[1]
- Desmopressin – a synthetic hormone (not a blood product) that enables VWF to be released into the blood circulation
  - given iv at specialist centres[1]
  - nasal spray is available
- Clotting factor concentrate – derived from human plasma, and used to treat severe cases of VWD[1]

Advice[1]

- **Avoid aspirin**
- Carry 'green card' from haemophilia centre at all times in case of accident or emergency
- For children, parents should inform the school
- Caution with certain holiday destinations, and a 'travel pack' of drugs may have to be issued
- Encourage exercise, but discourage contact sports
- Maintain a healthy lifestyle with an iron-rich diet

PRE-CONCEPTION ISSUES AND CARE

Women with a history of heavy menstrual bleeding since menarche, and a family history suggestive of a coagulation disorder, should be screened for coagulation disorders[10].

Von Willebrand's Disease

- There is no evidence that fertility is impaired[4]
- Pre-conception care aims to optimise maternal health
- The risk of a mother with Type 1 transmitting the condition to her child is 50% but only 33% of these will be clinically affected[7]
- Opportunity for pre-natal diagnosis for women with Type 3, whose genetic mutation is identifiable[7]
- If parents already have a child with Type 3, the chance of each subsequent child being affected is 25%[7]

Haemophilia

- Women with relevant family histories are assessed for carrier status and counselled over reproductive options[7]

Factor XI Deficiency

- Pre-natal diagnosis should be discussed if the woman's condition is severe[7]

Pregnancy Issues

There is considerable variability of the hae-mostatic response of VWD to pregnancy[7].

Both factor VIII and VWF levels rise in second and third trimesters[2] which may lead to a 'normalisation' of these levels with improve-ment in minor bleeding problems[8] but makes diagnosis of VWD difficult[8]. However, the first trimester retains a risk of bleeding. In severe VWD, levels remain low throughout[8].

VWD miscarriage risk is not significantly different from that of the general population[2].

Desmopressin is used with caution in preg-nancy due to concerns over inducing contrac-tions, placental insufficiency, hyponatraemia, and its antidiuretic effect[8]. It can be used once based on a risk–benefit assessment. It should not be used in the presence of pre-eclampsia[7].

Co-existing thrombocytopenia can worsen[8]

Medical Management and Care
- Pregnancy in women with VWD or other clotting disorders should be managed by a multidisciplinary team comprising obstetrician, hae-matologist, senior anaesthetist[7], specialist nurse or midwife
- Counsel about pre-natal diagnosis and options arising
- Chorionic villus sampling for fetal DNA analysis might be performed

Von Willebrand's Disease
- Check factor levels including VWF:Ag, VWF:AC and FVIII:C at booking, 28 and 34 weeks and prior to invasive procedures[7]
- Aim for factor VIII level ≥50% to cover delivery and postpartum[8]
- Prophylactic treatment when factor levels are <50 IU/dl to cover inva-sive procedures and delivery[7]
- Platelet count is monitored regularly with VWD Type 2b[7]
- Monitor clinically, advising the laboratory of haemorrhage potential[8]
- If desmopressin is used, advise to restrict fluid intake[8] and observe closely for water retention[7]
- Avoid external cephalic version for malpresentation

Midwifery Management and Care
- Ensure the mother is booked for antenatal care at a specialist haematological/obstetric clinic and delivery at a consultant unit
- Be aware 'booking bloods' will be augmented by the doctor to include FBC, bleeding time or platelet closure time[8]; these are repeated prior to invasive procedures[8]
- Report abnormal blood test results promptly, especially platelets
- Encourage parentcraft attendance, but advise that an epidural *might* be contraindicated and discuss alternative pain relief options

Labour Issues

Delivery is a significant haemostatic chal-lenge[8], hence staff should be alert for intra-partum and postpartum haemorrhage.

Von Willebrand's Disease
- Epidurals can be sited by a senior anaes-thetist for VWD Type 1 where VWF >50 IU/dl[7,8], but its use is debatable for Type 2[8], and contraindicated for Type 3[7]
- Prompt removal of epidural catheter reduces risk of bleeding[8]
- Effort should be made to ensure a prompt third stage with complete placenta[11]

Haemophilia carriers: for most haemophilia carriers labour and anaesthesia carry normal risk, but those with low factor levels should be identified and a plan agreed. Cord blood should be sent for clotting factor assay in male babies of haemophilia carriers[12].

Medical Management and Care
- In advance agree a delivery/anaesthetic plan, seek haematological advice, ascertain laboratory facilities, and order clotting factors[8]
- IVI, FBC, coagulation screen and group and save in labour[8,12]
- Avoid fetal blood sampling
- Avoid ventouse and mid-cavity rotational forceps delivery[7]
- Tranexamic acid can be used in the treatment of PPH, after obstetric causes have been treated[7]
- Avoid prolonged labour; early recourse to caesarean section should be considered[7] ensuring surgical haemostasis[8]
- If ristocetin cofactor remains low there may be a need for Alphanate infusion during labour, checking ristocetin levels (750%)

Midwifery Management and Care
- Avoid fetal scalp electrodes for continuous fetal monitoring
- Active management of third stage of labour is essential[7]
- If needed, give desmopressin *after* clamping of the umbilical cord[2]
- Ask the doctor if im injections, including Syntometrine, can be given
- Prompt and expert suturing of all perineal trauma
- Ascertain if cord bloods should be taken for fetal VWF[7]
- Prompt administration to the neonate of *oral* vitamin K[7,12]

Postpartum Issues
- Levels of factor VIII and VWF fall mark-edly 24 hours postpartum[8], putting mothers of all three types of VWD[2] at:
  - 22% risk of primary PPH[8]
  - 25% risk of secondary PPH[8], which can occur up to *5 weeks* postpartum[2]
- The safety of desmopressin in breast-feeding has not been studied[8]
- Neonates who inherit VWD Type 3 are at risk of intracranial haemorrhage, cephal-haematoma from labour[7] and umbilical stump bleeding postpartum

Medical Management and Care
- Check VWF level if there was a low pre-pregnancy baseline[7]
- Desmopressin can be used immediately postpartum[8]
- Tranexamic acid 1 g tds po if a risk of bleeding is predicted

Midwifery Management and Care
- This mother is not for early discharge
- Vigilant postnatal maternal observations, being alert for PPH[8]
- If desmopressin is used, confer with paediatrician over breast-feeding
- Vigilant daily neonatal examinations being alert for intracranial bleeding or umbilical cord stump bleeding
- Advise the parents that circumcision of the baby, or other invasive procedures, must be delayed until the haematologist is in agreement[7]
- When *heel prick* (Guthrie) tests are performed, apply local pressure for a full 5 minutes and report excess bleeding or bruising[7]

S. E. Robson and J. Waugh

14.5 Thrombocytopenia in Pregnancy

Incidence	Risk for Childbearing
Gestational: 5–8% of pregnancies[1]	High Risk
Immune: 0.1% of pregnancies[1,2]	

EXPLANATION OF CONDITION

Thrombocytopenia is a reduced platelet (thrombocyte) count which can lead to bleeding in the skin, called **purpura**, and can result in spontaneous bruising and post-injury bleeding[3]. Up to 50% of women with pre-eclampsia will also develop thrombocytopenia[4]. There are several categories, of which midwives and doctors are likely to encounter two.

Gestational Thrombocytopenia

Gestational thrombocytopenia is also known as incidental thrombocytopenia of pregnancy[4]. It is exclusive to pregnancy and presents in the late second or third trimesters. The decreased platelet count is associated with haemodilution, and with increased platelet 'trapping', and with destruction in the placenta[1]. Usually asymptomatic, diagnosis often arises from a routine antenatal FBC[5] or can be retrospective, after delivery[4]. The platelet levels gradually fall reaching $50–150 \times 10^9/l$ by term. It is considered a benign condition[6] and does not affect the fetus[1]. The platelet count usually returns to normal by 6 weeks postpartum[4].

Immune Thrombocytopenic Purpura

Immune thrombocytopenic purpura (ITP) was formerly called idiopathic thrombocytopenic purpura. It can have an acute presentation, often occurring in children, and may follow a viral infection[6]. Alternatively, it can be chronic[7] and mainly affects young to middle-aged women, with the incidence increasing with age[8]. It is this version the midwife may encounter in the pre-conception period. It may also present for the first time in pregnancy.

ITP results from the body producing IgG autoantibodies that act against the woman's own platelets[9], reducing their lifespan from 10 days to a few hours. As the bone marrow cannot keep pace with replacement, the count drops[9] from a normal value of $150–400 \times 10^9/l$ to $10–140 \times 10^9/l$, with the risk of purpura and haemorrhage. Most cases are idiopathic (unknown cause) but some are secondary to drugs, HIV infection and connective tissue disorders[4].

Diagnosis is difficult as it is based on excluding other illnesses, such as SLE or von Willebrand's disease[5], and side effects of drugs that cause a low platelet count. Additionally, 30% of patients do not have antibodies detected on laboratory investigation.

If thrombocytopenia presents for the first time in pregnancy, diagnosis is complex, as pregnancy symptoms 'overlap'[1], and it is difficult to differentiate between gestational and immune thrombocytopenia. For this reason gestational thrombocytopenia may be considered a high-risk condition as well as ITP. The small IgG antibodies cross the placental barrier sometimes initiating neonatal thrombocytopenia[4].

HELLP syndrome[1] can be an associated condition.

COMPLICATIONS

- Impaired haemostasis[4] when platelet count is less than 50
- Bleeding from nose and gums[7]
- Bruising[7]
- Menorrhagia[7] and secondary anaemia
- Splenomegaly is rare in isolated thrombocytopenia[7]
- Major haemorrhage is rare[7]
- Side effects of steroids, e.g. diabetes, hypertension

NON-PREGNANCY TREATMENT AND CARE

- Corticosteroids, e.g. prednisone, to reduce the production of autoantibodies and the removal of antibody-coated platelets; complete response in 20% of cases and no further treatment necessary[7]
- Intravenous gammaglobulin is given to prolong the clearance time of antibody-coated platelets[5]
- Immunosuppressant drugs, e.g. azathioprine, ciclosporin, vincristine, danazol (see Appendix 11.1.1)
- Consideration of platelet transfusion in life-threatening situations or immediately before surgery under the advice of a haematologist; only a short-term effect as transfused platelets also have short lifespan[5]
- Splenectomy if medical management has failed. Removal of the spleen improves condition in 90% of cases[7] because the spleen is the principal site for production of IgG autoantibodies, as well as being the location for sequestration of antibody-coated platelets[5]. This operation is not recommended for children[7] or HIV-positive adults[10], because of a subsequent risk of pneumococcal infection.

PRE-CONCEPTION ISSUES AND CARE

- Former advice to avoid pregnancy, or deliver by caesarean section, no longer applies due to modern management[11]
- When a woman had ITP in a previous pregnancy the course of the disease and the effect on the fetus is likely to be similar in future pregnancies
- If the woman is still on treatment, she should be referred back to the haematologist for a risk–benefit analysis to maintain or alter drug therapy
- The woman might be investigated for other immune conditions, such as pernicious anaemia
- Usual pre-conception care is given, with additional consideration of:
  - prophylactic antibiotics if post-splenectomy
  - encourage a healthy diet that is rich in iron and folates
  - advising the mother *not* to discontinue her maintenance therapy once she suspects she is pregnant, without prior discussion with the haematologist

Pregnancy Issues

- In immune thrombocytopenia the IgG autoantibodies can cross the placental barrier, causing fetal, and later neonatal, thrombocytopenia[4,12,13]
- The only reliable predictor of neonatal outcome is a prior affected pregnancy[13]
- There is a risk of severe thrombocytopenia in approximately 1% of neonates[11]
- Splenectomy in pregnancy can precipitate pre-term labour[13]
- Therapy for pregnant women is similar to that of non-pregnant women[11]
- Little correlation exists between maternal and fetal platelet counts, so it is not possible to predict fetal outcome from non-invasive tests[3]
- Thrombocytopenia can arise secondary to pre-eclampsia and HELLP syndrome[12]

Medical Management and Care

- Regular FBC for platelet count, frequency dependent upon the severity of the condition
- Adjust steroids in ITP (usually prednisolone) in relation to platelet count
- Intravenous immunoglobulins (IVIG) if required[11]
- Prophylactic antibiotics if a previous splenectomy[6]
- Splenectomy is best avoided, but if necessary should be performed in the second trimester[1,17]; alternatively it might be combined with caesarean section in third trimester[16] in very rare situations
- Maternal platelet transfusion only if severely compromised
- Avoid cordocentesis if possible[11,15]
- Iv Anti D is an experimental treatment used in specialist centres only
- Aim to optimise third trimester platelet count to maximise the prospect of a vaginal delivery near term

Midwifery Management and Care

- Book for hospital confinement and for antenatal care by the multidisciplinary team at a combined obstetric/haematology clinic
- Discuss with the mother a realistic care and birth plan, with consultation with haematologist and obstetrician
- Encourage healthy diet and lifestyle
- Iron and folate tablets throughout pregnancy
- Aim to keep pregnancy otherwise as normal as possible

Labour Issues

- Risk of intrapartum haemorrhage[1], especially from a surgical incision
- Higher chance of pre-term delivery[12]
- Theoretical risk of epidural haematoma[1]. However, epidural is considered safe if the platelet count >80–100 × 10^9/l[14]
- There is a small risk of fetal intracranial haemorrhage[11], with chance of fetal bruising and significant cephalhaematoma

Medical Management and Care

- Maintain iv access during labour
- Take blood for FBC and platelets, group and save
- Caesarean section only for obstetric reasons[11,14]
- Avoid ventouse and forceps delivery[14]
- Avoid fetal blood sampling[2,11,15]
- Risk–benefit analysis for epidural if platelet count <80 × 10^9/l
- The anaesthetist may prefer a spinal anaesthetic to an epidural[1]
- Avoid im injections if platelet count <40 × 10^9/l

Midwifery Management and Care

- Inspect iv cannulation site regularly for signs of bleeding
- Aim for normal vaginal delivery if all is otherwise well
- Active management of third stage of labour; consider use of iv Syntocinon if im injections are contraindicated (see above)
- Leave adequate length of umbilical cord below the cord clamp, to allow blood samples to be taken by the paediatrician
- All perineal trauma to be sutured promptly[14] and expertly
- At placental examination take placental cord blood for neonatal platelet count, and ascertain if other samples are required[14,16]
- Confirm with paediatrician if the neonatal vitamin K can be given im
- Neonatal assessment by paediatrician, and possible transfer to the neonatal unit for concerns about bleeding or general condition

Postpartum Issues

- Risk of postpartum haemorrhage if platelet count is low[12]
- ITP secondary to pre-eclampsia or HELLP syndrome often deteriorates immediately post delivery
- The risk of thrombocytopenia in the neonate cannot be predicted from clinical or laboratory test results in the mother[15] hence a cord blood sample should have been taken immediately after delivery[16]
- 6% risk of the neonate having severe thrombocytopenia with a limited risk of intracranial haemorrhage[13]

Medical Management and Care

- Avoid maternal non-steroidal drugs if platelet count <100 × 10^9/l[15,16]
- Review platelet count post delivery[14] and repeat regularly if pre-eclamptic

Midwifery Management and Care

- TED stockings may be used for women requiring specific thromboprophylaxis[16]
- The neonate is not for early discharge if daily platelet counts, from umbilical cord stump, are required[1,5]
- Vigilant postnatal examination to ascertain if vaginal loss is excessive and to ascertain if effective uterine involution is occurring
- Vigilant daily examination of the newborn to look for signs of bleeding from cord stump and other areas
- Be alert for intracranial bleeding symptoms such as seizures, bulging fontanelle or altered responses, especially if paediatric advice is that there is a risk of haemorrhage

14.6 Thalassaemia

Incidence	Risk for Childbearing
Over 16 000 healthy carriers[1] and approximately 700 people in UK estimated to have β-thalassaemia major[2,3]	High Risk – thalassaemia major Low or Variable Risk – all other thalassaemias

EXPLANATION OF CONDITION

Thalassaemia is an autosomal recessive inherited disorder of haemoglobin synthesis, prevalent in population groups that originate from Africa, the Caribbean, the Mediterranean, Southeast Asia and the Middle East[4].

Adult haemoglobin consists of two pairs of alpha (α) and beta (β) globin chains per haem complex. The α-globin chain production is controlled by four genes located on chromosome 16 and β-globin chain production is controlled by two genes located on chromosome 11. Individuals inherit two α genes and one β gene from each parent[5].

There are three types of haemoglobins present at birth, produced from the pairing of α, β, γ (gamma) or δ (delta) globin chains:

1. **Haemoglobin A** ($\alpha_2\beta_2$) – 97%
2. **Haemoglobin A$_2$** ($\alpha_2\delta_2$) – 2%
3. **Haemoglobin F** ($\alpha_2\gamma_2$) – 0.5%

Thalassaemia is caused by the inheritance of a defective α- or β-globin gene. This results in a reduced rate of globin chain formation and red blood cells (RBC) with inadequate haemoglobin (Hb) content. The thalassaemias are classified by the defective gene inherited[4] and further sub-classified by the reduction of globin chains produced.

α-Thalassaemias

Characterised by defective production and number of functional α-globin chains:

- **α-thalassaemia trait** (α-thal$^+$)
  - inheritance of one defective α gene
  - clinically undetectable
- **α-thalassaemia intermedia**
  - inheritance of two defective α genes
  - mainly asymptomatic
  - α-thal^0 trait: both defective genes inherited from one parent
  - homozygous α-thal$^+$ trait: one defective gene is inherited from each parent
- **Haemoglobin H disease (HbH)**
  - inheritance of three defective genes resulting in rapid RBC haemolysis and mild/moderate anaemia
- **Thalassaemia major** (homozygous α-thal^0)
  - all four α genes are absent and substituted by the four γ-globulin chains
  - the resultant Bart's haemoglobin (Hb Barts hydrops) is incapable of oxygen exchange at tissue level
  - this hydropic fetus requires intrauterine transfusions to survive and will be transfusion dependent for life

β-Thalassaemias

Characterised by defective production of β-globin chains:

- **β-thalassaemia minor**
  - a carrier state caused by the inheritance of one defective β
  - characterised by a mild microcytic anaemia
- **β-thalassaemia intermedia**
  - moderate homozygous β-thalassaemia where both inherited genes are defective
  - individuals are less likely to require blood transfusions
- Clinical findings include:
  - enlargement of heart, liver and spleen
  - bone deformities due to bone marrow expansion
- **β-thalassaemia major**
  - inheritance of both defective genes resulting in a severe homozygous β-thalassaemia
  - severe haemolysis of red blood cells
  - life-threatening anaemia requiring chronic blood transfusion therapy

Diagnosis

Diagnosis is by identifying high risk groups[6] and performing:

- Full blood count – reveals low mean corpuscular haemoglobin (MCH <27 pg) and a low MCV (<75 fl)
- Bone marrow examination – reveals microcytic, hypochromic red blood cells
- Haemoglobin analysis – elevated HbA$_2$ levels

COMPLICATIONS

- Severe haemolysis and anaemia
- Bone marrow expansion
- Elevated cardiac output and severe cardiac impairment
- Endocrine, splenic and hepatic dysfunction
- Megaloblastic anaemia, iron overload in organs

NB: Those with 'trait only' have anaemia of variable severity.

NON-PREGNANCY TREATMENT AND CARE

Screening involves the identification of at-risk groups from history taking – ethnicity of woman, family origins, medical history, paternal screening, full blood count, haemoglobin analysis[2,6]. Further investigations include cardiology assessment, blood-borne infection screening, maternal antibody and iron overload levels.

Treatment

- Oral iron if low ferritin levels; avoid parenteral iron
- 5 mg folic acid daily
- Transfusion therapy for severe anaemia
- Iron chelation therapy with desferrioxamine (25–50 mg/kg) infusion pump overnight for 10–12 hours; removes iron from tissues and reduces organ damage caused by iron overload
- Desferrioxamine is given daily through the abdominal wall subcutaneously

PRE-CONCEPTION ISSUES AND CARE

- Accumulation of iron stores in the heart, pancreas and thyroid can lead to cardiomyopathy, type 1 diabetes and hypothyroidism, hence screening is indicated
- Levels of iron overload are measured through gall bladder and biliary tract assessments
- Those with major thalassaemia infertility problems caused by chronic iron overload in the ovaries and pituitary gland can be treated with ovulation induction
- Assisted conception, pre-implantation, prenatal diagnosis and surgical termination of pregnancy should be discussed
- Multidisciplinary care from haematology, genetic counselling, partner screening, physiotherapy and maternal–fetal medicine
- Iron chelation programme should be optimised

Pregnancy Issues

There is a 1:4 chance of a child inheriting a major condition from parents who are both healthy α, β or sickle cell carriers.

Diagnostic Tests

Tests are offered to determine fetal risk and include:
- DNA analysis of chorionic villi
- Fetal blood sample or amniotic fluid[4]

Risk of Pregnancy Complications
- Thrombo-embolic disease
- Congestive heart failure caused by iron deposits in heart; increases maternal mortality by 50%[7]
- Damage to liver, renal and endocrine organs due to iron overload
- Diabetes more likely
- Increased transfusion requirements
- Haemolytic disease of the newborn
- Intrauterine growth restriction
- Spontaneous abortion caused by worsening de-oxygenation of placental tissue
- Maternal red blood cell allo-antibodies
- Anaemia
- Pre-eclampsia (Hb Bart's hydrops)
- For individuals with **thalassaemia trait** an **Hb** of 8.5–10.5 gd/l is considered **normal**

Medical Management and Care
- Counselling depends on whether the risks are fetal or maternal or both – discuss the potential perinatal outcomes of antenatal tests and available options for ongoing pregnancy and care
- Specialist haematologist involvement – discuss transfusion therapy for treatment of worsening Hb levels
- Iron chelation is contraindicated in pregnancy, therefore implement aggressive iron chelation programme prior to conception[8]
- Serial ultrasound assessments for fetal anaemia, growth and placental pathology[6,7]
- Maternal surveillance includes:
  - MRI scanning to assess iron overload in maternal organs[9]
  - echocardiography to exclude cardiomyopathy
  - regular assessment of blood antibody levels, liver and thyroid function tests
- Discuss risks for continuing pregnancy and birth options

Midwifery Management and Care
- Book at consultant unit, discussing high-risk care and birth options
- Assess for blood-borne infections, haemoglobin levels and full blood count to determine severity of maternal anaemia
- Assess for signs of pre-eclampsia – blood pressure measurements and urinary microscopy and culture
- Treat iron and folic acid deficiency anaemia as prescribed[10] to meet the increased demands of pregnancy and increased turnover of red blood cells in bone marrow; caution with the **use of iron** in β major or trait is advised[8] and should always be **guided by ferritin levels**
- Provide dietary advice to enhance folate intake (see Section 14.2)
- Be vigilant for signs and symptoms of a reaction to transfusion therapy, including an exacerbation of existing cardiac problems
- Physiotherapy may be required as chelation can cause arthritis
- Encourage full attendance to antenatal surveillance visits and provide stress-reduction strategies through supportive care and counselling of the couple

Labour Issues

Thalassaemia **major** mothers are at risk of:
- Pre-term labour
- Fetal hypoxia
- Maternal hypoxia and exhaustion
- Raised blood pressure
- Delivery difficulties – hydropic fetus and placenta and maternal bone deformities
- Potential for postpartum haemorrhage (PPH)

Medical Management and Care
- Individual plan of care based on outcomes of feto-maternal surveillance including maternal pelvic size

Midwifery Management and Care
- Adhere to above plan and local guidelines
- Continuous EFM and assess for signs of early fetal hypoxia
- Optimise oxygenation of mother and utero-placental perfusion through appropriate positioning
- Monitor blood pressure and fluid balance strictly to prevent cardiac compromise and maintain hydration using intravenous fluids
- Provide support and pain relief to avoid cardiopulmonary stress
- Active management of third stage of labour

Postpartum Issues

Neonate with thalassaemia **major** at risk of:
- Pre-term birth
- Low birth weight
- Fetal haemolytic anaemia
- Feeding problems
- Jaundice, enlarged liver and spleen
- Failure to thrive in first year

Mother at risk of:
- Poor wound healing
- Infection due to severe anaemia
- PPH and worsening of anaemia
- Depression

Medical Management and Care
- Individual plan of care based on outcomes of ongoing neonatal and maternal surveillance
- Multidisciplinary team working with neonatal, haematology and counselling professionals

Midwifery Management and Care
- Mother and infant are not for 6-hour discharge
- Affected neonate with failure to maintain body temperature, poor feeding or pallor is transferred to neonatal unit for investigation
- Universal newborn blood spot (Guthrie) screening test on sixth day[2]
- Monitor prescribed iv fluids and fluid balance/oral intake
- Provide supportive care and pain relief to prevent exacerbation of cardiopulmonary compromise
- Observe for signs of haemorrhage/infection with prompt referral
- Refer for appropriate types of counselling
- Arrange relevant maternal and neonatal follow-up[8]

14.7 Sickle Cell Disorders

Incidence
In the UK there are between 12 000–15 000 individuals[1,2] with sickle cell disease; the trait has a higher prevalence

Risk for Childbearing
High Risk

EXPLANATION OF CONDITION

Homozygous sickle cell disease includes sickle cell anaemia (HbSS), an autosomal recessive disease in which sufferers are homozygous (inherited from both parents) for the mutant gene while individuals with a trait are heterozygous (HbAS)[2].

Variants of the disease include sickle cell haemoglobin C disease (HbSC), sickle cell β^o thalassaemia (no normal β chains produced) and sickle cell β^+ thalassaemia (reduced amount of chains made). There are other, rarer variants of varying clinical significance.

HbSS results from an abnormality in the formation and quality of the adult haemoglobin molecule (HbA) caused by an error in the amino acid sequence. The amino acid glutamic acid is substituted for either valine (HbS) or lysine (HbC) on the beta globin chain.

HbSS is characterised by the distortion and slow movement of red blood cells which is exacerbated when oxygen levels drop, and leads to:

- Chronic haemolytic anaemia
- Metabolic acidosis
- Capillary stasis
- Increased blood viscosity
- Occlusion of blood vessels
- Resultant infarction and ischaemic necrosis of tissues in organs such as lungs, kidneys, spleen and bones[3]

Repeated deoxygenation of red blood cells (HbS) results in irreversible cell-membrane rigidity and damage and destruction within 17 days, compared with the 120-day lifespan of normal red blood cells (HbA). Damaged red blood cells are removed from the circulation by the reticulo-endothelial system (largely spleen and liver).

Acute episodes of deoxygenation in sickle cell disease can result in episodes called 'sickle cell crises', of which there are three types:

1. Sequestrative
2. Aplastic
3. Vaso-occlusive

Sickle cell crises are manifested by:

- Worsening of chronic anaemia (6.5–9.0 g/dl)
- Severe pain
- Breathlessness
- Weakness
- Pallor and fever[1]

HbSS is diagnosed by taking a thorough medical history, clinical examination and haemoglobinopathy investigations, which include:

- Hb electrophoresis
- Sickle-shaped red blood cells
- Hyperplastic, immature red blood cells in bone marrow aspirate if required

COMPLICATIONS

- Acute-on-chronic anaemia caused by blood loss, dehydration, cold or infection
- Excessive haemolysis and bone marrow suppression
- Acute chest syndrome, a life-threatening sickling in the lungs, manifests itself with:
  - cough
  - severe chest pain
  - difficulty breathing
  - severe anaemia
  - fever[4]
- Thrombo-embolic events including:
  - pulmonary embolism
  - cerebrovascular accident
  - seizures
  - liver and splenic autoinfarction
  - sequestration
- Vaso-occlusive or painful crisis exacerbated by stress, cold, infection, dehydration and exercise causing swelling to joints
- Cardiac failure due to chronic hypoxaemia and aplastic anaemia
- Sudden death

NON-PREGNANCY TREATMENT AND CARE

Prophylactic penicillin V by mouth daily, folic acid 1 mg daily both long term. Other measures may include hydroxyurea to induce increased levels of fetal haemoglobin (HbF), exchange blood transfusion, anti-thrombotic measures, family history to determine the requirement for partner haemoglobinopathy screening and counselling. Pneumococcal vaccine may be given. Renal, hepatic and retinal function are assessed regularly.

Other requirements include human immunodeficiency virus and hepatitis B or C screening following repeated transfusions[5].

PRE-CONCEPTION ISSUES AND CARE

- A thorough clinical and risk assessment; a family history of ancestors or relatives who originate from outside northern Europe is used as an indicator for screening; partners also require haemoglobinopathy screening and counselling
- The clinical assessment should identify immunisations to date, incidences of sickle cell crises (i.e. disease severity), past requirements for blood transfusion, iron status and levels of organ damage
- At-risk couples require information on: pre-implantation genetic diagnosis, which requires in-vitro fertilisation; pre-natal diagnostic tests, such as chorionic villus sampling, amniocentesis and fetal blood sampling[6]
- Folic acid should be increased to 5 mg per day when planning a pregnancy and hydroxyurea and iron chelation discontinued 3–6 months prior to conception due to possible teratogenicity
- Discuss analgesia for sickle pains and penicillin prophylaxis throughout pregnancy

Pregnancy Issues

- Hydroxyurea and iron chelation agents are contraindicated in pregnancy[7]
- Red cell antibodies may be present if previous multiple transfusions
- Hyperemesis may cause dehydration and sickle crisis
- Pregnancy is contraindicated with pulmonary hypertension due to increase in maternal mortality by 30–50%[1]
- At risk of:
  - haemolytic anaemia, with or without iron deficiency
  - IUGR
  - sickle crisis secondary to infection (particularly of the urinary tract)
  - increased risk of miscarriage
  - increased risk of pre-eclampsia
  - increased risk of stillbirth
  - increased risk of maternal mortality

Figure 14.7.1 gives an example of a management plan for pregnancy sickle crisis.

Medical Management and Care

- Women with pulmonary hypertension should consider termination of pregnancy because of high maternal mortality (see Section 4.9)
- Prescribe 5 mg folic acid per day orally[10,11]
- Provide iron supplements only if indicated
- Baseline investigations – FBC, blood group and antibody screen, reticulocyte count, serum ferritin levels, renal and liver function tests, HIV and hepatitis screening
- Ultrasound scans to confirm dates and for prompt detection of IUGR
- Monitoring of pregnancy – 2–4 weekly antenatal visits in first and second trimesters to assess blood pressure, urine microscopy and culture and an FBC
- **Third trimester**: serial growth scans, estimation of liquor volume, umbilical artery Doppler measurements
  - consider induction of labour for obstetric or medical indications, not as routine

Midwifery Management and Care

- Detailed booking history to refer at-risk couples to a specialist clinic
- Multidisciplinary management, including obstetrician, haematologist, anaesthetist, haemoglobinopathy specialist nurse and midwife
- Continue antibiotics and increase folic acid to 5 mg daily
- Give nutritional advice to enhance the management of chronic anaemia
- Encourage the woman to keep well hydrated, avoid both cold environments and excessive physical exertion
- Advise reporting of infection or crises for prompt medical treatment

Labour Issues

At risk of:

- Premature birth
- Pre-eclampsia[8]
- Placental abruption
- Sickle cell crises precipitated by immobilisation
- Blood loss hypoxia during labour and birth
- Hypertension
- Dehydration
- Infection
- Transfusion reactions

Medical Management and Care[10,11]

- Blood taken for FBC, group and save
- Refer to anaesthetist – discuss epidural analgesia as recommended for pain relief
- Keep warm and well hydrated – warmed iv fluids are essential
- Ensure optimal oxygenation
- Avoid prolonged labour with early recourse to caesarean section for slow progress
- Graduated compression stockings

Midwifery Management and Care

- Minimise stress in labour and provide one to one support
- Encourage alternative positions during labour and childbirth
- Maintain basic hygiene needs[12], adequate oxygen, hydration, pain relief and continuous monitoring of fetal heart rate[10]
- Cord blood taken at birth for haemoglobin electrophoresis
- Avoid opiates such as pethidine
- Maintain fluid balance with strict records of input and output[10]

Postpartum issues

Mother is at risk of:

- Postpartum haemorrhage
- Dehydration
- Tissue hypoxia
- Infections
- Thrombo-embolism
- Sickle cell crises

Recurrent pregnancies increase frequency of crises[9]. Intrauterine contraceptive devices are relatively contraindicated[8] due to risk of infections but maternal compliance with contraception is essential.

The baby requires:

- Universal screening of newborn
- Repeat electrophoresis at 6 weeks of age
- Prophylactic antibiotic therapy from 3 months of age is advised[5]

Medical Management and Care[10,11]

- Vigilant follow-up due to increased risk of sickle cell crisis
- Refer to paediatrician for results of neonatal screening and follow-up arrangements prior to discharge
- Prescribe antibiotics and thrombo-prophylaxis
- Early treatment of suspected endometritis

Midwifery Management and Care

- Early ambulation[10], good hydration and oxygenation encouraged in first 24 hours postpartum
- Four hourly temperature, pulse and respiration (TPR) observations[7]
- Use of thrombo-embolic deterrent stockings and daily subcutaneous heparin, because thrombo-embolic prophylaxis is recommended until fully mobile
- Discuss family planning options to space pregnancies[7]; includes progesterone only preparations, but ensure the choice is acceptable to the woman to ensure compliance
- Arrange relevant maternal and neonatal follow-up appointments[10]

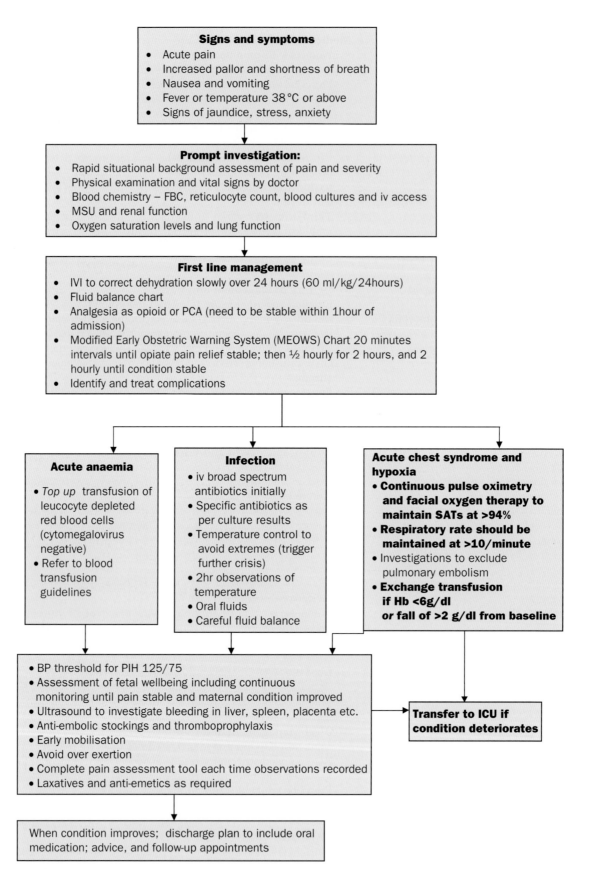

Signs and symptoms
- Acute pain
- Increased pallor and shortness of breath
- Nausea and vomiting
- Fever or temperature 38°C or above
- Signs of jaundice, stress, anxiety

Prompt investigation:
- Rapid situational background assessment of pain and severity
- Physical examination and vital signs by doctor
- Blood chemistry – FBC, reticulocyte count, blood cultures and iv access
- MSU and renal function
- Oxygen saturation levels and lung function

First line management
- IVI to correct dehydration slowly over 24 hours (60 ml/kg/24hours)
- Fluid balance chart
- Analgesia as opioid or PCA (need to be stable within 1hour of admission)
- Modified Early Obstetric Warning System (MEOWS) Chart 20 minutes intervals until opiate pain relief stable; then ½ hourly for 2 hours, and 2 hourly until condition stable
- Identify and treat complications

Acute anaemia
- *Top up* transfusion of leucocyte depleted red blood cells (cytomegalovirus negative)
- Refer to blood transfusion guidelines

Infection
- iv broad spectrum antibiotics initially
- Specific antibiotics as per culture results
- Temperature control to avoid extremes (trigger further crisis)
- 2hr observations of temperature
- Oral fluids
- Careful fluid balance

Acute chest syndrome and hypoxia
- **Continuous pulse oximetry and facial oxygen therapy to maintain SATs at >94%**
- **Respiratory rate should be maintained at >10/minute**
- Investigations to exclude pulmonary embolism
- **Exchange transfusion if Hb <6g/dl or fall of >2 g/dl from baseline**

- BP threshold for PIH 125/75
- Assessment of fetal wellbeing including continuous monitoring until pain stable and maternal condition improved
- Ultrasound to investigate bleeding in liver, spleen, placenta etc.
- Anti-embolic stockings and thromboprophylaxis
- Early mobilisation
- Avoid over exertion
- Complete pain assessment tool each time observations recorded
- Laxatives and anti-emetics as required

Transfer to ICU if condition deteriorates

When condition improves; discharge plan to include oral medication; advice, and follow-up appointments

Figure 14.7.1 Pregnancy sickle cell crisis – multidisciplinary team management[2,13–16]. This figure is downloadable from the book companion website at www.wiley.com/go/robson

14 Haematological Disorders

PATIENT ORGANISATIONS

Idiopathic Thrombocytopenia Support Association
http://www.itpsupport.org.uk

Women Bleed Too Project (The Haemophilia Society)
http://www.haemophilia.org.uk/uploads/guidetolivingvon-will.pdf

Hospital Information Services (for Jehovah's Witnesses)
his@wtbts.org.uk

SHOT – Serious Hazards of Transfusion (www.shotuk.org)
Dietary information sheets (normal diet, traditional Asian diet, Asian vegetarian diet) from:
Leicestershire Nutrition and Dietetic Service
Units 11 & 12 Warren Park Way
Enderby
Leicestershire LE19 4SA

UK Thalassaemia Society
19 The Broadway
Southgate Circus
London N14 6PH
E-mail: office@ukts.org

NHS Sickle cell/Thalassaemia Screening Programme, Kings
http://www.kcl-phs.org.uk/haemscreening/

Sickle Cell Society
www.sickecellsociety.org

Sickle Cell and Thalassaemia Centre
Haematology Department
Sandwell and West Birmingham NHS Trust
Lyndon
West Bromwich B71 4HJ
E-mail: Jayne.Swingler:swbh.nhs.uk

UK Forum on Haemoglobin Disorders
http://www.haemoglobin.org.uk

ESSENTIAL READING

Anionwu EN and Atkin K 2001 **The Politics of Sickle Cell and Thalassaemia**. UK; Open University Press

Anon 2007 **A Guide for Women Living with Von Willebrand's Disease**. London; Haemophilia Society
http://www.haemophilia.org.uk/Resources/HaemophiliaMain/Images/Project%20Images/Women%20Bleed%20Too/vW%20booklet.pdf

British Committee for Standards in Haematology Task Force 2003. Guidelines for the investigation and management of idiopathic thrombocytopenic purpura in adults, children and pregnancy. **British Journal of Haematology**, 120:570–596

Chi C, Shiltagh N, Kingman CEC, *et al.* 2006 Identification and management of women with inherited bleeding disorders: a survey of obstetricians and gynaecologists in the United Kingdom. **Haemophilia**, 12:405–412

Clarke P and Greer IA 2006 Chapters 3 and 9. **Practical Obstetric Haematology**. London; Taylor & Francis

Contreras M 2009 **ABC of Transfusion**, 4th Edn. Oxford; BMJ Books/Wiley-Blackwell

Dyson SM 2005 **Ethnicity and Screening for Sickle Cell/Thalassaemia. Lessons for Practice from the Voices of Experience**. Oxford; Churchill Livingstone

Green D and Ludham CA 2006 **Fast Facts: Bleeding Disorders**. Oxford; Health Press 90–92

Hoffbrand A and Moss P 2011 **Essential Haematology**, 6th Edn. Oxford; Wiley-Blackwell

Howard J and Oteng-Ntim 2011 The Obstetric management of sickle cell disease. **Best Practice and Research Clinical Obstetrics and Gynaecology**, doi: 10.1016/j.bpobgyn.2011.10.001

Lee CA, Chi C, Pavord S, *et al.* 2006 The obstetrical and gynaecological management of women with inherited bleeding disorders – review with guidelines produced by a taskforce of UK Haemophilia Centre Doctors' Organisation. **Haemophilia**, 12: 311–336

Okpala I 2004 **Practical Management of Haemoglobinopathies**. Oxford; Blackwell Publishing Ltd.

Pavord S and Hunt B (Eds) 2010 **The Obstetric Hematology Manual**. Cambridge; Cambridge Medicine

Strong J 2006 Von Willebrand disease and pregnancy. **Current Obstetrics and Gynaecology**, 16:1–5

Taskforce of UK Haemophilia Centre Doctors' Organisation 2006 Obstetric and gynaecological management of women with inherited bleeding disorders, review with guidelines. **Haemophilia**, 12:301–336

References

14.1 Iron Deficiency Anaemia

1. Mahomed K 2001 Iron and folate supplementation in pregnancy. **Cochrane Database of Systematic Reviews**, Issue 3. Oxford; Update Software
2. WHO/UNICEF/UNU 2001 Iron deficiency anaemia: assessment, prevention and control. A guide for programme managers. Geneva; World Health Organization 15 (WHO/NHD/01.3)
3. Skikne B and Baynes RD 1994 Iron absorption in Brock JH, Halliday JW, Pippard MJ, Powell LW (Eds) **Iron Metabolism in Health and Disease**. London; W.B. Saunders 151–187
4. Pavord S, Myers B, Robinson S, Allard S, Strong J, Oppenheimer C, (2011) **Uk Guidelines on Management of Iron Deficiency in Pregnancy**. London; British Society for Haematology
5. Milman N, Bergholt T, Eriksen L, *et al.* 2005 Iron prophylaxis during pregnancy – how much iron is needed? A randomized dose-response study of 20–80 mg ferrous iron daily in pregnant women. **Acta Obstetricia et Gynecologica Scandinavica**, 84:238–247
6. National Collaborating Centre for Women's Health 2003 **Antenatal Care: Routine Care for Healthy Women**. London; National Institute for Clinical Excellence
7. Lumley J, Watson L, Watson M, *et al.* 2001 Periconceptional supplementation with folate and/or vitamins for preventing neural tube defects. **Cochrane Database of Systematic Reviews**, Issue 3. Oxford; Update Software
8. Siegenberg D, Baynes RD and Bothwell TH 1994 Ascorbic acid prevents the dose-dependent inhibitory effects of polyphenols and phytates on nonheme-iron absorption. **American Journal of Clinical Nutrition**, 53:537–541
9. James DK, Steer PJ, Weiner CP and Gonik B 2011 **High Risk Pregnancy: Management Options**, 4th Edn. Philadelphia; Elsevier 683–687
10. Barron WM and Lindheimer MD 2000 **Medical Disorders During Pregnancy**, 3rd Edn. Missouri; Mosby Inc. 267–272
11. Hemminki E and Merilainen J 1995 Long-term follow-up of mothers and their infants in a randomized trial on iron prophylaxis during pregnancy. **American Journal of Obstetrics and Gynecology**, 173:205–209
12. National Health Service 2006 Healthy Start – Pregnancy www.healthystart.nhs.uk
13. NICE 2008 **Clinical Guideline: Antenatal care**. London; National Institute for Health and Clinical Excellence www.nice.org.uk/guidance/CG62.
14. WHO 2006 **Standards for Maternal and Neonatal Care 1.8 – Iron and Folate Supplementation – Integrated Management of Pregnancy and Childbirth**. Geneva; World Health Organization
15. Simmons WK, Cook JD and Bingham KC 1993 Evaluation of a gastric delivery system for iron supplementation in pregnancy. **American Journal of Clinical Nutrition**, 58:622–626
16. Klebanoff MA, Shiono PH, Selby JV, Trachtenberg AI, Graubard BI 1991 Anemia and spontaneous preterm birth, **American Journal of Obstetrics and Gynecology**, 164:59–63
17. Pasricha SS, Flecknoe-Brown SC, Allen KJ, *et al.* (2010) Diagnosis and Management of iron deficiency anaemia: **a clinical update Medical Journal of Australia**, 193: 525–532

14.2 Megaloblastic Anaemia

1. Chanarin I 1990 Folate deficiency in pregnancy in Chanarin I (Ed.) **The Megaloblastic Anaemias**, 3rd Edn. Oxford; Blackwell Publishing Ltd. 140–148
2. Letsky EA 2002 Blood volume, haematinics, anaemia in de Swiet M (Ed.) **Medical Disorders in Obstetric Practice**, 4th Edn. Oxford; Blackwell Publishing Ltd. 29–60
3. Barron WM and Lindheimer MD 2000 **Medical Disorders During Pregnancy**, 3rd Edn. Missouri; Mosby Inc. 274–275
4. Clark P and Greer IA 2006 **Practical Obstetrical Haematology**. London; Taylor and Francis 48–53
5. MRC Vitamin Study Research Group 1991 Prevention of neural tube defects: results of the medical research council vitamin study. **Lancet**, 228:131–137

6. Mahomed K 2001 Iron and folate supplementation in pregnancy. **Cochrane Database of Systematic Reviews**, Issue 3. Oxford; Update Software
7. Langley-Evans SC and Langley-Evans AJ 2002 Use of folic acid supplements in the first trimester of pregnancy. **Journal of the Royal Society of Health**, 122:181–186
8. Lumley J, Watson L, Watson M, *et al.* 2001 Periconceptual supplementation with folate and or multivitamins for preventing neural tube defects. **Cochrane Database of Systematic Reviews**, Issue 3. Oxford; Update Software
9. NICE 2008 **Antenatal Care: Routine Care for the Healthy Pregnant Woman**. London; National Institute for Health and Clinical Excellence http://www.nice.org.uk/guidance/CG62
10. Department of Health 2000 **Folic Acid and the Prevention of Disease: Report of the Committee on Medical Aspects of Food and Nutrition Policy**. London; The Stationery Office

14.3 Disseminated Intravascular Coagulation

1. Mattar F and Sibai BM 2000 Risk factors for maternal mortality. **American Journal of Obstetrics and Gynaecology**, 182:307–312
2. Treacher DF and Grant IS 2006 Chapt.8 Major organ failure in Boon NB, Colledge NR and Walker BR (Eds) **Davidson's Principles and Practice of Medicine**, 20th Edn. London; Elsevier 190
3. Craig JIO, McLelland DBL and Ludlam CA 2006 Chapt.24 Blood disorders in Boon NB, Colledge NR and Walker BR (Eds) **Davidson's Principles and Practice of Medicine**, 20th Edn. London; Elsevier 1060–1061
4. Bick RL 2000 Syndromes of disseminated intravascular coagulation in obstetrics, pregnancy and gynaecology. **Hematology/Oncology Clinics of North America**, 14:999–1044
5. Kumar P and Clarke M 2004 **Clinical Medicine**, 5th Edn. London; Saunders 463–464
6. Stables D 1999 **Physiology in Childbearing: With Anatomy and Related Biosciences**. London; Elsevier 398–399
7. Baglin T 1996 Fortnightly review: disseminated intravascular coagulation: diagnosis and treatment. **British Medical Journal**, 312:683–686
8. Steele D 2006 Chapt.7 Haemorrhagic disorders in Billington M and Stevenson M (Eds) **Critical Care in Childbearing for Midwives**. Oxford; Blackwell Publishing Ltd. 118–139
9. James DK, Steer PJ, Weiner CP and Gonik B 2011 **High Risk Pregnancy: Management Options**, 4th Edn. Philadelphia; Elsevier 1331–1345
10. Letsky EA 2001 Disseminated intravascular coagulation. **Best Practice and Research in Clinical Obstetrics and Gynaecology**, 15:623–644
11. Nelson-Piercy C 2002 **Handbook of Obstetric Medicine**. London; Martin Dunitz 264–265
12. Burrow GN, Duffy GN and Copel JA 2004 **Medical Complications During Pregnancy**, 6th Edn. Philadelphia; Saunders/Elsevier 82
13. Green D and Ludham CA 2006 **Fast Facts: Bleeding Disorders**. Oxford; Health Press 90–92
14. Sood M, Juneja Y and Goyal U 1995 Maternal mortality associated with clandestine abortions. **Journal of the Indian Medical Association**, 93:77–79

14.4 Von Willebrand's Disease and Other Bleeding Disorders

1. Haemophilia Society 2003 **Fact Sheet – Von Willebrand's: General Information**. London; The Haemophilia Society www.womenbleedtoo.org.uk/User_Files/vwillebrandsgeneral.pdf
2. Kouides PA 2001 Obstetric and gynaecological aspects of von Willebrand's disease. **Best Practice and Research in Clinical Haematology**, 2:381–399
3. Lee CA and Abdul-Kadir R 2005 Von Willebrand's disease and women's health. **Seminars in Haematology**, 42:42–48
4. Kujovich JL 2005 von Willebrand's and pregnancy. **Journal of Thrombosis and Haemostasis**, 3:246–253

5. Green D and Ludham CA 2006 **Fast Facts: Bleeding Disorders**. Oxford; Health Press 63–69
6. Kadir RA, Lee CA, Sabin CA, *et al.* 1998 Pregnancy in women with von Willebrand's disease or factor XI deficiency. **British Journal of Obstetrics and Gynaecology**, 105:314–321
7. Lee CA, Chi C, Pavord S, *et al.* 2006 The obstetrical and gynaecological management of women with inherited bleeding disorders: review with guidelines by a taskforce of UK Haemophilia Centre Doctors' Organisation. **Haemophilia**, 12:311–336
8. Strong J 2006 von Willebrand's disease and pregnancy. **Current Obstetrics and Gynaecology**, 16:1–5
9. Edland M, Blomback M, von Schoulz B and Andersson O 1996 On the value of menorrhagia as a predictor for coagulation disorders. **American Journal of Haematology**, 53:234–238
10. NICE 2007 **Clinical Guideline No.44 Heavy Menstrual Bleeding**. London; National Institute for Health and Clinical Excellence www.nice.org.uk/guidance/CG44
11. James DK, Steer PJ, Weiner CP and Gonik B 2011 **High Risk Pregnancy: Management Options**, 4th Edn. Philadelphia; Elsevier 717–752
12. Dhanjal M and Nelson-Piercy C 2009 Chapt. 21 Labour in women with medical disorders in Warren R and Arulkumaran S (Eds) **Best Practice in Labour and Delivery**, Cambridge; Cambridge University Press 233–234

14.5 Thrombocytopenia in Pregnancy
1. Kam PC, Thompson SA and Liew AC 2004 Thrombocytopenia in the parturient. **Anaesthesia**, 59:255–264
2. Stamilio DM and Macones GA 1999 Selection of delivery method in pregnancies complicated by autoimmune thrombocytopenic purpura. **Obstetrics and Gynaecology**, 94:41–47
3. Macpherson G 2004 **Black's Student Medical Dictionary**. London; Black Publishers
4. Strong J 2003 Bleeding disorders in pregnancy. **Current Obstetrics and Gynaecology**, 13:1–6
5. McFadden TM, Lerrieri L and Settler RW 1998 Immune thrombocytopenic purpura in pregnancy: the ongoing debate surrounding obstetric management. **Primary Care Update for Ob/ Gyns**, 5:300–305
6. Nelson-Piercy C 2002 **Handbook of Obstetric Medicine**. London; Martin Dunitz 259–264
7. Kumar P and Clarke M 2004 **Clinical Medicine**, 5th Edn. London; Saunders 458–459
8. Frederickson H and Schmidt K 1999 The incidence of idiopathic thrombocytopenic purpura in adults increases with age. **Blood**, 94:909–913
9. Higgins C 2000 **Understanding Laboratory Investigations**. Oxford; Blackwell Publishing Ltd. 243
10. Fisher M, Peters B, McBride M and Kitchen V 1994 Consider HIV infection in thrombocytopenia. **British Medical Journal**, 308 (6921):133–136
11. Webert KE, Mittal R, Sigouin C, Heddle NM and Kelton JG 2003 A retrospective analysis of obstetric patients with idiopathic thrombocytopenic purpura. **Blood**, 102:4306–4311
12. Parnas M, Sheiner E, Shoham-Vardi I, *et al.* 2006 Moderate to severe thrombocytopenia during pregnancy. **European Journal of Obstetrics and Gynaecology**, 127:163–168
13. Cines DB 2003 ITP and pregnancy. **Blood**, 102:4250–4251
14. Horn EH and Kean L 2006 in James DK, Steer PJ, Weiner CP and Gonik B (Eds) **High Risk Pregnancy: Management Options**, 3rd Edn. Philadelphia; Elsevier 901–908
15. British Committee for Standards in Haematology General Haematology Task Force 2003 Guidelines for the investigation and management of idiopathic thrombocytopenic purpura in adults, children and pregnancy. **British Journal of Haematology**, 120:570–596
16. James DK, Steer PJ, Weiner CP and Gonik B 2011 **High Risk Pregnancy: Management Options**, 4th Edn. Philadelphia; Elsevier 717–723
17. Gottlieb P, Axelson O, Bakos O and Rastad J 1999 Splenectomy during pregnancy: an option in the treatment of autoimmune thrombocytopenic purpura. **British Journal of Obstetrics and Gynaecology**, 106:373–377

14.6 Thalassaemia
1. NHS 2011 **Annual report 2009-2010 Sickle cell and Thalassaemia screening programme**. London; National Health Service
2. NHS Sickle Cell and Thalassaemia Screening Programme 2006 **NHS Sickle Cell and Thalassaemia Screening Programme Information for Midwives**. Kings College London www.kcl–phs. org.uk/haemscreening
3. Atkin K and Ahmad W 1998 Genetic screening and haemoglobinopathies; ethics, politics and practice. **Social Science and Medicine**, 46:445–458
4. Modell B, Harris R, Lane B, *et al.* 2000 Informed choice in genetic screening for thalassaemia during pregnancy: audit from a national confidential inquiry. **British Medical Journal**, 320: 337–341
5. Weatheral D and Clegg J 2001 **The Thalassaemia Syndromes**, 4th Edn. Oxford; Blackwell Publishing Ltd.
6. Weatherall D and Letsky E 1999 Genetic haematological disorders in Wald N (Ed.) **Antenatal and Neonatal Screening**, 2nd Edn. Oxford; Oxford University Press
7. Letsky E 2002 Anaemia in James D, Steer P, Weiner D and Gonik B (Eds) **High Risk Pregnancy: Management Options**, 2nd Edn. London; WB Saunders 729–747
8. James DK, Steer PJ, Weiner CP and Gonik B 2011 **High Risk Pregnancy: Management Options**, 4th Edn. Philadelphia; Elsevier 695–698
9. Billington M and Stephenson M 2006 **Critical Care in Childbearing for Midwives**. Oxford; Blackwell Publishing Ltd. 78–83
10. NICE 2008 **Clinical Guideline 62 Antenatal Care: Routine Care for the Healthy Pregnant Woman**. London; National Institute for Health and Clinical Excellence. www.nice.org.uk

14.7 Sickle Cell Disorders
1. Oteng-Ntim E, Cottee C, Bewley S and Anionwu E 2006 Sickle cell disease in pregnancy. **Current Obstetrics and Gynaecology**. London; Elsevier
2. Royal College of Obstetrics and Gynaecology (2011) **Management of Sickle Cell Disease in Pregnancy Green-top Guideline No. 61**. London; RCOG
3. Serjeant GR 2001 Historical review. The emerging understanding of sickle cell disease. **British Journal of Haematology**, 12:3–18
4. Vichinksy EP, Neumayr LD and Ealres AN 2000 Causes and outcomes of the acute chest syndrome in sickle cell disease: National Acute Chest Syndrome Study Group. **New England Journal of Medicine**, 342:1855–1865
5. NHS 2006 Sickle cell and thalassaemia screening programme – screening for sickle cell and thalassaemia in pregnancy. www.kcl–phs.org.uk/haemscreening
6. Streetly A 2006 Sickle cell screening makes genetic counselling everybody's business. **British Medical Journal**, 332:570–572
7. Charache S, Terrin ML and Moore RD 1995 Effect of hydroxyurea on the frequency of painful crises in sickle cell anaemia. **New England Journal of Medicine**, 332:1317–1322
8. Billington M and Stephenson M 2006 **Critical Care in Childbearing for Midwives**. Oxford; Blackwell Publishing Ltd. 72–78
9. Howard RJ, Lillis C and Tuck SM 1995 Contraceptives counselling and pregnancy in women with sickle cell disease. **British Journal of Obstetrics and Gynaecology**, 102: 945–951
10. James DK, Steer PJ, Weiner CP and Gonik B 2011 **High Risk Pregnancy: Management Options**, 3rd Edn. Philadelphia; Elsevier 692–696
11. Howard J and Oteng-Ntim 2011 The Obstetric management of sickle cell disease. **Best Practice and Research Clinical Obstetrics and Gynaecology**, doi: 10.1016/j.bpobgyn.2011.10.001
12. RCN 2011 **Caring for People with Sickle Cell Disease and Thalassaemia Syndromes: A Framework For Nursing Staff**. London; Royal College of Nursing
13. Lewis G (Ed.) 2011 Centre for Maternal and Child Enquiries (CMACE). **Saving Mothers' Lives: Reviewing Maternal Deaths to Make Motherhood Safer – 2006–2008. The Eighth Report on Confidential Enquiries into Maternal Deaths in the United Kingdom**. London: CMACE
14. Royal College of Obstetricians and Gynaecologists 2009 **Green Top Guidance 37. Reducing the risk of thrombosis and embolism**

during pregnancy and peurperium. London: Royal College of Obstetricians and Gynaecologists

15. Singh S, McGlennan A, England A and Simons R 2011 A validation study of the CEMACH recommended modified early obstetric warning system (MEOWS). **Anaesthesia**. doi: 10.1111/j.1365-2044.2011.06896.x

16. Department of Health 2008 **Competencies for Recognising and Responding to Acutely Ill Patients in Hospital**. London; Department of Health www.dh.gov.uk/en/Publicationsandstatistics/Publications/PublicationsPolicyAndGuidance/DH

Figure Reference
Hoffbrand A and Moss P 2011 **Essential Haematology**, 6th Edn. Oxford; Wiley-Blackwell

Appendix References

1. NPSA 2006 **Safer Practice Notice 14 – Right Patient, Right Blood**
2. SHOT 2012 Current Resources. http://www.shotuk.org/resources/current-resources [Accessed 10-07-2012]

Appendix 14.1.1 Blood and Blood Products Overview

BLOOD PRODUCTS

The following are blood and blood products for administration which could be encountered in a maternity context. Other products may be given in the care of a pregnant woman with a specific condition. All blood-derived products are organised and supplied by the blood transfusion services who can give expert and detailed advice.

Red Blood Cells

Packed Red Cells

This is the form of blood cell most commonly administered in obstetrics. Each unit is prepared from whole blood collected into an anticoagulant solution. Each unit is about 250 ml and has a haematocrit of 55–80% (normal haematocrit 35–50%).

- All units produced in the UK are *leucocyte depleted* as this has been shown to reduce viral and possibly prion transmission
- Red cells may be irradiated (for immunodeficient women) or CMV (cytomegalovirus) negative for immunosuppressed women and neonates
- Packed cells are indicated for women with symptomatic anaemia who require rapid alleviation of symptoms or women with Hb <7 g/dl in whom blood loss is a significant risk
- Also given for major blood loss when initial measures including volume expansion and cell salvage have been used
- Adverse reactions include:
  - raised temperature
  - rigors
  - allergic reaction (rashes, reduced BP)
  - haemolysis
- More severe, rarer, reactions include:
  - transfusion-related acute lung injury (TRALI)
  - graft versus host disease (GVH)
- In the longer term RBC antibody formation and viral infection (hepatitis, CMV, HIV, CJD) may occur

Whole Blood

Whole blood is now rarely used, but may be available in specific circumstances for resuscitation.

- Administration would be in conjunction with blood bank and the haematology services
- Red blood cell preparations such as these have a shelf life of approximately 35 days stored at the appropriate temperature
- Transfusion must be started within 30 minutes of removal from the fridge and completed within 4 hours
- Blood can be requested in different forms depending upon urgency:
  - uncrossmatched O negative
  - group specific (~30 minutes)
  - full cross-match (45–60 minutes)

Platelets

In obstetrics, platelet transfusion is most likely to be seen either in the acute situation of haemorrhage, disseminated intravascular coagulopathy (DIC) or in a woman with ITP and evidence of impaired haemostasis. Also given prophylactically in a woman with a platelet count of less than 10 000 at risk of bleeding.

- Most of the platelet units used in maternity care will be concentrates from whole blood
- Can be stored for up to 5 days at room temperature but must be continually agitated to prevent clumping
- It is usual to use ABO and Rh compatible platelets
- Side effects include:
  - temperature and rigors in 1% (rising to 30% in those who have had multiple platelet transfusions)
  - risk of viral transmission (higher than for red cells because platelets are pooled from a number of donors)
  - allergic reaction
- Pay close attention to surgical and obstetric causes of bleeding as part of the decision to transfuse platelets

Plasma Products

Intravenous Immunoglobulin (IVIg)

This may be given to women with a falling platelet count in immune thrombocytopenic purpura (ITP), prevention of fetal bleeding in feto-maternal alloimmune thrombocytopenia (FMAIT) and other immunologically based disorders. The dose is weight- and condition-based and is usually given once per week or 2 weeks. Infusion takes several hours.

- This is again a pooled plasma product associated with a small risk of infection transmission
- Headache and malaise are also reported
- Alternatives should be carefully considered before the use of IVIg because of monetary and convenience costs and side effects, as well as the risks of blood products

Cryoprecipitate

The main use of cryoprecipitates in obstetrics is replacement of fibrinogen and factors XII and VIII in massive haemorrhage, to complement transfusion of more than eight units of blood (red cell transfusion is poor in clotting factors), and as part of the management of DIC.

- It is prepared from a single rather than a multiple donation and is 20–40 ml/unit
- It is stored at −30 °C for up to 12 months and must be thawed to body temperature before use
- ABO compatible units should be used

Fresh Frozen Plasma (FFP)

This again is produced from a single donation. It is also used as an adjunct to massive transfusion and in the management of DIC. Each bag contains all the clotting factors, albumin and gamma globulin. It must be used immediately after thawing, and in maternity care should be Rhesus compatible.

Anti-D

Anti-D is a pooled plasma product, which is usually used for prevention of formation of anti-D antibodies. While there are no recorded cases of infection or prion transmission it must be remembered, and patients told, that it is a blood product.

THROMBO-EMBOLIC DISORDERS

Daksha Elliott and Sue Pavord

University Hospitals of Leicester NHS Trust

15.1 Thrombophilia and Inherited
Clotting Disorders
15.2 Deep Vein Thrombosis
15.3 Pulmonary Embolism
15.4 Thromboprophylaxis

Medical Disorders in Pregnancy: A Manual for Midwives, Second Edition. Edited by S. Elizabeth Robson and Jason Waugh.
© 2013 John Wiley & Sons, Ltd. Published 2013 by John Wiley & Sons, Ltd.

15.1 Thrombophilia and Inherited Clotting Disorders

Incidence	Risk for Childbearing
Approximately 10% of the general population have an inherited thrombophilia	Variable or High Risk – depending upon type of disorder

EXPLANATION OF CONDITION

The term thrombophilia refers to disorders of the haemostatic system that result in an increased risk of thrombosis. It includes inherited and acquired risk factors.

Inherited

- Factor V Leiden (FVL)
- Prothrombin 20210
- Protein C deficiency
- Protein S deficiency
- Antithrombin deficiency

Acquired

- Antiphospholipid syndrome (see Section 11.4)

Complex

- Raised factor VIII levels
- Hyperhomocysteinaemia

COMPLICATIONS

- The relative risk of VTE varies with the nature of the thrombophilia but is greatest for antithrombin deficiency and antiphospholipid syndrome
- Thrombophilias existing in combination act synergistically, with a resulting risk greater than would be expected for the sum of the individual factors
- There is increased risk for gestational venous thrombosis, recurrent miscarriage and late pregnancy complications

NON-PREGNANCY TREATMENT AND CARE

Women with a previous history of thrombosis should be screened for thrombophilia prior to pregnancy.
Other relative indications for testing include:

- Individuals with a first-degree family history of VTE or known thrombophilia who are planning pregnancy or intending to undergo a procedure or course of treatment that would greatly increase their risk of thrombosis:
  - orthopaedic surgery
  - hormone replacement therapy
  - combined oral contraceptive pill
  - invasive vascular procedures
- Previous history of unprovoked or minimally provoked thrombosis.
- Children or young adults with thrombosis
- Women with a history of unexpected pregnancy complications should be tested for antiphospholipid antibodies (see Section 11.4):

- three or more early miscarriages
- late fetal loss
- stillbirth
- early or severe pre-eclampsia
- placental abruption
- poor fetal growth
- Young patients with unexplained arterial thrombosis should be investigated for antiphospholipid antibodies

PRE-CONCEPTION ISSUES AND CARE

For potential childbearing there are:

- Increased thrombotic risks
- Potential associations with:
  - recurrent miscarriage
  - fetal loss
  - placental abruption
  - pre-eclampsia
  - poor fetal growth

Women with thrombophilia should be informed of their diagnosis and its implications. Counselling should be reinforced by written patient information where possible.

- Advise against using the combined oral contraceptive pill, which acts in synergy with FVL and other thrombophilia to greatly enhance thrombotic risk
- Precautions for travel should be highlighted and the importance of additional thromboprophylaxis for high-risk situations such as surgery, prolonged immobility and plaster casts should be emphasised
- Plans for pregnancy should be discussed before conception and should include thromboprophylactic measures and any need for heparin
- Ideally patients should be placed on a database and issued with a registration card bearing details of their condition and phone numbers for contact
- Women with previous thrombosis and who are on long-term warfarin should be made aware of the teratogenic risks. They should keep a diary of their menstrual cycle and seek immediate medical advice if they suspect that they are pregnant
- Anticoagulation should not be interrupted but provision made to ensure that warfarin is stopped and replaced with heparin no later than 6 weeks gestation

Pregnancy Issues

Thrombosis is usually a *multi-hit phenomenon*, with cumulative risk factors triggering a clinical event.

Pregnancy significantly increases the risk for patients with underlying thrombophilia, due to a combination of various physiological changes including:

- A further increase in hypercoagulability as pregnancy advances
- Decreased venous return secondary to compression of the pelvic veins by the gravid uterus
- Reduced vessel tone with venous pooling

Of those women with previous VTE, those with underlying thrombophilia are more at risk of recurrent thrombosis than those without. The relative risk varies according to the nature of the thrombophilia, with antithrombin deficiency and antiphospholipid syndrome being the highest.

Antiphospholipid syndrome is characterised by the presence of persistent antiphospholipid antibodies (lupus anticoagulant and anticardiolipin antibodies) in association with clinical complications. In addition to venous and arterial thrombotic events, it is associated with recurrent miscarriages and late fetal loss, as well as complications in advanced pregnancy including pre-eclampsia, stillbirth and IUGR (see Section 11.4). There is also recent focus on the association of inherited thrombophilia with poor pregnancy outcome.

Pregnant women with acquired thrombophilia, and those with inherited thrombophilia and a complex obstetric or thrombosis history, should be managed by a multidisciplinary team which includes a consultant obstetrician and consultant haematologist. Ideally, the women would be seen in a joint obstetric haematology clinic.

Medical Management and Care

All women should undergo an assessment of thrombotic risk in early pregnancy, taking into account their personal and family histories, the nature of their thrombophilia and any additional acquired risk factors, such as age and obesity. Repeat assessments should be made in the second and third trimesters and each time the circumstances and risk factors change. The risks for VTE, thromboprophylaxis and management for the pregnancy should be discussed with the mother.

Thrombophilia and a history of VTE – these mothers should be offered thromboprophylaxis with antenatal low molecular weight heparin (LMWH), and also for at least 6 weeks postpartum[1].

Antiphospholipid (Hughes) syndrome – this is associated with a recurrent thrombotic risk of up to 70%[2] and therefore women with antiphospholipid syndrome and previous venous thrombosis should receive heparin from the onset of pregnancy until 6 weeks postpartum. If the condition was diagnosed because of recurrent miscarriages, treatment may not be required in the postpartum period. The addition of aspirin has been shown to improve pregnancy outcome in antiphospholipid syndrome patients with a prior history of obstetric complications[3,4] (see Section 11.4).

Asymptomatic inherited or acquired thrombophilia – these women may require antenatal or postnatal thromboprophylaxis depending on the specific thrombophilia. Antithrombin deficiency carries a 30% increased risk of thrombosis in pregnancy and these women should always receive heparin in high prophylactic or treatment doses from the onset of pregnancy. Other thrombophilias requiring antenatal prophylaxis include combined defects and homozygous states. Women with protein C and protein S deficiency may need to start heparin antenatally.

Absent thrombophilia but previous VTE – these women should be offered postpartum prophylaxis with LMWH. It may be reasonable not to use antenatal prophylaxis with heparin for a previous single VTE associated with a temporary risk factor that has now resolved[1]. However, thromboprophylaxis has been advocated if the previous VTE was related to the combined oral contraceptive pill or if additional acquired risk factors are present[5]. Also, if there is a positive first-degree family history of VTE, recurrent VTE or a history of thrombosis affecting an unusual site LMWH should be offered antenatally and for at least 6 weeks postnatally[1].

Midwifery Management and Care

- The midwife should be a point of contact so that the woman can inform her regarding the onset of pregnancy. This contact should be continued throughout the pregnancy to report any concerns or changes in circumstances which increase the thrombotic risk
- The woman should be taught correct self-injection technique and educated regarding safe disposal of 'sharps'
- Potential side effects of heparin should be discussed:
  - osteoporosis
  - HIT
  - cutaneous allergy
- Reinforce general antithrombotic advice regarding hydration, mobility, travel and leg care
- Ensure that TED stockings have been provided, are a good fit and encourage compliance
- Ensure use of compression stockings where necessary
- Be aware of and report any signs and symptoms of complications
- Effective communication with the community midwife and other members of the multidisciplinary team

---

Labour Issues – as for DVT and PE (see 15.2 and 15.3)

Management and Care – as for DVT and PE (see 15.2 and 15.3)

Postpartum Issues – as for DVT and PE (see 15.2 and 15.3)

Management and Care – as for DVT and PE (see 15.2 and 15.3)

15.2 Deep Vein Thrombosis

Incidence	Risk for Childbearing
1 in 1000 in pregnancy[1]	High Risk

EXPLANATION OF CONDITION

Deep vein thrombosis (DVT) is the formation of a blood clot or thrombus in a deep vein, partially or completely occluding the flow of blood. It commonly affects the leg veins but can occur elsewhere. In pregnant women, 85% of DVT occurs in the left leg[2] due in part to compression of the left iliac vein by the right iliac artery as they cross[3]. Virchow described the factors that promote venous thrombosis:

- Reduction of blood flow (stasis)
- Alteration of the constituents of the blood (hypercoagulability)
- Abnormalities/damage to the vessel wall

All three elements of this triad are affected by pregnancy. Pressure of the gravid uterus on the inferior vena cava and pelvic veins, an increase in coagulation factors and reduction in natural inhibitors to anticoagulation and decreased venous tone all predispose to venous thrombo-embolism (VTE).

Symptoms of DVT

- Pain in area of clot
- Unilateral and occasionally bilateral swelling
- Redness or discolouration
- Difficulty weight bearing on the affected leg
- Low grade pyrexia
- Lower abdominal pain if the pelvic veins are affected

COMPLICATIONS

Pulmonary Embolus (PE)

This occurs when a fragment of thrombus breaks away, travels through the right side of the heart and lodges in the pulmonary arterial circulation. Approximately 25% of DVT will be complicated by PE if left untreated. The risk is higher with femoral or ileofemoral thrombus than for more distal DVT.

Post-Thrombotic (or Post-Phlebitic) Syndrome

This long-term complication of DVT arises due to damage of venous valves, resulting in incompetence with reflux and backflow of blood. This increases hydrostatic pressure below the damaged area and causes disruption of the more distal valves, which in turn become incompetent. The venous hypertension leads to oedema and hypoxia of the tissues. Symptoms range from mild to severe and include:

- Pain
- Oedema
- Eczematous dermatitis
- Pruritus
- Hyperpigmentation
- Skin ulceration
- Cellulitis

Post-thrombotic syndrome occurs in 50% of patients following a DVT[4-7], with onset of symptoms often several months or even years after the initial event.

NON-PREGNANCY TREATMENT AND CARE

Prompt treatment is necessary to reduce the risk of extension and propagation of the thrombus and to minimise the risk of post-thrombotic syndrome. Urgent referral is therefore required for all patients with a suspected DVT to confirm the diagnosis objectively. Diagnosis is made from a combination of clinical probability score and radiological imaging. Non-invasive techniques, such as Doppler ultrasound, should be used where possible.

Negative D-dimers associated with a low clinical probability score reliably excludes VTE[8]. D-dimers are breakdown products of cross-linked fibrin and are raised in inflammatory, infective or malignant conditions. They should not be used to aid positive diagnosis of venous thrombosis but have a high negative predictive value in patients whose clinical probability of VTE is low as assessed by a formal scoring system, as in Table 15.2.1.

There are different opinions regarding D-dimer testing in pregnancy as they are less likely to be negative in pregnancy. For this reason the Royal College of Obstetricians and Gynaecologists (RCOG)[9] do not recommend testing whereas the American College of Chest Physicians (ACCP) do recommend testing

Heparin is the initial treatment of choice, because of its fast onset of anticoagulation and evidence for reduced risk of further thrombo-embolic events[8]. LMWH has a number of advantages over unfractionated heparin, including predictable dose-response and longer half-life enabling once daily administration. In patients with moderate to high clinical probability scores, heparin should be commenced immediately and continued until the diagnosis is excluded by diagnostic imaging[10].

Once a DVT has been confirmed, oral anticoagulation is initiated, in non-pregnant patients, and should be overlapped with heparin therapy until the International Normalized Ratio is greater than 2.0 on two consecutive days[10].

The recommended duration of anticoagulation following a first episode of DVT is 3–6 months[8], but this needs to be continued depending upon on-going presence of risk factors.

PRE-CONCEPTION ISSUES AND CARE

Pregnancy increases the risk of VTE 10-fold, which increases to 25–fold in the puerperium[11]. Undetected proximal venous thrombosis can increase the risk of premature labour and abruption. Therefore, where possible, women should be encouraged to optimise health prior to undertaking a pregnancy:

- If overweight, advise on diet and exercise
- Stop smoking
- Reduce caffeine and alcohol intake

Warfarin is contraindicated in pregnancy, other than in exceptional circumstances, and women who are on long-term warfarin should be made aware of the teratogenic risks if taken at 6–12 weeks gestation.

Table 15.2.1 LVTE Risk Assessment Scale

RCOG Risk Assessment for Venous Thromboembolism[12]		
Pre-existing Risk Factors	**Tick**	**score**
Previous recurrent VTE		3
Previous VTE – unprovoked or oestrogen related		3
Previous VTE – provoked		2
Family history of VTE		1
Known thrombophilia		2
Medical comorbidities		2
Age (>35 years)		1
Obesity – Score 1 for BMI >30 kg/m^2; 2 for BMI >40 kg/m^2 (BMI based on booking weight)		½ to 2
Parity ≥3		1
Smoker		1
Gross varicose veins		1
Obstetric risk factors	**Tick**	**score**
Pre-eclampsia		1
Dehydration/hyperemesis/OHSS		1
Multiple pregnancy or conceived by Artificial Reproductive Technology		1
Caesarean section in labour		2
Elective caesarean section		1
Mid-cavity or rotational forceps		1
Prolonged labour (>24 hours)		1
PPH (>1 litre or transfusion)		1
Transient risk factors		
Current systemic infection		1
Immobility		1
Surgical procedure in pregnancy or ≤6 weeks postpartum		2
TOTAL		

Reproduced from RCOG (2009) with the permission of the Royal College of Obstetricians and Gynaecologists

Pregnancy Issues

The risk of thrombosis is present from the first trimester until at least 6 weeks postpartum.

All pregnant women should have thrombotic risk assessment at booking, taking into account their personal and family history, the presence of acquired risk factors and any known thrombophilia (see Table 15.2.1). This should be repeated if circumstances change, such as excessive weight gain, immobility or vomiting with dehydration.

Women should be given advice on ways to reduce thrombotic risk:

- Keep hydrated
- Remain as active as possible
- Avoid standing for long periods
- Elevate feet when sitting
- Leg care (massage legs gently with oil or cream)
- Avoid unnecessary, long journeys by aeroplane, bus or car

Women with a past history of venous thrombo-embolic disease must be booked for antenatal care and delivery at a consultant unit.

If a DVT arises for the first time during pregnancy, the care and place of delivery must be transferred to a consultant unit, if not already done so.

An objective confirmation of diagnosis in pregnancy is crucial, as appropriate treatment reduces morbidity and mortality[9], but a false diagnosis has implications for:

- The current pregnancy
- Subsequent pregnancies
- Contraceptive choices
- HRT decisions
- Family members

D-dimers are less likely to be helpful in excluding the diagnosis because levels increase as pregnancy advances. Where DVT is suspected, non-invasive testing by ultrasound should be performed.

In addition to warfarin embryopathy during the first trimester, the risks continue throughout pregnancy, with neurological complications in later stages and the risk of fetal intracranial haemorrhage during delivery[1,13,14]. Continued ongoing low molecular weight heparin (LMWH) is the treatment of choice for DVT in pregnancy.

Medical Management and Care

If there is a high index of suspicion then full anticoagulation should be initiated until thrombo-embolic disease is excluded[15].

- If a Doppler ultrasound is negative but signs and symptoms are persistent and highly suggestive of a DVT the investigations should be repeated after 7 days

Venography confers a small radiation risk to the fetus and should be avoided if possible. However, if on balance of risk it is felt that venography is necessary to obtain a diagnosis, then the fetus should be shielded from radiation.

In the absence of contraindications treatment is with LMWH[16]:

- Heparin does not cross the placenta and therefore does not affect the fetus
- LMWH is given subcutaneously and can be self-administered, allowing outpatient management
- LMWH has a more predictable dose response allowing the doses to be based upon patient weight
- For treatment of DVT, LMWH should be given 12 hourly to minimise peaks and troughs
- Aim for antiXa levels of 0.4–1.0 U/ml; may be variable between laboratories and depends on the type of LMWH used
- It may be possible to reduce the dose of LMWH to a high prophylactic dose once there has been complete resolution of symptoms.
- Heparin-induced thrombocytopenia (HIT) is rare in pregnancy but the platelet count should be checked 5–7 days after starting therapy[17]
- A small proportion of patients develop cutaneous allergy and may require changing to a different LMWH
- A degree of cross-reactivity exists[18] and alternative anticoagulants such as fondaparinux (Arixtra) may be required
- Anticoagulation should be continued for at least 6 months after the thrombotic event and should not be stopped before 6 weeks postpartum

Midwifery Management and Care

- The mother should be taught correct self-injection technique
- Ensure that she is given a sharps bin and knows how to dispose of sharps safely
- The side effects of heparin should be discussed:
  - osteoporosis
  - HIT
  - cutaneous allergy
- Reinforce general antithrombotic advice regarding hydration, mobility, leg care and avoidance of unnecessary long journeys
- Ensure that compression stockings have been prescribed, are a good fit and encourage compliance
- Graduated elastic compression stockings should be worn on the affected leg following proximal DVT for at least 2 years, to reduce the incidence of severe post-thrombotic syndrome[7,6,19]
- Ensure that the woman is seen by an anaesthetist prior to delivery
- Be aware of, and report any signs and symptoms of complications of this condition
- In particular be aware of the risk of a DVT causing pulmonary embolism

Labour Issues

The intrapartum period is associated with an increase in both thrombotic and bleeding risks, and a careful assessment of these risks needs to be undertaken when planning safe management for the patient.

Ideally women should be allowed to labour spontaneously, as this reduces the need for obstetric intervention. However, depending on staffing levels, some centres may prefer a planned delivery.

Regional anaesthesia carries a possible risk of significant spinal bleeding and should be avoided within 12 hours of a prophylactic dose of LMWH and within 24 hours of a treatment dose.

General anaesthesia is associated with a higher thrombotic risk due to immobility, but may have to be considered for a caesarean section if temporary interruption of heparin is not thought suitable.

Prolonged labour and dehydration increase thrombotic risk.

Medical Management and Care

An intrapartum care plan must be worked out on an individual basis with each patient, involving the consultant obstetrician, consultant haematologist and consultant anaesthetist.

Women who are admitted in spontaneous labour or for a planned delivery will have been advised to omit their LMWH injection at the onset of contractions. This should avoid the problem of having an anticoagulant effect at the time of delivery and facilitate the use of epidural anaesthesia.

Women who are considered to be at high risk of further veno-thrombotic events may need to be converted to intravenous unfractionated heparin. This allows more flexibility in controlling anticoagulation and minimises time with trough levels. The heparin would need to be interrupted temporarily for the second and third stages of labour. These women **should not** be given intramuscular injections or NSAIDs.

Midwifery Management and Care

- TED stockings
- Encourage mobility by changes of position in labour
- Passive leg exercises if mother has an epidural
- Ensure that the woman remains hydrated, and consider iv fluids if necessary
- Avoid prolonged use of lithotomy position
- Active management of third stage after vaginal delivery, including the use of intravenous oxytocin
- Early suturing of perineal tears/episiotomy

Postpartum Issues

The risk of thrombosis increases 25-fold in the puerperium[11], therefore particular vigilance should be given to:

- Leg care
- Hydration
- Mobility
- Use of compression stockings
- Consideration to the most suitable form for continued anticoagulation
- Length of time that treatment should be continued for postnatally

Breast-feeding is safe on heparin or warfarin treatment and should be promoted[20].

Reliable contraception should be advised. However, the combined oral contraceptive pill should be avoided in women with a history of thrombo-embolism.

- Depo-Provera, the progesterone-only pill (mini-pill) and condoms (with the addition of a spermicide) may be considered. Intrauterine devices, including intrauterine progestogen-only devices, are also suitable although are unlikely to be inserted in the immediate postpartum period
- There is interaction between warfarin and oral contraception. Note that oestrogen and progesterone antagonise the anticoagulant effect

Medical Management and Care

- A follow-up plan must be documented in the notes
- LMWH should be restarted 4 hours after removal of epidural catheter or 2 hours after vaginal delivery with no epidural, unless there are complications such as bleeding or the need for surgery
- Anticoagulation should always be continued until at least 6 weeks postpartum, when the coagulation status returns to pre-pregnancy levels
- If treatment is to be continued for longer than this, in order to complete 6 months anticoagulation for those with acute thrombosis, the woman may need to convert to warfarin

Midwifery Management and Care

- If converting to warfarin, counsel regarding safety issues with warfarin therapy, drug and food interactions
- Encourage and support breast-feeding
- Discuss contraception choices before discharge
- Make sure that follow-up appointments have been made including thrombophilia testing for those with acute VTE
- If further pregnancy is planned, ensure information is given regarding teratogenicity of warfarin therapy

S. E. Robson and J. Waugh

Patient Information Leaflet to Avoid Travel Related DVT

INTRODUCTION

Deep vein thrombosis (DVT) is a term used to describe the formation of a clot, or thrombus. The clot blocks up deep veins, usually in the legs. DVT occurs when blood flows too slowly through the veins.

Long periods of immobility can slow the blood flow from the lower legs which can result in pooling and coagulation. A thrombus may then form which can occlude the blood vessel. Reduced blood flow can be further compounded by pressure on the popliteal vein in the back of the knee, such as that caused by an airline or car seat. It is important for travellers to keep moving their legs to help the blood flow back to the heart

A serious complication of DVT is a pulmonary embolus (PE) caused by the thrombus dislodging and travelling to the lungs.

WHAT IS TRAVEL-RELATED DEEP VEIN THROMBOSIS?

Sitting motionless for long periods may put some travellers at an increased risk for DVT. The risk applies to any form of travel whether it is long haul air travel or long trips by car, coach or train.

BEFORE THE TRIP

Consult your doctor if you have

- Ever had a DVT or PE
- A family history of clotting conditions
- An inherited tendency to clot (thrombophilia)
- Cancer or had treatment for cancer in the past
- Undergone major surgery in the last 3 months
- Had hip or knee replacement within the last 3 months
- Ever suffered from a stroke
- Are being treated for heart failure and circulation problems
- Are pregnant
- Have recently had a baby
- Are taking the contraceptive pill
- Are on hormone replacement therapy or HRT

People can reduce their risk of getting DVT by taking some simple precautions.

- *Wear loose, comfortable clothes:* some clothes, such as jeans, are too tight at the groin and restrict the blood supply to the legs. If your feet normally swell on long journeys, wear some old comfortable shoes.
- *Consider buying flight socks (compression stockings):* any hosiery should be measured properly to ensure a suitable fit.
- *Store luggage overhead so you have room to stretch out your legs*
- *Do anti-DVT exercises:* raise your heels, keeping your toes on the floor, then bring them down. Do this 10 times.

Now raise and lower your toes 10 times. Do it at least every half an hour.

- *Walk around whenever you can*
- *Drink plenty of water:* this will keep you hydrated, increasing the number of times that you have to get up and go the toilet, thereby exercising your legs.
- *Don't drink alcohol or too much tea or coffee:* these can cause dehydration. If you do drink alcohol and coffee, drink an equal volume of water or juice to counteract the dehydration.
- *Don't take sleeping pills:* tempting as it may be to sleep for the whole of the journey, you will not be able to keep yourself hydrated or keep your legs moving
- *If travelling by car, take regular breaks to get a drink and stretch your legs*

AFTER THE TRIP

For the vast majority of air passengers there will be no problems upon disembarkation. However symptoms of DVT can appear after arrival. If you develop swollen painful legs, especially where one is more affected than the other, or if you have breathing difficulties, see a local doctor urgently or go to the nearest A&E department.

15.3 Pulmonary Embolism

Incidence	Risk for Childbearing
60–70/100 000 of the general population Risk increases to 0.5–3/1000 pregnancies	High Risk and Life Threatening Pulmonary embolism is a leading cause of direct maternal death in the UK[2]

EXPLANATION OF CONDITION

Pulmonary embolism (PE) is an occlusion of the pulmonary arterial circulation, usually occurring when a thrombus breaks free from a distant site, often the deep veins in the leg. More rarely they may originate in the pelvic or renal veins or upper extremities or in the right heart chambers.

Typical symptoms of PE include:

- Severe sudden onset of shortness of breath
- Sharp chest pain which is worse on inspiration (pleuritic pain)
- Cough with blood (haemoptysis)

Risk factors for venous thrombo-embolism include:

- Age (over 35 years)
- Increased body mass index ($>30 \, kg/m^2$)
- Immobility
- Surgery
- Pregnancy and particularly the puerperium
- Combined oral contraceptive pill
- Hormone replacement therapy
- A past history of venous thrombo-embolism
- A strong family history of venous thrombo-embolism
- An inherited clotting tendency (thrombophilia)
- An acquired clotting tendency, e.g. antiphospholipid syndrome or acquired activated protein C resistance
- Dehydration
- Myeloproliferative disorders
- Drugs such as tamoxifen
- Nephrotic syndrome

COMPLICATIONS

Large clots may lodge in the pulmonary artery or lobar branches and cause haemodynamic compromise including:

- Cardiac arrest and sudden death
- Heart failure or shock
- Severe breathing difficulty
- Arrhythmias
- Pleural effusion

Smaller clots continue travelling distally to occlude smaller vessels in the lung periphery. These are more likely to produce pleuritic chest pain by initiating an inflammatory response involving the pleura.

Chronic thrombo-embolic disease with recurrent pulmonary embolism and pulmonary hypertension is more unusual.

Untreated, there is a mortality of 30%[1].

NON-PREGNANCY TREATMENT AND CARE

Pulmonary embolus is potentially fatal and urgent referral is necessary for all women with a suspected PE to confirm the diagnosis objectively. Diagnosis is made from a combination of clinical probability score and radiological imaging.

A negative D-dimer test reliably excludes PE in patients with low clinical probability; such patients do not require imaging for VTE. Patients with raised D-dimers and/or moderate or high clinical probability score should have either a ventilation perfusion (VQ) scan or computed tomographic pulmonary angiography (CTPA) performed. CTPA provides a more definitive diagnosis and will detect any additional lung pathology, but is not available in all centres.

Heparin, usually LMWH, should be commenced at presentation. Once a PE has been confirmed, oral anticoagulation is initiated in non-pregnant patients and should be overlapped with heparin therapy until the International Normalized Ratio (INR) is within therapeutic range (usually 2–3) on two consecutive tests. Anticoagulation should be continued for 3–6 months, but a longer duration may be necessary depending on the presence of on-going risk factors.

Massive or sub-massive PE associated with cardiac compromise, require thrombolytics in addition to heparin. Resuscitative measures include oxygenation and supporting cardiac output.

PRE-CONCEPTION ISSUES AND CARE

Pregnancy increases the risk of PE 10-fold, which is further increased in the postpartum period[3]. Women should be encouraged to minimise their acquired risk factors and improve fitness prior to undertaking a pregnancy.

Women who are on long-term warfarin therapy should be made aware of the teratogenic risks. The risk is greatest when the daily warfarin dose exceeds 5 mg. If taken at 6–12 weeks' gestation, the risk of warfarin embryopathy is around 5% including:

- Chondrodysplasia punctata
- Nasal hypoplasia
- Growth restriction
- Short proximal limbs

Women should keep a diary of their menstrual cycle and seek immediate medical advice once pregnancy is suspected so that warfarin can be replaced by heparin within 2 weeks of the first missed menstrual period.

Pregnancy issues

All pregnant women should have thrombotic risk assessment at booking and again if circumstances, such as excessive weight gain, immobility or vomiting with dehydration, change[4]. Then advice should be given on ways to reduce thrombotic risk.

Additional Risk Factors

- Hyperemesis
- Parity >4
- Caesarean section, particularly if emergency
- Operative vaginal delivery
- Pre-eclampsia
- Ovarian hyperstimulation

Rare Causes of PE

- Amniotic fluid embolism, caused by entry of amniotic fluid and fetal antigen into the maternal circulation, invoking an anaphylactic reaction; associated with 80% mortality
- Air embolism caused by intrauterine manipulation or neck vein cannulation

Diagnosis of PE is much more problematic in pregnant patients, mainly due to the fears of the effects of harmful radiation on the fetus. However, the potential risks associated with the radiological tests used are minimal when compared with the consequences of inaccurate diagnosis.

Diagnostic difficulties are compounded by the relative frequency of chest pain and shortness of breath in pregnant patients and the rise with D-dimers as pregnancy advances, rendering them less useful for diagnostic exclusion in low-probability cases. As a consequence, only 10% of patients investigated for a suspected pulmonary embolism are confirmed thromboses.

Medical Management and Care

Objective confirmation of thrombo-embolism is crucial because of implications for the current pregnancy, subsequent pregnancies, contraceptive choices and HRT decisions. In addition, it is well established that treatment reduces morbidity and mortality[5].

Clinical suspicion of PE warrants a chest X-ray and Doppler ultrasound of the legs. If there is confirmation of DVT, lung scanning is not required, as the diagnosis of PE can be presumed.

A pulmonary ventilation/perfusion scan (VQ scan) is a sequenced nuclear scan test that uses inhaled and injected material to measure breathing (ventilation) and circulation (perfusion). Acute pulmonary embolism results in perfusion defects which are not matched by ventilation defects. VQ carries a slight increased risk of childhood cancer (1:280 000)[6].

CTPA involves multiple X-rays being passed through the lungs. This produces cross-sectional images, or 'slices', on a cathode-ray tube, to construct a three-dimensional image of the lungs. Intravenous iodine is used to highlight the structure of the lungs. The advantages are a more definitive result and identification of other lung pathology. However, it is associated with a life-time risk of breast cancer of 13.6%[7]. Women should be given full information where possible and consent obtained.

LMWH is the preferred option for use as it has clear advantages over unfractionated heparin. Reduced binding to non-specific plasma proteins provides a predictable dose-response effect, allowing doses to be based on patient weight, without the need for intense monitoring. The long half-life facilitates self-administration on an outpatient basis.

Anticoagulation should be the same as treatment for DVT.

Midwifery Management and Care

If a woman presents with the signs and symptoms of PE, she should be referred immediately to hospital. After diagnosis she should be informed of the result and the need to be treated with heparin.

- The woman should be taught correct self-injection technique
- Ensure that the woman is given a sharps bin and knows how to dispose of sharps safely
- The side effects of heparin should be discussed:
  - osteoporosis
  - heparin-induced thrombocytopenia
  - cutaneous allergy
- Reinforce general antithrombotic advice regarding hydration, mobility and leg care
- Ensure that compression stockings have been prescribed, are a good fit and encourage compliance
- Ensure that the woman is seen by an anaesthetist prior to delivery
- Be aware of and report any signs and symptoms of complications

Labour Issues

Labour and delivery are associated with a further increase in hypercoagulability as well as risks of uterine haemorrhage and bleeding from surgical sites. The balance between these risks needs to be carefully assessed and managed, to ensure safety of the patient during this unstable period.

Both thrombotic and bleeding risks are further increased by:
- Prolonged labour
- Interventional vaginal delivery
- Caesarean section, particularly when undertaken as an emergency

Ideally, patients on prophylactic or therapeutic anticoagulation should be allowed to labour spontaneously, as this reduces the need for intervention.

Inferior vena caval filters are rarely needed but may be required if anticoagulation is contraindicated and the risk of PE is felt to be significant. However, whilst the PE rate is reduced, the DVT risk is increased and only retrievable filters should be used.

Epidural should be timed to avoid bleeding complications[8] and general anaesthesia may have to be considered for caesarean section in women on full anticoagulation.

Medical Management and Care

An intrapartum care plan must be worked out on an individual basis with each patient, involving the consultant obstetrician, consultant haematologist and consultant anaesthetist.

Women who are admitted in spontaneous labour or for a planned delivery will have been advised to omit their low molecular weight heparin (LMWH) injection at the onset of contractions. This should avoid the problem of having an anticoagulant affect at the time of delivery and facilitate the use of epidural anaesthesia.

Women who are considered to be at high risk of further veno-thrombotic events may need to be converted to intravenous unfractionated heparin, as this allows more flexibility in controlling anticoagulation and minimises time with trough levels. The heparin would need to be temporarily interrupted for the second and third stages of labour. These women should *not* be given intramuscular injections or NSAIDs.

Midwifery Management and Care
- Encourage mobility with regular changes of position
- TED stockings
- Passive leg exercises if epidural given
- Attention to hydration and consideration to iv fluids if necessary
- Regular observations in labour
- Active management of third stage after vaginal delivery, including the use of intravenous oxytocin
- Early suturing of perineal tears/episiotomy

Postpartum Issues

The risk of thrombosis increases 25-fold in the puerperium[8]. Signs of PE, e.g. chest pain or breathlessness, need to be taken seriously and regarded as an emergency.

Particular vigilance should be given to:
- Leg care
- Hydration
- Mobility
- Use of compression stockings
- Most suitable form of continued anticoagulation
- Length of time that treatment should be continued postnatally

The mother should be informed of the safety of breast-feeding whilst on heparin or warfarin treatment[9].

Reliable contraception should be advised:
- The combined oral contraceptive pill is relatively contraindicated with a history of thrombo-embolism
- Depo-Provera, the progesterone-only pill (mini-pill) and condoms (with the addition of a spermicide) may be considered. Intrauterine devices, including intrauterine progestogen-only devices, are also suitable although are unlikely to be inserted in the immediate postpartum period
- There is interaction between warfarin and oral contraception. Note that oestrogen and progesterone antagonise the anticoagulant effect

Medical Management and Care
- A follow-up plan must be documented in the case notes
- LMWH should be restarted 4 hours after removal of epidural catheter or 2 hours after vaginal delivery with no epidural unless there are complications such as bleeding or need for surgery
- Anticoagulation should always be continued until at least 6 weeks postpartum
- If treatment is to be continued for longer than this, in order to complete 6 months anticoagulation, then the woman may need to convert to warfarin

Midwifery Management and Care
- If converting treatment to warfarin, counsel the mother regarding safety issues with warfarin therapy
- Before discharge make sure that follow-up appointments have been made, including thrombophilia testing for those with an acute VTE
- Discuss contraception choices before discharge
- If further pregnancy is planned, ensure information is given regarding teratogenicity of warfarin
- Pay attention to postnatal observations, including pulse, respiration and leg swelling
- Be aware that PE can present suddenly in the puerperium, necessitating emergency re-admission

15.4 Thromboprophylaxis

EXPLANATION OF CONDITION

Venous thromboembolism (VTE) may present as deep vein thrombosis (DVT) or pulmonary embolism (PE) but if untreated can result in fatal PE. Although fatal PE is clearly the most significant consequence of VTE in pregnancy, DVT also often leads to morbidity related to the development of post-thrombotic syndrome (PTS)[1–4]

PE used to be the leading cause of maternal death in the UK and the second most common cause overall, accounting for 11% of maternal deaths. It has long been recognised that many of these are preventable and through improved awareness and effective preventative measures, incidence has declined from 41 deaths in 2003–2005 to 18 in 2006–2008 and is now lower than deaths from infections[5]. It seems likely that the fall in deaths is the result of better recognition of at-risk women and more widespread thromboprophylaxis[6].

Pregnancy is an independent risk factor for VTE, with an approximate 10-fold increased relative risk. The risk begins in the first trimester and increases as pregnancy advances. The puerperium is the time of highest risk. Additional risk factors may be specifically related to the pregnancy or may be pre-existing, congenital or have developed prior to pregnancy.

When an individual has a venous thrombosis, it is usually because more than one risk factor is present at any one time. This is known as the *multi-hit hypothesis* (Figure 15.4.1). VTE risk increases with age. In this patient with thrombophilia, the caesarean section pushes them over the thrombotic threshold and causes a clinical VTE.

In its guideline[9] on reducing the risk of VTE in pregnancy, the RCOG has listed significant risk factors.

Pre-existing Risk Factors

- Previous VTE
- Thrombophilia (see table below)
- Age >35 years
- Obesity (BMI >30 kg/m^2) pre-, or early, pregnancy
- Parity >2
- Smoking
- Medical co-morbidities, e.g. sickle cell disease, cardiac disease, proteinuria >3 g/day, inflammatory bowel disease, joint disease or myeloproliferative disorders
- Intravenous drug user
- Gross varicose veins
- Paraplegia

Genetic/Inherited Risk Factors

- Antithrombin deficiency
- Protein C deficiency
- Protein S deficiency
- Factor V Leiden
- Prothrombin gene variant

Acquired Risk Factors

- Lupus anticoagulant

Obstetric Risk Factors

- Multiple pregnancy
- Assisted reproductive therapy
- Pre-eclampsia
- Prolonged labour
- Mid-cavity, rotational operative vaginal delivery
- Caesarean section
- Excessive blood loss (>1 litre) requiring transfusion

New Onset/Transient Risk Factors

- Hyperemesis/dehydration
- Ovarian hyperstimulation syndrome
- Admission, immobility (4 or more days of bed rest), e.g. symphysis pubis dysfunction restricting mobility
- Surgical procedure in pregnancy or puerperium

NON-PREGNANCY TREATMENT AND CARE

The House of Commons Health Select Committee Enquiry into VTE, which reported in 2005, agreed with the evidence presented by thrombosis experts and charities that up to 25 000 deaths each year can be attributed to VTE, and that VTE is the immediate cause of death in 10% of patients who die in hospital[7].

Subsequently in 2007, NICE produced guidelines on medical and surgical thromboprophylaxis. This guidance is about the care and treatment of people who are at risk of developing deep vein thrombosis (DVT) while in hospital in the NHS in England and Wales. The advice in the NICE guideline covers the care and treatment that should be offered to all adults, aged 18 and over, who are admitted to hospital in England and Wales[8]. Indeed the Department of Health has mandated risk assessment for every patient admitted to hospital.

Within local guidelines, individual prophylaxis should be chosen according to the balance of efficacy and risks (*especially bleeding*), and the patient's preferences.

PRE-CONCEPTION ISSUES AND CARE

Pregnancy is a risk factor for venous thromboembolism and is associated with a 10-fold increase compared with the risk for non-pregnant women. Women with a previous unprovoked or hormonally-related VTE should have a careful history documented and undergo screening for both inherited and acquired thrombophilia, ideally before pregnancy. Some women are at even higher risk during pregnancy because they have one or more additional risk factors. The level of risk associated with many of these factors is unclear. An individual assessment of thrombotic risk should be undertaken, ideally before pregnancy or in early pregnancy.

Women at high risk of VTE, including those with previous confirmed VTE, should be offered pre-pregnancy counselling with a prospective management plan[9]. This is important because the increase in thrombotic risk starts very early in pregnancy, usually before the antenatal booking has taken place. Section 15.2 provides information to avoid travel-related DVT.

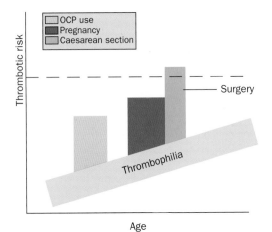

Figure 15.4.1 Schematic representation of the multi-hit theory of VTE. OCP, oral contraceptive pill. This figure is downloadable from the book companion website at www.wiley.com/go/robson

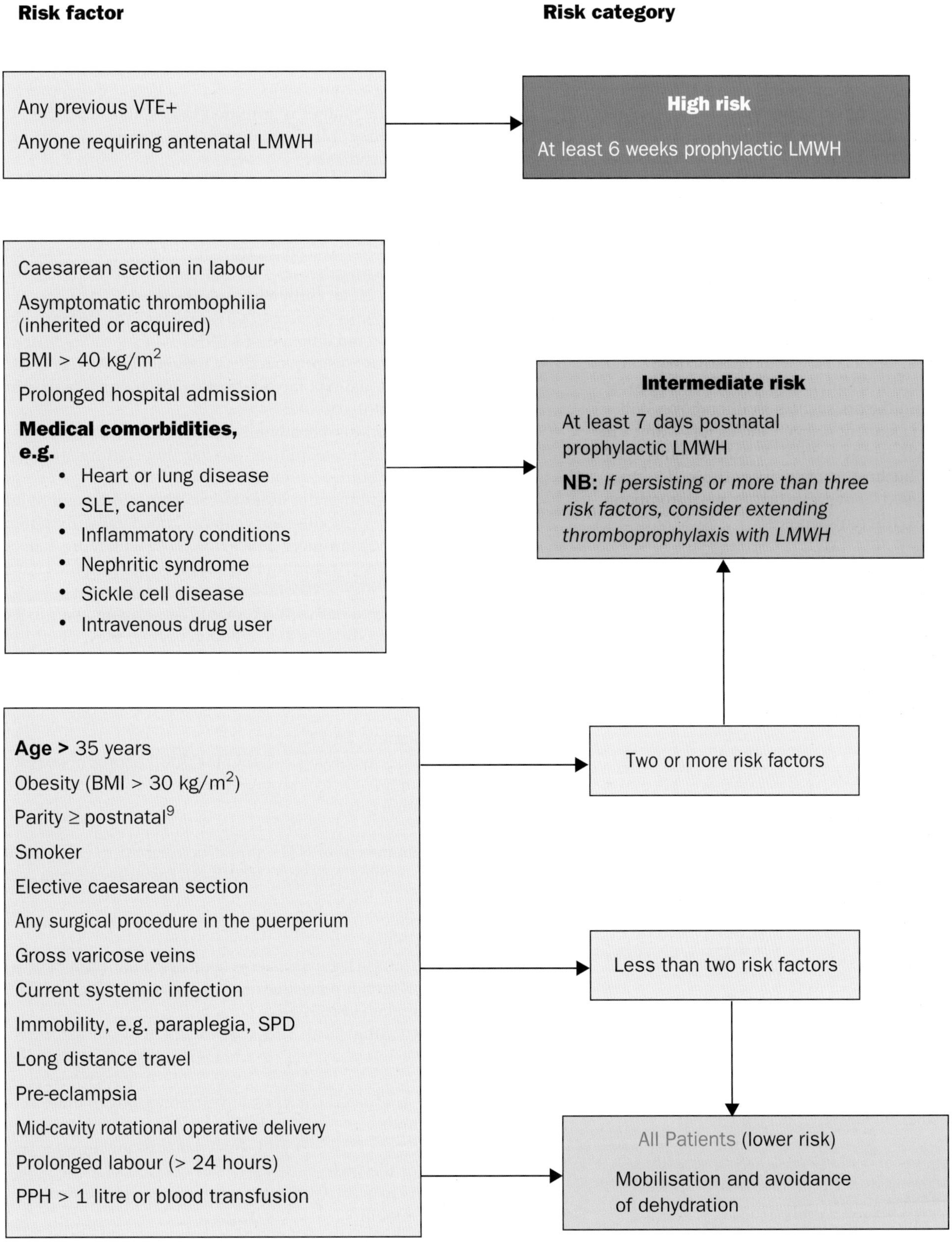

Risk factor

Risk category

| Any previous VTE+
Anyone requiring antenatal LMWH | → | **High risk**
At least 6 weeks prophylactic LMWH |

Caesarean section in labour

Asymptomatic thrombophilia (inherited or acquired)

BMI > 40 kg/m^2

Prolonged hospital admission

Medical comorbidities, e.g.
- Heart or lung disease
- SLE, cancer
- Inflammatory conditions
- Nephritic syndrome
- Sickle cell disease
- Intravenous drug user

→ **Intermediate risk**

At least 7 days postnatal prophylactic LMWH

NB: *If persisting or more than three risk factors, consider extending thromboprophylaxis with LMWH*

Age > 35 years

Obesity (BMI > 30 kg/m^2)

Parity ≥ postnatal[9]

Smoker

Elective caesarean section

Any surgical procedure in the puerperium

Gross varicose veins

Current systemic infection

Immobility, e.g. paraplegia, SPD

Long distance travel

Pre-eclampsia

Mid-cavity rotational operative delivery

Prolonged labour (> 24 hours)

PPH > 1 litre or blood transfusion

→ Two or more risk factors

→ Less than two risk factors

All Patients (lower risk)

Mobilisation and avoidance of dehydration

Figure 15.4.2 Algorithm for postnatal thromboprophylaxis risk assessment and management[9] (adapted from the RCOG Green Top Clinical Guideline 37a). Reproduced from RCOG (2009) with the permission of the Royal College of Obstetricians and Gynaecologists. This figure is downloadable from the book companion website at www.wiley.com/go/robson

Pregnancy Issues

The increased VTE risk in pregnancy is brought about by a combination of hypercoagulability, loss of venous tone and reduction of venous blood flow due in part to the gravid uterus. This is in keeping with Virchow's triad (Figure 15.4.3) which describes the three broad categories of factors that are thought to contribute to thrombosis:

- Hypercoagulability
- Haemodynamic changes (stasis, turbulence)
- Endothelial injury/dysfunction

The hypercoagulability has likely evolved to protect women against the bleeding challenges associated with miscarriage and childbirth. Changes include a rise in procoagulant factors such as FVIII and Von Willebrand factor, fibrinogen and factors X and VII as well as a reduction in natural anticoagulants such as protein S. Additional factors described above exacerbate the thrombotic risk to different degrees.

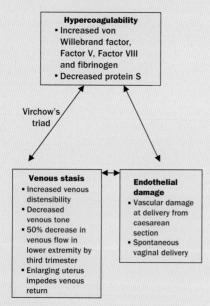

Figure 15.4.3 Prothrombotic changes associated with pregnancy and relationship to Virchow's triad. This figure is downloadable from the book companion website at www.wiley.com/go/robson

Patients at *very high* risk are those with;

- Previous VTE on long-term warfarin
- Antithrombin deficiency
- Antiphospholipid syndrome with previous VTE

Patients at *high* risk are those with:

- Previous recurrent or unprovoked VTE
- Previous oestrogen-provoked (pill or pregnancy) VTE
- Previous VTE + thrombophilia
- Previous VTE + family history of VTE
- Asymptomatic thrombophilia (combined defects, homozygous FVL)

Medical Management and Care

- A local thromboprophylaxis risk assessment proforma should be completed at:
  - antenatal booking
  - **and** repeated if the mother is admitted to hospital
  - **and** repeated if other intercurrent problems develop
- The RCOG[9] recommend that:
  - any woman with three or more current or persisting risk factors should be considered for prophylactic low molecular weight heparin (LMWH) antenatally
  - women with a previous single provoked (excluding oestrogen-related) VTE and no other risk factors require close surveillance; antenatal LMWH is not routinely recommended
  - women with previous recurrent VTE or a previous unprovoked VTE should be offered antenatal LMWH
  - women with a previous provoked DVT should be offered LMWH if there are additional risk factors, known thrombophilia or a first degree family history of VTE
  - women with previous hormonally-related VTE, including pregnancy, the contraceptive pill or ovarian hyperstimulation syndrome should be offered antenatal LMWH
  - women with asymptomatic inherited or acquired thrombophilia may be managed with close surveillance antenatally. Exceptions are women with antithrombin deficiency, those with more than one thrombophilic defect (including homozygosity for factor V Leiden) or those with additional risk factors
- Women receiving antenatal LMWH should be advised that, if they have any vaginal bleeding, or once labour begins, they should not inject any further LMWH
- They should be reassessed on admission to hospital and further doses should be prescribed by medical staff

Midwifery Management and Care

Complete a local risk assessment proforma for thromboprophylaxis at:

- Antenatal booking
- Each antenatal admission
- Post-delivery

Women who are at high risk of VTE should be referred to a consultant obstetrician or trust-nominated expert in thrombosis in pregnancy, early in pregnancy[9].

- Do not allow woman to become dehydrated
- Encourage to mobilise
- If immobilised, arrange leg exercises as soon as possible after surgery
- Consider using regional anaesthesia if appropriate (risk of VTE is higher with general anaesthesia)
- Risk assessment (using local VTE assessment tool) to ascertain if further measures necessary, e.g. graduated compression stockings, LMWH

On admission, offer graduated compression stockings (GCS) unless contraindicated (see below)

Staff trained in the use of GCS should show patients how to wear them correctly and monitor their use

Encourage patients to wear GCS from admission until they return to their usual levels of mobility

Be Aware of Contraindications to Graduated Compression Stockings

- Peripheral vascular disease
- Severe dermatitis
- Leg deformity
- Recent skin graft
- Peripheral neuropathy
- See Appendix 15.4.1 for further information on GCS/TED stockings

Labour Issues

LMWH is relatively contraindicated in labour because of bleeding risks and potential need for regional anaesthesia. Patients on antenatal heparin prophylaxis should omit their injection when labour starts.

The intrapartum period is associated with an increase in both thrombotic and bleeding risks, and a careful assessment of these risks needs to be undertaken when planning safe management for the patient.

Spontaneous labour is preferred where possible as this is associated with a lower incidence of obstetric intervention. Regional anaesthesia carries a possible risk of spinal bleeding and although this risk is extremely small, the consequences can be devastating and for this reason it is the usual recommendation to delay until 12 hours after a prophylactic dose of LMWH. Caesarean section, general anaesthesia, prolonged labour and dehydration increase thrombotic risk.

Medical Management and Care

As the duration and mode of delivery impact on thrombotic risk, reassessment is crucial within 6 hours of delivery so that all the delivery details can be taken into account. Particular risk factors include:

- Emergency caesarean section
- Mid-cavity instrumental delivery
- Development of pre-eclampsia
- Labour prolonged >24 hours
- Bood loss exceeding 1 litre
- Blood transfusion

Midwifery Management and Care

- Anti-embolic stockings
- Encourage mobility by changes of position in labour
- Passive leg exercises if mother has an epidural
- Ensure that the woman remains hydrated, and consider iv fluids if necessary
- Avoid prolonged use of lithotomy position
- Active management of third stage after vaginal delivery, including the use of intravenous oxytocin
- Early suturing of perineal tears/episiotomy

Postpartum Issues

The risk of thrombosis increases 25-fold in the puerperium[10] therefore particular vigilance should be given to:

- Leg care
- Hydration
- Mobility
- Use of compression stockings
- Length of time that treatment should be continued for postnatally

Medical Management and Care

See Figure 15.4.2 for postnatal thromboprophylaxis risk assessment and management algorithm.

High Risk Women

- Require 6 weeks postnatal prophylactic LMWH[9]
- If >3 persisting risk factors, consider giving thromboprophylactic LMWH for up to 6 weeks postnatal in addition to antiembolic stockings[9]

Intermediate Risk Women

- Consider 7 days postnatal prophylactic LMWH[9]
- If risk factors persist, consider extending LMWH for up to 6 weeks

Low Risk Women

- Women with less than two risk factors. Mobilisation and avoidance of dehydration[9]

Midwifery Management and Care

- The mother should be taught correct self-injection technique
- Ensure that she is given a sharps bin and knows how to dispose of sharps safely
- Advise to report any itching or skin changes
- Reinforce general antithrombotic advice regarding hydration, mobility, leg care and avoidance of unnecessary long journeys (see Section 15.2)
- Ensure that anti-embolic stockings are a good fit and encourage compliance (see Appendix 15.4.1)

15 Thromboembolic Disorders

PATIENT ORGANISATIONS

Hughes Syndrome Foundation
Louise Coote Lupus Unit
Gassiot House
St Thomas's Hospital
London SE1 7EH
http://www.hughes-syndrome.org

Thrombosis Research Institute
Emmanuel Kaye Building
Manresa Road
London SW3 6LR
http://www.tri-london.ac.uk

Lifeblood: The Thrombosis Charity
PO Box 1050
Spalding PE12 6YF
http://www.thrombosis-charity.org.uk

Electronic Quality Information for Patients:
Blood and Circulation Disorders
http://www.equip.nhs.uk/topics/blood.html

ESSENTIAL READING

Boyle M 2004 *Thromboembolism in pregnancy*. In: **Emergencies Around Childbirth**. Oxford; Radcliffe Medical Press

Dike P 2007 *Haematological disorders* part 2 in Billington M and Stevenson M (Eds) **Critical Care in Childbearing for Midwives**. Oxford; Blackwell Publishing Ltd. 83–88

Greer I, Nelson-Piercy C. and Walters B 2007 Chapt. 8 *Thrombosis and hemostasis* in **Maternal Medicine: Medical Problems in Pregnancy**. London; Elsevier

James D (Ed) 2011 **High Risk Pregnancy Management Options**, 4th Edn. London; Elsevier. Chapters 40 and 41

Lifeblood: The Thrombosis Charity, Fact Sheet: **Thrombosis and Pregnancy**.

www.thrombosis-charity.org.uk/Thrombosis_and_pregnancy_factsheet.pdf

NICE 2010 **Clinical Guideline 92**. Venous Thromboembolism. London; National Institute of Health and Clinical Excellence. http://guidance.nice.org.uk/CG46/quickrefguide/pdf/English

Pavord S, Hunt B 2010 *The Obstetric Hematology Manual*. Cambridge; Cambridge University Press

Powrie R, Greene M and Camman W (Eds) 2010 **de Swiet's Medical Disorders in Obstetric Practice**. 5th Edn. Oxford; Wiley-Blackwell, Chapters 40–42

RCOG 2007 Clinical Guideline (Green-top 37b) – **Thromboembolic Disease in Pregnancy and the Puerperium: Acute Management**. London; Royal College of Obstetricians and Gynaecologists

RCOG 2009 Clinical Guideline (Green-top 37a) **Thrombosis and Embolism during Pregnancy and the Puerperium, Reducing the Risk**. London; Royal College of Obstetricians and Gynaecologists

UK Thromboprophylaxis Forum
http://www.tpforum.co.uk

References

References

15.1 Thrombophilia and Inherited Clotting Disorders

1. RCOG 2004 **Clinical Guideline No.37 – Thromboprophylaxis during Pregnancy, Labour and after Vaginal Delivery**. London; Royal College of Obstetricians and Gynaecologists
2. Khamashata MA, Guadrado MJ, Mujic F, Taub NA, Hunt BJ and Hughes GR 1995 The management of thrombosis in the antiphospholipid-antibody syndrome. **New England Journal of Medicine**, 332:993–997
3. Pattison NS, Chamley LW, Birdsall M, Zanderigo AM, Liddel HS, McDougal J 2000 Does aspirin have a role in improving pregnancy outcome for women with the antiphospholipid syndrome? A randomised controlled trial. **American Journal of Obstetrics and Gynecology**, 183:1008–1012
4. Rai R 2000 Obstetric management of antiphospholipid syndrome. **Journal of Autoimmune Diseases**, 15:203–207
5. SIGN 1999 Report No.36 **Antithrombotic Therapy**. Edinburgh; Scottish Intercollegiate Guidelines Network

15.2 Deep Vein Thrombosis

1. Walker ID 1993 Guidelines on the prevention, investigation and management of thrombosis associated with pregnancy. Maternal and Neonatal Haemostasis Working Party of the Haemostasis and Thrombosis Task Force. **Journal of Clinical Pathology**, 46:489–496
2. Ginsberg JS, Brill-Edwards P, Burrows RF, *et al.* 1992 Venous thrombosis during pregnancy: leg and trimester of presentation. **Thrombosis and Haemostasis**, 67:519–520
3. Ikard RW, Ueland K, and Folse R. 1971 Lower limb venous dynamics in pregnant women. **Surgery, Gynecology and Obstetrics**, 132:483–488
4. Beyth RJ, Cohen AM, Landefeld CS 1995 Long-term outcomes of deep vein thrombosis. **Archives of Internal Medicine**, 155: 1031–1037
5. Prandoni P, Lensing AW, Cogo A, *et al.* 1996 The long term clinical course of acute deep vein thrombosis. **Annals of Internal Medicine**, 125:1–7
6. Brandejes DP, Buller HR, Heijboer H, *et al.* 1997 Randomised trial of effect of compression stockings in patients with symptomatic proximal-vein thrombosis. **Lancet**, 349(9054):759–762
7. Gorman WP, Davis KR and Donnelly R 2000 ABC of arterial and venous disease. Swollen lower limb – 1: general assessment and deep vein thrombosis. **British Medical Journal**, 320(7247): 1453–1456
8. Wells PS, Anderson DR, Rodger M, *et al.* 2003 Evaluation of D-dimer in the diagnosis of suspected deep-vein thrombosis. **New England Journal of Medicine**, 349:1227–1235
9. RCOG 2009 **Clinical Guideline No.37 – Thromboembolic Disease in Pregnancy and the Puerperium: Acute Management**. London; Royal College of Obstetricians and Gynaecologists
10. SIGN 1999 Report No. 36 – **Antithrombotic Therapy**. Edinburgh; Scottish Intercollegiate Guidelines Network
11. McColl MD, Ramsay JE, Tait RC, *et al.* Risk factors for pregnancy associated venous thromboembolism. **Journal of Thrombosis and Haemostasis**, 78:1183–1188
12. RCOG 2009 Clinical Guideline (Green-top 37a) **Thrombosis and Embolism during Pregnancy and the Puerperium, Reducing the Risk**. London; Royal College of Obstetricians and Gynaecologists.
13. Bick RL and Haas SK 1998 International consensus recommendations. Summary statement and additional suggested guidelines. **Medical Clinics of North America**, 82:613–633
14. British Committee for Standards in Haematology 1998 Guidelines on oral anticoagulation, 3rd Edn. **British Journal of Haematology**, 101:374–387
15. Lewis G and Drife J 2002 Confidential enquiries into maternal and child health. **CEMACH 6th report: Why Mothers Die 2000–2002**. London; RCOG Press
16. Weitz JI 1997 Low-molecular-weight heparins. **New England Journal of Medicine**, 337:688–698

17. Warkentin TE, Levine MN, Hirsh J, *et al.* 1995 Heparin induced thrombocytopenia in patients treated with low molecular weight heparin or unfractionated heparin. **New England Journal of Medicine**, 332:1330–1335
18. Wutschert R, Piletta P and Bounameaux H 1999 Adverse skin reactions to low molecular weight heparins: frequency, management and prevention. **Drug Safety**, 20:515–525
19. McCollum C 1998 Avoiding the consequence of deep vein thrombosis. Elevation and compression are important and too often forgotten. **British Medical Journal**, 317(7160):696
20. Ginsberg JS, Greer I and Hirsh J 2001 Use of antithrombotic agents during pregnancy. **Chest**, 119:122s–131s

15.3 Pulmonary Embolism

1. Barrit DW and Jordan SC 1960 Anticoagulant drugs in the treatment of pulmonary embolism: a controlled trial. **Lancet**, 1:1309–1312
2. Lewis G (Ed.) 2011 Saving Mothers' Lives: Reviewing Maternal Deaths to Make Motherhood Safer: 2006–2008. **British Journal of Obstetrics and Gynaecology**, 118(supplement). London; Centre for Maternal and Child Enquiries
3. McColl MD, Ramsay JE, Tait RC, *et al.* 1997 Risk factors for pregnancy associated venous thromboembolism. **Journal of Thrombosis and Haemostasis**, 78:1183–1188
4. RCOG 2004 **Greentop Clinical Guideline No. 37 – Thromboprophylaxis during Pregnancy, Labour and after Vaginal Delivery**. London; Royal College of Obstetricians and Gynaecologists
5. RCOG 2007 **Greentop Clinical Guideline No.28 – Thromboembolic Disease in Pregnancy and the Puerperium: Acute Management**. London; Royal College of Obstetricians and Gynaecologists
6. Cook JV and Kyriou J 2005 Radiation from CT and perfusion scanning in pregnancy. **British Medical Journal**, 331:350
7. Remy-Jardin M, Remy J and Spiral CT 1999 Angiography of the pulmonary circulation. **Radiology**, 212:615–636
8. Checketts MR and Wildsmith J 1999 Central nerve block and thromboprophylaxis: is there a problem? **British Journal of Anaesthesia**, 82:164–167
9. Ginsberg JS, Greer I and Hirsh J 2001 Use of antithrombotic agents during pregnancy. **Chest**, 119:122s–131s

15.4 Thromboprophylaxis

1. Beyth RJ, Cohen AM and Landefeld CS 1995 Long-term outcomes of deep vein thrombosis. **Archives of Internal Medicine**, 155:1031–1037
2. Prandoni P, Lensing AW, Cogo A, *et al.* 1996 The long term clinical course of acute deep vein thrombosis. **Annals of Internal Medicine**, 125:1–7
3. Brandejes DP, Buller HR, Heijboer H, *et al.* 1997 Randomised trial of effect of compression stockings in patients with symptomatic proximal-vein thrombosis. **Lancet**, 349(9054):759–762
4. Gorman WP, Davis KR and Donnelly R 2000 ABC of arterial and venous disease. Swollen lower limb – 1: general assessment and deep vein thrombosis. **British Medical Journal**, 320(7247):1453–1456
5. Lewis G (Ed.) 2011 Saving Mothers' Lives: Reviewing Maternal Deaths to Make Motherhood Safer: 2006–2008. **British Journal of Obstetrics and Gynaecology**, 118(supplement). London; Centre for Maternal and Child Enquiries
6. Drife J **Thrombosis and Thromboembolism, Saving Mothers' Lives, 2003–2005**. 7th report of Confidential Enquiries into Maternal Deaths in the UK
7. House of Commons Health Select Committee 2005 **The Prevention of Venous Thromboembolism in Hospitalised Patients**. London; The Stationery Office
8. *Implementation of Department of Health Guidance relating to Thromboprophylaxis and Anticoagulation* 2007. London; National Institute for Health and Clinical Excellence. http://www.nice.org.uk/usingguidance/sharedlearningimplementingniceguidance/examplesofimplementation/eximpresults.jsp?o=161

9. RCOG 2009 Clinical Guideline (Green-top 37a) **Thrombosis and Embolism during Pregnancy and the Puerperium, Reducing the Risk**. London; Royal College of Obstetricians and Gynaecologists.
10. SIGN 2010 **Prevention and Management of Thromboembolism**. Edinburgh; Scottish Intercollegiate Guidelines Network

Appendix References

Appendix 15.4.1 Thrombo-embolic Disease Stockings
1. Morris C 2009 **Guidelines for Best Practice: The Nursing Care of Patients Wearing Anti Embolic Stockings**. All Wales Tissue Viability Nurse Forum – in association with the **British Journal of Nursing**
2. NICE 2010 Venous thromboembolism: reducing the risk. **NICE Clinical guideline 92**. London; National Institute for Health and Clinical Excellence. www.nice.org.uk

Appendix 15.4.1 Thrombo-embolic Disease Stockings

Compression stockings are made from strong elastic material being designed to increase blood circulation by fitting tightly at the ankles, gradually become less tight at the knee/thigh. The pressure in the stockings is graded allowing the stockings to constantly squeeze the leg muscles. This motion helps to drive blood back to the heart, reduce swelling in the feet and prevent blood clot formation.

(a) **There are two types of compression stockings:**
   1. Anti-embolic – for thromboprophylaxis
   2. Class II – to treat VTE and prevent develop of post-thrombotic syndrome. They should be worn for at least 2 years after the event

(b) **Before Application of Stocking[1]**
   - Identify contraindications:
     - Peripheral vascular disease
     - Absent or weak foot pulses (vascular referral essential)
     - Slow capillary filling (pinched nail-bed taking more than three seconds to return to normal colour)
     - History of intermittent claudication or rest pain
     - Tropic skin changes (cold, pale, shiny, hairless leg)
     - Peripheral neuropathy
     - Leg, foot or heel ulceration
     - Fragile skin
     - Cellulitis
     - Allergies to the components or material of the stockings
     - Severe leg or pulmonary oedema from congestive cardiac failure
     - On noradrenalin
   - If the above are identified, do not fit the stocking and seek specialist advice.
   - Attain informed consent, and give an information leaflet if these are available.

(c) **Proper Fitting[1]**
   - Optimum therapy is dependent upon well-fitting hosiery so measurements should not be guessed
   - Over-large stockings have minimal effect on the circulation of blood through the leg
   - Tight stockings compromise the blood circulation and restrict blood returning to the heart
   - TED stocking provide 14–19 mmHg at the ankle reducing to 11–14 mmHg at the knee
   - Follow manufacturer's measurement and fitting instructions
   - Measure ankle and calf circumferences, and if necessary thigh circumference
   - The distance from the knee to the ankle will also be measured to determine proper sizing
   - Record measurements in the case notes
   - Legs should be re-measured by a midwife if either an increase or a decrease is size is noted.
   - An increase in leg diameter of 5 cm can double pressure applied by the stocking

(d) **Every Eight Hours[1]**
   - Observe the legs to identify any tissue ischaemia
   - Check the stockings to ensure they are not acting as a tourniquet anywhere, as this will increase the risk of DVT
   - Ascertain that the stocking fits comfortably with no wrinkles and there is absence of pain and discomfort
   - All anti-embolic stocking checks should be documented in the case notes
   - Report any increase in leg size to medical staff

(e) **Every Day[1]**
   - Anti-embolic stockings should be worn for 23 hours and 30 minutes per day
   - The stockings can be removed for 30 minutes in a 24-hour period to permit washing
   - At the same time observe to ascertain that the circulation and sensation are adequate, being alert for pressure sores

(f) **Other Considerations[1]**
   - Apply clean stockings every 3 days, or before if soiled
   - Patients who are known to have MRSA should have their stockings changed at cessation of the decolonisation programme

(g) **On Discharge**
   - Patients/mothers must not be discharged with anti-embolic stockings unless medically indicated[2]

ADDICTIVE DISORDERS

16

Paul Moran and Madeleine Findlay

Royal Victoria Infirmary, Newcastle upon Tyne, UK

Medical Disorders in Pregnancy: A Manual for Midwives, Second Edition. Edited by S. Elizabeth Robson and Jason Waugh.
© 2013 John Wiley & Sons, Ltd. Published 2013 by John Wiley & Sons, Ltd.

16.1 Substance Misuse

Incidence	Risk for Childbearing
≥10% pregnant women screened positive for illicit substances[1-3]	Low to High Risk – depends on the substances used, dose and route of administration

EXPLANATION OF CONDITION

The misuse of drugs during pregnancy encompasses both legal and illegal substances, prescribed and non-prescribed. Nicotine and alcohol are also often overlooked but their detrimental effects on maternal and fetal wellbeing are additive and even in isolation can be considerably harmful.

Women misuse substances for a whole variety of reasons during pregnancy. Some lack awareness of the potential harm it may cause, some are struggling against a psychological or physical dependency, some choose to continue to use substances but many are under pressure to use from their partners and restrictive social network.

Health is also compromised indirectly by the attendant risk-taking behaviour, neglect and adverse socioeconomic factors.

Many will fear stigmatisation from professionals or from family members if the drug use is disclosed. Revealing the extent of substance misuse risks social care involvement which many will simply view as increasing the risk of the baby 'being taken into care' after birth. This perception is in stark contrast to the professional's aim which is that all professionals aim to maximise the chances of the mother and partner safely parenting the child together.

Other barriers to accessing healthcare include:

- Misinterpreting the early symptoms of pregnancy as relating to drug use or withdrawal
- Mistakenly believing pregnancy is not possible due to drug use
- Guilt about current or past substance misuse and many women have used drugs or alcohol before pregnancy is confirmed
- A lack of awareness of the mainstream and specialist services and help available
- Psychiatric co-morbidity and drug-induced mental health problems, depression, psychosis, lethargy
- Arranging child care
- The cost of transport
- Chaotic lifestyle

Nevertheless, many women will be able to stop drug and alcohol use once pregnant and a further proportion will be able to limit their use. Even in those who continue there is often sound, simple and practical advice that can minimise the potential for harm. Pregnancy is seen as a catalyst for change and is a window of opportunity for health professionals. Whilst a minority of women may not be interested in harm reduction for themselves they are still likely to wish to protect their child[4].

COMPLICATIONS

- High risk health and social behaviours, whether current or past each contribute to vulnerability

- Injecting drug use can lead to infection, blood-borne viruses, thromboembolism and poor venous access
- Difficulties with informed consent if under the influence of drugs or alcohol at appointments
- Anaemia, malnutrition, under-nutrition and poor dental health
- Co-existing mental health problems particularly anxiety and depression[5]
- Social problems and housing difficulties with transient lifestyles
- Strong correlation between substance use and domestic abuse both current and historic[6-8]
- Social exclusion. Saving Mothers Lives 2007 highlighted that socially excluded women are at higher risk of death during or after pregnancy than other women[9]
- Complications specific to each drug (see later sections)

NON-PREGNANCY TREATMENT AND CARE

Education about the implications of pregnancy for mother and baby made available at various points of contact. Ensure contraceptive needs are met with clear responsibilities agreed and shared between the obstetric team, drug treatment providers and general practioners. Inconsistent or poor engagement with services

Harm minimisation[10]:

- Accessing any antenatal care
- Stabilising drug use
- Engaging with treatment services
- Where possible arrange for substitute prescribing
- Avoiding the intravenous route
- Using needle exchanges and not sharing needles
- Give contraceptive advice and encourage safe sex practices

PRE-CONCEPTION ISSUES AND CARE

Pregnancy is often unplanned. Consider all contact as an opportunity for pre-pregnancy counselling with harm minimisation as above.

- Offer information about the potential effects of substance misuse on her unborn baby[5]
- Liaison with specialist midwives if pregnancy planned
- Review prescribed medication with the future pregnancy in mind. Simplify multidrug regimens if possible

Pregnancy Issues
These are high risk pregnancies and from the outset there should be a named consultant for maternity care with expertise working with women who use drugs and alcohol[10].

Medical Management and Care[5]
- Use open and honest confidential questioning
- Provide regular surveillance with obstetric and midwifery team and assertive follow-up if non-engagement
- Serial scans from 28 weeks for fetal growth
- Information on the potential effects of substance misuse on the unborn baby and what to expect when the baby is born
- Offer referral to a substance misuse programme if indicated
- Offer referral to nutrition worker and consider supplementation of diet

Midwifery Management and Care[5]
- An empathetic service will enhance attendance[11]
- Take a comprehensive history to include health and social risk factors
- There should be a dedicated midwifery liaison post for continuity of care
- Work closely with substance misuse teams and community staff
- Offer support and information on the benefits of stability in drug use
- Be realistic about expectations and accept that abstinence does not always immediately improve the maternal situation
- Be aware that withdrawal from drugs can significantly impair capacity to tolerate stress or anxiety[12]
- Accept that the details given may not be entirely accurate
- Think about domestic violence and the significance of the partner in the women's ability to engage with services[6]
- Ensure that the substance use doesn't become the whole focus of encounters which can deflect from holistic assessment of midwifery care
- Work with local services to deliver a programme of parent education tailored to meet the client's needs
- Understand that safeguarding the baby begins at conception and early intervention and support is appropriate

Labour Issues
Specific issues will depend on the substances used and are addressed in later sections. Please see appropriate sections for individual risk factors.
- More likely to present in advanced labour or deliver unattended if chaotic drug use
- Less likely to have support for labour
- Fluctuating levels of consciousness depending on recent drug use will impact upon the comprehension of labour events

Multidisciplinary Management and Care
- Provide clear information in labour as less likely to have planned choices
- Support of clients and use a non-judgemental approach
- Be alert to any child protection concerns and plans
- Ensure informed consent for care planning for labour
- Provide support as often women are ill prepared for labour and birth
- Be sensitive to the woman's emotional state and potential difficulties in cases where child is to be placed with alternative carers after birth
- Act as woman's advocate and work on a basis of mutual trust

Postpartum Issues

Infant Safeguarding:
- Instigate programmes of education and support before the baby is born
- Encourage the future parents to set realistic goals
- Consider the added pressure of being parents on the parent's ability to remain drug free or stable on substitute medication
- Postpartum relapse rates are high and continuing support is very important
- Not all families need referral to social care but offer support following assessment
- Accurate and timely information and support throughout helps with safe decision-making and engagement with services
- Role of the male partner or absent father can be overlooked to the detriment of the assessment
- Do not presume abstinence will improve parenting skills as some parents use substance to maintain equilibrium[12]
- For a structured approach to care, use a formal assessment framework (see Appendix 16.1.1)
- Ensure relevant health care professionals are informed once the postnatal care plan is agreed

Medical Management and Care
- Use alternatives to drugs of abuse wherever possible.
- Women who misuse opiates develop tolerance to the analgesic effects rapidly
- Further opiate analgesia can be given postpartum but substitutes can usually be found
- Involve anaesthetic colleagues early for postpartum pain relief advice
- Clear, open discussion about family planning appropriate with follow-up

Midwifery Management and Care
- Support safe care of the infant
- Encourage the mother to care for baby whenever possible
- Breast-feeding as for all women and babies has many benefits not least the nutritional value, immunological benefits, maternal-child bonding and reduction of SIDS
- In the UK the only absolute contra-indication to breast-feeding is HIV positive status. However, chaotic and persistent drug use will impair conscious levels and affect the mother's ability to commit to successful breast-feeding
- Encourage breast-feeding if the mother is stable on prescribed medication and abstinent from illicit drug use
- In the immediate hours and days after delivery maternal exhaustion may compromise effective breast-feeding
- Use the full post-natal inpatient stay to teach and assess parenting skills

16.2 Alcohol Addiction

Incidence	**Risk for Childbearing**
>90% of UK population drink alcohol to some extent[1]	Variable
A third of women cease alcohol use when pregnancy is confirmed.	
The remainder cut down, but 1% drink more than 14 units per week[2]	

EXPLANATION OF CONDITION

Although legal, the social use of alcohol can evolve into dependency and even moderate levels of drinking in pregnancy may be harmful. Whilst the long -term health risks of alcohol misuse can seem distant, pregnancy can bring the associated risks sharply into focus and provides an opportunity for intervention.

The NHS recommends that non-pregnant women should not drink more than 2–3 alcohol units daily. Fifteen percent regularly drink more than this and overall rates of alcohol use have increased most rapidly amongst women[3,4].

During pregnancy the Royal College of Obstetricians and Gynaecologists recommend limiting use to 1–2 units taken 1–2 per week[5]. Whilst there is no conclusive evidence that drinking alcohol within this limit is harmful there is widespread confusion over the number of units within each drink and the clearest message is to recommend abstinence during pregnancy[3].

Box 16.2.1 Examples of Alcohol by Volume

1 litre of spirits, e.g. vodka, whisky, rum, gin with an AbV between 37.5% and 40% will contain 37.5–40 units
1 litre bottle of 12.5% wine will contain 12.5 units
500 ml bottle of beer 4.5% will contain 2.25 units
500 ml can of cider 4.5% will contain 2.25 units

Box 16.2.1 gives examples of how the number of units of alcohol relates to both the amount and the strength (AbV) of each drink.

COMPLICATIONS

Maternal Complications

- Alcohol intoxification leads progressively to disorientation, loss of consciousness and respiratory depression
- The effects are potentiated if accompanied by illicit drug use
- Vomiting and risk of aspiration
- Impaired fertility
- Obesity
- Domestic violence, social and financial harm
- Sexual risk taking and unwanted pregnancy
- Long-term risks include increased risk of head, neck, throat cancer; breast cancer risk increased up to 50%, liver cirrhosis, and hypertension

Fetal Alcohol Spectrum Disorder

In Western countries fetal alcohol spectrum disorder affects just under 1% of pregnancies and has been reported with apparently moderate amounts of alcohol[6]. Features include:

- Facial features are characteristic – subtle facial features of the condition such as a smooth philtrum, thin upper lip and flattened nasal bridge[2,8]. You will see from the list below that these features alone are unlikely to be the main concern and will often go unnoticed
- Disproportionately low height to weight

- Intellectual impairment
  - Structural brain anomalies such as agenesis of the corpus callosum and microcephaly
  - Poor language and comprehension skills, poor abstraction, memory, attention and judgement
- Increase rate of cardiac defects
- Behavioural difficulties
- Poor social skills persist and lead to secondary disabilities later in life that include:
  - depression
  - running away
  - anger and aggression
  - low self-esteem
  - mental health problems (90%)
  - disrupted school experience (60% of those over 12 years)
  - trouble with crime (60% charged or convicted)
  - substance abuse (30% over 12 years)
  - dependent living (over 80% 21 years and older are in dependent living situation)

NON-PREGNANCY TREATMENT AND CARE

- Provide information on long- and short-term effects of alcohol use
- Identify simple measures that can reduce or eliminate intake
- Those who abuse alcohol rarely drink weak alcoholic drinks
- Reduce units by substituting some alcohol for a mixer. e.g. adding soda to wine, lemonade to lager. This will mean the person can still have four 'drinks' but the number of units will decrease
- Address behavioural triggers for alcohol use
- Identify whether there is tolerance
- Identify whether there is dependency
- Once dependency has developed there is a risk of withdrawal if alcohol use is stopped suddenly
- Detoxification requires an individualised plan and multidisciplinary involvement with local treatment services. Admission to hospital for detoxification is often necessary

PRE-CONCEPTION ISSUES AND CARE

- Women need to be advised of the long-term health problems caused by alcohol
- The risk of fetal alcohol syndrome is as high as one in three at >18 units alcohol per day[5]. However, it also occurs with lower consumption: there is no proven safe drinking threshold
- Recognise that many of the children affected by alcohol in pregnancy will not manifest with a complete clinical diagnosis of fetal alcohol syndrome, but will exhibit some of the features particularly learning difficulties, behavioural and psychological symptoms. The broader term fetal alcohol spectrum disorder captures a continuum of permanent birth defects due to alcohol some of which will be quite subtle[5,7,8]
- Fetal alcohol spectrum disorder affects 1% of all newborns making it the leading cause of 'preventable' birth defects

Pregnancy Issues

There is no proven safe alcohol limit during pregnancy and abstinence is advised.

- Binge drinking may be especially harmful as is sustained, regular heavy drinking
- Miscarriage
- Pre-term delivery (doubled by heavy drinking)
- Growth restriction
- Fetal alcohol spectrum disorder
- Consider the partner and who may be a stabilising (or destabilising influence)
- Child protection issues (if any) should be addressed antenatally and a clear post-partum plan devised

Withdrawal: sudden withdrawal with dependency produces anxiety, sweating, trembling and delirium. Acute withdrawal may result in convulsions and death.

Medical Management and Care

As a high risk pregnancy, care is led by a Consultant Obstetrician with expertise in substance misuse in pregnancy. Key issues are:

- Serial growth scans: note particularly third trimester head circumference
- Gamma-GT (GGT)
- As part of the liver function test serial GGT measurements can be used to monitor alcohol use in much the same way that an HbA1C gives an indication of diabetic control. Measuring GGT is a tangible way of providing feedback to women and demonstrating a positive effect if alcohol consumption is reduced or discontinued. GGT, however, is a relatively insensitive marker and a normal GGT at booking may fail to highlight women who continue to drink
- FBC. Evidence of long-term alcohol misuse may result in a macrocytic anaemia (increased MCV)

Midwifery Management and Care

- Provide information on the effects of alcohol use in pregnancy to every pregnant woman and be prepared to discuss the impact of alcohol on the unborn baby
- Be alert to making assumptions on alcohol use based on culture, ethnicity or social class
- Assess every pregnant woman for alcohol use in pregnancy and be aware of local referral pathways
- Be alert for any child protection issues

Labour Issues

Alcohol is not tocolytic, it does not stop contractions or prevent pre-term labour which is a widely held mistaken belief.

Standard intrapartum guidelines are used.

Medical Management and Care

- Prior to labour the birth plan should be reviewed
- It is helpful to discuss views on treatment and investigations antenatally as intoxication may impair consent when labour starts

Midwifery Management and Care

- Fetal growth restriction may be present and continuous CTG monitoring is warranted
- Anaesthetic review if intoxicated, because of risk of further analgesia and respiratory depression

Postpartum Issues

If women have hidden their alcohol dependency and then stay in hospital for longer than they expected, they may present with features of withdrawal.

If a woman is known to be alcohol dependent forward planning should be made to prevent withdrawal occurring.

Medical Management and Care

- Where women have found it difficult to reduce or stop alcohol intake during the pregnancy offer further support and follow-up
- For those at risk of long-term health problems offer hepatitis C and BCG vaccinations
- Neonatal review is indicated but a diagnosis of fetal alcohol spectrum disorder cannot be confidently made in the neonate

Midwifery Management and Care

- Ideally social, financial and psychological issues will have been identified antenatally and support can continue into the postnatal period
- If a woman is suspected to be withdrawing from alcohol it is important to get a clear sensitive history of how much she has been drinking in order to offer medication and support if appropriate
- An extended postnatal stay offers the chance for parenting skills to be reviewed and supported

16.3 Tobacco and Cannabis Use

Incidence	Risk for Childbearing
Tobacco – 33% smoked in the 12 months before/during pregnancy; half cease, then only 10% of the remainder reduce the amount[1–3] Cannabis – 3.5% in pregnancy[4]	Mother – Low to Moderate Fetus – Low to Moderate

EXPLANATION OF CONDITION

Cannabis is the most commonly used illicit drug in pregnancy, estimated at 3.5%[4] but under-reporting renders percentage estimates and pattern of use in pregnancy as unreliable.

Cigarette smoking in adults is addictive and while legal and socially acceptable in some communities it remains the greatest single preventable cause of illness and premature death in the UK[5].

Smoking amongst women has continued to rise over the last decade and this is reflected in high rates of smoking whilst pregnant despite advice to stop and an increasing awareness of the associated health risks.

Women who use illicit substances are more likely to smoke tobacco. The impact of smoking, however, can easily be overlooked although it has the potential to cause as much direct harm through maternal ill health and placental damage as the illicit substances themselves.

Almost all women who smoke cannabis also smoke tobacco and this is a major confounder when analysing the effects of cannabis on the pregnancy and after birth. Cannabis may be smoked with tobacco as a 'joint', or inhaled through a pipe or 'bong'. Occasionally it may be baked and eaten within cakes or biscuits. Cannabis comes in several forms: a resin (hash or hashish); dried leaves (marijuana, grass or weed); 'skunk' is its strongest form. The effects are immediate and last for one or more hours. Cannabis strength has increased over recent years and placental transfer to the fetus of the active cannaboids is one-third that of the maternal plasma levels[6].

COMPLICATIONS

Smoking tobacco increases the risk of infant mortality by an estimated 40% due to:

- Fetal growth restriction
- Placental abruption
- Pre-term labour
- Stillbirth
- SIDS

Both SIDS and growth restriction are directly correlated to the amount smoked. The increase of SIDS and neonatal death may be attributed both to smoking in pregnancy but also to exposure after birth by either parent or carer. The Foundation for the Study of Infant Deaths (FSID) estimated that in the UK if no woman smoked in pregnancy over 100 babies each year could be saved[7].

Smoking cannabis:

- Cannabis does not appear to increase the risk of low birth weight, pre-term delivery or placental abruption beyond the risk of any concurrent tobacco use[8]

- Cannabis has been shown to increase anxiety, panic and paranoia and can lead to dependence
- Cannabis increases the likelihood of developing a psychotic illness where there is a family history

Smoking tobacco

- Women who smoke are at increased risk of chest infections, respiratory problems and DVT
- Smoking cigarettes does not alter consciousness. However, smoking cannabis or other drugs does so and needs to be factored in to any assessment of parenting

NON-PREGNANCY TREATMENT AND CARE

The NICE public health guideline on smoking suggests everyone who smokes should be advised to stop unless there are exceptional circumstances[9]. This guidance may be downloaded at www.nice.org.uk/nicemedia/live/11375/31864/31864.pdf

In the UK the NHS Stop Smoking Service has a comprehensive menu of services and support available to people who wish to stop and the public health guideline outlines the process.

If a woman is smoking cannabis, she should be offered referral to a specialist stop smoking advisor or a substance misuse treatment centre as she may anticipate increased challenges in stopping use.

PRE-CONCEPTION ISSUES AND CARE

- The current UK position is clear and any woman planning a pregnancy should be encouraged and supported to stop smoking
- For women who do not wish to stop smoking advice should be given and appropriate information offered by a specialist advisor

Pregnancy Issues

All pregnant women who have used tobacco in the past 2 weeks should be referred to the NHS Stop Smoking service[10]. Although the primary care team are often best placed to raise the issue, their input cannot be assumed and further discussion continues to highlight the health benefits of stopping or reducing smoking.

Medical Management and Care
- Nicotine replacement therapy (NRT) is only recommended if other interventions have failed. Evidence surrounding the use of NRT is mixed, but there is currently no convincing evidence that it is effective or improves birth weight
- A 2-week course is prescribed solely for daytime use. The prescription is only repeated if concurrent smoking has ceased[10]

Midwifery Management and Care
- The community midwife should follow the NICE guideline in early discussion and appropriately monitor carbon monoxide readings from the first visit and refer to the stop smoking service
- Inform about the risks associated with smoking in pregnancy and exposure to second hand smoke, including the health message to stop rather than cut down
- If a woman is also dependent on other substances, sometimes stopping smoking is the only thing she feels she can do for her baby and the benefits of doing so should be highlighted and encouraged
- Studies have shown that motivational interviewing, structured self-help and support from stop smoking services and cognitive behavioural therapy are all effective interventions in pregnancy
- Evidence also shows that giving pregnant women feedback on the effects of smoking on their health and that of the fetus is not an effective tool in smoking cessation although giving informed choice[10]
- If a woman is smoking cannabis then safeguarding assessment and information should be available from the outset and safety planning commenced. It needs to be considered that while cannabis use is very common in some communities, use to the point of intoxication when in charge of a child is a safeguarding issue. Use of cannabis is to be discouraged and abstinence encouraged
- Bed sharing should be discouraged due to the increased risk of SIDS[11]
- All of the advice and the benefits from smoking cessation also apply to partners

Labour Issues

Although used for its relaxing properties cannabis can increase heart rate and produce hypertension.

Women under the influence of cannabis may be panicky, suspicious and anxious and have poor co-ordination.

Occasionally it may invoke a short-lived psychotic state with delusions and confusion.

Of those who use cannabis 10% become dependent on the drug and experience physical withdrawal symptoms similar to nicotine withdrawal. These symptoms may present in labour or postpartum.

Medical Management and Care
- Care should be managed as for any other woman
- Recent cannabis use may impair alertness and concentration and therefore the ability to consent to treatment
- If there is fetal growth restriction then continuous CTG monitoring is appropriate

Midwifery Management and Care
- All smoking should be discouraged once labour has commenced
- Remain supportive throughout
- Refer to medical staff if concerned about cannabis use and maternal mental health or if evidence of maternal withdrawal

Postpartum Issues

SIDS
Sudden unexpected infant death in the first 2 years of life affects approximately 1 in 2000 babies born in the UK. There is now strong evidence that the advice given in Appendix 16.3.1 can reduce (but not eliminate) the risk of SIDS[8].

Breast-Feeding
- Milk production may be reduced by smoking[12]
- If cigarette smoking continues the benefits of breast-feeding still outweigh the potential for harm

If cannabis use continues then active cannaboids are present in breast milk. Also, cannabis induces drowsiness and impairs safe parenting skills.

Medical Management and Care
- Craving for cigarettes can lead to early mobilisation and this can risk wound breakdown after caesarean section
- Smoking is an independent risk factor for thromboembolism; if immobilisation after operative delivery is expected then thrombopropyhlaxis is indicated

Midwifery Management and Care
- Relapse rates are high so postnatal support and encouragement is crucial for the mother in her efforts to continue to stop smoking[10]
- Almost half of all children are exposed to tobacco smoke in the home. Continue to provide information on the benefits of remaining smoke free
- Advise against co-sleeping and bed sharing from the outset and explain the risks involved
- Provide written information on reducing the risk of SIDS or 'cot death'[11]
- Strongly advise against smoking cannabis to aid sleep
- Cannabis use has the potential to affect judgement and mental functioning therefore extended stay on the postnatal area may benefit any parenting assessment

16.4 Cocaine Addiction

Incidence	Risk for Childbearing
Cocaine powder use (2.4%) was second only to cannabis use (6.6%) in the UK 2009–2010 British Crime Survey	Variable Risk

EXPLANATION OF CONDITION

Cocaine was the only class of drug in which use increased from 1996 to 2010[1]. In its commonest form, cocaine hydrochloride is a creamy white powder that is then chopped into a finer powder to snort through the nose or rub onto gums. The purity is rarely greater than 50% and white powders, such as glucose, may be used by suppliers to increase volume. Local anaesthetic drugs and amphetamines are also substituted as they are cheaper and mimic cocaine's numbing sensation on the nostril lining.

Cocaine may be injected producing almost immediate effects. It may be injected in combination with heroin as a 'speedball' with unpredictable results. To smoke cocaine it needs to be released from its base – 'freebasing'. One method mixes cocaine with sodium bicarbonate and when heated small but potent rocks of crack cocaine result.

All routes produce central nervous system stimulant effects resulting in arousal, exhilaration, indifference to pain and fatigue, wellbeing and mental alertness. These effects are intense but short-lived, lasting only 20–40 minutes with a strong compulsion to repeat the experience. Feeling of anxiety and panic may predominate especially during binges of quickly repeated doses. Cocaine is also used as a recreational drug associated with the 'party' scene. Increase in use can quickly lead to addiction. Regular users must take escalating amounts to derive the same effects and although physical dependency does not develop the psychological dependency, especially to crack cocaine, can be considerable.

Dose: episodic weekend use might be 0.25 g whilst daily use with sufficient resources can be 1–2 g.

Detection: cocaine metabolites can be identified in the urine for up to 3–5 days.

COMPLICATIONS

Severe maternal complications are rare but include:

- Cerebrovascular accident, including subarachnoid and intracerebral haemorrhage and cerebral infarcts
- Cardiovascular complications, myocardial infarction, ventricular arrhythmias and cardiac arrest
- Intestinal ischemia
- Respiratory failure

Chronic maternal complications

General: hypertension, tachycardia, anorexia, nausea, weight loss, malnutrition, dehydration, tremor, severe depression and isolated convulsions. Anaesthetic effects can lead to increased risk of physical harm; numbness on the mucus membranes of the vagina can lead to an increased risk of tears and therefore a greater risk of contracting HIV/Hep C.

Smoking: haemoptysis, black sputum, chest pains, lung damage.

Snorting: loss of smell, increased susceptibility to upper respiratory tract infections, sinusitis, erosions and nasal perforations.

Injecting: local abscess formation, the injecting site becomes anaesthetised, veins collapsing and increased risk-taking behaviour. There is also an increased risk of septicaemia due to impaired immune system.

Psychiatric co-morbidity: psychosis with coexisting substance misuse can be especially challenging[2]. Forty percent of stimulant users have psychiatric symptoms. With chronic use it is the unwanted psychological effects that persist: anxiety and agitation, insomnia, persecutory beliefs, psychotic illnesses classically indistinguishable from schizophrenia, depression and suicidal ideation.

NON-PREGNANCY TREATMENT AND CARE

Cocaine is frequently misused with other stimulants as well as alcohol. Persistent use is associated with a variety of other substances to counteract the over-activity, agitation and other adverse effects of stimulants. Over time users can acquire complex multiple dependencies. Substitute prescribing is not available for cocaine and users may not engage with treatment services. Some can and do stop use when pregnant with no perceived ill effects. Polydrug users, however, or those with long standing and heavy use are unlikely to be successful unless the underlying causes of drug taking are explored.

In the UK cocaine is a class 'A' drug carrying a maximum custodial sentence for possession of 7 years and an unlimited fine. The maximum penalty for cocaine supply or dealing is life and an unlimited fine.

PRE-CONCEPTION ISSUES AND CARE

Cocaine misuse is especially risky during pregnancy and an understanding of the implications may provide motivation to change. Cocaine metabolism is reduced in pregnancy and it easily diffuses across the placenta to the fetus which has only a limited capacity to metabolise cocaine.

Take a full drug history, determine the level of cocaine use (as frequency and cost) and whether smoked, injected, snorted or ingested. Explore how the drug use is funded. The history is likely to reveal additional complex needs including social, financial, housing needs, as well as criminal and risk taking behaviour.

Harm reduction: abstinence is recommended. Abstinence is safe and physical withdrawal symptoms if they occur at all will be mild. If abstinence is unlikely then the intravenous route should be replaced by other routes. Needles and syringes should never be shared. Cocaine should not be taken with alcohol or other drugs.

Pregnancy Issues

It is rare for cocaine to be the only substance misused and the effects of other drugs as well as smoking, alcohol, poor diet, general physical health and risk taking behaviour all need to be considered.
- Not thought to be teratogenic
- Miscarriage
- Abruption (approximately fourfold increase)[3]
- Low birth weight <2500 g (approximately twofold increase)[4]

The potential fetal effects have been extensively studied. Of 33 studies, only the risk of abruption and premature rupture of the membranes (but not preterm delivery) were statistically associated with cocaine use itself. Many of the other adverse outcomes were attributable to multiple confounders[5].

The prospective Maternal Life Style Study followed over 700 infants exposed to cocaine *in utero*. They found no increased risk of congenital anomalies but all growth parameters were affected[6]. These children were also 49 times more likely to be involved with child protection services and 17 times more likely to be placed into foster care. Of all growth parameters, head circumference is the most consistently reduced but this does not appear to lead to associated deficits at 3 years[7]; instead it is the home environment that is a better predictor of long-term development[8].

Early fears of a 'crack syndrome' have not been realised. Many findings once thought to be specific effects of *in utero* cocaine exposure can be explained in whole or in part by other factors, including pre-natal exposure to nicotine, cannabis, or alcohol as well as the quality of the child's environment.

Medical Management and Care

Overdose:
- Overdose is a risk. Purity fluctuates and the metabolism of cocaine not only varies between individuals, but is variably reduced in pregnancy. Similarly polydrug use produces unpredictable results
- Binge use lasting longer than 24 hours is especially hazardous[9]

If you know or fear that a woman has ingested a large amount of cocaine then she needs to be taken to the Accident and Emergency services as quickly as possible. Treatment with 50–100 g of activated charcoal is recommended within 1 hour of ingesting and the patient closely observed.

Withdrawal:
- Cocaine withdrawal is not life threatening to mother or fetus. However, babies can exhibit symptoms of withdrawal which are unpleasant. But as cocaine is rarely taken in isolation close monitoring and extreme caution is required with evidence of neonatal withdrawal
- Hallucinations may occur as part of withdrawal, but are more commonly seen during intoxication

Multidisciplinary Management and Midwifery Care
- Encourage early engagement with all aspects of antenatal care
- As these are high risk pregnancies care should be led by a consultant obstetrician with expertise in substance misuse
- A non-judgemental approach across the team is crucial
- Document all drug use, frequency, cost and administration route
- Inform of the risks of the drug taking and the unpredictable effects on the pregnancy
- Consider the role and influence of the partner
- Advise that all cocaine use should cease
- Toxicology screen is obtained with consent wherever possible
- Additional STD screening may be indicated
- Serial fetal growth scans offered
- Determine whether there is current or previous involvement with treatment agencies and psychiatric services. Refer as appropriate
- Explore the need for social care and previous involvement of social care services
- The anaesthetist and neonatal team need to be aware

Labour Issues

Care during labour may follow standard pregnancy guidelines. There may be placental insufficiency and fetal growth restriction so continuous CTG monitoring is warranted.

Medical Management and Care
- Deliver in consultant led unit
- Inform anaesthetist and neonatal team
- Analgesic requirements

Midwifery Management and Care
- Care follows standard intrapartum midwifery guidelines
- CTG interpretation is unaltered. Although cocaine may reduce long-term variability and lessen the frequency of accelerations there is no consistent effect on the CTG
- Opiates may be used and there is no contraindication to an epidural. Discuss pain relief early with the mother and the anaesthetist

Postpartum Issues

A clear postpartum care plan should be in place during the antenatal period and the women fully informed of its requirements. The plan needs to consider:
- There is a risk of withdrawal, the baby may be jittery, agitated and be difficult to manage (Appendix 16.4.1)
- Child protection issues (if any)

Medical Management and Care
- Postpartum analgesia can follow standard guidelines
- Neonatal review prior to discharge

Midwifery Management and Care
- Mother and baby should remain together and supported on the postnatal ward wherever possible
- If abstinent then breast-feeding is to be encouraged
- A 4–5 day postnatal stay is helpful. This is an opportunity to establish care and feeding routines and address any new or unexpected concerns, particularly if the baby is unsettled
- Inform all necessary professionals of the delivery and discharge plan so that seamless care continues into the community setting

16.5 Opiate Addiction

Incidence	Risk for Childbearing
Use varied between 0.3 and 0.1% over the previous year in the British Crime Survey 2009–2010[1]	Variable Risk

EXPLANATION OF CONDITION

Misuse of opiates as a group includes not only heroin (diamorphine) but also prescribed medications (codeine phosphate, dihydrocodeine and tramadol) and the substitution treatments buprenorphine and methadone. Heroin powder may be heated and the fumes smoked, swallowed (rarely), sniffed like cocaine powder or dissolved in water and injected. Injection provides the most intense effect – the 'rush'. Heavy or chronic users usually inject.

All opiates are analgesic. At high doses they produce detachment, relaxation, euphoria and eventually sedation[2]. Tolerance can develop after a few weeks requiring increasing amounts for the same effect or conversion from smoking to the intravenous route. Eventually little effect is obtained from further use and use persists merely to feel 'normal' and prevent the features of withdrawal.

Polydrug use is common. Other cheaper depressants such as benzodiazepines and alcohol are used to ameliorate the effects of fluctuating heroin use.

Dose: heroin is sold rarely purer than 50%. A small bag might cost £20 and contain a 0.25 g dose used gradually over a day.

COMPLICATIONS

Much of the harm caused by opiates is linked to the associated lifestyle, the need to fund drug use and the inherent risks of intravenous administration.

General: poor nutrition, apathy, self-neglect, poor dentition, constipation

Injecting: abscess formation at injection sites, deep vein thrombosis, thromboembolism, septicaemia, endocarditis, blood-borne infections HIV and hepatitis.

Smoking: respiratory infections, 'asthma'.

Respiratory depression presents the greatest risk of mortality. Fortunately tolerance also develops to the respiratory depressant effects, but fatal dosage can occur if there has been a drug-free period and use reverts to their prior level of use.

NON-PREGNANCY TREATMENT AND CARE

Although users wish to avoid the physical symptoms of withdrawal they usually underplay the importance of the psychological features of dependency. Successful treatment of opiate addiction needs to address these psychological needs as well as the complex social and habitual behavioural patterns that are the background to the drug taking.

As a highly addictive drug, a significant proportion of heroin abuse leads to dependence. Treatment services are able to encourage and support abstinence or offer substitute prescribing with methadone. The dosage is titrated against symptoms to achieve a maintenance dose. The maintenance dose may be subsequently taken all at once or as divided doses during the day. For those who are well motivated gradual dose reductions are used to detoxify or, more usually, the maintenance dose may continue to prevent relapse. The majority of people will rely upon methadone maintenance for a number of years and the common misconception that it is a short-term solution leading to rapid abstinence is unrealistic. Methadone has a longer half-life than heroin; it does not provide euphoria or other pleasurable effects but does act as an analgesic. Tolerance develops to its analgesic, euphoric, sedative, respiratory depressant and nauseating effects but not the constipating effect. Methadone withdrawal starts at 24–48 hours, peaks at 3–21 days and lasts up to 6–7 weeks[3].

Buprenorphine is increasingly used as an alternative to methadone. It is a partial opiate agonist/antagonist. A recent Cochrane review compared 24 randomised clinical trials of buprenorphine maintenance versus placebo or methadone maintenance. Buprenorphine was superior to placebo in retention of patients in treatment at all doses However, only medium and high dose buprenorphine suppressed heroin use significantly above placebo[4].

PRE-CONCEPTION ISSUES AND CARE

- A non-judgemental approach is vital[5]
- Determine the pattern and type of drug misuse. Note the frequency and route of each substance used. Heroin use can be usefully documented in terms of cost per day
- Identify current links with other agencies and inform the client of the range of support services and help that is locally available
- Give clear information of the potential risks of persistent drug taking on a future pregnancy
- It is natural to hope to be free of opiates by the end of the pregnancy and many women will request detoxification. This may not be achievable, however, and stabilisation on prescribed substitute medication is usually the more realistic option
- Referral to treatment agencies is encouraged to allow an approach tailored to the woman's needs
- Supervision of detoxification or maintenance treatment is the role of the treatment agency
- Substitute prescribing negates the health risks of a chaotic lifestyle and direct risks of injecting or smoking heroin
- Offer screening for blood-borne viruses and be open and honest about the reasons for screening and treatment options available in pregnancy and in the postnatal period
- As for all pre-conception care, address any other health care concerns

Pregnancy Issues
- Opiates are not teratogenic
- Prematurity rates are increased
- Low birth weight rates are increased
- Acute fetal withdrawal risks stillbirth
- Neonatal abstinence syndrome may occur

Because of the risk of fetal withdrawal pregnant women should not abruptly stop their opiate use. Unsupervised withdrawal is discouraged as it risks miscarriage or preterm delivery.

Withdrawal: physical symptoms of heroin withdrawal resemble bad flu starting 8–24 hours after the missed dose. Symptoms improve after 7–10 days. Abrupt withdrawal is not life threatening to the mother, but must be avoided in pregnancy as it can precipitate fatal withdrawal in the fetus.

Overdose: overdose may result from
- Loss of tolerance when restarting use after a period of abstinence
- Heroin more concentrated than expected
- The combination of opiates with other respiratory depressants
- Injecting rather than smoking heroin

Respiratory support is required in overdose. Naloxone should not be given to reverse the opiate effects as it may precipitate fetal distress.

Medical Management and Care
- Care should be led by a consultant with expertise in substance misuse
- Substitute prescribing is well documented as beneficial during pregnancy and initially aims for stabilisation on an individualised maintenance dose[6,7]
- A stepwise sequence of harm minimisation can follow which involves switching away from intravenous heroin use to smoking, reducing risk taking behaviour and engagement with treatment services
- Once stabilised, treatment agencies may consider detoxification for highly motivated individuals who have stopped all additional substance misuse[8]

Multidisciplinary Management and Midwifery Care
- Consider the role and influence of the partner
- Toxicology screen is obtained with consent wherever possible and the results discussed in an open non-judgmental way with clients
- Additional STD screening may be indicated and one needs to be mindful of the possibility of continued high risk sexual behaviours in order to fund illicit drug use which is often hidden from support services
- Serial fetal growth scans offered from 28 weeks
- Determine whether there is current or previous involvement with treatment agencies and psychiatric services. Refer into treatment services as appropriate
- Treatment agencies should lead on substitute prescribing
- Methadone maintenance is the preferred option during pregnancy as detoxification is unsuccessful in all but the most motivated and carries the risk of relapse[9-11]. Too low a maintenance dose risks additional drug use on top and high-dose regimens do not appear to increase the risk of neonatal abstinence syndrome. The methadone dose may need to be increased as pregnancy progresses due to increased hepatic clearance[12]

Labour Issues
Devise delivery care plan antenatally.
- Need for social care and social care services should have already been addressed
- Anaesthetist and neonatal team to be aware
- Care during labour may follow standard pregnancy guidelines. There may be placental insufficiency and fetal growth restriction so continuous CTG monitoring is warranted

Analgesia: opiates are not contra-indicated but receptors may be saturated so opiate analgesia is less effective. Opiate misuse itself will not provide adequate analgesia for labour.

Medical Management and Care
- Deliver in consultant led unit
- Inform anaesthetist and consider analgesic requirements
- Continue substitute medication (confirm dose with usual prescriber)

Midwifery Management and Care
- Care follows standard intrapartum midwifery guidelines
- CTG interpretation is unaltered
- Opiates may be used and there is no contraindication to an epidural. Discuss pain relief early with the mother and the anaesthetist
- There is no evidence that intramuscular opiate use for labour analgesia will precipitate relapse of drug misuse
- It is important to continue with any prescribed opiate replacement. This will not provide analgesia and is in addition to any analgesic requirements

Postpartum Issues
Risk of neonatal withdrawal is 1 in 3. Risk is not strongly linked to antenatal opiate or substitute dose but may increase with chaotic use. A clear postpartum care plan should be in place during the antenatal period, which should consider:
- Child protection issues (if any)
- Contact details for all services involved and a clear plan of care and liaison is essential
- The likely postnatal opiate substitute dose – typically the pre-pregnancy dose
- Arrangements for uninterrupted substitute prescribing need to continue when in hospital and after discharge to prevent withdrawal or conversely duplication of prescription
- Indicate the arrangements for contraception and involve community outreach services

Medical Management and Care
- Postpartum analgesia can follow standard guidelines
- Neonatal review prior to discharge. Respiratory support is indicated rather than naloxone (Narcan) for neonatal respiratory depression after birth

Midwifery Management and Care
- Mother and baby should remain together and supported on the postnatal ward wherever possible
- Encourage breast-feeding if the mother is stable on prescribed medication
- A 4–5 day postnatal stay is helpful. This is an opportunity to establish care and feeding routines, identify early withdrawal symptoms and address any new or unexpected concerns
- Ensure the mother is aware of signs of neonatal withdrawal such as irritability and failure to settle after a feed
- Maternal Hepatitis B and BCG vaccines may be given
- Inform all necessary professionals of the agreed delivery and discharge plan so that seamless care continues into the community setting

16.6 Stimulant Addiction

Incidence	Risk for Childbearing
16–24 age group: amphetamines 2.4 %; amyl nitrate 3.2%; ecstasy 1.6%[1]	Maternal: Low to moderate with heavy use Fetal: Low risk (but extremely limited data)

EXPLANATION OF CONDITION

The British Crime Survey 2009–2010 reported that amphetamine use in the past year continues to fall from 3.6% in 1996 to 1.0% and methamphetamine use was less than 0.05%. Stimulant use, however, remains a concern for women of childbearing age.

Amphetamines (speed) and its crystalline form methamphetamine (ice) are synthetic compounds similar to the naturally occurring CNS neurotransmitter norepinephrine. They are manufactured illegally but also legally sold as Ritalin and Dexedrine. They may be smoked, dissolved in drinks or taken as a powder which is snorted or injected. They produce effects similar to adrenaline making the user feel more alert, energetic and exhilarated. They are also abused as appetite suppressants. Effects last a few hours but end in tiredness from which it can take days to recover. Prolonged use and high doses take their toll on mental health inducing anxiety, panic and psychosis[2].

Amyl and butyl nitrates are inhaled from a small bottle or popped open from a vial 'poppers'. They loosen inhibitions and boost the effects of other stimulants. They cause a 'rush' of vasodilatation and relax smooth muscle which can result in hypotension and collapse. The effects are immediate and last only a few minutes. Tolerance develops after a few weeks of continual use but is regained if discontinued for a few days.

Ecstasy or MDMA is a hallucinogenic amphetamine. One or two tablets are taken or may be crushed and snorted. Stimulant effects start within an hour and can last for several hours. Death has resulted although the precise mechanism remains unclear.

Psychological dependency to the effects of stimulant use can develop but there is no physical withdrawal syndrome other than the tiredness and hunger that has been postponed by the drug use.

Amphetamines share the vasoconstriction properties of cocaine which is covered in the section on cocaine addiction.

Dose: occasional use is 0.5 g amphetamine over a few weeks, heavy use with tolerance is up to several grams each day. Purity is low, typically 10% or less, so a 0.5 g wrap may only contain 50 mg amphetamine.

COMPLICATIONS

- Harm as a consequence of risk-taking behaviour whilst under the drug's influence
- Purity is low and intravenous use risks thrombophlebitis, thrombosis, ulcer and abscess formation, endocarditis and blood-borne viruses
- Weight loss and neglect
- Poor dentition particularly with methamphetamine (meth mouth)

- Psychological sequelae are usually short lived but may include dangerous delusions or suicidal ideation.
- Chronic heavy users are restless, with paranoia and anxiety symptoms possibly persisting for months
- Chronic use risks pulmonary hypertension and dilated cardiomyopathy

NON-PREGNANCY TREATMENT AND CARE

- Inform of the dangers of stimulant use
- Encourage engagement with treatment agencies
- Lifestyle and psychosocial interventions remain the key approach to address stimulant addiction
- There is no pharmacological substitute identified to treat stimulant dependence
- Antidepressants have been used to treat amphetamine withdrawal but none reported any significant benefit[3,4]

PRE-CONCEPTION ISSUES AND CARE

Growth restriction and neurological sequelae in the newborn are potential risks specific to stimulant use and pregnancy; this may provide motivation to change.

- Take a full drug history. Determine the level of use (as frequency and cost) and whether injected, snorted or ingested
- Explore how the drug use is funded
- The history is likely to reveal additional complex needs including social, financial, housing needs, as well as criminal and risk taking behaviour

Harm reduction: abstinence is recommended. Immediate abstinence is safe. There may be psychological reluctance to stop but physical withdrawal symptoms will not occur. If abstinence is unlikely then the intravenous route should be replaced by other routes, needles and syringes should never be shared and stimulants should not be taken with alcohol or other drugs.

Pregnancy Issues
- Growth restriction threefold increase[5]. Growth restriction is most pronounced if misuse is continued into the third trimester especially with concurrent nicotine use[6]. Maternal weight gain is encouraging but may be misleading as amphetamines suppress appetite and when stopped can lead to a rebound in maternal weight gain that is not always reflected in improved fetal weight[6].
- Neurotoxic effects[5]. Methamphetamine has a longer half-life potentially increasing the risk of newborn neurotoxic effects. Subtle neurological sequelae similar to those seen with cocaine and nicotine use have also been identified although there is no amphetamine 'syndrome' as such[7].
- Teratogenicity. Amphetamines are teratogenic when used in very high doses in animal studies. Convincing human evidence for teratogenicity is lacking, but a role in cardiac defects, talipes and cleft lip and palate have all been suggested[8]

Medical Management and Care
Withdrawal: treatment is supportive. On rare occasions symptomatic relief of severe agitation using short-acting benzodiazepines may be used. Withdrawal may be associated with severe depression and this should be monitored[3].

Overdose: acute overdose can result in seizures, hypertension, tachycardia, hyperthermia, psychosis, hallucinations, stroke, and fatality. Transfer to accident and emergency. Recent oral ingestion can be treated with activated charcoal; sedation, cardiovascular support and monitoring, and body cooling may all be required.

Multidisciplinary Management and Midwifery Care
- A non-judgemental approach across the team is crucial
- Encourage early engagement with all aspects of antenatal care
- As high risk pregnancies their care is led by a consultant obstetrician with expertise in substance misuse
- Document all drug use, frequency, cost and administration route
- Inform of the risks of the drug taking and advise abstinence
- Consider the role and influence of the partner
- Toxicology screen is obtained with consent wherever possible
- Additional STD screening may be indicated and serial fetal growth scans offered
- Determine whether there is current or previous involvement with treatment agencies and psychiatric services. Refer as appropriate
- Explore the need for social care and previous involvement of social care services
- Establish whether there are child protection concerns
- The neonatal team needs to be aware

Labour Issues
Care during labour may follow standard pregnancy guidelines. There may be unrecognised fetal growth restriction so continuous CTG monitoring is warranted.

Medical Management and Care
- Deliver in a consultant-led unit
- Inform neonatal team
- Analgesic requirements are unaltered
- Amphetamine-induced convulsions and hypertension have been mistaken for eclampsia[9]

Midwifery Management and Care
- Care follows standard intrapartum midwifery guidelines
- CTG interpretation is unaltered
- Opiates may be used and there is no contraindication to an epidural. Discuss pain relief early with the mother and the anaesthetist

Postpartum Issues
A clear postpartum care plan should be in place during the antenatal period and the women fully informed of its requirements.
The plan needs to consider:
- The risk of neonatal withdrawal
- Child protection issues (if any)

Medical Management and Care
- Postpartum analgesia can follow standard guidelines.
- Neonatal review prior to discharge

Midwifery Management and Care
- Mother and baby should remain together and supported on the postnatal ward wherever possible
- Breast-feeding is to be encouraged, unless there is on-going erratic drug use
- Neonatal withdrawal is usually mild restlessness and irritability
- A 4–5 day postnatal stay is helpful. This is an opportunity to establish care and feeding routines and address any new or unexpected concerns
- Inform all necessary professionals of the delivery and discharge plan so that seamless care continues into the community setting

16 Addictive Disorders

PATIENT ORGANISATIONS

http://www.lifelineproject.co.uk
Lifeline provides a range of drug and alcohol services and works alongside service users, communities and professionals. Lifeline has a track record of working alongside the hardest to reach client group.

http://www.talktofrank.com
FRANK is a UK government-funded website, giving information and advice on drug use. Information is easy to read and offers 24 hour help-lines for anyone worried about themselves or others.

http://www.addaction.org.uk
'UK's leading specialist drug and alcohol charity.' Services are free and confidential. Addaction aims to help transform the lives of people affected by drug and alcohol problems.

http://www.barnardos.org.uk
Whatever the issue from drug misuse to disability; youth crime to mental health; sexual abuse to domestic violence; child poverty to homelessness; Barnardo's aims to bring out the best in every child and runs 415 projects across the UK.

www.alcoholics-anonymous.org.uk
'Alcoholics Anonymous is a fellowship of men and women who share their experience, strength and hope with each other to solve their common problem and help others to recover from alcoholism.' Regular support meetings held in the UK and internationally.

http://www.adfam.org.uk
'Our mission is to improve the quality of life for families affected by drug and alcohol use.' Adfam is a UK organisation which runs projects linked to drugs, alcohol and families.

http://www.turning-point.co.uk
'Turning Point is the UK's leading health and social care organisation. We provide services for people with complex needs, including those affected by drug and alcohol misuse, mental health problems and those with a learning disability.'

http://www.ukna.org
Narcotics Anonymous is a non-profit society of men and women for whom drugs had become a major problem. Staffed by recovering addicts who meet regularly to help each other stay clean

http://www.nta.nhs.uk
The National Treatment Agency for substance misuse is a NHS Special Health Authority established to improve the service provision of drug treatment in England in terms of capacity, effectiveness and availability.

http://www.harmreductionworks.org.uk/
This website provides harm reduction information and resources in order to make drug use safer in the UK in terms of reducing the dangers associated with abuse. There are information leaflets on a variety of harm reduction topics, such as safer injecting.

http://www.avaproject.org.uk
'Against Violence and Abuse' charity website, with good practice and advice guidance.

ESSENTIAL READING

Advisory Council for the Misuse of Drugs 2003 **Hidden Harm: Responding to the Needs of Children of Problem Drug Users: The Report of an Inquiry by the Advisory Council on The Misuse Of Drugs**. London: Home Office

BMA 2007 **Fetal Alcohol Spectrum Disorders: A Guide for Healthcare Professionals**. A publication from the BMA Science and Education Department and the Board of Science. www.bma.org.uk

Hart D and Powell J 2006 **Adult Drug Problems, Children's Needs: Assessing the Impact of Parental Drug Use – A Toolkit For Practitioners**. National Children's Bureau, 8 Wakley Street London EC1V 7QE. www.ncb.org.uk

NICE 2007 Interventions to reduce substance misuse among vulnerable young people: NICE Public Health Guidance 4. London; National Institute for Health and Clinical Excellence. www.nice.org.uk

RCOG 2010 Pregnancy and complex social factors: a model for service provision for pregnant women with complex social factors NHS Evidence provided by NICE. www.rcog.org.uk

Whittaker A 2011 **The Essential Guide to Problem Substance Use in Pregnancy: a Resource book for Professionals**. DrugScope Publications. www.drugscope.org.uk

References

16.1 Substance Misuse

1. Lester BM, ElSohly M, Wright LL, *et al.* 2001 The Maternal Lifestyle Study: drug use by meconium toxicology and maternal self report. **Pediatrics**, 107:309–317
2. Sanuallah F, Gillian M and Lavin T 2006 Screening of substance misuse during early pregnancy in Blyth: an anonymous unlinked study. **Journal of Obstetrics and Gynaecology**, 26:187–190
3. Sherwood RA, Keating J, Kavvadia V, *et al.* 1999 Substance use in early pregnancy and relationship to fetal outcome. **European Journal of Pediatrics**, 158:488–492
4. Walker J and Walker A 2011 Chapt. 33 Substance Abuse in James D, Steer PJ, Weiner CP, Gonik B, Crowther CA and Robson SC (Eds) **High Risk Pregnancy: Management Options**, 4th Edn. London; Elsevier Saunders 565–577
5. NICE 2010 Pregnancy and complex social factors: a model of service provision for pregnant women with complex social factors NICE clinical guidance 110. London; National Institute for Health and Clinical Excellence. http://guidance.nice.org.uk/CG110 [Accessed 1-5-2011]
6. Humphreys C, Regan L, River D and Thiara RK 2005 Domestic violence and substance use: tackling complexity. **British Journal of Social Work**, 35:1303–1320
7. Velez ML, Montoya ID, Jansson LM *et al.* 2006 Exposure to violence amongst substance-dependent women and their children **Journal of Substance Abuse Treatment**, 30:31–38
8. Galvani S 2011 **Supporting Families Affected by Substance Use and Domestic Abuse**. Research Report, University of Bedfordshire. [Accessed 1-5-2011] www.avaproject.org
9. Lewis G (Ed) 2007 **The Confidential Enquiry into Maternal and Child Health (CEMACH). Saving Mothers Lives: Reviewing Maternal Deaths to Make Motherhood Safer 2003–2005**. The Seventh Report on Confidential Enquiries into Maternal Deaths in the UK. London: CEMACH
10. Centre for Maternal and Child Enquiries 2011 Saving mothers lives 2006–2008. **British Journal of Obstetrics and Gynaecology**, 118(suppl. 1)
11. Mitchell E, Hall J, Campbell D and Van Tejlingen E 2003 Specialist care for drug using pregnant women. **British Journal of Midwifery**, 11:7–11

16.2 Alcohol Addiction

1. Drug abuse briefing 2002 **A Guide to the Non Medical Use of Drugs In Britain**. London; Drugscope
2. Fetal Alcohol Spectrum Disorders 2007 **A Guide for Healthcare Professionals**. British Medical Association Board of Science.
3. Crome IB and Kumar MT 2007 Epidemiology of drug and alcohol use in young women. **Seminars in Fetal and Neonatal Medicine**, 12:98–105
4. Elliott EJ, Payne J, Morris A, Haan E and Bower C 2008 Fetal alcohol syndrome: a prospective national surveillance study. **Archives of Disease in Childhood**, 93:732–737
5. Fraser RB 2006 **Alcohol Consumption and the Outcomes of Pregnancy** (RCOG Statement No. 5). London; Royal College of Obstetricians and Gynaecologists
6. Autti-Rämö I 2002 Foetal alcohol syndrome – a multifaceted condition. **Developmental Medicine and Child Neurology**, 44:141–144
7. Stromland K 2004 Fetal alcohol syndrome a birth defect recognized worldwide. **Fetal and Maternal Medicine Review**, 15:59–71
8. Barrow M and Riley EP 2011 Diagnosis of fetal alcohol syndrome: emphasis on early detection in Preece PM and Riley EP (Eds) **Alcohol, Drugs and Medication in Pregnancy. The Long-term Outcome for the Child**. London; Mac Keith Press

16.3 Cannabis and Tobacco Use

1. British Market Research Bureau 2007 **Infant feeding survey 2005**. A survey conducted on behalf of the Information Centre for Health and Social Care and the UK Health Departments. Southport; The Information Centre
2. Lawrence T, Aveyard P, Cheng KK, *et al.* 2005 Does stage-based smoking cessation advice in pregnancy result in long-term quitters? 18-month postpartum follow-up of a randomised controlled trial. **Addiction**, 110:107–116
3. Owen L and McNeill A 2001 Saliva cotinine as an indicator of cigarette smoking among pregnant women. **Addiction**, 96:1001–1006
4. SAMHSA 2005 **Results from 2004 National Survey on Drug Use and Health: National Findings**. US Department of Health and Human Services. Publication number SMA 05-062
5. Peto R, Lopez AD, Boreham J and Thun M 2006 **Mortality from Smoking in Developed Countries 1950–2000**, 2nd Edn. www.deathsfromsmoking.net
6. Behnke M and Eyler FD 1993 The consequence of prenatal substance use for the developing fetus, newborn and young child. **International Journal of the Addictions**, 28:1341–1391
7. **Research Background to Reduce the Risk of Cot Death, Advice by the Foundation of the Study of Infant Deaths**. 2009 Factfile 2. London; Foundation for the Study of Infant Deaths. http://fsid.org.uk/document.doc?id=42
8. Walker J and Walker A 2011 Chapt. 33 Substance Abuse in James D, Steer PJ, Weiner CP, Gonik B, Crowther CA and Robson SC (Eds) **High Risk Pregnancy: Management Options**, 4th Edn. London; Elsevier 565–578
9. NICE Public Health Intervention Guidance 2006 **Brief Interventions and Referral for Smoking Cessation in Primary Care and Other Settings**. London; National Institute for Health and Clinical Excellence
10. NICE Guidance 26 2010 **Quitting Smoking in Pregnancy and Following Childbirth**. London; National Institute for Health and Clinical Excellence www.nice.org.uk/guidance/PH26
11. Department of Health 2009 **Reduce the Risk of Cot Death**. http://fsid.org.uk/document.doc?id=25
12. Einarson A and Riordan S 2009 Smoking in pregnancy and lactation: a review of risks and cessation strategies. **European Journal of Clinical Pharmacology**, 65:325–330

16.4 Cocaine Addiction

1. Hoare J and Moon D (Eds) 2010 **Drug Misuse Declared: Findings from the 2009/10 British Crime Survey England and Wales**. Home Office Statistical Bulletin
2. NICE Clinical Guideline 120. **Psychosis with Co-existing Substance Misuse: Assessment and Management in Adults and Young People**. London; National Institute for Health and Clinical Excellence. www.nice.org.uk
3. Hulse GK, Milne E, English DR and Holman CD 1997 Assessing the relationship between maternal cocaine use and abruptio placentae. **Addiction**, 92:1547–1551
4. Little BB, Snell LM, Trimmer KJ, *et al.* 1999 Peripartum cocaine use and adverse pregnancy outcome. **American Journal of Human Biology**, 11:598–602
5. Addis A, Moretti ME, Ahmed Syed F, Einarson TR and Koren G 2001 Fetal effects of cocaine: an updated meta-analysis. **Reproductive Toxicology**, 15:341–369
6. Bauer CR, Langer JC, Shankaran S, *et al.* 2005 Acute neonatal effects of cocaine exposure during pregnancy. **Archives of Pediatric and Adolescent Medicine**, 159:824–834
7. Behnke M, Eyler FD, Warner TD, Garvan CW, Hou W and Wobie K 2006 Outcome from a prospective, longitudinal study

of prenatal cocaine use: preschool development at 3 years of age. **Journal of Pediatric Psychology**, 31:41–49

8. Frank DA, Augustyn M, Knight WG, Pell T and Zuckerman B 2001 Growth, development, and behavior in early childhood following prenatal cocaine exposure: a systematic review. **Journal of the American Medical Association**, 285:1613–1625

9. Burkett G, Yasin SY, Palow D, LaVoie L and Martinez M 1994 Patterns of cocaine binging: effect on pregnancy. **American Journal of Obstetrics and Gynaecology**, 171:372–378

16.5 Opiate Addiction

1. Hoare J and Moon D (Eds) 2010 **Drug Misuse Declared: Findings from the 2009/10 British Crime Survey England and Wales**. Home Office Statistical Bulletin

2. Drug Abuse Briefing 2002 **A Guide to Non- Medical Use of Drugs in Britain**. London; Drugscope

3. Ward J, Mattick PR and Hall W (Ed.) 1998 **Methadone Maintenance Treatment and Other Opioid Replacement Therapies**. Harwood Academic Publishers

4. Mattick RP, Kimber J, Breen C and Davoli M 2008 Buprenorphine maintenance versus placebo or methadone maintenance for opioid dependence. Cochrane Database of Systematic Reviews (Online). CD002207

5. NICE 2010 **Pregnancy and Complex Social Factors: A Model of Service Provision for Pregnant Women with Complex Social Factors**. NICE Clinical Guidance 110. London; National Institute for Health and Clinical Excellence. http://guidance.nice.org.uk/CG110 [Accessed 1-5-2011]

6. Winklbaur B, Kopf N, Ebner N, Jung E, Thau K and Fischer G 2008 Treating pregnant women dependent on opioids is not the same as treating pregnancy and opioid dependence: a knowledge synthesis for better treatment for women and neonates. **Addiction**, 103:1429–1440

7. Minozzi S, Amato L, Vecchi S and Davoli M 2008 **Maintenance Agonist Treatments for Opiate Dependent Pregnant Women**. Cochrane Database of Systematic Reviews (Online). CD006318

8. NICE 2007 **Drug Misuse and Dependence. UK Guidelines on Clinical Management**. London: National Institute for Health and Clinical Excellence. www.nice.org.uk

9. Burns L, Mattick RP, Lim K and Wallace C 2007 Methadone in pregnancy: treatment retention and neonatal outcomes. **Addiction**, 102:264–270

10. Jones HE, O'Grady KE, Malfi D and Tuten M 2008 Methadone maintenance vs methadone taper during pregnancy: maternal and neonatal outcomes. **American Journal of Addiction**, 17:372–386

11. McCarthy JJ, Leamon MH, Parr MS and Anania B 2005 High-dose methadone maintenance in pregnancy: maternal and neonatal outcomes. **American Journal of Obstetrics and Gynecology**, 193:606–610

12. Wolff K, Boys A, Rostami-Hodjegan A, Hay A and Raistrick D 2005 Changes to methadone clearance during pregnancy. **European Journal of Clinical Pharmacology**, 61:763–768

16.6 Stimulant Addiction

1. Hoare J and Moon D (Eds) 2010 **Drug Misuse Declared: Findings from the 2009/10 British Crime Survey England and Wales**. Home Office Statistical Bulletin

2. Drug Abuse Briefing 2002 **A Guide to Non- Medical Use of Drugs in Britain**. London; Drugscope, London

3. Department of Health 2007 **Drug Misuse and Dependence. UK Guidelines on Clinical Management**. London: Department of Health (England), the Scottish Government, Welsh Assembly and Northern Ireland Executive

4. Srisurapanont M and Jarusuraisin N, Kittirattanapaiboon P 2001 Treatment for amphetamine dependence and abuse. Cochrane Database of Systematic Reviews (Online).

5. Smith LM, LaGasse LL, Derauf C, *et al.* 2006 The infant development, environment, and lifestyle study: effects of prenatal methamphetamine exposure, polydrug exposure, and poverty on intrauterine growth. **Pediatrics**, 118:1149–1156

6. Smith L, Yonekura ML, Wallace T, Berman N, Kuo J and Berkowitz C 2003 Effects of prenatal methamphetamine exposure on

fetal growth and drug withdrawal symptoms in infants born at term. **Journal of Developmental and Behavioral Pediatrics**, 24:17–23

7. Smith LM, Lagasse LL, Derauf C, *et al.* 2008 Prenatal methamphetamine use and neonatal neurobehavioral outcome. **Neurotoxicology and Teratology**, 30:20–28

8. Schaefer C, Peters P and Miller RK (Eds) 2007 **Drugs during Pregnancy and Lactation. Treatment Options and Risk Assessment**, 2nd Edn. New York; Academic Press

9. Elliott RH and Rees GB 1990 Amphetamine ingestion presenting as eclampsia. **Canadian Journal of Anesthesia**, 37:130–133

Appendices References

Appendix 16.1.1 Applying a Formal Assessment Framework

1. Hart D, Powell J 2006 **Adult Drug Problems, Children's Needs: Assessing the Impact of Parental Drug Use**. London; National Children's Bureau

Appendix 16.4.1 Care of the Baby Who Experiences Withdrawal

1. Abdel-Latif ME, Pinner J, Clews S, Cooke, F, Lui K, Oei J 2006 Effects of breast milk on the severity and outcome of neonatal abstinence syndrome among infants of drug dependent mothers. **Pediatrics**, 117:e1163–e1169 DOI: 10.1542/peds.2005-1561

Appendix 16.1.1 Applying a Formal Assessment Framework

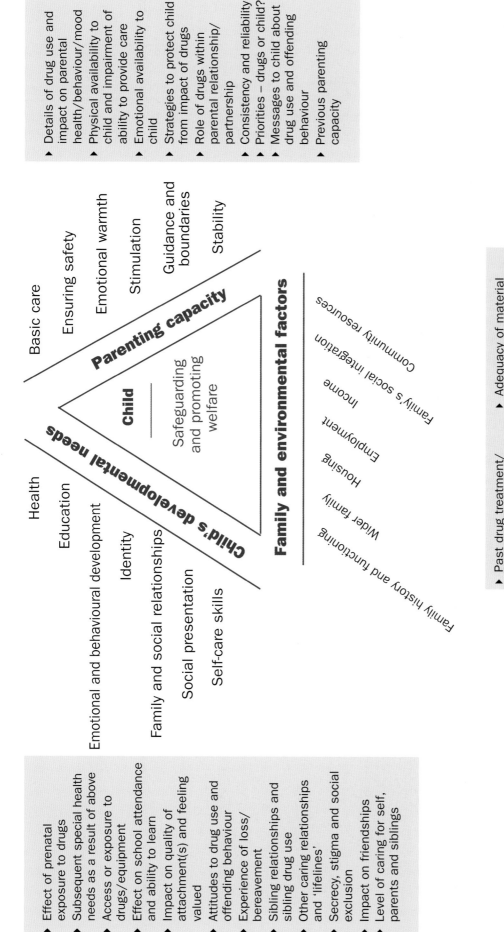

- Details of drug use and impact on parental health/behaviour/mood
- Physical availability to child and impairment of ability to provide care
- Emotional availability to child
- Strategies to protect child from impact of drugs
- Role of drugs within parental relationship/ partnership
- Consistency and reliability
- Priorities – drugs or child?
- Messages to child about drug use and offending behaviour
- Previous parenting capacity

Parenting capacity

- Basic care
- Ensuring safety
- Emotional warmth
- Stimulation
- Guidance and boundaries
- Stability

Child

Safeguarding and promoting welfare

Child's developmental needs

- Health
- Education
- Emotional and behavioural development
- Identity
- Family and social relationships
- Social presentation
- Self-care skills

Family and environmental factors

- Family history and functioning
- Wider family
- Housing
- Employment
- Income
- Family's social integration
- Community resources

- Past drug treatment/ engagement
- Offending behaviour and convictions
- Who knows about drug use? and implications for wider family relationships
- Extended family able to act as carers
- Adequacy of material resources – money and housing
- Home is exposed to risky adults or activities
- Community attitudes and stigma
- Support network outside the home

- Effect of prenatal exposure to drugs
- Subsequent special health needs as a result of above
- Access or exposure to drugs/equipment
- Effect on school attendance and ability to learn
- Impact on quality of attachment(s) and feeling valued
- Attitudes to drug use and offending behaviour
- Experience of loss/ bereavement
- Sibling relationships and sibling drug use
- Other caring relationships and 'lifelines'
- Secrecy, stigma and social exclusion
- Impact on friendships
- Level of caring for self, parents and siblings

From Hart and Powell, 2006[1]. This figure is downloadable from the book companion website at www.wiley.com/go/robson

Appendix 16.3.1 Preventing SIDS: Advice to Parents

Cut smoking in pregnancy – fathers too!

And don't let anyone smoke in the same room as your baby

- Place your baby on the back to sleep (and not on the front or side)
- Do not let your baby become too hot, and keep your baby's head uncovered indoors
- Place your baby with their feet to the foot of the cot, to prevent them wriggling down under the covers, or use a baby sleep bag
- Never sleep with your baby on a sofa or armchair
- The safest place for your baby to sleep is in a crib or cot in a room with you for the first 6 months
- It's especially dangerous for your baby to sleep in your bed if you or your partner:
  - are a smoker, even if you never smoke in bed or at home
  - have been drinking alcohol
  - taken medication or drugs that make you drowsy
  - or if you feel very tired
  - or if your baby was born before 37 weeks, and/or weighed less than 2.5 kg (5½ lbs) at birth
- Don't forget, accidents can happen: you might roll over in your sleep and suffocate your baby, or your baby could get caught between the wall and the bed, or could roll out of an adult bed and be injured
- Breast-feeding your baby protects from SIDS
- Settling your baby to sleep with a dummy, even for naps, can reduce the risk of cot death, even if the dummy falls out while your baby is asleep

Appendix 16.4.1 Care of the Baby Who Experiences Withdrawal

Infants can experience withdrawal from a range of substances, both prescribed and illicit.

SYMPTOMS

Symptoms of withdrawal can range from periods of discomfort, jitteriness and being unsettled through to a comprehensive neonatal abstinence syndrome often (but not always) seen in babies whose mothers have regularly taken opiate and narcotic drugs in pregnancy. These include but are not restricted to:

- Heroin
- Methadone
- Codeine
- Dihydrocodeine
- Buprenorphine

In some cases this drug use is illicit and in other cases prescribed by GPs or drug treatment agencies. Many of the affected babies will be born to women who have stable prescribed drug use, so symptoms are not a sign of, or restricted to, those with chaotic, illicit drug use.

In many cases withdrawal is transient and mild, so comfort measures such as cuddling, gentle rocking and skin to skin contact, along with optimising the environment (e.g. quiet surroundings, avoidance of bright light etc.) may suffice.

NEONATAL ABSTINENCE SYNDROME

Neonatal abstinence syndrome describes a collection of symptoms seen when a baby experiences abrupt discontinuation of opiates in the early postnatal period. Some babies do not appear to be affected other than very mild symptoms and the severity of the withdrawal may be unanticipated. It is very difficult to predict with any degree of certainty which babies will experience withdrawal. So some babies exposed to very high levels of maternal methadone occasionally experience only mild withdrawal, whereas babies exposed to maternal codeine use can experience prolonged withdrawal.

The symptoms of neonatal abstinence include:

Central Nervous System
- High pitched cry
- Restlessness
- Jitteriness and tremors
- Hypertonia

Gastrointestinal Problems
- Excessive, vigorous sucking
- Not settling after a feed
- Vomiting
- Loose and watery stools
- Abdominal cramps

Metabolic and Respiratory Problems
- Sweating and pyrexia
- Sneezing and nasal flaring
- Rapid respirations

PARENTS

It is often stressful for the parents to see their baby suffering and the associated guilt may impact on their ability to cope, which could in turn lead to destabilisation of their drug use. The staff working in this environment will also be vulnerable to the stress associated with caring for a withdrawing baby and may need support.

Assessment of parent's coping strategies is vital to the health of the child and support should be offered to increase their ability to care for their child. Baby and mother should not be separated unless there are over-riding medical or social reasons. Maintaining a quiet environment will help keep the baby calmer which in turn will help the parents.

BREAST-FEEDING

Evidence suggests that substantial breast-milk intake may offer some protection against the severity of neonatal abstinence syndrome and may delay the onset[1]. Therefore breast-feeding should be encouraged unless there are definitive medical or social contraindications (e.g. HIV positive, continuing illicit drug use, especially if intravenous).

MEDICATION

If the baby exhibits symptoms of neonatal abstinence to opiates and is unwell a full paediatric review is needed. This may result in a decision to commence medication which is usually oral morphine solution. If the baby is unable to sleep and feed, then without the appropriate care the baby would become ill quickly.

Onset of symptoms most often occurs in the first 3–5 days of life (slightly later in those breast fed). However, some babies present as late as day 7–10.

Most babies who require pharmacological therapy require it for a few weeks. Once the baby is on a stable dose, parents can be taught how to administer, and further management can take place in the outpatient setting. Careful attention to dosage and strength of solution is of utmost importance.

Mothers must never use their own prescribed methadone to treat neonatal withdrawal as this may led to fatal neonatal overdose.

PSYCHIATRIC DISORDERS

17

Renuka Lazarus[1] and
Kathryn Gutteridge[2]

[1]Leicestershire Partnership Trust, Leicester, UK
[2]Sandwell and West Birmingham Hospitals NHS Trust, UK

17.1 Antenatal Psychiatric Disorders
17.2 Postnatal Psychiatric Disorders
17.3 Eating Disorders
17.4 Post-Traumatic Stress Disorder

Medical Disorders in Pregnancy: A Manual for Midwives, Second Edition. Edited by S. Elizabeth Robson and Jason Waugh.
© 2013 John Wiley & Sons, Ltd. Published 2013 by John Wiley & Sons, Ltd.

17.1 Antenatal Psychiatric Disorders

Incidence	Risk for Childbearing
Depression: 10–15%	Variable risk – high risk if severe

EXPLANATION OF CONDITION

Childbirth is a significant life event resulting in profound and permanent changes in a woman's role and responsibilities. It is a time when a woman is at greatest risk for developing a psychiatric disorder. This risk is further increased if she has previously suffered from a serious mental illness. Mental illness is one of the leading causes of maternal deaths[1].

Pregnancy is not protective against mental illness[2]. In fact, mental health problems during pregnancy are at least as common as they are after childbirth and are increasingly recognised as important forerunners of postnatal illness[3,4]. Socio-cultural expectations often make it difficult for women to seek help for perinatal mental health problems.

Some degree of emotional lability and anxiety during pregnancy is normal. Sleep problems are also common. However, it is important to be able to differentiate these from the signs of mental illness. Early detection and treatment of mental illness is crucial[5,6].

Any psychiatric disorder may present in pregnancy. The clinical issues to note are:

- New psychiatric disorders as well as relapses and recurrences of previous disorders may occur both during pregnancy and after chilbirth[7]
- Most first-onset conditions are mild depressive and anxiety disorders and the cause is commonly psychosocial[6]
- Relapses of the following disorders may occur: depressive and anxiety disorders, obsessive compulsive disorder, schizophrenia, bipolar disorder and substance misuse
- It is important to enquire for a previous history of serious mental illness at the booking visit, to be able to predict and possibly prevent a relapse
- Identifying women with a past or family history of bipolar disorder or puerperal psychosis is particularly important because of the high risk of postpartum relapse (one in two).
- Psychiatric medication should not automatically be discontinued once the woman becomes pregnant[7]. This is a frequent cause of relapse.
- Mild to moderate disorders may be managed in primary care. Past or current severe illness should be referred to specialist psychiatric services, preferably to a perinatal psychiatric service[7,8]
- Good communication between all health professionals both in primary and secondary services is crucial[1]

COMPLICATIONS

Antenatal psychiatric disorders may be associated with[9–12]:

- Poor attendance in antenatal clinic
- Smoking and substance misuse
- Poor general health and nutrition
- Deliberate self-harm and suicide
- Low birth weight and pre-term deliveries
- Problems with mother–infant attachment
- Neglect or harm to infant and other children; safeguarding issues
- Possible long-term developmental and behavioural problems in the child
- Mental health problems in the woman's partner

NON-PREGNANCY TREATMENT AND CARE

Mild to moderate mental illness may be managed in primary care. Severe mental illness is managed by psychiatric services either in the community or in hospital.

Management of mental illness may include:

- Advice on lifestyle, exercise and coping with stress
- Psycho-education
- Talking therapies (psychotherapy)
- Psychotropic medication (e.g. antidepressants and antipsychotics)
- Rarely, electroconvulsive therapy (ECT)

PRE-CONCEPTION ISSUES AND CARE

Women with previous mental illness should receive advice about the following issues in a manner that is socially and culturally sensitive:

- Contraception
- Risk of recurrence of mental illness in perinatal period
- Risks and benefits of medication in pregnancy
- Some psychiatric medications reduce fertility and should be changed if pregnancy is planned
- Avoid certain drugs (especially sodium valproate) due to high rates of birth defects

Pregnancy Issues

Persistent anxiety and depressive symptoms have an impact on the woman's general health. They may prevent her from seeking antenatal care and engaging with services. If severe, they could put her life at risk.

Anxiety and depression may also have effects on the baby, probably related to the increased levels of cortisol.

These include[9,10]:

- Fetal growth retardation
- Low birth weight
- Prematurity
- Long-term developmental and behavioural problems in the child

Mental illness may be associated with other behaviours that could indirectly affect her health and that of the baby. These include:

- Smoking
- Alcohol and substance misuse
- Poor dietary habits
- Lack of exercise
- Self-harming behaviour
- Lack of engagement with services

Medical Management and Care

Early detection of perinatal serious mental illness is crucial. There should be clearly defined care pathways and good communication between all professionals. The psychiatric care plan is recorded in the woman's hand-held maternity records and the woman receives shared care with obstetrician, psychiatrist and midwifery services. If there is a risk to the baby, a referral to the safeguarding team and a pre-birth multi-agency meeting is indicated.

Medical care

- Mild to moderate depressive and anxiety symptoms are the most frequent psychiatric problems in pregnancy and may be managed in primary care
- Psychological therapies such as cognitive behaviour therapy, interpersonal therapy or self-help strategies may be indicated
- Advice may be sought from specialist psychiatric services if needed, regarding continuing or commencing medication
- All women with serious mental illness (past or current) should be referred to specialist services, preferably to a specialist perinatal psychiatry team[7]
- The risk–benefit ratio of psychotropic medication is assessed and decisions regarding medication during pregnancy are made after discussion with the woman
- For treatment guidance see Appendix 17.1

Midwifery Management and Care

- At the booking visit, the midwife will screen for past or present serious mental illness in the woman and her family. If positive, refer to perinatal psychiatric services
- Establish a trusting relationship with the woman that is socially and culturally sensitive
- Advice regarding smoking cessation, diet and exercise, breast-feeding, birth preparation and support services

Labour Issues

- There are no physical reasons why the birth should be managed differently
- Anxiety management techniques may be useful in anxious women
- Neonatologists should be contacted if the woman is currently receiving psychotropic medication

Medical Management and Care

- Labour should be managed from a normal perspective
- Discuss methods of support for labour pain to reduce anxiety
- Support throughout labour is important
- Consent should be obtained throughout labour

Midwifery Management and Care

- Advice regarding continuation or discontinuing psychotropic medication prior to labour should be entered in the pre-birth care plan
- Drugs should be used judiciously in view of possible effects on the baby

Postpartum Issues

Symptoms of pre-existing illness might worsen or relapse; new symptoms might emerge. These include:

- Increased anxiety and agitation
- Low mood, excessive tearfulness or apathy
- Poor handling or attachment to baby
- Bizarre or unusual behaviour
- Delusions and hallucinations
- Thoughts or acts of harming herself or baby

Medical Management and Care

- Specialist perinatal psychiatry team should be contacted if symptoms are severe
- Appropriate treatment takes precedence over breast-feeding. Many psychotropic drugs are safe in breast-feeding and need not be discontinued
- Transfer to a specialist psychiatric mother and baby unit may be indicated if the woman's mental state deteriorates

Midwifery Management and Care

- Observe mother and baby interaction
- Discuss rest, diet and self-care, assess how mother is coping
- Reassure if mood change is due to postnatal blues
- Observe baby if breast-feeding mother is on medication
- Assess risk to baby
- If symptoms indicate serious mental illness, liaise and refer to specialist perinatal psychiatric service

17.2 Postnatal Psychiatric Disorders

Incidence	Risk for Childbearing
Depression: 10–15%[1,2]	Variable risk for depression; high risk if severe
Puerperal psychosis: 0.2%[3]	High risk for puerperal psychosis

EXPLANATION OF CONDITION

Psychiatric disorders following childbirth are common, and include both new episodes specific to the postpartum period, as well as recurrences of previous illnesses[1]. Depression and puerperal psychosis will be described here.

Depression

The term 'postnatal depression' is often used inappropriately to describe all postnatal psychiatric disorders, and is best avoided[2]. The relative risk of depression in the postnatal period is five. The symptoms do not differ from depression outside of childbirth[3-5]. Severe depression occurs in 3–5% of postpartum women and commonly presents within 1–3 months postpartum. Normal emotional changes following childbirth may mask or be mistaken for depressive symptoms.

'Postnatal blues' are experienced by 50–80% of women. Symptoms are transient and occur between 3 and 7 days after delivery[6,7], including irritability, tearfulness, low mood, euphoria and sleep disturbance. Symptoms resolve spontaneously and the woman and her family need reassurance and support.

General Symptoms

In the postnatal period depression may range from mild to severe. Prediction and early detection are important. The key features of depressions are:

- Low mood, loss of interest and enjoyment, and reduced energy
- Associated symptoms such as: reduced concentration and self-esteem, ideas of guilt, hopelessness, thoughts or acts of self-harm or suicide and sleep and appetite disturbance

At the booking visit and at all subsequent visits the midwife should screen for depression. Ask the following questions[2]:

- During the past month, have you often felt low, depressed or hopeless?
- During the past month, have you had little interest or pleasure in doing things?

Puerperal Psychosis

This is a severe mood disorder with delusions and hallucinations. The onset is sudden, usually within the first 2 days postpartum. The illness is closely related to bipolar disorder. Women with a personal history or family history of bipolar disorder are particularly at risk[8]. There is also an association with primiparity and association with obstetric complications[9].

The clinical picture includes:

- Mood changes: elation, depression or irritability
- Perplexity and confusion
- Agitation and abnormal behaviour
- Delusions and hallucinations
- Thoughts or acts of harm to self or others
- Difficulty in caring for self and baby

COMPLICATIONS

Complications include:

- Self-harm and suicide[3]
- Neglect of baby and rarely, infanticide
- Problems with mother–infant attachment and interaction[8,10,11]
- Long-term emotional, behavioral and cognitive problems in the child[12]
- Relationship problems and family breakdown
- Social, occupational and financial complications
- Depression in the partner[13]

NON-PREGNANCY TREATMENT AND CARE

Depression in the non-pregnant population is managed in primary care if it is mild to moderate, and referred to psychiatric services if severe[2]. The following management options are available:

- Advice on lifestyle, exercise and coping with stress
- Talking therapies, e.g. cognitive behaviour therapy
- Antidepressant medication
- Mood stabilisers, e.g. lithium
- Electroconvulsive therapy (ECT)

PRE-CONCEPTION ISSUES AND CARE

Women with a past history of severe depression or puerperal psychosis should be counselled regarding relapse rates (about 50%) in future pregnancies. Medication should not be discontinued abruptly. Many psychiatric drugs are safe in pregnancy. The risk–benefit ratio should be assessed to decide whether or not to continue medication[14,15].

Some drugs are associated with birth defects and should be avoided. Sodium valproate (an anti-epileptic drug that is used as a mood stabiliser) should not be prescribed to childbearing women because of the high risk of birth defects. Issues that may be associated with depression are as follows and require further advice and support:

- Poor diet and nutritional status
- Smoking
- Substance/alcohol abuse
- Self-harming behaviour
- Relationship problems

Pregnancy Issues

Psychosocial risk factors play a role in mild to moderate depression. However, in severe depression and in puerperal psychosis, biological factors are more important. At antenatal visits, women should be screened particularly for biological risk factors and for symptoms suggestive of serious mental illness.

Biological risk factors:
- Past history of severe depression
- Past or family history of bipolar disorder or puerperal psychosis

Psychosocial factors:
- Lack of social support
- Recent stressful life events
- Longstanding difficulties in coping
- Sexual abuse
- Domestic violence

Medical Management and Care
- Antenatal depression may be treated either with talking therapies or antidepressants
- Psychotropic medication need not be discontinued
- For treatment guidance see Appendix 17.1
- Women at risk should have access to a specialist perinatal psychiatry service for advice or assessment if needed

Midwifery Management and Care
At the booking visit, the midwife will screen for past or present severe mental illness in the woman and her family[10]. If positive:
- Communication with other professionals is important
- Refer to obstetrician
- Refer to perinatal service
- A trusting relationship should be established that is socially and culturally sensitive
- General advice on smoking cessation, diet and exercise, breast-feeding, birth preparation and support services
- If there is an identified risk to the baby, safeguarding referral and pre-birth multi-professional meeting is held

Labour Issues
- There are no physical reasons why the birth should be managed differently
- Obstetric complications may increase the risk for developing postnatal psychiatric disorders
- Specialist perinatal psychiatric team may need to be contacted for advice or assessment
- Neonatologists should be contacted if the mother is on psychotropic medication

Medical Management and Care
- Psychotropic medication may be indicated in women with past or present psychiatric illness
- Drugs should be used judiciously during labour in view of possible effects on the baby

Midwifery Management and Care
- Discuss all carefully with the woman and birth partner
- Ensure that any plan has the woman's full consent
- Psychological and physical support is important throughout labour
- Avoid unnecessary interventions
- Encourage skin to skin contact between mother and baby
- Breast-feeding to be encouraged if not pharmacologically contraindicated

Postpartum Issues
- Postnatal blues and normal emotional changes should be distinguished from depression
- Depression usually presents within the first 12 weeks postpartum; one-third to one-half of these are severe and tend to present early, usually by 4–6 weeks postpartum
- Puerperal psychosis presents acutely, usually within 2 days postpartum
- Severe depression and puerperal psychosis needs referral to specialist perinatal psychiatric services
- Suicide is one of the leading causes of maternal mortality; hence early detection and treatment of mental illness are crucial

Medical Management and Care
- Specialist perinatal psychiatry team should be contacted if there are symptoms of serious mental illness
- Risk assessment and safeguarding issues are important
- Psychotropic medication may be indicated. Medication that is safe in breast-feeding can be prescribed
- Admission to a specialist psychiatric mother and baby unit may be indicated if the mother is severely ill

Midwifery Management and Care
- Observe mother and baby interaction
- Discuss sleep, diet and self-care, and how she is coping
- Reassure if mood change is due to postnatal blues
- Observe baby if breast-feeding mother is using medication
- Ask screening questions for depression; scales, e.g. EPDS[16] may be used but only as part of a thorough clinical assessment[2]
- Communicate with specialist services and refer if needed
- Refer to Social Services if there are safeguarding issues

17.3 Eating Disorders

Incidence	Risk for Childbearing
Anorexia nervosa – 8 per 100 000 Bulimia nervosa – 12 per 100 000 Prevalence: anorexia nervosa 0.3 %; bulimia nervosa 1%	Low Risk

EXPLANATION OF CONDITION

Eating disorders (ED) are characterised by severe disturbances in eating behaviour[1]. The two main diagnostic categories are anorexia nervosa (AN) and bulimia nervosa (BN).

In anorexia there is a deliberate attempt to lose weight whereas bulimia is characterised by repeated episodes of binge eating followed by compensatory behaviours (self-induced vomiting or purging)[2]. Atypical anorexia and bulimia do not fully meet the diagnostic criteria, but present with some of these symptoms[3]. Eating disorders are associated with complex psychological and medical complications[4].

Eating disorders affect menstruation and fertility[5]. Pregnancy is a particularly difficult time for women with eating disorders because of the associated changes in body shape and weight[6–8]. Eating disorders are associated with antenatal and postnatal complications for the woman and baby and management in pregnancy is challenging. Close liaison between maternity and eating disorders services is needed.

Both biological and psychosocial factors are involved. Genetic factors are important, and eating disorders have a higher prevalence in some families[9,10]. Psychosocial factors include stressful life events, personality traits, cultural factors and social pressures that link attractiveness to being thin[11–14].

Anorexia Nervosa

In AN, women restrict their weight and perceive themselves as being overweight in spite of evidence to the contrary. The diagnostic criteria are as follows:

* Body weight maintained at least 15% below that expected, or BMI less than 17.5 (BMI is outlined in Appendix 13.1.1)
* Weight loss, self-induced vomiting, purging, excessive exercise, appetite suppressants/diuretics
* Body-image distortion; dread of fatness
* Widespread endocrine disorder involving the hypothalamic-pituitary-gonadal axis causing amenorrhoea
* If onset is pre-pubertal, puberty is delayed or even arrested

Associated clinical features:

* Amenorrhoea, infertility, loss of sexual interest
* Lethargy, weakness, anaemia
* Hypotension, peripheral oedema, cardiac arrhythmias
* Constipation, abdominal pain, enlarged salivary glands
* Dry skin, alopecia, lanugo hair, brittle nails, osteoporosis
* Tooth decay, erosion of dental enamel

Onset of AN typically occurs between 14 and 18 years and may follow a stressful life event. Personality problems are common. Depression, self-harming behaviour and suicide may also occur. The course of the disorder is variable. Some women recover completely; others relapse or recover partially. Severe medical complications can be fatal and early diagnosis and treatment are crucial[15].

Antenatal visits provide a good opportunity to check for eating disorders. Thorough physical examination and relevant tests are needed to detect medical complications. A referral to a psychiatric eating disorders service should be made as early in pregnancy as possible so that treatment can be commenced.

Bulimia Nervosa

BN is characterised by repeated bouts of overeating and excessive preoccupation with control of body weight leading to extreme measures to counteract effects of overeating (such as self-induced vomiting or purging). The preoccupations in bulimia are similar to those seen in anorexia.

Diagnostic criteria are:

* Persistent preoccupation with eating; craving for food; eating large quantities of food within a short time period.
* Counteracting the fattening effects of food by self-induced vomiting, purgative abuse, periods of starvation, or use of drugs (e.g. appetite suppressants/diuretics)
* Morbid dread of fatness
* Inappropriately low target weight
* Often, but not always, an earlier episode of AN

Onset of bulimia usually occurs in late adolescence. Most women are within normal weight range. Impulsivity, self-harming behaviour and alcohol or drug misuse are often associated. Depression may also occur. The course may be chronic or intermittent.

Associated clinical features:

* Irregular periods; amenorrhoea
* Dependence on laxatives, diarrhoea; constipation
* Dehydration, fluid and electrolyte disturbances
* Tooth erosion; loss of dental enamel
* Enlarged salivary glands

NON-PREGNANCY TREATMENT AND CARE[16–19]

* Psychotherapies:
  * Cognitive behaviour therapy
  * Interpersonal therapy
  * Psychodynamic psychotherapy
* Medication – antidepressants
* Assess and treat medical and psychiatric complications
* Admission to a specialist eating disorder inpatient unit if needed

PRE-CONCEPTION ISSUES AND CARE

* Counselling and support: regarding amenorrhoea and infertility; discuss complications related to pregnancy
* Dietary and nutritional assessment and advice
* Polycystic ovaries more common in BN

Pregnancy Issues
- Midwife , GP and obstetrician can detect eating disorders early
- Maternal worries about change in body shape and weight
- Self-induced vomiting; hyperemesis
- Symptoms may be disguised as hyperemesis gravidarum
- Nutritional deficiencies
- Intrauterine growth restriction
- Poor maternal weight gain
- Increased rate of miscarriage and stillbirth
- Premature labour
- Associated depression
- Self-harming behaviour
- Associated alcohol or drug misuse
- Medical complications of eating disorders
- Failure to attend antenatal clinics

Medical Management and Care
- Multidisciplinary care plan needed; refer to psychiatric (ED) service
- Monitor weight and check for IUGR
- Serial scans may be needed to observe fetal growth
- Expected weight gain in pregnancy may be used as incentive
- Check for nutritional/electrolyte abnormalities and correct them
- Assess vitamin and mineral deficiencies and treat
- Check for cardiac complications
- Multidisciplinary care plan is needed
- Liaise closely with GP and ED service
- If antidepressants are prescribed, liaise with neonatal team. For treatment guidance see Appendix 17.1

Midwifery Management and Care[18,19]
- At the booking visit the midwife will check the woman's weight and BMI; enquire for other symptoms of ED if BMI is low
- If presence of ED, discuss the complications in pregnancy
- Explain the importance of weight gain in pregnancy
- Monitor weight regularly; reassure especially in third trimester
- Screen for past or current serious mental illness as usual
- Develop a supportive and trusting relationship
- Give support with changing body shape and weight
- Dietary advice; correct vitamin and mineral deficiencies
- General advice regarding smoking cessation, diet and exercise, breast-feeding, birth preparation and support services
- Encourage antenatal preparation for parenthood
- Refer to ED service for management
- If ED is detected, refer to obstetrician for medical care plan
- Be alert for pre-term labour and advise mother of the warning signs

Labour Issues
- Labour will proceed as normal unless there are complications
- Pre-term labour can occur
- Higher rate of caesarean sections
- Neonatologists should be informed if the mother is on psychotropic medication

Medical Management and Care
- Advice regarding psychotropic medication during labour should be entered in the pre-birth care plan
- Drugs should be used judiciously in view of possible effects on the baby

Midwifery Management and Care[20]
- Labour should be managed from a normal perspective if pregnancy allows[2,3]
- Discuss methods of support for labour pain to reduce anxiety

Postpartum Issues
A relapse or worsening of ED symptoms can occur. There may also be other medical or psychiatric complications of ED.
Check for:
- Preoccupation with weight gained in pregnancy
- Exaggerated weight loss after birth
- Excessive exercise
- Depression
- Self-harming behaviour
- Alcohol or substance misuse
- Mother–infant attachment

Medical Management and Care
- Normal postnatal care indicated unless problems occurred during labour
- Watch for signs of relapse of ED; refer to ED service
- Check for associated symptoms of depression
- Assess risks to mother and baby
- If the woman is breast-feeding and is taking psychotropic medication, monitor the baby
- Liaise with other professionals involved in her care

Midwifery Management and Care[21]
- Observe mood, attachment and interaction with baby
- Monitor weight and BMI of the woman
- Assess and advise on nutritional status
- Observe attachment and caring for infant, being alert for risks to mother and baby
- If relapse of ED occurs, refer to ED service
- If there are safeguarding issues, refer to Social Services

17.4 Post-Traumatic Stress Disorder

Incidence	Risk for Childbearing
3–7.7%[1]	Low risk

EXPLANATION OF CONDITION

Post-traumatic stress disorder (PTSD) is a delayed or protracted response to a stressful event of an exceptionally threatening or catastrophic nature, affecting individuals at any age or time of life including childbearing[2]. The stressful event may, or may not, be related to the birth itself or to traumatic experiences surrounding it. Previous PTSD may be exacerbated during pregnancy or following childbirth. About 3–7.7% of all postnatal women experience symptoms of PTSD within the first year after delivery[1].

Features include repeated reliving of the trauma in flashbacks, dreams or nightmares. Hypervigilance and anxiety symptoms occur, with avoidance of activities and situations that are reminiscent of the trauma. Emotional numbing and detachment are common, and depression with suicidal thoughts might occur. Symptoms follow a life-threatening event and involve re-experiencing the event in the form of nightmares or flashbacks[3]. Other symptoms include:

- Avoidance of situations similar to the stressful event
- Inability to recall the event
- Increased arousal or hyper-vigilance
- Sleep problems
- Irritability and/or anger outbursts
- Poor concentration
- Exaggerated startle response
- Dissociation or emotional numbing

Onset is usually within a few weeks after the traumatic event but occasionally may be delayed by months or years[4]. Women may not initially admit to the trauma, but present instead with unexplained physical symptoms, depression or complications such as substance misuse.

Risk Factors for PTSD in Childbirth

Previous psychological problems, anxiety, obstetric procedures, loss of control and lack of partner support are known risk factors for PTSD[5–7]. Other risk factors include:

- Miscarriage and stillbirth[8]
- Emergency procedures such as cord prolapse
- Complicated deliveries and emergency caesarean section
- Catheterisation or other procedures
- Intimate clinical procedures, e.g. vaginal examinations
- Attitude and behaviour of healthcare professionals
- Survivor of disaster or accident[2,9]

COMPLICATIONS

If unrecognised, PTSD can have serious consequences[9–11], with sufferers often developing low self-esteem, anxiety, depression, and other psychological symptoms. Employment problems, relationship breakdown and social isolation may result. Alcohol, illicit drugs and nicotine misuse might also follow. About one-third of women report thoughts of self-harm. Self-harming behaviour may occur and the incidence of suicide is also increased[10].

Women who develop PTSD symptoms after childbirth become preoccupied with the birth and develop anxiety, flashbacks and nightmares possibly avoiding situations that remind them of the event[8]. Symptoms may present, or worsen, in childbirth.

PTSD can also occur after the following situations:

- Rape, sexual assault, childhood sexual abuse
- Victim of violent crime or domestic violence
- Victim of torture, war, disaster or accident[2,9]
- Refugee or asylum seeker
- Previous female genital mutilation
- Occupation – armed forces, emergency services

PTSD frequently follows sexual abuse in childhood or rape in later life[6,12]. Women who experience PTSD following childbirth are likely to give negative accounts of the birth and to describe caregivers as lacking empathy and failing to meet their needs[13]. They may find breast-feeding difficult. They may struggle to cope with infant care whilst preoccupied with the trauma and may develop secondary depressive or anxiety symptoms. Consequences include[12,14–21]:

- Depression, anxiety, self harm, suicide
- Avoidance of intimate and sexual relationships
- Impaired mother–infant attachment
- Fear and avoidance of future pregnancies (tokophobia)
- Avoidance of vaginal examinations
- Termination of pregnancy
- Requests for caesarean section without medical reason
- Requests for sterilisation/removal of reproductive organs
- Social, physical and psychological problems

NON-PREGNANCY TREATMENT AND CARE

Thorough assessment to elicit symptoms as sensitively as possible is the first step in management. PTSD shows substantial natural recovery over months or years following the traumatic event[2]. Watchful waiting may be indicated with support from appropriate healthcare professionals, family and friends. A single episode of 'debriefing' should *not* be routinely offered; it can cause re-traumatisation and worsen the symptoms.

Trauma-focused Cognitive Behaviour Therapy (CBT) and Eye Movement Desensitisation and Reprocessing Therapy (EMDR) are effective. Medication such as antidepressants may be helpful. Depression secondary to PTSD is unlikely to respond to medication unless the PTSD is treated first. Management of complications such as alcohol/drug use is important. If the trauma is ongoing, such as domestic violence, the symptoms will persist.

PRE-CONCEPTION ISSUES AND CARE

PTSD has implications for future pregnancy. Reluctance to attend health screening[6], and avoidance of cervical screening[22], are common, increasing the risk of underlying comorbidity[12].

A full history should identify anxiety and depressive symptoms. Principles of preconception management should include:

- Detection of PTSD symptoms
- Identification of complications
- Discussion of plans for pregnancy
- Referral for psychological therapies (CBT, EMDR)
- Medication may be indicated for complications

Pregnancy Issues

Identification of a woman with current or pre-existing PTSD is vital to achieve a positive outcome for both the woman and her baby.

Women might find it difficult to build a rapport and develop a trusting relationship with health professionals. A woman may delay or refuse antenatal care if she is fearful of hospitals or of being examined. She might request a termination. Rather than disclosing the trauma initially, she might present with other symptoms of PTSD. It is imperative that healthcare professionals respond with empathy and compassion at the first meeting and develop a trusting relationship with the woman.

The birth plan should include her specific fears and wishes. It is helpful to have a multi-disciplinary meeting to discuss and formulate the birth plan.

Failure to detect and address the condition may result in:

- Poor attendance at antenatal clinic
- Exacerbation of PTSD symptoms
- Use of illicit drugs and alcohol
- Self-harming behaviour
- Secondary depression

Medical Management and Care

- PTSD may be managed in primary or secondary care depending on its severity and complications
- Psychological therapies such as trauma-focused CBT and EMDR are preferred in pregnancy and should be delivered by trained professionals
- Medication may also need to be considered in some cases
- The diagnosis and management should be communicated to the multi-disciplinary team and documented in the woman's maternity notes

Midwifery Management and Care

- A midwife will establish a relationship with the woman early in the pregnancy and offer continued support
- Booking history is important. It is essential that a full history is taken in a sensitive and empathic manner
- Consider factors that might contribute towards developing PTSD
- If the woman is preoccupied with a previous traumatic birth, the possibility of PTSD should be considered and other symptoms explored
- If symptoms are significant and interfere with level of functioning, appropriate referrals for further treatment are made
- Reassurance that efforts will be made to avoid a recurrence of the birth trauma as far as possible
- Desensitisation by arranging visits to the labour room and meeting staff
- Including fears and wishes in the birth plan and preparation
- Referral to trained professionals for psychological therapy
- Communication with health visitor, GP and other professionals
- Referral to Social Services if safeguarding issues identified

Labour Issues

Care in labour may be the critical event to either repair the trauma or increase previous symptoms.

- Continuity of care and support is vital whatever the mode of delivery
- Familiarisation with the staff and setting of the labour ward in advance may be helpful
- The specific fears and wishes of the woman are incorporated into the birth plan[12,14–16]
- Care should be empathic and sensitive and avoid recurrence of specific traumatic events

If the woman is on medication, neonatology involvement is necessary[2].

Medical Management and Care

- For the best outcome, the woman should be offered shared obstetric consultant and midwifery care
- Psychiatric medication may need to be discontinued prior to delivery following advice from the GP or psychiatrist

Midwifery Management and Care

- Birth plan should be developed as early as possible
- Sensitive avoidance of specific anxiety triggers during labour
- Labour care should be managed from a normal perspective unless there have been any indications otherwise
- Arrange for antenatal visit to labour ward and to meet staff
- Discussion of available analgesia for labour to reduce anxiety
- Arrange meeting with anesthetists to discuss requests for epidural
- Birth support and continuity of care is important
- Inform neonatology if woman is on medication

Postpartum Issues

PTSD symptoms could recur or worsen following delivery. Mother–infant attachment may be impaired if symptoms are severe. Complications such as depression or self-harm might follow.

Observe for:

- Escalation of anxiety symptoms[2]
- Handling and attachment to baby[8]
- Depression or irritability
- Self-harming behaviour
- Alcohol or illicit drug use
- Social, relationship and work problems
- Difficulty in coping with care of baby
- PTSD symptoms often resolve spontaneously over time and watchful waiting may be all that is needed initially

Medical Management and Care

- If the birth is uneventful, further obstetric follow-up may not be needed
- New-onset symptoms of PTSD initially require watchful waiting and support
- Symptoms that persist or worsen may be managed in primary care by trained professionals or may require a psychiatry referral
- Psychotherapy is helpful and medication may be needed in some cases

Midwifery Management and Care

- Identification of any abnormal mood changes after birth
- Observe mother–infant interaction and attachment
- Observe and discuss how mother is feeling and coping
- Avoid de-briefing sessions
- Discuss rest, diet and self-care
- Be prepared for breast-feeding difficulties and support accordingly
- Observe the infant if mother is breast-feeding and taking medication
- Communicate with other health professionals
- Referral to Social Services if safeguarding issues are identified

17 Psychiatric Disorders

PATIENT ORGANISATIONS

PNI-UK
http://www.pni-uk.com/pniuk.html

ForParentsbyParents
http://www.depression-in-pregnancy.org.uk/

Meet a Mum Association
http://www.mama.co.uk/default.asp?nc=4104&id=1
0845 120 3746

Mind
www.mind.org.uk
Tel: 08457 660 163

National Childbirth Trust (NCT)
www.nctpregnancyandbabycare.com
Tel: 0870 444 8707

Association for Postnatal Illness
www.apni.org
Tel: 020 7386 0868

Perinatal Illness UK
www.pni-uk.com

Action on Puerperal Psychosis
www.app-network.org

Birth Trauma Association
www.birthtraumaassociation.org

PaNDa
www.vicnet.net.au/-panda
Royal College of Psychiatrists

Perinatal Special Interest Group
www.rcpsych.ac.uk/college/sig/peri.htm

CRY-SIS
www.cry-sis.com
Tel: 0207 404-5011

ESSENTIAL READING

Policy and Guidelines

Royal College of Obstetricians and Gynaecologists 2011 **Confidential Enquiry into Maternal Deaths in the United Kingdom. Saving Mothers' Lives 2006–2008**. London; Royal College of Obstetricians and Gynaecologists

NICE 2007 **Clinical Guideline 45: Antenatal and Post natal Mental Health**. London; National Institute for Health and Clinical Excellence. http://guidance.nice.org.uk/CG45/niceguidance/

The Scottish Intercollegiate Guidelines Network (SIGN) 2002 **Guidelines: Postnatal Depression and Puerperal Psychosis** (includes screening, diagnosis, management for a multidisciplinary team).http://www.sign.ac.uk/guidelines/fulltext/60/index.html

WHO UK Collaborating Centre 2005 **Introduction to Postnatal Disorders**. http://www.libraries.nelh.nhs.uk/mentalhealth

Evidence and Best Practice

The Cochrane Library has systematic reviews on: **Antidepressant Prevention of Postnatal Depression**. http://dx.doi.org/10.1002/14651858.CD004363.pub2

Dennis C-L and Creedy D 2004 **Psychosocial and psychological interventions for preventing postpartum depression**. Cochrane Database.http://dx.doi.org/10.1002/14651858.CD001134.pub2

MIDIRS Informed Choice Leaflet 20: **Postnatal Depression**. http://www.clinicalevidence.com/ceweb/conditions/pac/1407/1407.jsp

Books

Dalton K 2001 **Depression after Childbirth: How to Recognize, Treat, and Prevent Postnatal Depression**, 4th Edn. Oxford; Oxford University Press

Edwards G and Byrom S 2007 **Essential Midwifery Practice: Public Health**. Oxford; Blackwell Publishing Ltd.

Gutteridge KEA and Waheed W 2007 *Maternal mental health: working in partnership* in Byrom S and Edwards G (Eds) **Essential Midwifery Practice: Public Health**. Oxford; Blackwell Publishing Ltd.

Hanzak E 2005 **Eyes without Sparkle: A Journey through Postnatal Illness**. Oxford; Radcliffe

Lazarus R, in press *Perinatal psychiatry* in Guthrie E, Rao S and Temple M (Eds) **Seminars in Liaison Psychiatry**, 2nd Edn. RC Psych Publications. 118–134

Littlewood J and McHugh N 1997 **Maternal Distress And Postnatal Depression**. Basingstoke; Macmillan

Price S (Ed.) 2007 **Mental Health in Pregnancy and Childbirth**. Oxford; Blackwell Publishing Ltd.

Raphael-Leff J 1991 **Psychological Processes of Childbearing**. London; Chapman and Hall

Shaw F 2001 **Out of Me**. London; Virago Press

17.1 Antenatal Psychiatric Disorders

1. Royal College of Obstetricians and Gynaecologists 2007 **Confidential Enquiry into Maternal and Child Health Saving Mothers' Lives 2003–2005**. London; Royal College of Obstetricians and Gynaecologists
2. Appleby L 1991 Suicide during pregnancy and the first postnatal year. **British Medical Journal**, 302:137–140
3. Evans J, Heron J, Oke S and Golding J 2001 Cohort study of depressed mood during pregnancy and after childbirth. **British Medical Journal**, 323:257–260
4. Freeman M, Smith K, Freeman S, *et al.* 2002 The impact of reproductive events on the course of bipolar disorder in women. **Journal of Clinical Psychiatry**, 63:84–87
5. Cantwell R and Cox JL 2003 Psychiatric disorders in pregnancy and the puerperium. **Current Obstetrics and Gynaecology**, 13:7–13
6. Oates MR 2009 The Confidential Enquiry into Maternal Deaths 1997–2005: implications for practice. **Psychiatry**, 8:13–16
7. NICE 2007 **Clinical Guideline 45 – Antenatal and Postnatal Mental Health**. London; National Institute for Health and Clinical Excellence. www.nice.org.uk
8. Royal College of Psychiatrists 2000 **Perinatal Maternal Mental Health Services** (Council Report CR88)
9. Rice F, Jones I and Thapar A 2007 The impact of gestational stress and prenatal growth on emotional problems in offspring: a review. **Acta Psychiatrica Scandinavica**, 115:171–183
10. Brand S and Brennan P 2009 Psychiatric disorders in pregnancy: impact of antenatal and postpartum maternal illness: how are the children? **Clinical Obstetrics and Gynaecology**, 52:441–445
11. Hay DF, Asten P, Mills A, Kumar R, Pawlby S and Sharp D 2001 Intellectual problems shown by 11-year-old children whose mothers had postnatal depression. **Journal of Child Psychology and Psychiatry**, 42:871–889
12. Manning C and Gregoire A 2009 Effects of parental mental illness on children. **Psychiatry**, 8:7–9

17.2 Postnatal Psychiatric Disorders

1. Oates MR 2009 The Confidential Enquiry into Maternal Deaths 1997–2005: implications for practice. **Psychiatry**, 8:13–16
2. NICE 2007 **Clinical Guideline 45 – Antenatal and Postnatal Mental Health**. London; National Institute for Health and Clinical Excellence. www.nice.org.uk
3. O'Hara MW and Swain AM 1996 Rates and risk of postnatal depression – a meta-analysis. **International Review of Psychiatry**, 8:37–54
4. Royal College of Psychiatrists 2000 **Perinatal Maternal Mental Health Services** (Council Report CR88)
5. SIGN 2002 **Postnatal Depression and Puerperal Psychosis – A National Clinical Guideline**. Edinburgh; Scottish Intercollegiate Guidelines Network
6. Cantwell R and Cox JL 2003 Psychiatric disorders in pregnancy and the puerperium. **Current Obstetrics and Gynaecology**, 13:7–13
7. Raynor M 2003 Pregnancy and the puerperium: the social and psychological context. **Psychiatry**, 2:2(1–3). The Medicine Publishing Company
8. Jones I and Craddock N 2005 Editorial. Bipolar disorder and childbirth: the importance of recognising risk. **British Journal of Psychiatry**, 186:453–454
9. Brand S and Brennan P 2009 Psychiatric disorders in pregnancy: impact of antenatal and postpartum maternal illness: how are the children? **Clinical Obstetrics and Gynaecology**, 52:441–445

10. Martins C and Gaffan EA 2000 Effects of early maternal depression on patterns of infant–mother attachment: a meta-analytical investigation. **Journal of Child Psychology and Psychiatry**, 41:737–746
11. Ramchandani P, Stein A, Evans J and O'Connor TG 2005 Paternal depression in the postnatal period and child development: a prospective population study. **Lancet**, 365:2201–2205
12. Jones I, Doshi M, Haque S, Holder R, Brockington I and Craddock N 2006 Obstetric variables associated with bipolar affective puerperal psychosis. **British Journal of Psychiatry**, 188:32–36
13. Blackmore E, Jones I, Doshi M, *et al.* 2006 Obstetric variables associated with bipolar affective puerperal psychosis. **British Journal of Psychiatry**, 188:32–36
14. Paton C. 2008 Prescribing in pregnancy. **British Journal of Psychiatry**, 192:321–322
15. Weick A and Gregoire A 2009 Pharmacological management and ECT in childbearing women with psychiatric disorders. **Psychiatry**, 8:33–37
16. Cox JL, Holden JM and Sagovsky R 1987 Detection of postnatal depression. Development of the 10-item Edinburgh postnatal depression scale. **British Journal of Psychiatry**, 150:782–786

17.3 Eating Disorders

1. WHO 1992 **The International Classification of Diseases (ICD 10): Classification of Mental and Behavioural Disorders: Clinical descriptions and Diagnostic Guidelines**. Tenth Revision. Geneva; WHO
2. Fairburn CG and Harrison PJ 2003 Eating disorders. **Lancet**, 361:407–416
3. Strober M, Freeman R and Morrell W 1999 Atypical anorexia nervosa: separation from typical cases in course and outcome in a long-term prospective study. **International Journal of Eating Disorders**, 25:135–142
4. Herzog DB, Keller MB, Sacks NR, Yeh CJ and Lavori PW 1992 Psychiatric comorbidity in treatment-seeking anorexics and bulimics. **Journal of the American Academy of Child and Adolescent Psychiatry**, 31:810–818
5. Key A, Mason H and Bolton J 2000 Reproduction and eating disorders: a fruitless union. **European Eating Disorders Review**, 8:98–107
6. Ward VB 2008 Eating disorders in pregnancy. **British Medical Journal**, 336:93–96
7. Lacey JH and Smith G 1987 Bulimia nervosa: the impact of pregnancy on mother and baby. **British Journal of Psychiatry**, 150:777–781
8. Lemberg R and Phillips J 1989 The impact of pregnancy on anorexia nervosa and bulimia. **International Journal of Eating Disorders**, 8:285–295
9. Micali N, Treasure J and Simonoff E 2007 Eating disorders symptoms in pregnancy: a longitudinal study of women with recent and past eating disorders and obesity. **Journal of Psychosomatic Research**, 63:297–303
10. Stice E 2002 Risk and maintenance factors for eating pathology: a meta-analytic review. **Psychological Bulletin**, 128:825–848
11. Fairburn CG, Cowen PJ and Harrison PJ 1999 Twin studies and the aetiology of eating disorders. **International Journal of Eating Disorders**, 26:349–358
12. Paxton SJ, Schutz HK, Wertheim EH and Muir SL 1999 Friendship clique and peer influences on body image concerns, dietary restraint, extreme weight-loss behaviors, and binge eating in adolescent girls. **Journal of Abnormal Psychology**, 108: 255–266

13. Sriegel-Moore R, Silberstein LR and Rodin J 1986 Toward an understanding of risk factors for bulimia. **American Psychologist**, 41:246–263

14. Wentz E, Gillberg IC, Anckarsater H, *et al.* 2009 Adolescent-onset anorexia nervosa: 18-year outcome. **British Journal of Psychiatry**, 94:168–174

15. McKnight Investigators 2003 Risk factors for the onset of eating disorders in adolescent girls: results of the McKnight longitudinal risk factor study. **The American Journal of Psychiatry**, 160:248–254

16. NICE 2004 **Eating Disorders Core Interventions in The Treatment and Management of Anorexia Nervosa, Bulimia Nervosa and Related Eating Disorders**. NICE Clinical Guideline 9. London; National Institute for Health and Clinical Excellence. www.nice.org.uk

17. Cooper PJ and Steere JA 1995 Comparison of two psychological treatments for bulimia nervosa: implications for models of maintenance. **Behaviour Research and Therapy**, 33:875–885

18. Cantrell C, Kelley T and McDermott T 2009 Midwifery management of the woman with an eating disorder in the antepartum period. **Journal of Midwifery and Women's Health**, 54:503–507

19. NICE 2010 **Dietary Interventions and Physical Activity Interventions for Weight Management Before, During and After Pregnancy**. London; NICE

20. NICE 2007 **Intrapartum care: care of healthy women and their babies during childbirth**. NICE Clinical Guideline 55. London; National Institute for Health and Clinical Excellence. www.nice.org.uk

21. NICE 2006 **Routine postnatal care of women and their babies**. NICE clinical guideline 37. London; National Institute for Health and Clinical Excellence. www.nice.org.uk

17.4 Post-Traumatic Stress Disorder

1. Lewin J 2010 Perinatal psychiatric disorders in Cohen D (Ed.) **Oxford Textbook of Women and Mental Health**. Oxford; Oxford University Press 161–168

2. NICE 2005 **Post-Traumatic Stress Disorder (PTSD) – The Management of PTSD in Adults and Children in Primary and Secondary Care**. Clinical Guideline 26: NICE. London; National Institute for Health and Clinical Excellence. www.nice.org.uk

3. WHO 1992 **The International Classification of Diseases (ICD 10): Classification of Mental and Behavioural Disorders: Clinical descriptions and Diagnostic Guidelines**. Tenth Revision. Geneva; WHO

4. Schnurr PP and Green BL (Eds) 2003 **Trauma and Health: Physical Consequences of Exposure to Extreme Stress**. Washington, DC; American Psychological Association

5. Olde E, van der Hart O, Kleber R and Van Son MJM 2006 Posttraumatic stress disorder following childbirth: a review. **Clinical Psychology Review**, 26:1–16

6. Menage J 1993 Post-traumatic stress disorder in women who have undergone obstetric and/or gynaecological procedures. **Journal of Reproductive and Infant Psychology**, 11:221 – 228

7. Crompton J 1996a Post-traumatic stress disorder and childbirth. **British Journal of Midwifery**, 4:290–294

8. Turton P *et al.* 2001 Incidence, correlates and predictors of post-traumatic stress disorder in the pregnancy after still birth. **British Journal of Psychiatry**, 178:556–560

9. Crompton J 1996b Post-traumatic stress disorder and childbirth: 2. **British Journal of Midwifery**, 4:354–356 and 373

10. Smith MV *et al.* 2006 Symptoms of post traumatic stress disorder in a community sample of low-income pregnant women. **American Journal of Psychiatry**, 163:881–884

11. Creedy D 2000 Development of acute trauma symptoms: incidence and contributory factors. **Association for Improvements in Maternity Services**, 12:19

12. World Health Organisation 2009 **Mental Health Aspects of Women's Reproductive Health: A Global Review of the Literature**. Geneva:WHO

13. Mayer L 1995 The severely abused woman in obstetric and gynaecological care. guidelines for recognition and management. **Journal of Reproductive Medicine**, 40:13–18

14. Goldbeck-Wood S 1996 PTSD may follow childbirth. **British Medical Journal**, 313:774

15. Ballard CG, Stanley AK and Brockington IF 1995 Posttraumatic stress disorder (PTSD) after childbirth. **British Journal of Psychiatry**, 166:525–528

16. Reynolds JL 1997 Posttraumatic stress disorder after childbirth: the phenomenon of traumatic birth. **Canadian Medical Association Journal**, 156:831–835

17. O'Driscoll M 1994 Midwives, childbirth and sexuality. **British Journal of Midwifery**, 2:39–41

18. Hofberg K and Brockington I 2000 Tokophobia: an unreasoning dread of childbirth. **British Journal of Psychiatry**, 176:83–85

19. Ryding EL, Wijma B and Wijma K 1997 Posttraumatic stress reactions after emergency caesarean section. **Acta Obstetrica et Gynaecologica Scandinavica**, 76:856– 861

20. Sjogren B 1997 Reasons for anxiety about childbirth in 100 pregnant women. **Journal of Psychosomatic Obstetrics and Gynaecology**, 18:266–272

21. Bailham D and Joseph S 2003 Post-traumatic stress following childbirth: a review of the emerging literature and directions for research and practice. **Psychology, Health and Medicine**, 8:159–168

22. Frieder A, Dunlop AL, Culpepper L and Bernstein P 2008 The clinical content of preconception care: women with psychiatric conditions. **American Journal of Obstetrics and Gynaecology**. Supplement December 328–322

Appendix Reference

1. NICE 2007 **Clinical Guideline 45 – Antenatal and Postnatal Mental Health**. London; National Institute for Health and Clinical Excellence 8–9. http://guidance.nice.org.uk/CG45/niceguidance/pdf/English/download.dspx

Appendix 17.1 Treatment Guidance for Depression

MEDICAL MANAGEMENT OF DEPRESSION

When choosing an antidepressant for pregnant or breast-feeding women, NICE recommend that prescribers should, while bearing in mind that the safety of these drugs is not well understood, take into account that[1]:

- Tricyclic antidepressants, such as amitriptyline, imipramine and nortriptyline, have lower known risks during pregnancy than other antidepressants
- Most tricyclic antidepressants have a higher fatal toxicity index than selective serotonin reuptake inhibitors (SSRI)
- Fluoxetine is the SSRI with the lowest known risk during pregnancy
- Imipramine, nortriptyline and sertraline are present in breast milk at relatively low levels
- Citalopram and fluoxetine are present in breast milk at relatively high levels
- SSRI taken after 20 weeks' gestation may be associated with an increased risk of persistent pulmonary hypertension in the neonate
- Paroxetine taken in the first trimester may be associated with fetal heart defects
- Venlafaxine may be associated with increased risk of high blood pressure at high doses, higher toxicity in overdose than SSRI and some tricyclic antidepressants, and increased difficulty in withdrawal
- All antidepressants carry the risk of withdrawal or toxicity in neonates; in most cases the effects are mild and self-limiting

For a woman who develops mild or moderate depression during pregnancy or the postnatal period, the following should be considered[1]:

- Self-help strategies (guided self-help, computerised cognitive behavioural therapy, exercise)
- Brief cognitive behavioural therapy or interpersonal psychotherapy

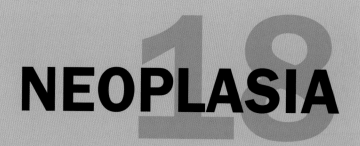

NEOPLASIA

Caroline Farrar[1] and Francis J.E. Gardner[2]

[1]De Montfort University, Leicester, UK
[2]Portsmouth Hospitals NHS Trust, Portsmouth, UK

18.1 Gestational Trophoblastic Disease (Hydatidiform Mole and Choriocarcinoma)
18.2 Cervical Cancer
18.3 Cervical Screening
18.4 Breast Cancer
18.5 Non-Hodgkin's Lymphoma
18.6 Hodgkin's Lymphoma
18.7 Ovarian Neoplasia
18.8 Malignant Melanoma

Medical Disorders in Pregnancy: A Manual for Midwives, Second Edition. Edited by S. Elizabeth Robson and Jason Waugh.
© 2013 John Wiley & Sons, Ltd. Published 2013 by John Wiley & Sons, Ltd.

18.1 Gestational Trophoblastic Disease

Incidence[8]	**Risk for Childbearing**
1 in 714 live births in UK[1]	Current choriocarcinoma – High Risk
	Previous GTD – Low Risk

EXPLANATION OF CONDITION

Gestational trophoblastic disease (GTD) is a spectrum of pregnancy related tumours arising from trophoblastic proliferative disorders without a viable fetus. At the benign end of the disease spectrum there is **hydatidiform mole** and at the malignant end of this continuum spectrum there is the metastatic **gestational trophoblastic neoplasia** (GTN).

- **Complete hydatidiform mole (CM)** – is associated with a chromosomal anomaly. This is often diploid and androgenetic in origin. This condition develops from abnormal fertilisation and abnormal development of the placental tissue. It presents as a collection of fluid-filled cysts that develop when the chorion surrounding the embryo degenerates in early pregnancy
- **Partial hydatidiform mole (PM)** – they are usually paternally derived triploid conceptions in which embryonal development occurs in association with trophoblastic hyperplasia
- **Choriocarcinoma** – this is an invasive hydatidiform mole that has the potential to metastasise
- **Placental site trophoblastic tumours** – only complete hydatidiform mole have been shown to develop into tumours. These are extremely rare but have a variable prognosis

Risk factors:

- Increased maternal age[2]
- Previous hydatidiform mole[3]
- Grand multiparas[3]
- Ethnicity (women from Asia have a higher incidence)[4]
- Socioeconomic status[2]
- Environmental exposure[3]

COMPLICATIONS

Abnormal trophoblastic tissue is commonly associated with vaginal bleeding, particularly in the first trimester[5]. The medical history and examination often reveals an excessive nausea and vomiting (hyperemesis gravidarum) associated with an abnormally high beta human chorionic gonadotrophin (βhCG) level and a uterus which is larger than expected for the gestational age. Other associated complications may include anaemia, thromboembolism or hyperthyroidism, but these are less commonly seen, especially in developed countries because there is widespread use of sensitive pregnancy tests and early diagnosis of pregnancy and viability by high quality ultrasound. However, early onset of pre-elampsia in the second trimester is a recognised presentation in developing countries in particular where access to these facilities is limited.

With the availability of ultrasonography and in particular transvaginal sonography in the first trimester[6] such abnormalities can usually be confirmed. However, the diagnosis of complete hydatidiform moles is more reliable ultrasonographically than diagnosing partial moles as this can be more complex[1]. Approximately 50% of women with an abnormal ultrasound scan will have a hydatidiform mole confirmed by histology[7].

Molar pregnancy recurs in about 1 in 80 subsequent pregnancies[8].

TREATMENT AND CARE

Suction curettage is the preferred method of evacuation regardless of the size of the uterus in women, who desire to preserve their fertility[9], and precautions need to be taken against massive blood loss. A second evacuation is not usually required unless the woman has persistent bleeding and ultrasound shows significant abnormal residual tissue. The avoidance of oxytocic agents should be considered due to speculative risk of causing disseminated trophoblastic disease. Histological examination of the products of conception is recommended in both the cases where a diagnosis of GTD is suspected but also from medical or surgical management of all failed pregnancies[1].

Hysterectomy is a reasonable option for women who do not wish to preserve their fertility[10]. However, women should be counselled that although this procedure stops the risk of local invasion, it does not eliminate the possible need for chemotherapy or the need for monitoring of βhCG concentrations after the procedure.

All women in the UK with GTD should be registered with the Trophoblastic Disease Registration and Surveillance scheme[11]. Women are followed up with serial serum and urinary βhCG levels to identify those women with persistent trophoblastic tissue either localised to the uterus or disseminated elsewhere such as in choriocarcinoma. This tissue is highly sensitive to chemotherapy with high rates of remission expected.

Chemotherapy is the treatment of choice especially for choriocarcinoma. The need for chemotherapy following a complete mole is 15% and after a partial mole is 0.5%[12]. Treatment is used based on the International Federation of Obstetricians and Gynaecologists (FIGO) scoring system[13].

Women who receive chemotherapy treatment for choriocarcinoma are likely to have an earlier menopause and are at risk of developing secondary cancers if their choriocarcinoma is classified as high risk[1].

Psychological support is important for women with a diagnosis of GTD as this can have a profound effect on a woman and therefore when discussing the management and care required it is also essential to acknowledge this disease is associated with not only the loss of a pregnancy but also the concerns regarding malignancy[14]. Women may experience feelings of anxiety, anger, confusion, sexual dysfunction and concerns for future pregnancies[10].

PRE-CONCEPTION ISSUES AND CARE

The risk to women of having a further molar pregnancy is relatively low at a rate of 1 in 80[1]. If a further molar pregnancy occurs it is usually of the same histological type[8]. Women are advised to avoid conception while they are on active follow-up because the monitoring process relies on the use of βhCG levels to detect persistent trophoblastic disease. Obviously if a further pregnancy occurs the βhCG levels will rise, causing confusion in the follow-up process.

Both early pregnancy and hormonal contraception may increase the risk of persistent trophoblastic disease and choriocarcinoma so effective use of barrier methods of contraception is recommended[1].

Pregnancy Issues

Vaginal bleeding in the first trimester is common. The common aetiologies are early pregnancy failure or miscarriage, ectopic pregnancy and less commonly GTD. Other sources of bleeding unrelated to pregnancy need to be ruled out such as cervical pathologies whether inflammatory or neoplastic. Thus careful assessment utilising information from a detailed history and examination facilitated by serial βhCG levels and ultrasound assessments can lead to accurate diagnosis and appropriate management supported by appropriate counselling for the woman[15].

Complete molar pregnancy may rarely co-exist with a normal twin pregnancy. In this situation, the woman may wish to continue with the pregnancy despite a potential risk of developing persistent trophoblastic disease; however, the outcome of chemotherapy, if required is unaffected. Clearly this pregnancy would be considered high risk with an increased rate of early miscarriage, second trimester loss and pre-eclampsia. However, the reported literature suggests there is a 40% chance that a live birth is possible without radically increasing the risk of choriocarcinoma[4].

Medical Management and Care

- Pregnancy viability can be determined using a combination of ultrasound (transvaginal) and serial βhCG levels for management of first trimester bleeding[15]
- Significant fetomaternal haemorrhage may occur following an early pregnancy loss or threatened miscarriage of a viable fetus. In this situation rhesus negative women should have anti-D immunoglobulin administered to reduce the risk of iso-immunisation
- Obviously a twin pregnancy that is affected by GTD will be classified as high risk and a multidisciplinary approach will be taken

Midwifery Management and Care

- It is important to be alert to the signs and symptoms of GTD but at the same time be mindful that such symptoms could be related to a multiple pregnancy
- The majority of pregnancies following a molar pregnancy can be managed as low risk under the care of community midwifery.
- Accurate record keeping is essential to make sure subsequent pregnancies are observed closely with a referral mechanism if required

Labour Issues

Anticipation of a normal birth following a previous molar pregnancy should be considered under the management of the woman's obstetric and midwifery team.

If in the rare situation a twin pregnancy has been confirmed with one viable fetus and one molar pregnancy it is important that the care and treatment is managed by a multidisciplinary team including obstetricians, midwives, radiologists and oncologists[16].

Medical Management and Care

- If a subsequent pregnancy has continued uneventfully to term after a molar pregnancy it is not necessary for obstetric input into the labour provided progress and fetal monitoring are satisfactory[17].

Midwifery Management and Care

- Normal midwifery care in labour is appropriate following a molar pregnancy
- The placenta and membranes should be sent for histological assessment after birth to rule out evidence of GTD

Postpartum Issues

Women who have previously been diagnosed with GTD are at increased risk of further GTD compared with the general population[11].

Following a normal pregnancy with no previous history of GTD there can be on a rare occasion the development of GTD. This should be considered in any postnatal women with persistent irregular vaginal bleeding. A positive serum βhCG with no evidence of a new intra- or extra-uterine pregnancy on ultrasound imaging may indicate a new diagnosis GTD. Long-term prognosis is worse for this group of women perhaps because of delay in diagnosis being associated with advanced disseminated disease being present at diagnosis or alternatively it may be due to biology of this type of GTD being naturally more aggressive[16,17].

Medical Management and Care

- The regional Trophoblastic Disease Screening Centre should be informed of the fact that a woman who has previously been registered with them has delivered so they may organise for her to provide postnatal urine samples for βhCG concentrations to rule out any recurrence of the disease[11]
- If there is any suspicion of recurrent GTD the obstetric team should liaise appropriately with the regional Trophoblastic Disease Screening Centre[17]
- Appropriate contraceptive advice should be offered with avoidance of hormonal contraception and utilisation of barrier contraception encouraged until βhCG levels are within normal limits

Midwifery Management and Care

- To provide information regarding contraception and refer to the woman's GP
- Normal postnatal care should be provided with careful monitoring of uterine involution and lochia as poor involution and excessive lochia or irregular bleeding could indicate evidence of GTD
- Women may require extra support if there is a need to attend the regional Trophoblastic Disease Screening Centre if serial βhCG levels are not returning to normal at an appropriate rate

S. E. Robson and J. Waugh

18.2 Cervical Cancer

Incidence	Risk for Childbearing
2830 new cases in 2007 in the UK[1]	1 in 4500–9000 pregnancies[2]
960 women died in 2008 in the UK[1]	
Worldwide, 275 000 women died in 2008[1]	

EXPLANATION OF CONDITION

Cervical cancer is the eleventh most common cancer in women in the UK and the third most common gynaecological cancer[1]. In the UK it is rare for young women to die from cervical cancer; over 80% of all cervical cancer deaths are women over 45 years old. Incidence has almost halved in the last 20 years[1]. However, mortality rates increase with age, with the highest number of deaths occurring over 75. Less than 6% of cervical deaths occur in women under 35[1].

Types

Cervical cancer is malignant neoplasm of the cervix uteri or cervical area. There are two main types:

- Squamous cell cancer
- Adenocarcinoma[2]

The most common type of cervical cancer, squamous cell cancer, arises in the squamous cells covering the outer surface of the cervix whilst adenocarcinoma arises in the glandular cells which are normally in the cervical canal. While the overall incidence of cervical cancer is falling in the UK as a result of an effective screening programme, adenocarcinoma is becoming relatively more common. Cervical cancer if left untreated invades the normal tissue of the cervix, the tissues around the cervix and vagina, the body of the uterus, the bladder towards the front and the rectum behind. If the tumour is allowed to grow to the pelvic side wall it will obstruct the ureters causing hydronephrosis and obstructive renal failure. The more extensive the tumour the greater is the chance the lymph glands in the pelvis and para-aortic chain will be involved with metastatic cancer.

Symptoms

Cervical cancer is often asymptomatic at an early stage and detected when women attend the colposcopy service with an abnormal smear. Most of these women can have local treatment to the cervix which is curative. As cervical cancer becomes more established abnormal vaginal bleeding such as post-coital bleeding (bleeding after intercourse), intermenstrual bleeding (unprovoked bleeding between periods) or postmenopausal bleeding is common[3,4].

Other symptoms may include an offensive vaginal discharge or discomfort or pain during sex. However, both of these symptoms are more likely to be due to other causes not related to cancer.

In advanced cervical cancer there may be symptoms of systemic malaise such as tiredness, lethargy and nausea. This may be related to obstructive renal failure causing uraemia and electrolyte disturbances.

Human papillomavirus (HPV)

Oncogenic (cancer forming) human papillomavirus (HPV) infection is believed to be the cause of both invasive cervical cancer and the premalignant change in the cervical epithelium (cervical intraepithelial neoplasia, CIN). There are more than 150 types of HPV acknowledged to exist although not all of these predispose to cervical cancer[2]. Some HPVs cause benign skin warts or papillomas, which is the origin of the name of the virus.

There are approximately 40 types that affect the genital area and these are sub-divided into two groups; low risk and high risk cervical cancer. Low risk types are responsible for genital warts (serotype HPV-6 and HPV-11) and high risk types occurring most frequently in cervical cancer are mainly serotypes HPV-16 and HPV-18. Together these account for over 70% of squamous cell cervical cancers[3]. HPV-18 is also thought to account for approximately 50% of all adenocarinomas[2].

HPV is transmitted sexually but is not considered a sexually transmitted disease so women who have been treated for CIN or cervical cancer should not feel stigmatised. Eighty percent of sexually active people will show serological evidence of exposure to oncogenic HPV during their lifetimes but it is believed that it is only those individuals who have persistent infection who develop CIN and then cervical cancer[5]. The majority of people exposed to oncogenic HPV just have a transient infection which does not cause long-term harm. It is reassuring that there is a long latent period between exposure to oncogenic HPV and developing cervical cancer. Because most infections are transient cervical screening (Figure 18.2.1 and Table 18.2.1) is not recommended in England before the age of 25 years as it is expected this will reduce the incidence of treatment in young women who would otherwise have reverted back to normality spontaneously.

Clearly, factors which affect the immune response are critical to the development of CIN and cervical cancer. Smoking is associated with increased risk in the development of pre-malignant and malignant changes in the cervix, although it is unclear as to which compounds in cigarette smoke are actually responsible for this action. A number of pre-scribed drugs, including long-term use of steroids for various autoimmune diseases or immunosuppressive drugs administered in transplantation patients, are associated with an increased risk of CIN and cervical cancer. Systemic illness such as HIV infection causes immunosuppression and increases the risk of cervical cancer. This link is so well established that diagnosis of cervical cancer in an HIV-positive patient is considered to be an AIDS defining condition.

There appears to be other factors that could also increase the risk of cervical cancer:

- Experiencing sexual intercourse from an early age
- Multiple sexual partners
- Having intercourse with a male partner who has had multiple sexual partners
- Oral contraceptive pill for more than 4 years has a theoretical link[6]

Staging

Staging is by the International Federation of Gynecology and Obstetrics (FIGO)[7]. This is based on clinical findings rather than surgical findings. Once cervical cancer has been identified it is then divided into stages.

A broad overview is below:

- **Stage I** – Carcinoma is strictly confined to the cervix
  1a – is microscopically invasive
  1b – is clinically visible
- **Stage II** – Carcinoma invades beyond the cervix into the immediate surrounding tissues including the upper two-thirds of the vagina
- **Stage III** – Carcinoma extends to the pelvic wall and involves the lower third of the vagina
- **Stage IV** – Carcinoma extends beyond the pelvis with involvement of the bladder and rectum, or more distant organs such as the lungs

NON-PREGNANCY TREATMENT AND CARE

Treatment for Abnormal Cells

There are several different treatments for pre-cancerous/abnormal changes (CIN) in the cervix. They all aim to remove or destroy abnormal cells. This can be done by freezing (cryotherapy), with heat from a laser (laser ablation) or a hot probe (cold coagulation – this is a misnomer, the probe is regulated to 140 °C), or by treating the abnormal area with electric cautery. Either electric diathermy may be used to ablate an area or a large loop excision of the transformation zone (LLETZ) may be used with electric cautery. This later technique has the benefit of providing a sample of tissue which can be sent for histological assessment to confirm the exact nature of the lesion.

Treatment for Cervical Cancer

Stage 1a cervical cancer (microinvasive disease) is mostly treated with local excision of the lesion from the cervix which, provided there is evidence of normal tissue from around the area of invasive disease, should not require further treatment. To rule out evidence of early spread of disease full cancer staging is performed with magnetic resonance imaging (MRI) and examination under anaesthetic in most cancer centres. These women retain normal fertility but may be at increased risk of pre-term birth in pregnancy.

Clinically visible cancers confined to the cervix (stage Ib) mostly require more extensive treatment. The risks of lymph node metastases increases with the grade of tumour and size of the primary. Patients who have lymph node metastases diagnosed on MRI, laparoscopic lymph node sampling or after radical surgery are recommended to have combination treatment with chemotherapy and radiotherapy. Those women who are lymph node negative who wish to retain fertility with small cervical cancers may be offered a radical trachelectomy operation. The cervix is resected with the surrounding tissues, including a cuff of vagina, and pelvic lymphadenectomy is performed. The body of the uterus is retained and an artificial cervix is created with a permanent non-absorbable suture inserted in the base of the body of the uterus. For women not wishing to retain fertility or those with larger tumours either confined to the cervix or just extending outside the cervix into the surrounding tissues or vagina (stage IIa) the standard treatment is radical hysterectomy with pelvic lymphadenectomy. The benefit of this over combination treatment with chemotherapy and radiotherapy

in premenopausal women is the women can retain their ovaries. They will remain premenopausal and could potentially provide eggs for IVF and a surrogacy program if they wished to have a baby in the future which is of their own biological make up. For women with more advanced disease, combination treatment with chemotherapy and radiotherapy is recommended but this treatment renders premenopausal women infertile, postmenopausal and with a high incidence of sexual dysfunction due to vaginal narrowing and dryness.

PRE-CONCEPTION ISSUES AND CARE

Pre-invasive abnormalities (CIN) should *not* preclude a pregnancy but repeated treatments put the woman at risk of pre-term birth. If there has been conservative fertility sparing treatment for early cervical cancer, pregnancy is possible but again the women should be counselled to the risks of premature labour.

Pregnancy is not an option for women who have undergone a hysterectomy or radiotherapy for invasive cervical cancer. If the ovaries have been retained and the woman remains premenopausal ovulation induction for an IVF cycle and surrogacy could be possible.

Pregnancy Issues

- Women with cervical cancer during pregnancy often present with vaginal bleeding. Despite vaginal bleeding usually being associated with pregnancy, this should not be presumed and cancer should be considered a possibility
- If there are any early stages of cervical cancer, these can be treated in the form of a suitably tailored cone biopsy. Although LLETZ is a more conservative method it has been shown to cause less complications[8]
- Colposcopic and cytological surveillance of cervical lesions during pregnancy appears to be safe in pregnancy
- If the tumour is at an advanced stage, radical surgery, chemotherapy or radiotherapy may need to be considered. Therefore this will depend on the stage of the disease and gestation, and appropriate delivery considered

Medical Management and Care

- A detailed medical and obstetric history should be documented
- On vaginal examination ensure the cervix and vagina can be visualised to identify any abnormalities
- Cervical cytology is not usually performed in pregnancy, unless there are specific reasons such as a 'poor attender' in which case they might be performed up to 12 weeks gestation
- If confirmed vaginal bleeding consider anti-D prophylaxis in cases of Rhesus negative women beyond 10 weeks gestation
- Cervical cerclage to prolong the pregnancy may be necessary if there is evidence of cervical shortening on serial cervical length measurements
- If possible delay any treatment until after 32 weeks to minimise the risk of prematurity

Midwifery Management and Care

- Ensure a thorough booking history, that identifies past or present gynaecological symptoms and treatment, and a referral should be made for obstetric review
- In the event of vaginal bleeding this should warrant referral for a medical examination and review
- Women who feel stigmatised by the link between sexual activity and cervical cancer should be supported, counselled and educated to the reality of risk of exposure of oncogenic HPV in our society

Labour Issues

- Vaginal delivery is possible if CIN is under surveillance, but there is a higher risk of haemorrhage if there is a cervical tumour[9]. There is also risk of cervical dystocia due to scar tissue, and caesarean section may be necessary for failure to progress in labour
- In cases of advanced cancer, which are rare in pregnancy, a caesarean-radical hysterectomy may be necessary. At the time of surgery the ovaries may be preserved

Medical Management and Care

- Active monitoring of progress in labour is important as cervical dystocia may cause poor progress in labour. Augmented labour in this situation with oxytoxic drugs could increase the risk of uterine rupture
- Obstetrician and oncology team should consider timing and type of caesarean section. A classical caesarean section under certain circumstances would minimise the risk of disturbing the tumour; this could be followed by a radical hysterectomy or combination treatment with chemotherapy and radiotherapy depending on the stage of disease

Midwifery Management and Care

- A multidisciplinary approach is imperative in the woman's care
- In cases of CIN only, the labour can be managed normally by the midwife if vaginal delivery is anticipated
- Be aware that slow progress in the first stage of labour could be due to cervical dystocia, hence regular assessment of the progress of labour should be made with judicious completion of the partogram
- Be alert for intra-partum bleeding, particularly in established labour

Postpartum Issues

- There should be an increased awareness that a cervical lesion could be the cause of postpartum haemorrhage particularly if the uterus is found to be well contracted
- The puerperium could be a period of anxiety, as the woman may have concerns about future cancer treatment and prognosis. There may be relationship tensions if the woman has experienced post-coital bleeding or feels traumatised
- In pregnancy and puerperium the cervical cytology (if they were deemed necessary) should be interpreted and evaluated as in a non-pregnant state[10]
- Contraception is advised and prescribed as normal

Medical Management and Care

Follow-up for Women Treated for Abnormal Cells in Pregnancy
- Seen within 3 months post-delivery
- Review every 3 months for 1 year post-treatment
- Review every 4 months for second year post-treatment
- Review every 6 months for third, fourth and fifth year post treatment
- Women should be informed about the potential impact of cervical procedures on future pregnancies/fertility

Follow-up for Women Treated for Cervical Cancer in Pregnancy
- After the treatment of a caesarean-radical hysterectomy women will need to be seen at regular intervals by the oncology team. Complex management is necessary, which cannot be addressed within the confines of this textbook and further sources should be consulted

Midwifery Management and Care

- Normal postpartum care, being alert for secondary postpartum haemorrhage
- Midwifery care of any surgical procedures as above
- Observe blood loss
- Encourage and support the woman to attend follow-up appointments
- Consider thrombo-prophylaxis

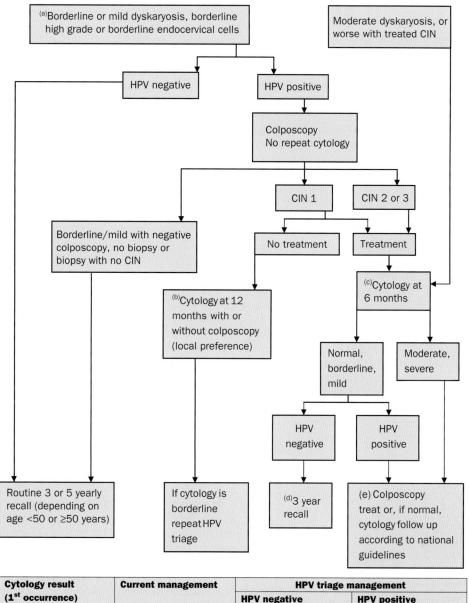

Figure 18.2.1 Human papilloma virus (HPV) triage and test protocol for women aged 25–64 years (reproduced with kind permission from the NHS Cancer Screening programme, August 2011. This algorithm may be updated at regular intervals, so check the NHSCSP website). (a) If sample is unreliable/inadequate for the HPV test, refer mild and recall borderline for 6 month repeat cytology. At repeat cytology HPV test if negative/borderline/mild. If HPV negative return to routine recall: if HPV positive, refer. Refer moderate or worse cytology. (b) Follow up of 12 month cytology only should follow normal NHSCSP protocols. (c) Women in annual follow up after treatment for CIN are eligible for the HPV test of cure at their next screening test. (d) Women >50 who have normal cytology at 3 years will then return to 5 yearly routine recall. Women who reach 65 must still complete the protocol and otherwise comply with national guidance. (e) Women referred owing to borderline or mild or normal cytology who are HR-HPV positive and who then have a satisfactory and negative colposcopy can be recalled in 3 years. This figure is downloadable from the book companion website at www.wiley.com/go/robson

Result	Percentage
Inadequate	2.8
Negative	90.0
Borderline changes	3.9
Mild dyskaryosis	2.1
Moderate dyskaryosis	0.5
Severe dyskaryosis	0.6
?Invasive carcinoma	0.0
?Glandular neoplasia	0.1

Table 18.2.1 NHS Cervical Screening Programme: percentage of tests in the year by type of invitation and result, 2010–2011 (all ages)

18.3 Cervical Screening

Incidence	**Risk for Childbearing**
Screening coverage – 78.6% in 2011[1]	Variable

EXPLANATION OF SCREENING

Cervical cancer is preventable and curable if detected in its pre-malignant stage or at an early stage of invasive disease[2]. Cervical screening does not test for cancer but, using cervical cytology, detects pre-malignant changes which, if untreated, could lead to cervical cancer. Women who have abnormal cells identified are referred to the colposcopy service for further assessment and if necessary treatment (Figure 18.2.1). HPV is transmitted through sexual activity but is not considered a traditional sexually transmitted disease because 80% of people have serological evidence of exposure to the virus. Persistent infection can result in cervical intraepithelial neoplasia (CIN) a premalignant condition which over a long latent period may progress to invasive carcinoma. Primary prevention is aimed at prophylactic vaccines against high risk HPV[3].

The UK NHS Cancer Screening Programme[4] announced it would introduce human HPV testing in 2012 to supplement the existing cervical cytology testing. The benefit is that those women with low grade cytological abnormalities, if found to be negative for oncogenic HPV, may return to routine cytology screening. Previously they would have attended colposcopy services for repeat assessments until cervical cytology returned to normality. This new development is based on evidence resulting from extensive research and assessment into the utility of HPV testing[4].

For any screening programme to be successful it relies on the targeted population to respond to an invitation to be screened. In the case of the cervical screening programme there is a long latent phase which lends itself to repeated opportunities for the pre-malignant changes to be detected and acted upon. Through a combination of public awareness campaigns and support from primary health care providers there has been a high uptake of screening in eligible women. This has facilitated the success of a screening programme reducing overall morbidity and mortality in the general population.

Despite HPV being common within the first 10 years[5] of women becoming sexually active, the NHS in England raised the age of commencement of screening from 21 to 25 years[6] to acknowledge the long latent phase between HPV infection and development of cervical cancer. Many will have a transient infection with associated changes on the cervix (CIN) which in many cases resolves spontaneously. The delay in commencement of screening will reduce the number of colposcopy treatments in this group reducing potential morbidity relating to cervical incompetence and pre-term labour.

The Process of Cervical Sampling

The cervical screening programme consists of a cytopathological examination of a cell sample taken from the cervix. Liquid-based cytology (LBC) is a relatively new way of preparing cervical samples for examination in the laboratory. The original technique described by Papanicolaou used a wooden spatula to sample cells on the cervix which were smeared onto a microscopic slide. Liquid-based cytology uses a specially designed brush to sample cells from the cervix. The head of the brush, where the cells are lodged from the sampling, is detached and placed into a small vial containing preservative fluid. The sample is sent to the laboratory where the cells are re-suspended. A sample of the fluid is used to prepare a glass slide. This method provides a more even preparation of cells which can be stained and assessed by the cytologist. This method is superior to the original technique because the fixation process causes the red blood cells to lyse reducing the chance of the sample being unsuitable for assessment. The cellular preparation is more uniform with less cellular grouping, lending itself to easier and more accurate assessment and potentially more automated assessments.

Cervical cytology is used to identify abnormal or dyskaryotic cervical cells which may indicate the presence of CIN, an established precursor for cervical cancer. Women who have abnormal cervical cytology are requested to attend the colposcopy service where any areas of abnormality can be further assessed and if necessary treated. Any tissue removed is sent for histological assessment to confirm the presence of CIN and to identify any evidence of invasive cancerous disease. Although not all CIN progresses to invasive cancer, persistent mild abnormalities increase the risk of developing cervical cancer in later life[7].

The Statistics

NHS cervical screening statistics[1] for 2010–2011 indicate that in almost 98% of cases English women are receiving results more quickly than before. However, only 79% of eligible women were screened, indicating that 21% of women are unscreened.

Effectiveness of a screening programme is the percentage of women in the target group who have been screened in the last 3 years (under 50s) or 5 years (under 50–64 years old). *The NHS Screening Programme Annual Review 2010–2011*[1] states 'the overall number of 3 351 127 women taking part has increased by over 70 000 compared with 2009–2010'. However, this number is still lower than the figure in 2008–2009 which reached a peak of 3 607 373 due to the high profile of celebrity Jade Goody's death. Table 18.2.1 illustrates the results of adequate tests for women aged 25–64 years (2010–2011)[8].

NON-PREGNANCY AND PRE-CONCEPTION CARE

- A primary prevention programme involves HPV vaccination for two groups, all 12–13-year-old girls (ideally before they are sexually active) and a 'catch-up' group of 17–18-year-old girls. This later group will be discontinued when the vaccinated 12–13-year-old girls reach 17–18 years. This caused controversy with issues of parental consent. Gillick competence was raised, and some groups complaining this promotes a promiscuous society
- UK eligibility for NHS cervical screening is:

Age Group (Years)	Frequency of Screening
25	First invitation
25–49	3 yearly
50–64	5 yearly
65+	Those who have not been screened since 50 years or have had recent abnormal tests

If a woman is planning to become pregnant, her GP should check that her cervical screening is up to date, to enable pre-pregnancy treatment.

Pregnancy Issues

- Mechanisms that compromise cervical function such as cervical excisional procedures may be associated with cervical incompetence and adverse pregnancy outcomes[9]
- Pregnancy after cervical surgery has a theoretical risk of a pre-term birth, but the risk only becomes significant if more than one excisional treatment has been performed
- Women who have CIN in pregnancy have a very low risk of progression to cancer during the pregnancy so a conservative approach is usually agreed with surveillance followed by any necessary treatment approximately 12 weeks post-delivery
- Only if there is a very high suspicion of invasive cancer would a biopsy be considered because during pregnancy there is a risk of haemorrhage and infection with a small chance of miscarriage or pre-term birth[10]

Medical Management and Care

- Cervical cerclage is still an option if cervical incompetence has been demonstrated usually by serial cervical length measurement by ultrasound
- Counselling of women who require cervical procedures must include the risks and benefits of ablative and excisional methods
- Accurate dating of the pregnancy is important as this information may be critical later in the pregnancy in the decision-making process

Midwifery Management and Care

- A thorough booking history is taken and a referral is made to be delivered within a consultant lead unit
- Midwifery support ideally in a specialist pre-term birth clinic is essential as many women who have had more than one colposcopy treatment are very anxious about the risks of pre-term birth during the antenatal period

Labour Issues

- If CIN has been diagnosed in pregnancy this should not significantly affect labour
- If cervical cancer has been diagnosed in pregnancy early, and is believed to be at an early stage without lymphovascular invasion a vaginal delivery is acceptable with therapeutic conisation in the postpartum period
- If the stage is IB1 or IB2 a caesarean-radical hysterectomy should be considered or caesarean followed by chemoradiotherapy
- A caesarean section is the preferred route of delivery to prevent fatal recurrences in the episiotomy scar[11] and catastrophic life threatening haemorrhage

Medical Management and Care

- To develop a plan of management and treatment in respect of cervical findings

Midwifery Management and Care

- Establish a multidisciplinary team approach
- Ensure there is good communication between all disciplines
- Discuss birth plan and provide optimal care as previous cervical treatment may affect the ability of the cervix to dilate in labour

Postpartum Issues

Following birth, counsel the woman about the risks and benefits of screening after the postnatal period; after 6 weeks but before 3 months. This is especially important before further pregnancies are considered.

Medical Management and Care

- Obstetric team to liaise with the oncology team if required
- Patients who have been diagnosed with CIN should have further colposcopy and possible further treatment but not before 3 months postpartum

Midwifery Management and Care

- Normal midwifery postpartum care
- Organise any follow-up appointments, explaining the benefits of screening and prompt commencement of treatment if required

18.4 Breast Cancer

Incidence	**Risk for Childbearing**
1:9 lifetime risk[1]	Variable Risk
1:3000 pregnancies[2]	

EXPLANATION OF CONDITION

Breast cancer is the most common cancer in women and is the leading cause of death in women aged between 35 and 54 years. Fifteen percent of cases are diagnosed before the age of 45 years and therefore this affects almost 5000 women of child-bearing age.

Pregnancy associated breast cancer is defined as a carcinoma that is diagnosed during pregnancy or within one year postpartum. The median age of these women is 33 years, ranging from 23 to 47 years[3].

Pregnant women are at a higher risk of presenting with more advanced disease than non-pregnant women as small lumps cannot be detected as well due to natural tenderness and engorgement of the breasts during pregnancy and lactation.

Most women present with painless masses, with up to 90% of cases being detected by self-examination. Other symptoms may be enlarging masses, nipple or skin retraction, other skin changes or axillary lymphadenopathy.

Screening by mammography detects around 68% of cancerous changes but this can be challenging in pregnancy. The use of ultrasound can detect around 93% of changes in pregnant women.

Diagnosis may be confirmed by using fine needle aspiration under local anaesthesia. However, the normal hyperplastic epithelial changes in breast tissue during pregnancy make interpretation of the specimen more difficult requiring a pathologist with particular expertise to make an accurate assessment.

In the absence of a positive fine needle aspiration a diagnostic excisional biopsy with either general or local anaesthetic is performed. Once a diagnosis of cancer is confirmed an assessment of stage of the disease is required.

Breast Cancer Stage Grouping[4]

- **Stage 0:** non-invasive breast cancer with no invasion of surrounding tissue
- **Stage I:** invasive breast cancer whereby the tumour measures less than 2 cm with no lymph node involvement
- **Stage IIA/IIB:** tumour measures a minimum of 2 cm and maximum of 5 cm or cancer has spread to the lymph nodes in the axilla on the same side as the affected breast
- **Stage IIIA:** tumour size is greater than 5 cm or there is significant lymph node involvement
- **Stage IIIB:** tumour has spread to the breast skin, chest wall or internal mammary lymph nodes
- **Stage IIIC:** tumour can be any size and has spread to the clavicle area including lymph node involvement
- **Stage IV:** tumour can be any size and may have spread to both nearby lymph nodes and also to distant organs; most common sites are bone, liver, brain or lung

COMPLICATIONS

Breast cancer may be associated with several signs and symptoms including fatigue, anaemia, anorexia, depression, sepsis, pain and metastasis.

The common treatments of breast cancer may also exacerbate these signs and symptoms:

- **Radiotherapy:** lethargy, anorexia and localised skin reactions
- **Chemotherapy:** hair loss, nausea, vomiting, fatigue, sepsis and menstrual dysfunction
- **Hormonal therapy:** depression, mood swings, weight gain, feelings of bloating, hot flushes and early menopause

NON-PREGNANCY TREATMENT AND CARE

After a diagnosis has been made and staging has also been confirmed there are several treatments that can be offered and recommended depending on the severity of the cancer.

- **Surgery:** breast conserving surgery (wide local excision), mastectomy, lumpectomy, or/and lymphadenectomy
- **Radiotherapy:** utilises high energy rays which although painless can cause significant side-effects. This treatment is given over several sessions which may last over several weeks. It preferentially destroys rapidly growing cells in the targeted area such as cancer cells minimising damage of normal cells which have a greater ability to repair themselves
- **Chemotherapy:** a course of drug treatment that aims to focus on cancer cells which are actively dividing creating new lethal mutations. There are many cytotoxic agents used with varying regimes depending on the staging of the disease
- **Hormonal Therapy:** if a woman's breast cancer is oestrogen receptor-positive[5] then adjuvant hormonal therapy may be prescribed to reduce risk of recurrence. Rapidly growing recurrent or metastatic breast cancer may also be tested for human epidermal growth factor receptor (HER2). If there are high levels of expression of these receptors then women may be prescribed trastuzumab.

PRE-CONCEPTION ISSUES AND CARE

Women who wish to plan for a pregnancy after breast cancer treatment should consult their clinical oncologist, breast surgeon and obstetrician[1].

Women are generally advised to wait for at least 2 years after treatment before conception[6] as this is the time period of early relapse, although, late relapses can occur up to 10 years or more from diagnosis[7].

There is debate around the duration of hormonal therapy as it is suggested that treatment should be carried out for 5 years[1]. However, other published data recommends delaying pregnancy has an impact on the outcome[8]. Therefore with a good prognosis women need not wait more than 2 years to become pregnant[8].

Pregnancy Issues

Cancer complicates between 0.02 and 0.1% of all pregnancies[9]. Some studies have shown an average delay of 5 months between the first symptoms and diagnosis[10]. There is no conclusive evidence that breast cancer during pregnancy is more aggressive than breast cancer occurring at other times[11].

Treatment

Surgery: this treatment can be undertaken in all trimesters including loco-regional clearance. Breast reconstruction or mastectomy can be considered dependent on the tumour characteristics and breast size[1].

Radiotherapy: this treatment is mainly delayed until after delivery but in some circumstances such as the preservation of organ function or life, fetal shielding can be discussed depending on the gestation.

Chemotherapy: this treatment is contraindicated in the first trimester because of a high rate of fetal abnormality. However, chemotherapy appears safe in the second and third trimester but there is a suggested link to IUGR and low birth weight[12].

Medical Management and Care

- Pregnant women with breast cancer should be treated with the same intentions as for non-pregnant women, i.e. optimal control of the disease
- Early termination of pregnancy has not been shown to improve the maternal outcome for breast cancer[13]
- Within pregnancy completing a modified radical mastectomy is the standard surgical treatment as radiotherapy may deliver potentially damaging high doses of radiation to the developing fetus. Breast conservation may be considered if it is possible to schedule the radiotherapy after delivery without an excessive potentially damaging delay
- If chemotherapy is to be considered this should be based on stage, age and pathological findings as for non-pregnant women
- Chemotherapy should be delayed at least until the second trimester as this reduces the risk of fetal loss and teratogenesis
- Hormonal therapy such as with tamoxifen or trastuzumab is not used until after delivery as there have been reported adverse fetal outcomes[14].

Midwifery Management and Care

- Ensure continuity of care is provided and therefore advocacy is paramount
- Ensuring effective communication between the multidisciplinary team is of vital importance not only for the woman and her family but equally for members of the healthcare team
- It is important when completing regular antenatal checks to observe fetal growth and discuss fetal movements
- If there has been any surgery, wound care may require basic nursing care by midwife or other disciplines such as a district nurse

Labour Issues

Majority of women may proceed to full term in pregnancy and have a normal delivery.

Birth should have a recommendation of more than 2–3 weeks after the last chemotherapy session to allow maternal bone marrow recovery and to minimise problems such as neutropenia[1].

Medical Management and Care

- If a pre-term delivery is to be considered, then use of corticosteroids may minimise the effect of prematurity on the fetal lung function
- A request for the placenta and membranes to be sent to histology should be recommended to examine for evidence of placental metastases

Midwifery Management and Care

- Care in labour needs to be discussed and planned with reference to mobility, especially if the woman has received recent surgery and therefore pain and weakness may be apparent in the upper arms

Postpartum Issues

Breast-feeding is contraindicated during chemotherapy, radiotherapy or hormonal therapy[1].

There is no evidence to suggest that the offspring of a woman having breast cancer whilst pregnant will have an increased risk of developing cancer in later life[11].

The prognosis from breast cancer when associated with a further pregnancy is predominately related to the stage of the disease at original diagnosis.

Stage 0, I, II: show no difference of overall 5-year survival rates regardless of the presence of a further pregnancy.

Stage III: women should defer further pregnancy for at least 5 years after treatment.

Stage IV: women should be advised to avoid future pregnancy[2].

Medical Management and Care

- Women should use effective contraception to avoid unwanted pregnancy particularly during treatment for breast cancer. Hormonal contraception is contraindicated in women with current or recent breast cancer thus effective use of barrier contraception and intrauterine devices may be considered

Midwifery Management and Care

- Discuss and support infant feeding concerns. Breast-feeding is dependent upon current treatment, and advice from a paediatrician or pharmacist is likely to be necessary. Alternative options may need to be discussed such as artificial feeding, milk bank, or even the possibility of a surrogate (wet nurse)
- Ensure adequate postnatal support is available, and ensure effective communication between the multidisciplinary team members is maintained to avoid undue delays in the treatment pathways

18.5 Non-Hodgkin's Lymphoma

Incidence	Risk for Childbearing
10500 cases are diagnosed each year in the UK 1:6000 diagnosed during pregnancy[1]	Low risk

EXPLANATION OF CONDITION

Lymphoma is the fourth most common malignancy diagnosed during pregnancy[1]. The disease is becoming more frequent as a result of late age of first pregnancy. There is also a suggested high incidence of AIDS-related non-Hodgkin's lymphoma (NHL) in developing countries[2]. There are a number of other risk factors that need to be considered; Epstein-Barr virus, human T-cell lymphotropic virus, hepatitis C have all been associated with late development of NHL[3].

In addition there are also autoimmune conditions that have been associated with NHL, as pregnancy is considered as an immunosuppressed condition and therefore can present itself at a more advanced stage. This could be either due to autoimmune changes or possibly a delay in diagnosis.

Non-Hodgkin's lymphoma comprises a heterogeneous group of lymphoid malignancies that originate in lymphoreticular tissues. NHL is distinctly different to Hodgkin's lymphoma by the absence of Reed Sternberg cells. These tumours can be T- or B-cell origin. Their presentation, stage at diagnosis and prognosis can be variable. The mean age at diagnosis for NHL is 42 years compared with Hodgkin's lymphoma which occurs during the reproductive years[4,5].

There are two main types of lymphomas[5]:

High Grade or Aggressive Non-Hodgkin Lymphoma
- Cells appear to be dividing quickly and therefore grow faster
- Most common high grade NHL is diffuse large B-cell lymphoma or Burkitt's lymphoma, lymphoblastic lymphoma and peripheral T-cell lymphoma
- More common in people over 50 years. However, as stated above, it can occur at any age
- This disease does respond well to treatment and can be cured in many cases

Low Grade or Indolent Non- Hodgkin Lymphoma
- Cells appear to be dividing slowly and therefore NHL can take a long time to develop.
- Most common low grade NHL is called follicular lymphoma. Other lymphomas are known as small lymphocytic lymphoma or chronic lymphocytic leukaemia, lymphplasmocytoid lymphoma and low grade mucosa-associated lymphoid tissue (MALT) lymphoma
- Most individuals have advanced low grade NHL by the time a diagnosis is made
- Advanced low grade NHL particularly stage 3 or 4 (see 18.6 Hodgkin's Lymphoma) are more difficult to cure completely

COMPLICATIONS

Fertility complications can still be an issue for both men and women. However, there are now advances in reproductive technologies that can assist preservation of fertility prior to undergoing cancer treatment.

The impact of chemotherapy drugs on sperm production in men is similar in many ways to the effect of radiation. Women having radiation therapy in the pelvic area may stop having menstrual periods and develop symptoms of the menopause. Treatment can also result in vaginal itching, burning and dryness.

NON-PREGNANCY TREATMENT AND CARE

Most people who have high grade NHL will be cured; treatment is almost always with intravenous combination chemotherapy.

Early stage low grade NHL is treated with radiotherapy to the enlarged lymph nodes. It is possible to cure the disease alone with this treatment. However, early stage disease is difficult to diagnose.

By the time symptoms occur the disease will be in an advanced stage and therefore difficult to cure completely. The aim of treatment with advanced low grade NHL is to control the disease while maintaining a good quality of life. Individuals can live for many years and feel well for the majority of the time.

Other treatments may be bone marrow or stem cell transplant – these treatments are under on-going investigation.

There are many side-effects of these treatments: nausea, hair loss, sore mouth, sore skin, change in taste, peripheral neuropathy and fatigue.

PRE-CONCEPTION ISSUES AND CARE

It is important not to become pregnant during radiation therapy as radiation can harm the fetus causing teratogenic affects and fetal death. Women should discuss how contraception is to be managed and to discuss how fertility can be affected.

For men, radiation can reduce both the number of sperm and their quality. One possible option may be to bank sperm before treatment commences.

Pregnancy Issues

Treatments such as chemotherapy and radiotherapy during the first trimester are associated with an increased risk of congenital malformations. However, this risk diminishes as the pregnancy advances.

The approach to treatment for NHL is similar to Hodgkin's lymphoma and is based on the Ann Arbor staging (see 18.6 Hodgkin's Lymphoma).

It is important to stage, classify and use the International Prognostic Index to be able to determine treatment choices.

Generally women diagnosed in the third trimester and those with early stage disease have a better prognosis[6].

Unfortunately many women present with aggressive, advanced stage disease so it is vital that treatment is delayed. Those women who are unwilling to accept the potential risk to the fetus should consider a termination.

Maternal to fetal transmission of non-Hodgkin's lymphoma is seen as a potential risk in pregnancy[6].

Medical Management and Care

- When lymphoma is diagnosed during the first trimester it is recommended that treatment should be carried out with a standard chemotherapy regimen. This is to be followed immediately by a pregnancy termination
- For patients that have indolent NHL, therapy can be delayed until the end of the first trimester
- When lymphoma is diagnosed during the second and third trimesters, evidence suggests that full-dose chemotherapy can be administered without causing a severe risk to the fetus[1]
- Although exposure to multi-agent chemotherapy in the second and third trimesters has been reported to be associated with fetal growth restriction and myelosuppression, conversely other studies indicate the risk of these complications may be lower than previously suggested[7]
- It is important to perform CT scans of the chest, abdomen and pelvis for staging even in the pregnant woman
- MRI can also provide additional information such as bone marrow involvement. MRI scanners are considered safe in pregnancy

Midwifery Management and Care

- Ensure excellent communication is established between the multidisciplinary team
- A precise booking history account needs to be obtained for an accurate plan of care
- It is important to ensure continuity of care
- Be aware of signs of infection and refer appropriately and promptly to the woman's obstetrician
- Organise a visit to the neonatal unit in advance just in case the pregnancy needs to be expedited

Labour Issues

Delivery should be delayed until corticosteroids have been administered to optimise fetal lung maturity.

A plan of care for such women can change dramatically depending on signs and symptoms.

All disciplines need to be aware of any sudden change of care management.

Medical Management and Care

- If possible delivery should be arranged to minimise the risks of prematurity as well as the risk of neonatal myelosuppression, which could occur in the first few weeks after administration of chemotherapy

Midwifery Management and Care

- Pathologic investigation of the placenta should be routinely performed with any maternal haematologic malignancies, hence the placenta should be sent to the laboratory
- Cord blood should be collected for a potential source of HLA-comparable progenitor cells which may be used for future bone marrow transplantation

Postpartum Issues

The central nervous system continues to develop throughout gestation, hence there are concerns regarding long-term neurodevelopmental issues in the outcome of children exposed *in utero* to chemotherapy.

There is limited research data regarding childhood malignancy and long-term fertility in the offspring of women treated for lymphoma during pregnancy. However, studies have shown that offspring have normal sexual development and the risk of development of childhood cancer was no higher than the general population[8].

As it is unclear how much toxicity can be attributed to chemotherapy drugs during lactation most authorities would advise against breast-feeding[9].

Medical Management and Care

- To safeguard mothers who have either had treatment or will pursue treatment, ensure up-to-date evidence and research is provided to enable women to make an informed choice about their care
- These women are susceptible to infection, so ensure they have open access to medical care at all times
- There is a critical need for multicentre co-operation and a central registry to collect data. This would facilitate better studies of treatment during pregnancy

Midwifery Management and Care

- Ensure support and continuity of care is provided and liaise closely with the multidisciplinary team
- Be supportive knowing that breast-feeding is not advised but still demonstrate skin to skin contact and the importance of this in relation to bonding with the baby

18.6 Hodgkin's Lymphoma

Incidence	Risk for Childbearing
1600 cases diagnosed in the UK each year[1] Incidence during pregnancy is 1:1000–1:6000[2]	Variable Risk

EXPLANATION OF CONDITION

Broadly lymphomas are known as a heterogeneous group of malignant disorders that affect the lymphoid tissue. These disorders are further subdivided into two main categories:

1. Hodgkin's disease
2. Non-Hodgkin lymphoma

Hodgkin's disease is an uncommon lymphoid malignancy[2].

The age distribution is most apparent around the childbearing years, this disease being the most common type of lymphoma seen in pregnancy and the fourth most common cancer overall in pregnancy[3]. The average age at diagnosis is 25.5 years. The presentation of this disease does not appear to differ from that in a non-pregnant woman. However, Hodgkin's disease appears to be less common in multiparous women[4].

Clinical findings are lymphadenopathy, usually of the cervical (neck), submaxillary or axillary nodes (groin). In some cases other symptoms can be experienced such as unexplained weight loss, unexplained fever and soaking night sweats.

The aetiology is unknown[5] but most probably multifactorial including environmental and genetic factors. Diagnosis can only occur from a biopsy of the affected tissue. Clonal malignant Hodgkin cells or multinucleated Reed Sternberg cells that are representative of this condition are present. These cells are derived from the B-cell lineage[6,7].

Staging of the disease is an important process as this will determine the appropriate treatment and therefore affects prognosis for the individual. The Ann Arbor system is still the most commonly used staging system together with the woman's age. However, none of the commonly used prognostic scoring systems have been validated in pregnancy[4].

Staging System (4 Stages)

1. **Stage I** – The lymphoma is in a lymph node in only one region, such as the neck
2. **Stage II** – The lymphoma is in two or more groups **on the same side of the diaphragm**
3. **Stage III** – The lymphoma is found in lymph node areas on both sides of the diaphragm
4. **Stage IV-** The lymphoma has spread outside the lymph system into an organ that is not right next to an involved node
5. Patients that have stage I and II and without symptoms are considered to have an early stage neoplasia with a good prognosis[7]
6. Most recurrences occur within 3 years. Despite this the 5-year disease-free survival rate in women with advanced disease treated with a combination of chemotherapy is 70–80%[8]

COMPLICATIONS

The majority of women who have been successfully treated for Hodgkin's disease usually return to a normal or nearly normal, quality of life. Many women who receive treatment such as chemotherapy remain fertile. However, there is a risk of premature menopause[9].

NON-PREGNANCY TREATMENT AND CARE

Such women should be counselled about the risks of pregnancy and therefore appropriate contraception measures should be considered[9].

When lymphoma is suspected, a complete history and a thorough examination of all node-bearing areas should be carried out.

A full range of blood tests including blood cell count, erythrocyte sedimentation rate, liver and renal function tests, lactate dehydrogenase and alkaline phosphatase should be determined. Supplementary radiographic studies include MRI of the chest, abdomen and pelvis.

Treatment can vary depending on the stage of the disease. However, the choice of treatment can include radiotherapy or chemotherapy or a combination of both therapies.

PRE-CONCEPTION ISSUES AND CARE

Following treatment it is suggested to delay conception by at least 2 or 3 years as the majority of recurrences tend to occur within this time period.

It is suggested that there is no increase in the rate of maternal complications or fetal abnormalities in subsequent pregnancies after a combination of chemotherapy[9].

Pregnancy Issues

Pregnancy does not appear to affect the stage of the disease, response to therapy, or overall survival compared with age and stage equivalent of non-pregnant patients[10].

A delay of treatment after delivery is unlikely to show significant differences with birth weight, gestational age or even mode of delivery compared with a healthy woman[11].

There appears to be a mixture of opinions of the risk of treatment in the first trimester that intensive chemotherapy increases the risk of fetal abnormalities, growth restriction and premature delivery. Therefore it could be prudent to wait for treatment until the second or third trimester; or to allow intensive treatment to commence. Termination of pregnancy is an option that should be discussed, although some studies suggest that termination of pregnancy does not improve maternal outcome.

Medical Management and Care

- To delay treatment for women with advanced disease in an early stage of pregnancy may adversely affect survival. Therefore, consideration of risk factors, treatment and an appropriate chemotherapy regime should be introduced
- Consideration of a therapeutic abortion should be considered due to the potential teratogenic effects of chemotherapy particularly within the first trimester[13]
- Patients with early staging in the first trimester can be followed up at short intervals for signs of disease progression without any treatment until the second trimester
- With limited data it can be suggested that women can be safely treated in the second and third trimester with chemotherapy[14]
- Additionally, infants born to women with Hodgkin's lymphoma[11] do not have a higher risk of prematurity or intrauterine growth restriction
- There also appears to be no reports of metastases to the placenta or the fetus
- Cancer is a risk for thrombosis; thromboprophylaxis should be considered

Midwifery Management and Care

- Women diagnosed in the first trimester should be counselled about the risks of continuing with the pregnancy
- A precise booking history needs to be obtained for an accurate plan of care
- Ensure the multidisciplinary team are aware of this patient and communications have been made with the woman's physician to ensure a well-structured care pathway has been created and is also acknowledged and understood by the woman and her family
- Be aware of signs of infection and refer appropriately and promptly to the woman's obstetrician

Labour Issues

For treatment to commence or continue at a more intense level the option to deliver before term maybe considered.

The gestation for an early delivery should be after 32 weeks particularly after corticosteroids have been administered to accelerate fetal lung maturity.

Medical Management and Care

- If expediting delivery of the fetus is required the mode of delivery will be dependent on gestation, parity, maternal and fetal well being
- Ensure neonatal support is sufficient in relation to the baby's gestation and obviously consider corticosteroids, a minimum 24 hours prior to delivery

Midwifery Management and Care

- Care for patients who will deliver prematurely
- Administer corticosteroids to the woman as prescribed taking into account the skill of administration as well as the role and responsibilities of a midwife
- Inform neonatal services and provide support to the woman/family

Postpartum Issues

There is no evidence to suggest the mode of delivery has any relevance. However, it is important to assess the placenta for evidence of metastases. Although this is rare it would give an indication to inspect the newborn more closely.

Women undergoing active treatment with a combination of chemotherapy should be advised not to breast-feed[12].

Medical Management and Care

- To ensure thrombo-prophylaxis assessment has been carried out
- Counselling about prognosis and preservation of fertility should be provided
- Cord blood banking should be considered as possible source of stem cells
- Women who maintain their fertility should be advised not to get pregnant for a minimum of 2–3 years due to the risk factors of a relapse

Midwifery Management and Care

- Supportive postnatal care should be provided for the woman and her family
- Encourage continuity of care from a small group of midwives rather than many carers therefore ensuring a good rapport can be established
- Consider further nursing support once midwifery care is no longer required

S. E. Robson and J. Waugh

18.7 Ovarian Neoplasia

Incidence	Risk for Childbearing
UK – 6000 cases per year[1]	In pregnancy – 1:18 000–1:48 000[2]

EXPLANATION OF CONDITION

Ovarian cancer is the second most common gynaecological cancer[1]. Eighty percent of ovarian cancer is classified as epithelial ovarian carcinoma[1]. It is more common in women after the menopause with a mean age of 64 years at presentation[1]. However, ovarian cancer may occur in pre-menopausal women with an incidence of 1 in 15 000 at the age of 30, 1 in 10 000 at the age of 40 years and 1 in 1500 at the age of 60 years after the menopause. The incidence is higher among caucasian women than Asian women[3].

Approximately 10% of ovarian cancers have a genetic link. Women with hereditary cancers have an earlier presentation with a mean age of 54 years[1]. Mutations in the Breast Cancer Gene (BRCA) have been characterised and so women with a family history of ovarian cancer can have their personal risk assessed by testing for the mutations in the BRCA gene. Women who have a confirmed BRCA gene mutation have a 40–50% life-time risk of ovarian cancer and so may elect to have prophylactic surgery to minimise this risk after completion of their families.

Epithelial ovarian cancers are due to a malignant transformation of the ovarian epithelium. There are less common forms of non-epithelial cancers: these include germ cell and sex cord-stromal cancers. The molecular events leading to malignancy are poorly understood but there appears to be a link to the number of ovulations and the risk of ovarian cancer. Ovulation suppression for example with the contraceptive pill or pregnancies reduces the risk of ovarian cancer even in those with family history and potential genetic risk. Table 18.7.1 lists the risk factors associated with ovarian cancer.

Primary ovarian cancers most commonly arise from the epithelium (epithelial cancers 70%), but may also arise from the connective tissue of the ovary (sex cord stromal) or the germ cells.

An ultrasound scan or cross-sectional imaging with either CT or MRI for another indication or for investigation of bloating or abdominal swelling may incidentally identify a cystic mass on the ovary which may be associated with fluid within the abdominal cavity in those women with no symptoms. This fluid commonly contains viable malignant cells which can seed onto the peritoneal covering of other organs in the abdomen developing metastatic deposits. Seventy percent of ovarian cancers present with evidence of disease spread in the abdomen. Ovarian cancer may also spread through the lymphatic system causing retroperitoneal lymph node enlargement particularly of the lymph node chain associated with the aorta. Less commonly there may be spread of ovarian cancer through the blood vessels causing secondary deposits within the liver or lungs.

Staging of Ovarian Cancer

Staging is by the International Federation of Gynaecology and Obstetrics (FIGO). A broad overview is below:

I Ovarian cancer limited to ovaries:

- Ia Ovarian cancer limited to one ovary
- Ib Ovarian cancer limited to both ovaries
- Ic Ovarian cancer affecting one or both ovaries with either capsule rupture or positive cytology in abdominal washings or ascites

II Ovarian cancer involving one or both ovaries with pelvic extension:

- IIa Ovarian cancer deposits involving one or both ovaries and affecting the uterus or fallopian tubes
- IIb Ovarian cancer deposits involving one or both ovaries and affect other pelvic organs
- IIc Ovarian cancer deposits involving one or both ovaries and any other pelvic organ with either capsule rupture or positive cytology in abdominal washings or ascites

III Ovarian cancer involving one or both ovaries with peritoneal deposits outside the pelvis or involvement of retroperitoneal or inguinal lymph nodes or peritoneal deposits on surface of the liver:

- IIIa Ovarian cancer visibly limited to the pelvis but with histologically confirmed microscopic deposits outside the pelvis
- IIIb Ovarian cancer not limited to the pelvis with visible deposits outside the pelvis less than 2 cm in diameter
- IIIc Ovarian cancer not limited to the pelvis with visible deposits outside the pelvis greater than 2 cm in diameter or positive retroperitoneal or inguinal nodes

IV Ovarian cancer involving one or both ovaries not limited to the pelvis but involving the parenchyma of the liver and or causing a cytologically proven malignant pleural effusion.

SYMPTOMS

Most women with ovarian cancer have vague non-specific symptoms such as bloating, abdominal and pelvic discomfort, increasing abdominal girth and reduced appetite. As these symptoms are often minor and non-specific, women commonly present with advanced disease which is associated with an overall poor prognosis[4]. The overall 5-year survival rate for women with ovarian cancer is below 35%[5].

When an ovary becomes enlarged it is at an increased risk of twisting on its own blood supply. This twisting or torsion

Table 18.7.1 Risk Factors Associated with Ovarian Cancer

Decreased Risk Factors	Increased Risk Factors
• Multiparity	• Nulliparity
• Oral contraceptive pill	• Endometriosis
• Tubal ligation	• Obesity
• Hysterectomy	• Infertility

Pregnancy Issues

Ovarian cancer in pregnancy is rare, affecting an estimated one in 10 000 pregnancies[7]. Pregnancy does not increase the mortality associated with ovarian cancer[8]. The dilemma it causes for women in pregnancy is a conflict between optimal maternal therapy and fetal wellbeing. Subsequently this will have an effect on the wellbeing of the mother, the fetus or both. However, in order not to jeopardise maternal outcome, standard cancer treatment should be aimed for.

In the rare situation that a woman presents in early pregnancy with advanced ovarian cancer then termination of the pregnancy would have to be discussed as delay in treatment until the third trimester when the fetus became viable could adversely affect the maternal outcome regarding the cancer. Standard treatment would involve a hysterectomy with removal of the ovaries and removal of the omentum. Chemotherapy prior to surgery (an alternative strategy in advanced ovarian cancer) is contraindicated in early pregnancy as this could cause fetal demise or teratogenic affects.

Medical Management and Care

- Ultrasound in early pregnancy has resulted in an increased detection of ovarian masses which would have not been clinically apparent
- Most ovarian masses resolve spontaneously
- Pregnancy may continue until full term in order to prevent prematurity issues. However, a decision may be made to expedite delivery ideally after 32 weeks gestation to minimise delay in treating the ovarian cancer. If an isolated complex ovarian mass is identified in early pregnancy this should be assessed with a detailed ultrasound examination and if demonstrating features of malignancy or significant symptoms then it should be removed by open surgery in the second trimester ideally around 19–20 weeks
- Removal of cysts in the first trimester should be avoided as the corpus luteum may haemorrhage giving complex features on ultrasound. Removal of this would cause the pregnancy to fail as the corpus luteum is the source of progesterone which supports an early pregnancy prior to the establishment of the placental tissue
- If a woman presents with symptoms of ovarian torsion (severe abdominal pain often causing vomiting) in pregnancy this should be considered as an emergency and urgent assessment with ultrasound and early surgical intervention is important to minimise the risk of early pregnancy failure or pre-term delivery

Midwifery Management and Care

- Midwives and oncology nurses need to be proactive in supporting women and their families in collaboration with the other multidisciplinary members to develop an individualised plan of care.

Labour Issues

If it is deemed necessary to commence chemotherapy during the later part of pregnancy for biopsy proven advanced ovarian cancer planned delivery should occur more than 2–3 weeks after the last dose of chemotherapy. This will minimise the risks of maternal sepsis secondary to post-chemotherapy neutropenia[1].

If the diagnosis of ovarian cancer is made in the second and third trimesters consideration could be given to delaying treatment until the risks of prematurity have diminished (ideally beyond 32 weeks) when the fetus could be delivered by caesarean section.

Medical Management and Care

- Debulking surgery may be performed after a vaginal delivery in the early postnatal period or at the same time as a caesarean section[9]
- Mode of delivery will be decided depending on factors such as the woman's overall health, gestation, parity, fetal wellbeing and maternal wishes
- If a pre-term delivery is necessary consideration of corticosteroids for fetal lung maturation may be required

Midwifery Management and Care

- The input of midwifery care during labour should be managed with a normal regime approach closely liaising with the woman's medical team

Postpartum Issues

- If treatment has been delayed until after the pregnancy this can now commence immediately or in the early postnatal period
- Women should be advised not to breast-feed during any chemotherapy treatment

Medical Management and Care

- Normal postpartum care with the input of the gynaecological oncology team where appropriate
- Thrombo-prophylaxis measures should be commenced as there is a high risk of thromboembolic events associated with both pregnancy and malignant disease

Midwifery Management and Care

- Supportive postnatal care should be provided for the woman and her family. To encourage continuity of care from a small group of midwives rather than many carers therefore ensuring a good rapport
- Consider further nursing support once midwifery care is no longer required
- Ensure support and continuity of care is provided and that there is close liaison with the multidisciplinary team
- Be supportive knowing that breast-feeding maybe not advised but still demonstrate skin to skin contact and the importance of this in relation to bonding with the baby

causes severe pain which inevitably causes the woman to seek medical assistance. This can ironically lead to the diagnosis of an ovarian cancer at an early stage and a good prognosis.

NON-PREGNANCY TREATMENT AND CARE

Due to the condition most commonly presenting at an advanced stage it is imperative that there is a greater public awareness of ovarian cancer and its symptoms. It is hoped that this will facilitate women to present earlier for initial investigations by their GP so that an onward referral may be expedited for further investigation and treatment. To optimise the treatment for those women with suspected ovarian cancer, cases should be referred to a cancer centre for treatment as long-term outcomes after specialist treatment in a cancer centre are better than if the woman is treated in a non specialist centre.

The primary aim of treatment is to remove or eradicate all suspected or confirmed cancerous tissue. This is achieved with a combination of surgical excision and if necessary chemotherapy. In a postmenopausal woman standard surgical treatment would include a hysterectomy with removal of both ovaries and fallopian tubes, the fat pad in the abdomen called the omentum, any enlarged lymph nodes and any other cancer deposits identified at the time of surgery which may include the appendix, segments of bowel, the spleen, the peritoneal surface of the liver or other organs. In a premenopausal woman in whom fertility conservation is important and if the disease is thought to be at an early stage (confined to the ovary) conservative surgery may be considered with removal of the affected ovary, biopsy of the other ovary, with sampling of fluid in the abdomen to assess for evidence of malignant cells and removal of the omentum. On completion of surgery all tissues removed would be subjected to thorough histological assessment with evidence of disease spread outside the ovary indicating a role for chemotherapy to minimise the risk of re-growth or recurrence of the disease.

PRE-CONCEPTION ISSUES AND CARE

Benign ovarian cysts are common during pregnancy. Fortunately ovarian cancer is rare in pregnancy with the incidence estimated between 1 in 10000 and 1 in 100000 deliveries[6].

Screening for ovarian cancer is problematic because there is no well- established premalignant phase in which to identify those individuals who are at high risk of developing ovarian cancer. However, in premenopausal women screening for ovarian cancer is not necessary in the general population as ovarian cancer is very rare in this age group[3].

Small functional ovarian cysts (<5cm) which are completely asymptomatic are a common finding in premenopausal women when assessed by ultrasound either prior to pregnancy or in early pregnancy. They are mostly related to the secretory phase of the menstrual cycle (after ovulation) and early pregnancy and are related to the physiological development of the corpus luteum cyst. These cysts will resolve spontaneously and should not be treated.

Other persistent simple ovarian cysts (<5cm) may also be left untreated if asymptomatic, e.g. benign serous cystadenomas. However, women should be aware that over time these may grow to a size where they will cause symptoms requiring treatment. If a cyst grows larger than 5cm then considera-

tion should be given to removing it laparoscopically by ovarian cystectomy to resolve the risk of ovarian torsion.

Complex cysts with solid and cystic components may have characteristics of dermoid cysts (contain tissues such as hair, skin, teeth). If <5cm these may be simply monitored by serial ultrasound scans and serial serum Ca 125 assessments. Larger cysts, that do not have features of a dermoid cyst, or symptomatic cysts, should be removed before pregnancy ideally. If there is a concern that there could be an underlying malignancy then the cyst should be removed by open operation to avoid spillage of the contents potentially upstaging an early ovarian cancer. This procedure should be associated with careful assessment of the pelvic and abdominal organs, with pelvic washing taken for cytological assessment and an omental biopsy.

18.8 Malignant Melanoma

Incidence	Risk for Childbearing
11767 new cases in the UK (latest figures for 2008)[1]	Variable Risk
2067 deaths in the UK (latest figures for 2008)[1]	

EXPLANATION OF CONDITION

Malignant melanoma is a malignant tumour of melanocytes. Melanocytes are cells that produce a dark pigment known as melanin which provides variable degrees of pigmentation of the skin depending on both the individual's skin type and the degree of exposure to various stimulating factors such as sunlight. Malignant melanoma commonly develops in the skin, but may arise in other parts of the body where melanocytes are present, including the bowel and the eye.

As with other cancers the condition is caused by changes or mutations to the DNA which makes up the genes which control cellular function. These changes may be either inherited genetic mutations which predispose the individual to malignant melanoma or acquired due to environmental factors such as exposure to ultraviolet (UV) light from the sun or from sunbeds[2]. Established risk factors for malignant melanoma include presence of moles (a pigmented naevus), pale or fair skin, history of episodic sunburn, prolonged sun exposure such as when living in hot climates and personal utilisation of sun beds.

A suspicion of malignant melanoma may be raised if a mole increases in size, particularly if it becomes irregular in shape, if its colour becomes irregular with the development of satellite lesions in the surrounding skin or if it becomes itchy or painful, with spontaneous bleeding.

Types of Malignant Melanoma

There are three common types of melanoma[3], that make up 90% of all malignant melanoma and the remaining 10%, known as **acral lentiginous melanoma**, are a rare form of melanoma.

1. **Superficial spreading melanoma** (Figure 18.8.1): this common melanoma accounts for 70% of melanoma in the UK population. These are common in middle age and

grow lateral and then vertical. They are at a low risk of producing metastases or until they develop the 'vertical' growth phase.

2. **Nodular melanoma** (Figure 18.8.2): this type of melanoma is more common in men and is associated with rapid growth. They are often found on the skin of the back or chest and demonstrate evidence of deep 'vertical' invasion at presentation with evidence of bleeding and ulceration. This type of melanoma has the poorest prognosis.

3. **Lentigo maligna melanoma** (Figure 18.8.3): this type accounts for at least 10% of malignant melanoma in the UK population. Most commonly found on the face and other areas that are exposed to the sunlight. This is very slow growing and is associated with the best prognosis.

4. **Acral lentiginous melanoma** (Figure 18.8.4): this type is most commonly found on the skin of the palms of the

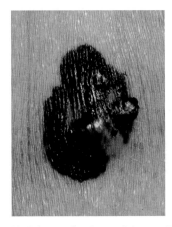

Figure 18.8.2 Nodular malignant melanoma (Buxton 2009). This figure is downloadable from the book companion website at www.wiley.com/go/robson

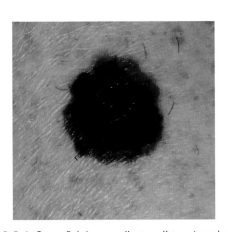

Figure 18.8.1 Superficial spreading malignant melanoma (Buxton 2009). This figure is downloadable from the book companion website at www.wiley.com/go/robson

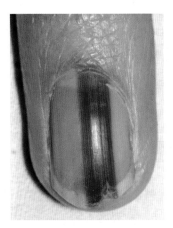

Figure 18.8.3 Melanonychia in a person with white skin. Could be a naevus or a subungal melanoma (Buxton 2009). This figure is downloadable from the book companion website at www.wiley.com/go/robson

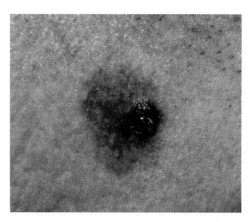

Figure 18.8.4 Lentigo maligna melanoma (Buxton 2009). Reprinted with permission of John Wiley & Sons. This figure is downloadable from the book companion website at www.wiley.com/go/robson

hands and soles of feet and under nails. These grow vertically and are the hardest tumours to diagnose especially around the nail-bed and therefore provide the poorest prognosis.

Staging Of Malignant Melanoma

A number of staging systems have been described including the 'Breslow scale' and 'Clark level' which are linked to long-term prognosis. They all encompass assessment of depth of tumour invasion. These systems have been used by the American Joint Committee on Cancer (AJCC)[4] to develop the staging system outlined below:

i.   <1 mm, no ulceration
ii.   >1–4 mm and >4 mm no ulceration/with ulceration
iii. Above thickness and lymph node involvement
iv.   Skin, subcutaneous or distant nodal disease and lung metastases

Malignant melanoma may be cured if it is identified and treated at an early stage with no spread to the lymph nodes or any other part of the body[3]. Within England and Wales 91% of women and 78% of men will live at least 5 years after diagnosis[3].

NON-PREGNANCY TREATMENT AND CARE

A multidisciplinary team approach as recommended and defined by the National Institute for Health and Clinical Excellence (NICE)[5]. All lesions suspected of being a melanoma should be urgently referred under the 2 week rule. A suspicious lesion should be photographed and excised completely. The excision biopsy should include the whole tumour with a clinical margin of 2 mm of normal skin and a cuff of fat. This will enable accurate assessment of the lesion based on the criteria described by Breslow thickness[6].

The majority of melanomas are treated surgically with wide local excision providing adequate surgical margins and there should be assessment of surrounding skin and regional lymph nodes for the presence of detectable metastatic disease. After treatment follow-up should be considered in both the short term and long term to identify evidence of recurrent disease.

Depending on the stage of disease at diagnosis further treatment may be required such as regional lymph node dis-

section, chemotherapy, radiotherapy and interferon therapy. If there is distant metastasis, the cancer is generally incurable and therefore the overall survival rate in this situation is less than 10%[7]. Therefore treatment is palliative focusing on symptom control and quality of life.

PRE-CONCEPTION ISSUES AND CARE

It is generally recommended that conception should be delayed for 2 years after the initial treatment unless there are exceptional circumstances[8]. However, individualised counselling should be provided based on the clinical features and stage of the initial lesion, the woman's age and desires for children[9].

Women with a recurrent disease or presence of metastases should be advised to avoid pregnancy due to the need for further treatment which could be harmful to a pregnancy. Recurrent disease or metastases is associated with a poor prognosis and thus consideration of termination of an early ongoing pregnancy would have to be discussed[10].

Pregnancy Issues

Malignant melanoma accounts for 8% of all malignancies occurring during pregnancy. However, the incidence has been consistently increasing year on year. It accounts for about 35% of all deaths in women of child-bearing age[12].

It was thought for the past 50 years that pregnancy increased the risk of development of malignant melanoma and also caused the disease to progress rapidly, and recur more commonly in those women who had a history of malignant melanoma[11]. However, further recent studies have not supported this, and it is now believed pregnancy does not have an impact on incidence or prognosis of malignant melanoma[13].

Placental metastasis from maternal cancer is extremely rare but malignant melanoma is the most likely type of cancer to metastasise to the placenta[14].

Medical Management and Care

- Any skin lesions with suspicious features should be referred for further assessment in pregnancy
- Excisional biopsy should not normally be delayed in pregnancy if a skin lesion is deemed suspicious enough to warrant a biopsy. Consideration should be given to the type of anaesthetic to be utilised and when possible or reasonable local anaesthetic should be considered as this poses little risk to the woman or fetus[11]
- Termination of the pregnancy is not indicated in early stage disease[10] but metastatic disease requires further consideration of termination due to the poor long-term prognosis

Midwifery Management and Care

All-Purpose Issues

- Discuss and encourage the observation of pre-existing moles and their changes during pregnancy (see also Chapter 2.1 Physiological Skin Changes)
- Immediate referral should be considered for any suspicious lesion in pregnancy
- Sun burn should be avoided but sensible exposure to sun should be encouraged to prevent vitamin D deficiency

Melanoma in Pregnancy

- Offer support groups
- Good communication between members of the multidisciplinary team
- Psychological support for women and their families should mention support groups

Labour Issues

Labour and delivery is to be managed as normal with a previous history of melanoma[10].

It has been noted that the incidence of placental metastasis may be underestimated because the placenta appears normal to the naked eye. Therefore histological assessment of the placenta should be encouraged to ensure metastases are not missed[15]. Metastasis to the placenta is indicative of stage IV of the disease in accordance with the AJCC[4].

Medical Management and Care

- Plan for a normal labour for women who have previously had the disease and for women with early stages of the disease
- Consider any medications required in labour particularly if the woman is or has received recent treatment for malignant melanoma

Midwifery Management and Care

- Normal intrapartum care
- Protective dressings for any damaged skin areas that have received treatment
- Ensure placenta has been sent to histopathology for a thorough assessment from women who are receiving treatment and who have previously received treatment for malignant melanoma

Postpartum Issues

In the rare situation that placental metastases are confirmed it should be noted there is clearly a potential risk to the fetus but this is also a poor prognostic factor for the woman as well[14]. In the infant it commonly manifests itself as skin lesions or abdominal swelling. Therefore, extremely careful follow-up of the neonate is essential to identify evidence of disease in the neonate so that treatment may be commenced to optimise the outcome for the baby. Unfortunately malignant melanoma in babies is associated with a high mortality rate.

Medical Management and Care

- Advice given to women diagnosed with a malignant melanoma during pregnancy is that future pregnancies are not contraindicated
- Counselling women on subsequent pregnancies should be based upon prognostic factors
- There are no standard guidelines, hence decisions are made on case by case basis

Midwifery Management and Care

- Normal postpartum care
- Encourage breast-feeding unless receiving ongoing treatment such as chemotherapy or radiotherapy
- Organise appropriate follow-up appointments

18 Neoplasia

PATIENT ORGANISATIONS

Breast Cancer Care
Kiln House
210 New Kings Road
London SW6 4NZ
www.breastcancercare.org.uk

Cancerbackup
3 Bath Place
Rivington Street
London EC2A 3JR
www.cancerbackup.org.uk

CancerHelp UK (aligned to Cancer Research UK)
www.cancerhelp.org.uk

Cancer Research UK
PO Box 123
Lincoln's Inn Fields
London WC2A 3PX
www.cancerresearchuk.org

Gynae C (Gynaecological cancer)
1 Bolingbroke Road
Swindon
Wiltshire SN2 2LB
www.communigate.co.uk/wilts/gynaec

Hydatidiform Mole and Choriocarcinoma Support Service
www.hmole-chorio.org.uk

Lymphoma Association
PO Box 386
Aylesbury
Buckinghamshire HP20 2GA
www.lymphoma.org.uk
www.lifesite.info

The Miscarriage Association
c/o Clayton Hospital
Northgate
Wakefield
West Yorkshire WF1 3JS
www.miscarriageassociation.org.uk

Macmillan Cancer Support
89 Albert Embankment
London SE1 7UP
www.macmillan.org.uk

Marie Curie Cancer Care
89 Albert Embankment
London SE1 7TP
www.mariecurie.org.uk

ESSENTIAL READING

BJOG 2012 Special Issue: Gynaecological Oncology. **British Journal of Obstetrics and Gynaecology**, 119:225–62 http://onlinelibrary.wiley.com/doi/10.1111/bjo.2011.119.issue-2/issuetoc

Collins G, Hatton C and Sweetenham J 2008 **Fast Facts – Lymphoma**. Oxford; Health Press

Del Priore G, Shahabi S and Smith JR 2010 **Fast Facts: Gynecologic Oncology**, 2nd Edn. Oxford; Health Press

James D (Ed.) 2011 Chapt. 39 *Malignancies of the hematologic and immunologic systems* in **High Risk Pregnancy Management Options**, 4th Edn. London; Elsevier

Kehoe S *et al.* 2008 **Cancer and Reproductive Health Concensus Views from the 55th study group**. Royal College of Obstetricians and Gynaecologists. Available online from the RCOG

Powrie R, Greene M and Camman W (Eds) 2010 *Chapter 22 Cancer in Pregnancy* in **de Swiet's Medical Disorders in Obstetric Practice**, 5th Edn. Oxford; Wiley-Blackwell

RCOG 2011 **Guideline No. 12: Pregnancy and Breast Cancer**. London; Royal College of Obstetricians and Gynaecologists. http://www.rcog.org.uk/files/rcog-corp/GTG12PregBreastCancer.pdf

RCOG 2010 **Guideline No. 38: The Management of Gestational Neoplasia**. London; Royal College of Obstetricians and Gynaecologists

RCOG 2011 **Guideline No. 62: Management of Suspected Ovarian Masses in Premenopausal Women**. London; Royal College of Obstetricians and Gynaecologists

References

18.1 Gestational Trophoblastic Disease

1. RCOG 2011 **Guideline no 38: The Management of Gestational Trophoblastic Disease**. London; Royal College of Obstetricians and Gynaecologists
2. Steigrad SJ 2003 Epidemiology of gestational trophoblastic diseases. **Best Practice and Research in Clinical and Obstetric Gynaecology**, 17:837–847
3. Alteri A, Franceschi S, Ferlay J, Smith J and La Vecchia C 2003 Epidemiology and aetiology of gestational trophoblastic diseases. **Lancet Oncology**, 4:670–678
4. Ngan HYS, Chan KKl and Tam KF 2006 Gestational trophoblastic disease. **Current Obstetrics and Gynaecology**, 16:93–99
5. Calleja-Agrus J 2008 Vaginal bleeding in the 1st trimester. **British Journal of Midwifery**, 16:656–661
6. Soto-Wright V, Bernstein M, Goldstein DP, *et al*. 1995 The changing clinical presentation of complete molar pregnancy. **Obstetric Gynecology**, 865:775–779
7. Kirk E, Papageorghion AT, Condous G, BoHomley C and Bourne T 2007 The accuracy of first trimester ultrasound in the diagnosis of hydatidiform mole. **Ultrasound in Obstetrics and Gynecology**, 29:70–75
8. Sebire NJ, Fisher RA, Fostett RA, Rees H, Secki MJ and Newlands ES 2003 Risk of recurrent hydatidiform mole and subsequent pregnancy outcome following complete or partial hydatidiform molar pregnancy. **British Journal of Obstetrics and Gynaecology**, 110:22–26
9. Berkowitz RS, Goldstein DP 2009 Molar pregnancy. **New England Journal of Medicine**, 360:1639–1645
10. Bertowitz RS, Goldstein DP 2009 Current management of gestational trophoblastic diseases. **Gynecologic Oncology**, 112:654–662
11. Seckl MJ, Sebire N and Bertowitz RS 2010 Gestational trophoblastic disease. **The Lancet**, 376:717–729
12. Newlands ES 2003 Presentation and management of persistent gestational trophoblastic disease and gestational trophoblastic tumours in the UK in Hancock BW, Newlands ES, Berkowitz RS, Cole LA (Eds) **Gestational Trophoblastic Disease**, 3rd Edn. London; International Society for the Study of Trophoblastic Disease
13. Petru E, Luch HJ, Stuart G, Gaffrey D, Millan D and Vergote I 2009 Gynecologic Cancer Intergroup GCIG proposals for changes of the current FIGO Staging System. **European Journal of Obstetrics and Gynaecology and Reproductive Biology**, 143:69–74
14. Sebire MD, Foskett MA, Paradinas FJ, *et al*. 2002 Outcome of twin pregnancies with complete hydatidiform mole and healthy co-twin. **The Lancet**, 359:2165–2166
15. Snell BJ 2009 Assessment and management of bleeding in the first trimester of pregnancy. **Journal of Midwifery and Women's Health**, 54:483–491
16. Mace K 1995 Hidden misery of hydatidiform mole. **Modern Midwife**, 5:5–17
17. Goddard J, Matharu J and Robson SE 2008 Neoplasia in Robson SE and Waugh J (Eds) **Medical Disorders in Pregnancy: A Manual for Midwives**. Oxford; Blackwell Publishing Ltd.

18.2 Cervical Cancer

1. **Cancer Research UK** 2011 Cancer Stats Key Facts – Cervical Cancer 2011. http://info.cancerresearchuk.org/cancerstats/types/cervix/uk-cervical-cancer-statistics [Accessed 17-11-11]
2. Cadman L 2006 **Human Papillomavirus (HPV) and Cervical Cancer – The Facts**. London: Royal College of Nursing. www.rcn.org.uk [Accessed 17-11-11]
3. Kumar VA, Abul K *et al*. 2007 **Robbins Basic Pathology** 8th Edn. London; Saunders Elsevier 718–721
4. Munoz N, Bosch FX, Castellsague X, *et al*. 2004 Against which human papillomavirus types shall we vaccinate and screen? The International Perspective. **International Journal of Cancer**, 111:278–285
5. Monga A and Dobbs S (Eds) 2011 **Gynaecology by Ten Teachers**. London; Hodder Arnold
6. Castellsagne X and Munoz N 2003 Cofactors in human papillomavirus xaranogenesis – role of parity, oral contraceptives and tobacco smoking. **Journal of the National Cancer Institute Monograph**, 31:20–28
7. Petru E, Luch HJ, Stuart G, Gaffrey D, Millan D and Vergote I 2009 Gynecologic Cancer Intergroup GCIG proposals for changes of the current FIGO Staging System. **European Journal of Obstetrics, Gynaecology and Reproductive Biology**, 143:69–74
8. Paraskevaidis E, Davidson EJ, Koliopoulos G, Alamanos Y, Lolis E and Martin-Hirsch P 2002 Bleeding after loop electrosurgical excision procedure performed in either the follicular or luteal phase of the menstrual cycle: a randomised trial. **Obstetrics and Gynecology**, 99:997–1000
9. Saeed Z and Shafi M 2011 Cancer in pregnancy. **Obstetrics and Gynaecology and Reproductive Medicine**, 21:183–189
10. Sadanandan S, Hurley T, Muller C, *et al*. 2010 Cancer in pregnancy in Powrie R, Greene M and Camann W (Eds) **de Swiet's Medical Disorders in Obstetric Practice**, 5th Edn. Oxford; Wiley-Blackwell

18.3 Cervical Screening

1. NHS Cervical Screening Programme Annual Review 2011. http://www.cancerscreening.nhs.uk/cervical/publications/cervical-annual-review-2011.pdf [Accessed 24-12-11]
2. Averian M, Noureddine S and Kabakian-Khasholian T 2006 Raising awareness and providing free screening improves cervical cancer screening among economically disadvantaged Lebanese/American women. **Journal of Transcultural Nursing**, 17:357–365
3. Bloomfield P 2007 Management of cervical cancer. **Australian Family Physician**, 36:122–125
4. NHS Cancer Screening Programmes 2010 **HPV Triage and Test of Cure Protocol**. http://bit.ly/qq313f [Accessed 24-12-11]
5. Heley S 2007 Pap test update. **Australian Family Physician**, 36:112–115
6. Bano F, Kolhe S, Zamblera D, *et al*. 2008 Cervical screening in under 25s: a high risk young population. **European Journal of Obstetric Gynecology and Reproductive Biology**, 139:86–89
7. Cadman L 2011 The cervical screening programme: HPV triage. **Practice Nursing**, 22:494–497
8. The NHS Information Centre, Public Health Indicators and Population Statistics Team 2011. Cervical Screening Programme England 2010–2011. http://www.ic.nhs.uk/statistics-and-data-collections/screening/cervical-screening/cervical-screening-programme–england-2010-11 [Accessed 24-12-11]
9. Chase DM, Angelucci M, DiSaia PJ 2011 Fertility and pregnancy after cervical procedures: the challenge of achieving good outcomes. **SRM-ejournal.com**, 9:3–9
10. Van Calsteren K, Vergote I and Amant F 2005 Cervical neoplasia during pregnancy: diagnosis, management and prognosis. **Best Practice and Research: Clinical and Obstetric Gynaecology**, 19:611–614.
11. Neumann G, Rasmussen KL and Peterson LK 2007 Cervical adenosquamous carcinoma: tumor implantation in an episiotomy scar. **Obstetrics and Gynecology**, 110:467–469

18.4 Breast Cancer

1. Royal College of Obstetricians and Gynaecologists 2011 **Green Top Guideline no 12: Pregnancy and Breast Cancer**. London; Royal College of Obstetricians and Gynaecologists
2. Pavlidis N 2002 Coexistence of pregnancy and malignancy. **The Oncologist**, 7:279–287
3. Zemlickis D, Lishner M and Degendorfer P 1992 Maternal and fetal outcome after breast cancer in pregnancy. **American Journal of Obstetrics and Gynecology**, 166:781–787
4. Sadanandan S, Hurley T, Muller C, *et al*. 2010 Cancer in pregnancy in Powrie R, Greene M and Camann W (Eds) **de Swiet's Medical Disorders in Obstetric Practice**, 5th Edition. Oxford; Wiley-Blackwell
5. Grosser L 2004 Breast cancer during pregnancy. **British Journal of Midwifery**, 12:299–304
6. Petrek J and Seltzer V 2003 Breast cancer in pregnant and postpartum women. **Journal of Obstetrics and Gynecology Canada**, 25:944–950
7. Early Breast Cancer Trialists Collaborative Group 2005 Effects of chemotherapy and hormonal therapy for early breast cancer on recurrence and 15 year survival: an overview of the randomised trials. **Lancet**, 365:1687–1717
8. Ives A, Saunders C, Bulsara M and Semmens J 2007 Pregnancy after breast cancer population based study. **British Journal of Medicine**, 334:194
9. Lishner M 2003 Cancer in pregnancy. **Annals of Oncology**, 14(Suppl 3):31–36

10. Max TK 1983 Pregnancy and breast cancer. **Southern Medical Journal**, 76:1088–1090
11. Breast Cancer during Pregnancy 2005 Breast Cancer Fact Sheet. **Breast Cancer Care**
12. Bernik SF, Bernik TR, Whooley BP, *et al*.1998 Carcinoma of the breast during pregnancy: a review and update on treatment options. **Surgical Oncology**, 7:45–49
13. Petrek J 1994 Breast cancer during pregnancy. **Cancer**, 74:518–527
14. Miv O, Berveiller P, Ropert S, Goffinet F, Poris G and Treluyer JM 2008 Emerging therapeutic options for breast cancer chemotherapy during pregnancy. **Annals of Oncology**, 19:607–613

18.5 Non-Hodgkin's Lymphoma

1. Pereg D, Koren G and Lishner M 2007 The treatment of Hodgkin's and non-Hodgkin's lymphoma in pregnancy. **The Haematology Journal**, 92:1230–1237
2. Diamond C, Taylor TH, Aboumrad T and Anton-Culver H 2006 Changes in acquired immunodeficiency syndrome-related non-Hodgkin lymphoma in the era of highly active antiretroviral therapy: incidence, presentation, treatment, and survival. **Cancer**, 106:128–135
3. Weinshel EL and Peterson BA 1993 Hodgkin's disease. **CA: A Cancer Journal for Clinicians**, 43:327–346
4. Selvais PL, Mazy G, Gosseye S, Ferrant A and van Lierde M 1993 Breast infiltration by acute lymphoblastic leukemia during pregnancy. **American Journal of Obstetricians and Gynecologists**, 169:1619–1620
5. Sadanandan S, Hurley T, Muller C, *et al.* 2010 Cancer in pregnancy in Powrie R, Greene M, Camann W (Eds) **de Swiet's Medical Disorders in Obstetric Practice**, 5th Edn. Oxford: Wiley-Blackwell
6. Hurley TJ, McKinnell JV and Irani MS 2005 Hematologic malignancies in pregnancy. **Obstetric and Gynecology Clinics of North America**, 32:595–614
7. Cardonick E and Iacobucci A 2004 Use of chemotherapy during human pregnancy. **Lancet Oncology**, 5:283–291
8. Nulman I, Laslo D, Fried S, Uleryk E, Lishner M and Koren G 2001 Neurodevelopment of children exposed in utero to treatment of maternal malignancy. **British Journal of Cancer**, 85:1611–1618
9. Koren G, Lishner M and Santiago S 2005 **The Mother Risk Guide to Cancer in Pregnancy and Lactation**, 2nd Edn. Toronto; Canada Mother Risk Program

18.6 Hodgkin's Lymphoma

1. Lymphoma Association 2010 4th Edn. www.lymphoma.org.uk.
2. Patel A, Camacho J and Stevenson J 2008 Hodgkin's lymphoma during pregnancy. **Community Oncology**, 5:389–391
3. Macfarlane GJ, Evstifeeva T, Boyle P, *et al.* 1995 International patterns in the occurrence of Hodgkin's disease in children and young adult males. **International Journal of Cancer**, 61:165–169
4. Smith LH, Danielsen B, Allen ME and Cress R 2003 Cancer associated with obstetric delivery: results of linkage with the California cancer registry. **American Journal of Obstetrics and Gynecology**, 189:1128–1135
5. Maelor Davies J and Kean L 2011 Malignancies of the hematologic and immunologic systems in James D, *et al.* (eds) **High Risk Pregnancy**, 4th Edn. St Louis; Elsevier Saunders
6. Sadanandan S, Hurley T, Muller C, *et al.* 2010 Cancer in pregnancy in Powrie R, Greene M, Camann W (Eds) **de Swiet's Medical Disorders in Obstetric Practice**, 5th Edn. Oxford: Wiley-Blackwell
7. Jox A, Zander T, Kornacker M, *et al.* 1998 Detection of identical Hodgkin-Reed Sternberg cell specific immunoglobulin gene rearrangements in a patient with Hodgkin's disease of mixed cellularity subtype at primary diagnosis and relapse two and a half years later. **Annals of Oncology**, 9:283–287
8. Connors JM 2004 **Hodgkin's Lymphoma**, 3rd Edn. Philadelphia; Elsevier
9. Joshing A, Wolf J and Diehl V 2000 Hodgkin's disease: prognostic factors and treatment strategies. **Current Opinion in Oncology**, 12:403–411
10. Aisner J, Wiernik PH and Pearl P 1993 Pregnancy outcome in patients treated for Hodgkin's disease. **Journal of Clinical Oncology**, 11:507–512
11. Lishner M, Zemlickis D and Degendorfer P 1996 Maternal and fetal outcome following Hodgkin's disease in pregnancy in Korean G, Lishner M and Farine D (Eds) **Cancer in Pregnancy: Maternal and Fetal risk**. Cambridge; Cambridge University Press,.107–115
12. Aviles A and Neri N 2001 Hematological malignancies and pregnancy: a final report of 84 children who received chemotherapy in utero. **Clinical Lymphoma**, 2:173–177
13. Pereg D, Koren G and Lishner M 2007 The treatment of Hodgkin's and non-Hodgkin's lymphoma in pregnancy. **The Haematology Journal**, 92:1230–1237

14. Koren G, Lishner M and Santiago S 2005 **The Mother Risk Guide to Cancer in Pregnancy and Lactation**, 2nd Edn. Toronto; Canada Mother Risk Program

18.7 Ovarian Neoplasia

1. Monga A and Dobbs S (Eds) 2011 **Gynaecology by Ten Teachers**. London; Hodder Arnold
2. Zhao XY, Huang HF, Lian LJ and Lang JH 2006 Ovarian cancer in pregnancy: a chinicopathologic analysis of 22 cases and review of the literature. **International Journal of Gynaecological Cancer**, 16:8–15
3. Shahabi S, Smith J and Del Priore G 2010 **Fast Facts: Gynecologic Oncology**, 3rd Edn. Oxford; Oxford Health Press Ltd
4. Impey L and Child T 2008 **Obstetrics and Gynaecology**, 3rd Edn. Oxford; Wiley-Blackwell
5. NICE 2011 **Ovarian Cancer. NICE Guideline 122**. Developed by the National Collaborting Centre for Cancer
6. Sadanandan S, Hurley T, Muller C, *et al.* 2010 Cancer in pregnancy in Powrie R, Greene M and Camann W (Eds), **De Swiet's Medical Disorders in Obstetric Practice**, 5th Edn. Oxford; Wiley-Blackwell
7. Paterson G 2004 Cancer in pregnant women. **British Journal of Midwifery**, 12:496–501
8. Blackwell DA, Elams S and Blackwell JT 2000 Cancer and pregnancy: a health care dilemma. **Journal of Obstetrics, Gynecology and Neonatal Nursing**, 29:405–412
9. Amant F, Calsteren K, Vergote I and Otteranger N 2008 Gynecologic oncology in pregnancy. **Critical Reviews in Oncology Hematology**, 67:187–195

18.8 Malignant Melanoma

1. Cancer Research UK 2011 **Cancer Stats. Key Facts** http://publications.cancerresearchuk.org [Accessed 10-11-11]
2. Elwood J and Koh H 1994 Etiology, epidemiology, risk factors and public health issues of melanoma. **Current Opinion Oncology**, 6:179–187
3. Cancer Research UK 2011 **About Melanoma Skin Cancer – A Quick Guide**. http://cancerhelp.cancerresearch uk.org [Accessed 10-11-11]
4. Marsden JR, Newton-Bishop JA, Burrows L, *et al.* 2010 Revised UK guidelines for the management of cutaneous melanoma 2010. **British Journal of Dermatology**, 163:238–256
5. NICE 2006 **Guidance on Cancer Services: Improving Outcomes for People with Skin Tumours including Melanoma – The Manual**. London; National Institute for Health and Clinical Excellence. www.nice.org.uk
6. Lees VC and Briggs JC 1991 Effect of initial biopsy procedure on prognosis in stage I invasive cutaneous malignant melanoma: review of 1086 patients. **British Journal of Surgery**, 78:1108–1110
7. Balch C, Buzaid A, Soong S, *et al.* 2001 Final version of the American Joint Committee on Cancer staging system for cutaneous melanoma. **Journal of Clinical Oncology**, 19:3635–3648
8. Mackie RM 1998 Pregnancy and exogenous female sex hormones in melanoma patients in Balch CM, Houghton AN, Sober AJ and Soong S-J (Eds) **Cutaneous Melanoma**, 3rd Edn. St Louis: QMP Publishing 187–193
9. Lens MB, Rosdahl I, Ahlbom A, *et al.* 2004 Effect of pregnancy on survival in women with cutaneous malignant melanoma. **Journal of Clinical Oncology**, 22:4369–4375
10. Goddard J, Matharu J and Robson SE 2008 Neoplasia in Robson SE and Waugh J (Eds) **Medical Disorders in Pregnancy: A Manual for Midwives**. Oxford; Blackwell Publishing Ltd.
11. Miller E, Burnea Y, Lesham D, *et al.* 2010 Malignant melanoma and pregnancy: second thoughts. **Journal of Plastic, Reconstructive and Aesthetic Surgery**, 63:1163–1168
12. Johnston SRD, Broadley K, Henson G, *et al.* 1998 A difficult case: management of metastatic melanoma during pregnancy. **BMJ**, 316:848
13. Youns H, Lee YW, Seung NR, *et al.* 2010 Rapidly progressing malignant melanoma influenced by pregnancy. **International Journal of Dermatology**, 49:1318–1320
14. Anderson JF, Kent S, Machin GA 1989 Maternal malignant melanoma with placental metastases: a case report with literature review. **Pediatric Pathology**, 9:35–52
15. Shanklin DR 1990 **Tumours of the Placenta and Umbilical Cord**. Philadelphia; Marcel Decker, 154–159

Figure Reference

Buxton PK and Morris Jones R (Eds) 2009 **ABC of Dermatology**, 5th Edn. Oxford; Wiley-Blackwell

Index

Medical Disorders in Pregnancy: A Manual for Midwives, Second Edition. Edited by S. Elizabeth Robson and Jason Waugh.
© 2013 John Wiley & Sons, Ltd. Published 2013 by John Wiley & Sons, Ltd.